Second Edition

DADH

Dental Anatomy | Dental Histology

Made Easy

Exam Oriented Questions–Answers
and
Practical Guide to Tooth Carving

for First Year BDS Students

- LAQs
- SAQs
- MCQs
- Carving
- Identification of Teeth
- Age Determination of Casts

Second Edition

DADH

Dental Anatomy | Dental Histology

Made Easy

Exam Oriented Questions–Answers and Practical Guide to Tooth Carving

for First Year BDS Students

- LAQs
- SAQs
- MCQs
- Carving
- Identification of Teeth
- Age Determination of Casts

Jayshree Daiya Mavani
Ex-Lecturer
Dental Anatomy
Yerala Dental College and Hospital
Navi Mumbai

Sheetal Korde Choudhari
Associate Professor
Department of Oral Pathology and Microbiology
Yerala Dental College and Hospital
Navi Mumbai

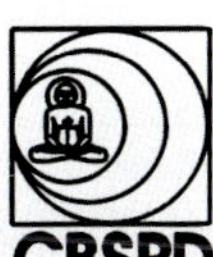

CBS Publishers & Distributors Pvt Ltd
New Delhi • Bengaluru • Chennai • Kochi • Kolkata • Lucknow • Mumbai
Hyderabad • Jharkhand • Nagpur • Patna • Pune • Uttarakhand

Disclaimer

Science and technology are constantly changing fields. New research and experience broaden the scope of information and knowledge. The authors have tried their best in giving information available to them while preparing the material for this book. Although, all efforts have been made to ensure optimum accuracy of the material, yet it is quite possible some errors might have been left uncorrected. The publisher, printer and the authors will not be held responsible for any inadvertent errors or inaccuracies.

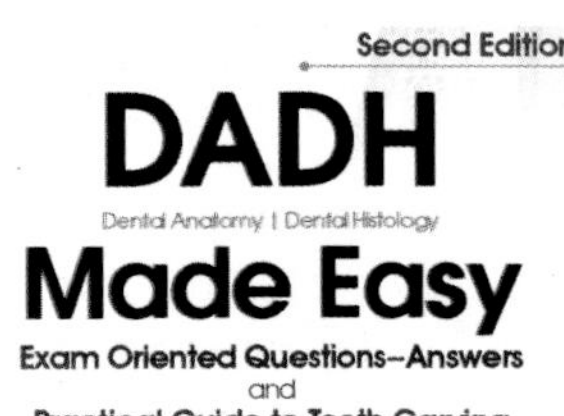

ISBN: 978-93-5466-574-5

Second Edition: 2023

First Edition: 2019

Published by Satish Kumar Jain and produced by Varun Jain for

CBS Publishers & Distributors Pvt Ltd

4819/XI Prahlad Street, 24 Ansari Road, Daryaganj, New Delhi 110 002, India.

Ph: 011-23289259, 23266861 Website: www.cbspd.com

e-mail: delhi@cbspd.com

Corporate Office: 204 FIE, Industrial Area, Patparganj, Delhi 110 092

Ph: 011-49344934 Fax: 011-49344935 e-mail: publishing@cbspd.com; publicity@cbspd.com

Branches

- **Bengaluru:** Seema House 2975, 17th Cross, K.R. Road, Banasankari 2nd Stage, Bengaluru 560 070, Karnataka, India
  Ph: +91-80-26771678/79 Fax: +91-80-26771680 e-mail: bangalore@cbspd.com
- **Chennai:** 7, Subbaraya Street, Shenoy Nagar, Chennai 600 030, Tamil Nadu, India
  Ph: +91-44-26680620, 26681266 Fax: +91-44-42032115 e-mail: chennai@cbspd.com
- **Kochi:** 42/1325, 1326, Power House Road, Opp KSEB, Ernakulum, Kochi 682 018, Kerala, India
  Ph: +91-484-4059061-65,67 Fax: +91-484-4059065 e-mail: kochi@cbspd.com
- **Kolkata:** 147, Hind Ceramics Compound, 1st Floor, Nilgunj Road, Belghoria, Kolkata-700056, West Bengal, India
  Ph: 033-25633055/56 e-mail: kolkata@cbspd.com
- **Lucknow:** Basement, Khushnuma Complex, 7 Meerabai Marg (Behind Jawahar Bhawan), Lucknow-226001, UP, India
  Ph: +91-522-4000032 e-mail: tiwari.lucknow@cbspd.com
- **Mumbai:** PWD Shed, Gala no 25/26, Ramchandra Bhatt Marg, Next to JJ Hospital Gate no. 2, Opp. Union Bank of India, Noorbaug, Mumbai-400009, Maharashtra, India
  Ph: +91-22-66661880/89 e-mail: mumbai@cbspd.com

Representatives

• **Hyderabad**	0-9885175004	• **Jharkhand**	0-9811541605	• **Nagpur**	0-9421945513
• **Patna**	0-9334159340	• **Pune**	0-9923910676	• **Uttarakhand**	0-9716462459

Printed at HT Media Ltd, Greater Noida

Foreword

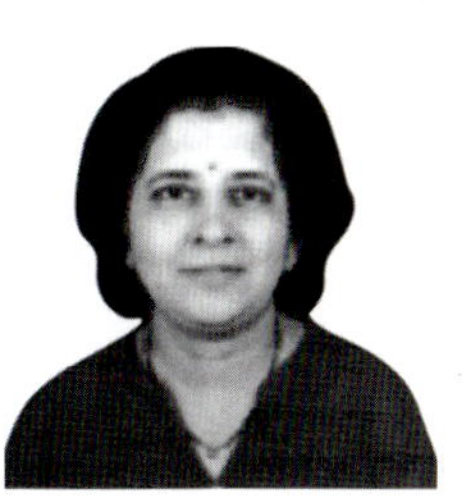

It gives me immense pleasure to foreword the book titled *DADH Made Easy—Exam Oriented Questions–Answers and Practical Guide to Tooth Carving* pertaining to the subject of Dental Anatomy and Dental Histology. This book is authored by Dr Jayshree Daiya Mavani and Dr Sheetal Korde Choudhari which is presented in question and answer format. It gives basic understanding of the subject and caters to the needs of the students for preparation of examination. I appreciate their efforts in striving towards this particular endeavour primarily keeping student welfare in mind.

The subject DADH warrants extensive reading for which various reference textbooks are available but due to limited time for preparation of examination, it is often difficult for the students to frame appropriate answers. In view of this difficulty and keeping in mind the overall significance of this subject in dental curriculum, I believe that this book, will be of great help to the students. Section III of this book, *The Practical Guide to Tooth Carving* would help both as a technique and as a hands-on to remember the details of morphology of each tooth.

I congratulate the authors for this venture and wish them all success.

Sangeeta Patankar
Professor and Head
Department of Oral Pathology
Yerala Dental College and Hospital
Navi Mumbai

Preface to the Second Edition

We take great pleasure in presenting this book titled the second edition of *DADH Made Easy Exam Oriented Questions–Answers and Practical Guide to Tooth Carving* for the first year BDS students. The subject of dental anatomy and dental histology is an important subject in the dental curriculum which forms the basis for understanding of various aspects of dentistry.

It is our observation that understanding this voluminous subject within a limited time-space is indeed a challenge especially in concising the information for exam oriented answers. This book has been compiled to help the students acquire comprehensive knowledge of the subject while familiarizing them with the questions frequently asked in university examination.

Section III of this book, *The Practical Guide to Tooth Carving* includes schematic representations that are easy to follow. This will also serve as a valuable aid to perfect the technique of carving. Along with carving, guidelines for identification of teeth and age determination of dental casts have also been included.

It is our earnest belief that our objectives will be accomplished and that the book will help the students to acquire comprehensive knowledge of the subject and deal with the exams confidently.

Jayshree Daiya Mavani
Sheetal Korde Choudhari

Acknowledgements

Our sincere gratitude to all those who have traversed with us in the making of this book.

We thank Dr Sangeeta Patankar, Professor and Head, Department of Oral Pathology, Yerala Dental College & Hospital for her scholarly and practical insights towards contents and format of the book.

We appreciate and acknowledge the assistance and efforts of Dr Komal Khot, Dr Sheeba Alex, Dr Kriti Bagri Manjrekar, Dr Gokul Sridharan and Dr Vaishali Joshi, faculty, Department of Oral Pathology, Yerala Dental College and Hospital.

Our sincere gratitude to Dr Rajkumar Maurya for his willing cooperation and contributory efforts.

We extend our sincere thanks to the DTP operator Sunita Tikare, artist Wadekar and CBS Publishers & Distributors of this book for bringing this matter to print.

Jayshree Daiya Mavani

Sheetal Korde Choudhari

Contents

Section III—Practical Guide

Jayshree Daiya Mavani and Sheetal Korde Choudhari

Abbreviations

ABBREVIATIONS USED IN THE BOOK ARE FOR EASE OF REPRESENTATION ONLY

Class of Teeth

Incisor	I
Canine	C
Premolar	PM
Molar	M

Side/Surface

Incisal	I
Mesial	M
Distal	D
Occlusal	O
Cervical	C
Labial	La
Lingual	Li
Buccal	B
Palatal	P

Angle

Mesioincisal angle	MIA
Distoincisal angle	DIA
Dimension/distance	Dd
Cervicoincisal	CI
Mesiodistal	MD
Labiolingual	LaLi
Buccolingual	BL
Buccopalatal	BP

Outline

Distolabial	DL
Mesiolabial	ML

Ridges

Labial ridge	LaR
Lingual ridge	LiR
Buccal ridge	BR
Palatal ridge	PR
Cervical ridge	CR
Triangular ridge	TR
Mesial marginal ridge	MMR
Buccal triangular ridge	BTR
Oblique ridge	OR
Lingual triangular ridge	LiTR
Palatal triangular ridge	PTR

Grooves

Central groove	CG
Buccal groove	BG
Lingual groove	LG
Palatal groove	PG
Mesiolingual groove	MLG
Mesial marginal ridge groove	MMRG
Mesiobuccal developmental groove	MBDG
Distobuccal developmental groove	DBDG
Mesiolingual developmental groove	MLDG
Distolingual developmental groove	DLDG

Fossa

Central Fossa	CF
Canine Fossa	CF
Mesial triangular fossa	MTF
Distal triangular fossa	DTF

Cusps

Mesiobuccal	MB
Mesiopalatal	MP
Mesiolingual	ML
Distobuccal	DB
Distopalatal	DP
Distolingual	DL

Other

Mesial Cusp Slope/Ridge	MCS/MCR
Distal Cusp Slope/Ridge	DCS/DCR

Section I

Dental Anatomy

1. Terminology Related to Tooth Morphology
2. The Permanent Incisors
3. The Permanent Canines
4. Premolars
5. The Permanent Molars
6. Differences between Deciduous and Permanent Dentition
7. Occlusion
8. Blood and Nerve Supply to Teeth and Tongue
9. Muscles of Mastication
10. Deglutition
11. Temporomandibular Joint
12. Maxillary Sinus

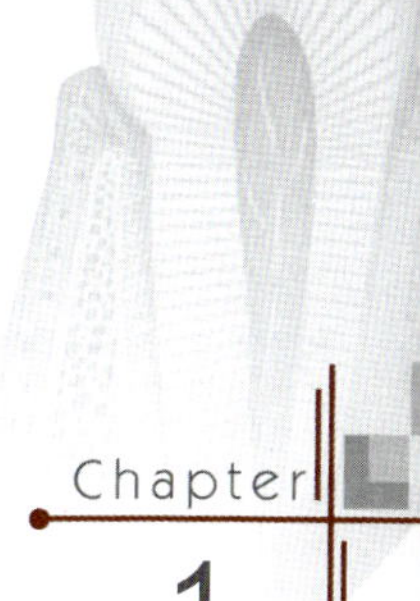

Terminology Related to Tooth Morphology

SAQs (3 Marks)

Q 1. What are elevations on the surface of the tooth?

(Oct. 2003, May 2008, 2013, Nov. 2010, 2015)

Ans. Elevations on the surface of the tooth are cusps, tubercle, cingulum, lobe, ridge, and mamelons.

Cusp (Fig. 1.4)

- It is an elevation or mound on the crown portion of a tooth making up a divisional part of the occlusal surface.
- A cusp can also be defined as an elevation or a point or a peak on the chewing surface of a molar or a premolar and on the incisal edge of the canine.
- Cusps are named according to their location on the tooth surface.
- The number of cusps varies according to the type of the tooth. Canine has one cusp, maxillary first premolar has two cusps, mandibular second premolar may have three cusps. Maxillary first molar has four cusps and the mandibular first molar has five cusps.
- Maxillary first molar has an accessory cusp on the palatal surface of the mesiopalatal cusp called "cusp of Carabelli".
- The cusp includes the ridges that form an angle at the cusp tip.
- Each cusp has four sides or four ridges which run down from the cusp tip.
  Mesial and distal cusp ridges or slopes.
  Buccal and lingual cusp ridges or triangular ridges.
- The cusp ridges are named according to the direction in which they extend from the cusp tip.

Tubercle

- It is a smaller elevation on some portion of a crown formed by enamel only.
- It can be called a mini cusp.
- It is deviation from typical form. It is variable in size and shape. *For example*: Cusp of Carabelli on the maxillary first molar is a tubercle. On the lingual surface of some maxillary anterior teeth especially deciduous canine a tubercle may be present.

Cingulum (Fig. 1.1)

- It is a Latin word for girdle since it encircles the cervical third of the lingual surface of the tooth mesiodistally in the form of a girdle.
- It is the lingual lobe of the anterior teeth.
- It is a bulge, a rounded **protuberance** or an elevation on the lingual surface of the anterior teeth in the cervical third of the crown.
- It makes up the bulk of the cervical third of the lingual surface of anterior teeth.

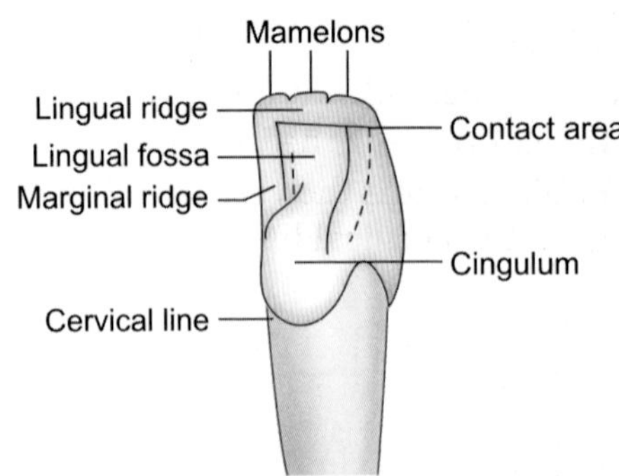

Fig. 1.1: Cingulum

Lobe (*SAQ, May 2007*) (Fig. 1.2)

- It is one of the primary sections of formation in the development of the crown of the tooth.
- Development of tooth takes place by formation of 3 or 4 centres. Each centre proceeds until there is coalescence of all of them. Each of these centres is called lobe.
- In terms of evolution of dentition, tooth crowns are said to have developed from lobes or primary centres or primary anatomic divisions on teeth separated by primary grooves. Cusps and mamelons are representive of lobes.
- Cingulum represents the lingual lobe on anterior teeth and mamelons represent the labial lobes on anterior teeth.
- All normal permanent teeth develop from minimum of 4 lobes.
- Permanent anterior teeth, maxillary premolars, and mandibular first premolar develop from four lobes (3 labial, 1 lingual).
- Mandibular second premolars and mandibular first molars develop from five lobes (3 buccal, 2 lingual).
- Permanent maxillary molars develop from four lobes (2 buccal, 2 lingual).
- Exception is some maxillary third molars which develop from 3 lobes.
- **Peg-shaped** maxillary lateral incisors develop from less than 3 lobes.

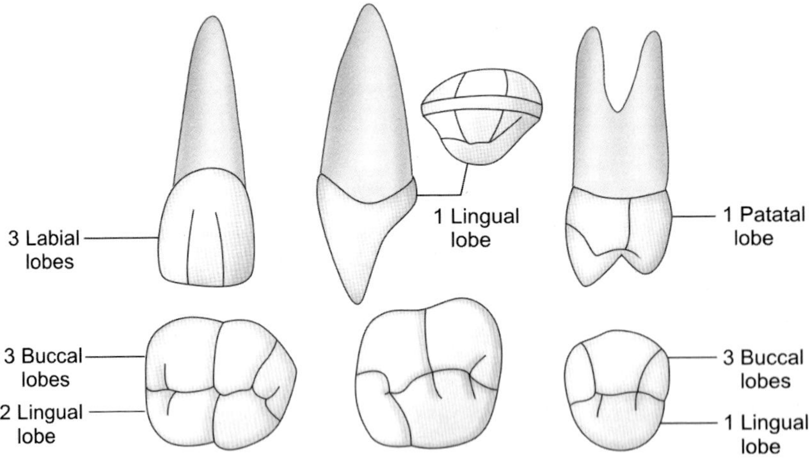

Fig. 1.2: Lobes

Ridge (*SAQ, May 2009*) (Fig. 1.6)

It is any linear elevation on the surface of a tooth and is named according to its location.

- **Incisal ridge** is the incisal edge of the incisor.
- **Labial ridge** is the vertical ridge on the labial surface of the canine that runs cervico-incisally from the cervical line to the cusp tip.
- **Cusp ridge:** Each cusp has four ridges. They are named by the direction in which they extend from the cusp tip.
  - Mesial and distal cusp ridges extend from the cusp tip in mesial and distal direction.
  - Buccal cusp ridge extends from the cusp tip towards the cervical line on the buccal surface of the cusp of premolars and molars.
  - Lingual cusp ridge extends on the lingual surface from the cusp tip.
- **Cervical ridge** extends mesiodistally in the cervical one-third of the facial surface of the crown. It is found on all deciduous teeth but in permanent teeth it is more prominent on mandibular second molars.
- **Marginal ridges** are rounded borders of enamel on mesial and distal borders of the lingual surface of the incisors and canines and on mesial and distal borders of the occlusal surface of premolars and molars (Fig. 1.1).
- **Triangular ridge** is the ridge from the tip of the cusp of premolars and molars towards the centre of the occlusal surface (Fig. 1.4).
- It is so named because the slopes of each side of the ridge are inclined to resemble two sides of a triangle.
  - It is named after the cusp to which it belongs. *For example*: Triangular ridge of buccal cusp, triangular ridge of lingual cusp.
  - Triangular ridge which extends from the cusp tip to the centre of the occlusal surface is same as one of the four cusp ridges (lingual cusp ridge).
  - All posterior teeth cusps have one triangular ridge each, except for the mesiolingual cusp of maxillary first molar which has two triangular ridges, mesial and distal separated by Stuart groove.
- **Transverse ridge** is the ridge that extends in buccolingual direction on the occlusal surface of the posterior teeth. It is formed by the union of triangular ridge of the buccal cusp and the lingual cusp.
- **Oblique ridge (SAQ, 2001, May 2007, 2012)** is a special type of transverse ridge, which extends buccolingually in oblique direction. It crosses the occlusal surface of the maxillary first molar of both the dentitions in an oblique direction from the mesiolingual cusp to the distobuccal cusp.
  - ***Function of oblique ridge:*** Central fossa of mandibular molar and oblique ridge of maxillary molar act as mortar-pestle and aid in mastication.

Mamelons (*SAQ, 2000*) (Fig. 1.3)

- Mamelons represent the lobes.
  Mamelons are the three rounded protuberances found on the incisal ridge of the newly erupted permanent incisor.
- They are normally worn away rather soon after eruption if the teeth are in normal occlusion.

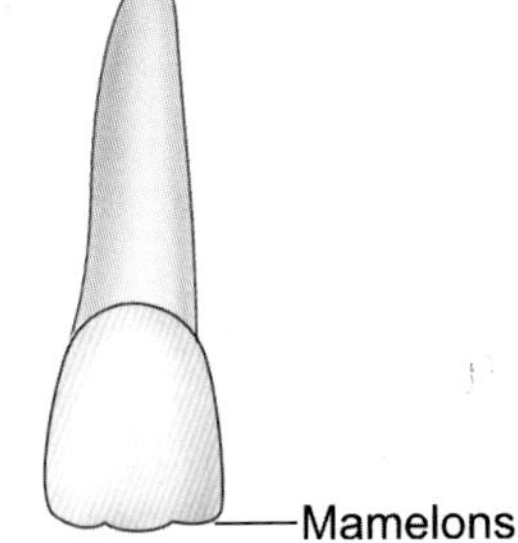

Fig. 1.3: Mamelons

- Mamelons occasionally do not wear out when the teeth are malaligned, e.g. when there is an anterior open-bite relationship.
- Mamelons are extensions made of enamel with no dentin layer underneath and because of their thinness they appear more translucent as opposed to the rest of the clinical crown which is always more opaque than the mamelons.

Q 2. What are depressions on the surface of the tooth? *(SAQ, Nov. 2011, 2014, 2015)*

Ans. Depressions on the surface of the tooth are sulcus, groove, fissure, fossa, and pit.

Sulcus (Fig. 1.4)

- It is a broad and long depression or valley between the ridges and cusps on the occlusal surface of posterior teeth, the inclines of which meet at an angle and extends outward to the cusp tip.
- Sulcus is an elongated valley or depression on the surface of the tooth formed by the inclines of adjacent cusps or ridges, e.g. a central sulcus is a major linear depression that traverses the occlusal surface of a posterior tooth from mesial triangular fossa to distal triangular fossa.
- A sulcus has a developmental groove at the junction of its inclines. (The term sulcus must not be confused with the term groove).
- It is the occlusal depression between cusps (valley) that is seen on all posterior teeth.

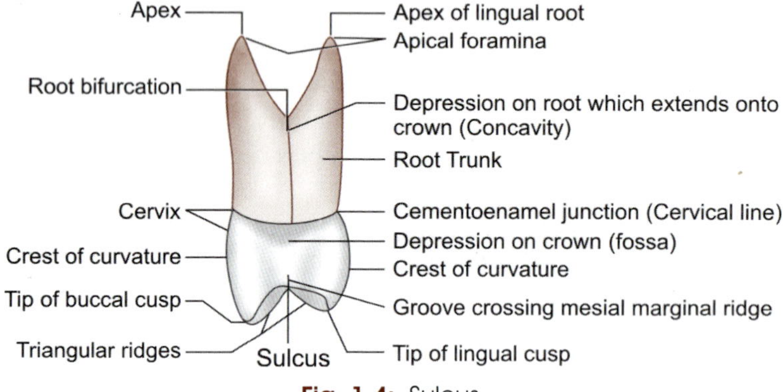

Fig. 1.4: Sulcus

Groove (*SAQ, Nov. 2004*) (Fig. 1.5)

Developmental Groove

- It is a shallow groove or line between the primary parts of the crown or root.
- It is a shallow groove, narrow or linear depression, short or long formed during tooth development, and usually separating lobes or major portions of the tooth.

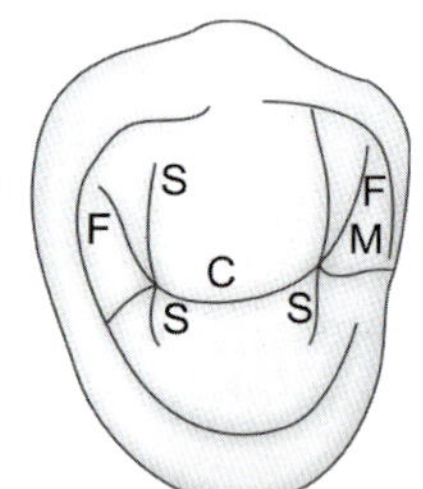

Fig. 1.5: Grooves

The major grooves are named according to their location.

Grooves are important escape-ways for cusps during lateral and protrusive jaw movement and for food morsels during mastication.

Buccal and lingual developmental grooves are present on the B and L surfaces of posterior teeth.

Central groove is present on the occlusal surface of posterior teeth.

Supplemental Grooves

- A supplemental groove, less distinct is also a shallow linear depression on the surface of the tooth but it is supplemental to a developmental groove and does not mark the junction of primary parts.

- They are small, irregularly placed grooves, not at the junction of lobes or major portions of a tooth, found usually on occlusal surfaces.

Fissure

Fissure is a narrow crevice, sometimes deep, present at the depth of the developmental groove formed during development and extending inward toward the pulp from the groove.

Decay begins in a deep fissure.

Fossa

Fossa is an irregular depression or concavity found on the surface of the tooth.

Lingual Fossa (Refer Fig. 1.1)

Lingual fossa is present on the incisal two-thirds of the lingual surface of the anterior teeth.

It is bounded by incisal ridge, mesial and distal marginal ridges, and cingulum.

The lingual fossa of canine is divided into mesial and distal lingual fossae by the prominent lingual ridge running cervico-incisally from the cingulum to the tip of the cusp.

Central fossa is present on the occlusal surface of the molars and premolars. It is formed by the covergence of the ridges terminating at a central point in the bottom of the depression where there is junction of grooves (Fig. 1.7).

Triangular fossae: They are present on the occlusal surfaces of the posterior teeth towards the mesial and distal marginal ridges.

The mesial triangular fossa is present distal to mesial marginal ridge (MMR) and the distal triangular fossa is present mesial to distal marginal ridge (DMR) (Fig. 1.7). They are sometimes found on the lingual sufaces of maxillary incisors at the edge of the lingual fossae where the marginal ridges and cingulum meet.

Canine fossa is a small concavity present on the mesial surface of the crown of the maxillary first premolar just above the cervical line to accomodate the distoincisal angle of the canine or It is a mesial developmental depression on the mesial surface of the maxillary first premolar where distal rounded surface of the canine rests. It is believed to be produced due to the pressure of the distal aspect of maxillary canine as it develops earlier than the first premolar (Fig. 1.4).

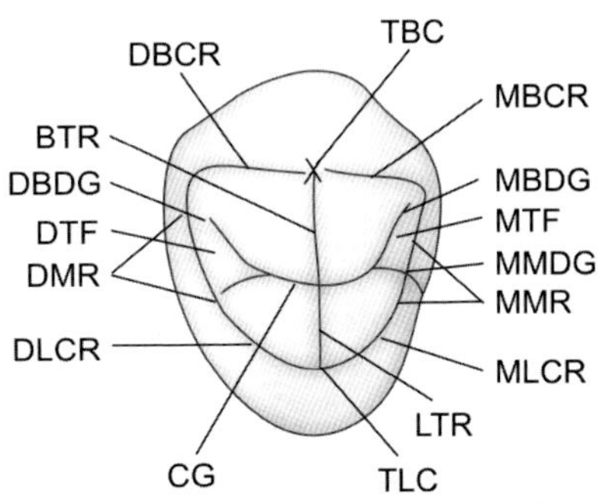

Ridges and Fossae: Maxillary first premolar, occlusal aspect TBC. Tip of buccal cusp; MBCR, mesiobuccal cusp ridge MBDG mesiobuccal developmental groove; MTR, mesial triangle fossa, MMDG, mesial marginal development groove; MMR, mesial marginal ridge; MLCR, mesiolingual cusp ridge; LTR, lingual triangular ridge; TLC, tip of lingual cusp CR, central groove; DLCR, distolingual cusp ridge; DMR, distal marginal ridge; DTF, distal triangular fossa, DBDG, distobuccal development groove; BTR, buccal triangular ridge, DBCR, distobuccal cusp ridge.

Fig. 1.6

Pit

Pits are small pinpoint depressions located at the junctions of developmental grooves or at terminals of those grooves. Pit is the deepest portion of the fossa.

Central pit is at the depth of the central fossa where developmental grooves join.

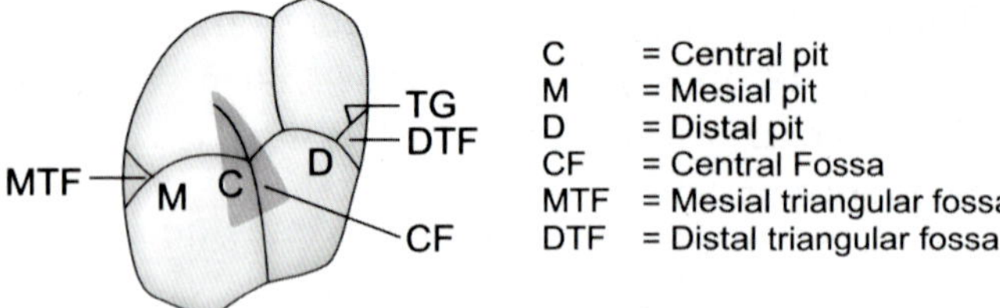

Fig. 1.7: Pits and fossae

Buccal pit is on buccal surface of molars at the terminal end of buccal developmental groove.

Lingual pit is on lingual surface of molars.

Lingual pit is also present on lingual surface of maxillary lateral incisor.

Q 3. What are inclined planes? *(SAQ, 2000, May 2002, 2011, Nov. 2010)*

Ans. Inclined planes are the sloping areas found between the two cusp ridges.

Each cusp has four inclined planes. They take the name of the two cusp ridges between which they lie.

Inclined planes **of buccal cusp are (Fig. 1.8):**

Mesiobuccal inclined plane (MBIP)

Mesiolingual inclined plane (MLIP)

Distobuccal inclined plane (DBIP)

Distolingual inclined plane (DLIP)

Functions: They give stability to the posterior teeth during lateral movement of the mandible.

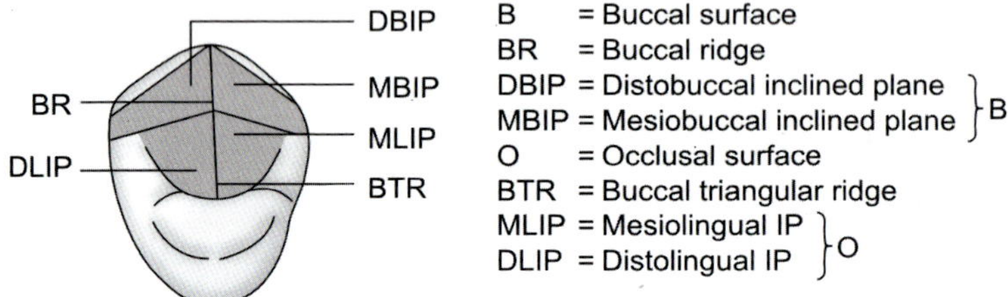

Fig. 1.8: Inclined planes

Q 4. What is human dentition?

Ans.

- Dentition means a set of teeth.
- The human dentition is termed **heterodont** which means it comprises of different classes of teeth to perform different functions in the mastication process.

  Human dentition has two sets of teeth—the primary set of teeth and the permanent set of teeth. Such a condition where two sets of teeth exist is known as **diphyodont.**
- **The primary teeth** are small in size, milky white in colour, 20 in number. 10 teeth in upper jaw and 10 teeth in lower jaw.

  They are also called deciduous teeth, baby teeth, lacteal teeth, milk teeth, temporary set, and first set of teeth.

  The primary teeth begin to form at about 6 weeks *in utero*.

  They begin to calcify between 4–6 months *in utero*.

  The crown is completed within first year after birth.

The root formation is complete one year after eruption.

They erupt between 6 months and 24 months of age.

Pattern of eruption is from anterior to posterior.

Sequence of eruption is A B D C E.

Primary dentition period is from 6 months to 6 years of age.

The first teeth to erupt are the mandibular central incisors between 6–10 months and the rest of the teeth follow.

The primary teeth are shed to be replaced by the permanent teeth. The permanent teeth that replace the primary teeth are called **succedaneous** teeth.

At around 6 years the permanent first molars erupt distal to the primary second molars. Permanent molars are called **accessional** teeth.

Primary maxillary canines are the last primary teeth to be shed.

- **The permanent teeth** are larger in size, yellowish white in colour and 32 in number. 16 teeth in each jaw.

  The permanent teeth are also called **secondary teeth.**

  They begin to form at birth and calcify between birth and 3 years of age except third molars which begin to calcify between 7–10 years.

  The crowns of permanent teeth are completed between 4 and 8 years except third molars which are completed between 12 to 16 years.

  Root is completed 3 years after eruption.

  Pattern of eruption is from posterior to anterior.

  Sequence of eruption in mandibular arch is 6 1 2 3 4 5 7 8 and in maxillary arch is 6 1 2 4 5 3 7 8 or 6 1 2 4 3 5 7 8.

  Permanent dentition period is 12 years onward.

  The first permanent tooth to erupt is the first molar at around 6 years of age.

  The central incisor is the second permanent tooth to emerge in the oral cavity. Eruption time occurs quite close to that of the first molar, i.e. 6–7 years.

  The mandibular permanent teeth tend to erupt before the maxillary permanent teeth.

  Before the permanent central incisor can come into position, the primary CI must be exfoliated. This is brought about by the resorption of the roots of the primary CI.

  Second molars erupt at around 12 years of age distal to the first molars.

  The maxillary canines occasionally erupt along with the second molars, but in most instances they precede the eruption of second molars.

  The third molars erupt at around 17 years or later.

Mixed Dentition (*SAQ 2000*)

- In human beings there are three periods or stages of dentition.
  - The primary dentition period from 6 months to 6 years. During this period oral motor behaviour and speech are established.
  - The mixed dentition period from 6 years to 12 years.
  - The permanent dentition period from 12 years onwards.
- During **mixed dentition** period both primary and permanent teeth are present in the oral cavity.
- It begins with the eruption of permanent first molars distal to the primary second molars.

- It is a transition stage when primary teeth are exfoliated in a sequential manner, followed by the eruption of their permanent successors.
- In the first transitional stage eruption of permanent first molars and replacement of primary incisors by the permanent incisors occurs.
- In the second transitional stage replacement of the primary molars and canines by the premolars and permanent canine occurs. It also involves the eruption of permanent second molars.
- Significant changes in occlusion occur during this stage.

Q 5. What is clinical and anatomical crown. *(SAQ, May 2002)*

Ans. Each tooth features two components the crown and the root **(Fig. 1.9)**.

- The crown is that portion of the tooth which is above gum line and projects into the oral cavity.
- The root is that portion of the tooth which is anchored into the socket and under the gingiva and not exposed to the oral cavity.
- **Anatomic crown** is that part of the tooth which is covered by enamel.
- **Anatomic root** is that part of the tooth which is covered by cementum.
- A **cervical line** separates anatomic crown from anatomic root. It signifies the cemento-enamel junction. This relationship does not change with age.
- Clinical crown and clinical root definition is applicable only when the tooth is in the oral cavity and at least partially erupted.
- **Clinical crown** is that part of tooth which is visible in the oral cavity. The clinical crown may be larger or smaller than the anatomical crown.
  In newly erupted tooth the clinical crown is shorter than the anatomic crown.
  In case of gum recession the clinical crown is longer than the anatomic crown because part of exposed root is also visible.
  Clinical root is that part of tooth which is not visible in the oral cavity and is covered by gingiva.
  This also could be either shorter than the anatomic root or longer than the anatomic root.
- The clinical crown and clinical root are separated by gingival margin (gum line).

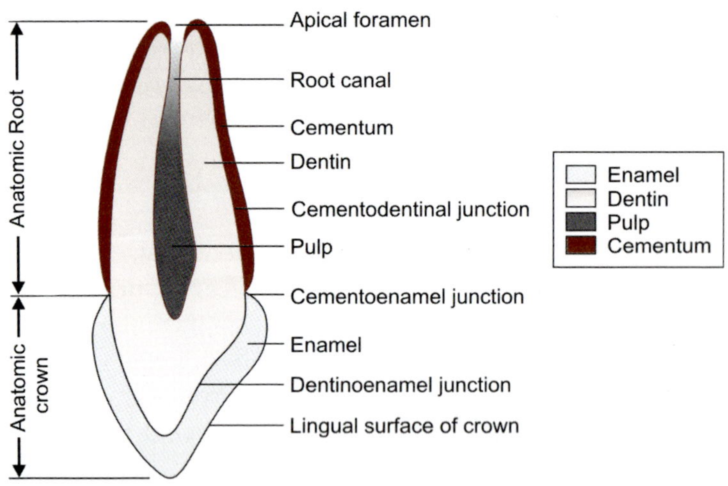

Fig. 1.9: Tissues of a tooth

Q 6. What is contact point and contact area? (*SAQ, July 2005*)

Ans. Contact Areas/Points (Refer Fig. 1.12)

Contact areas or points are the crests of curvatures on the proximal surfaces of the tooth crowns where the adjacent teeth contact each other in the same arch and when the teeth are in proper alignment.

Contact areas may be in the incisal third, middle third, or at the junction of incisal and middle third. They are never located more cervically than the middle of the tooth crown.

Mesial surfaces of all teeth face (approximate) the distal surfaces of the adjacent teeth except for the central incisors where the mesial surfaces approximate another mesial surface.

Every tooth in the dental arch except-third molar has two contact points.

Distal surfaces of permanent third molars and distal surfaces of primary second molars until 6 years of age have no teeth distal to them.

The contact of each tooth with adjacent tooth has important functions.

1. It stabilizes the tooth within the bony socket which thereby stabilizes the dental arch.
2. It helps prevent food impaction which can lead to decay and periodontal problem.
3. It protects the interdental papilla by shunting food towards buccal and lingual areas.

Contact areas of teeth are at first contact points, then as the teeth rub together in function they become flattened and become contact areas.

Q 7. What are developmental lobes? (*May 2007*)

Ans. Answer is same as in elevation on tooth surface.

Q 8. Define bifurcation and trifurcation. (*SAQ, Dec. 2005*)

Ans. Furcation (Fig. 1.4)

It is a place or area on multirooted teeth where the root trunk divides into two or three separate roots.

Bifurcation is two root branches from the root trunk. *For example,* maxillary first premolar and mandibular molars.

Trifurcation is three root branches from the root trunk. *For example,* maxillary molars.

The spaces between the roots at the furcation are called "furcation crotches".

Teeth with two roots have two furcation crotches.

Teeth with three roots have three furcation crotches.

Such crotches can be facial and lingual or mesial and distal depending on tooth type.

It may be close to CEJ or far from it.

Root concavities are also found on many root branches as well as on the furcal surfaces.

Q 9. State human dental formula. (*SAQ, Dec. 2005*)

Ans. Dental Formula

- Dental formula is the number-letter designation of various teeth in a dentition.
- The number and type of teeth present in a dentition can be expressed in the form of a dental formula.
- The denomination and number of all mammalian teeth are expressed by formulae that are used to differentiate the human dentition from that of other species.
- Since the right and left halves of the dental arches are exact mirror images, the dental formula includes the teeth in both the arches but of one side of the mouth only.
- Dental formula is different for both primary and permanent dentition.

- The class of each tooth is represented by its initial letter – I for incisors, C for canine, PM for premolars, M for molars.
  Each letter is followed by a horizontal line and the number of each class of tooth is placed above the line for the upper jaw and below the line for lower jaw. The formula is indicative of **one side only.**
  The dental formula for primary teeth in humans

$$I\frac{2}{2} \quad C\frac{1}{1} \quad M\frac{2}{2} \quad = 10$$

  The dental formula for permanent teeth is

$$I\frac{2}{2} \quad C\frac{1}{1} \quad PM\frac{2}{2} \quad M\frac{3}{3} \quad = 16$$

  This formula should be read as incisors two maxillary and two mandibular; canines, one maxillary and one mandibular; premolars, two maxillary and two mandibular; molars, 3 maxillary and 3 mandibulars.

Q 10. What is eruption sequence?

Ans. Eruption Sequence

- The emergence of **primary teeth** takes place between the 6th and 13th months of postnatal life.
- The sequence of eruption of primary teeth in each jaw is central incisor A, lateral incisor B, 1st molar D canine C, 2nd molar E.
- The lateral incisors, first molars and canines tend to erupt earlier in maxilla than in mandible.
- The eruption sequence of primary dentition can be represented as follows:

$$\frac{\text{AB D C E}}{\text{A B D CE}}$$

- In general, the teeth erupt earlier in females than in males.
- The mandibular **permanent teeth** tend to erupt before their maxillary counterparts.
- The sequence of eruption of permanent dentition is more variable than that of the primary dentition.
  There is a significant difference in the sequence of eruption between the two arches.
- Most common sequence of eruption in the maxillary arch is
  6-1-2-4-3-5-7-8 or
  6-1-2-4-5-3-7-8
- Most common sequence of eruption in the mandibular arch is
  6-1-2-3-4-5-7-8
- Mandibular canines usually erupt before the mandibular premolars.
- Maxillary canines erupt after the eruption of maxillary premolars, due to which very often they erupt labially or palatally because of loss of space due to mesial shift of erupted premolars.
- Usually the first permanent teeth to erupt are the first molars around 6 years of age. They are thus called **6 years** molars also.
- The mandibular central incisors erupt simultaneously or immediately after the first molars at around 6–7 years.

- Maxillary central incisors erupt next at around 7–8 years.
- Maxillary first premolars and mandibular canines follow the maxillary lateral incisors at around 10 years.
- Second premolars follow the next year and then the maxillary canines.
- The next are the second molars around 12 years of age. They are also called as **12 years** molar.
- The third molars erupt between 17–21 years. They may be impacted or even absent.

Q 11. Explain nomenclature system.

Ans. Nomenclature System/Tooth Numbering System/Notation System (NS)

- Tooth numbering system has been developed in order to have a standard way of referring to particular teeth.
- When identifying a specific tooth one has to list the dentition, the dental arch, the quadrant and the tooth name. Listing all this information in words is cumbersome and time-consuming.
- The numbering system acts like a dental 'short hand' used in the clinic to simplify tooth identification providing a standard and easy way of communication among dental professionals, students and care providers.
- It also gives a convenient method of record keeping in dental practice.
- Although there have been many different numbering systems, three systems are in common use.
- It is necessary to be familiar with all the three notation systems (NS) so that communication between the dental offices is efficient. However, it is important to stick to one NS in a dental practice so as to avoid confusion. Also it is important to specify which system is used.

The three numbering systems in common use are:

1. Palmer notation or Zsigmondy's NS/quadrant system/grid system.
2. FDI International NS is Federation Dentaire Internationale.
3. Universal NS.

Palmer notation is the oldest method in use and most papular system.

- In palmer NS the symbol for the quadrant is derived from an imaginary cross, with the horizontal bar placed between the upper and lower teeth and the vertical bar running between the right and left central incisors (quadrants).
- Each quadrant is assigned a specific symbol.

UR	UL
LR	LL

UR = Upper right
UL= Upper left
LL = Lower left
LR= Lower right

- Permanent teeth are numbered 1 to 8 in each quadrant from midline.
- Deciduous teeth are lettered A to E in each quadrant from the midline where A represents central incisor and E represents second molar.
- Only one digit is used.

6| is maxillary right first molar.

1| is mandibular right central incisor.

- In this notation: 1 represents the central incisor and 8 represents the third molar.
- Palmer NS is not accepted by computer.
  In this system verbal communication is difficult.

Federation Dentaire Internationale (FDI) NS: (*SAQ, June 2004, May 2009*)

- In FDI system, the quadrants are represented by numbers and no letters of alphabet are used.
- For permanent and deciduous dentition the quadrants are numbered as:
  - Permanent dentition
    UR = 1, UL = 2, LL = 3, LR = 4
  - Deciduous dentition
    UR = 5, UL = 6, LL = 7, LR = 8
- In this system permanent teeth are numbered 1 to 8 starting from midline and deciduous teeth are numbered 1 to 5 from the midline.
- This system uses two digits.
  The **first digit** always denotes the **dentition, arch, and side.**
- The **second digit** denotes the **tooth number:** For example, 51 symbolizes deciduous maxillary right central incisor and 26 symbolizes permanent maxillary left first molar.
- The notation is read as five one and two six.
- FDI NS is accepted by WHO and by computer.
- In this system verbal communication is easier.

Universal NS:

- In permanent dentition the teeth are numbered 1 to 32 starting with maxillary right third molar.
- **In UR** quadrant the teeth are numbered 1 to 8
  where 1 represents maxillary right third molar, and
  8 represents maxillary right central incisor.
- **In UL** quadrant the teeth are numbered 9 to 16,
  where 9 represents maxillary left central incisor, and
  16 represents maxillary left third molar.
- **In LL** quadrant the teeth are numbered 17 to 24,
  where 17 represents mandibular left third molar, and
  24 represents mandibular left central incisor.
- **In LR** quadrant the teeth are numbered 25 to 32,
  where 25 represents mandibular right central incisor, and
  32 represents mandibular right third molar.
- In **deciduous dentition** the teeth are lettered A to T starting with maxillary right second molar.
- **In UR** quadrant the teeth are lettered A to E,
  where A represents maxillary right second molar, and
  E represents maxillary right central incisor.
- **In UL** quadrant the teeth are lettered F to J,
  where F represents maxillary left central incisor, and
  J represents maxillary left second molar.

- **In LL** quadrant the teeth are lettered K to O,
  where K represents mandibular left second molar, and
  O represents mandibular left central incisor.
- **In LR** quadrant the teeth are lettered P to T,
  where P represents mandibular right central incisor, and
  T represents mandibular right second molar.

NUMBERING SYSTEMS

PERMANENT DENTITION/MAXILLA/UPPER JAW/MAXILLARY ARCH

	RIGHT									LEFT							
	Quadrant 1									Quadrant 2							
U Universal NS	1	2	3	4	5	6	7	8		9	10	11	12	13	14	15	16
F FDI NS	18	17	16	15	14	13	12	11		21	22	23	24	25	26	27	28
P Palmer	8	7	6	5	4	3	2	1		1	2	3	4	5	6	7	8
Class of Teeth	M	M	M	PM	PM	C	LI	CI	Mid-line	← Mesial			Distal →				
P Palmer	8	7	6	5	4	3	2	1		1	2	3	4	5	6	7	8
F FDI NS	48	47	46	45	44	43	42	41		31	32	33	34	35	36	37	38
U Universal	32	31	30	29	28	27	26	25		24	23	22	21	20	19	18	17
										CI	LI	C	PM	PM	M	M	M
	Quadrant 4									Quadrant 3							

Mandible/lower jaw/mandibular arch

e.g. Maxillary Left Central incisor

P	FDI	U
|1	21	9

DECIDUOUS DENTITION/SET

Maxillary Teeth

Universal	A	B	C	D	E	F	G	H	I	J
FDI NS	55	54	53	52	51	61	62	63	64	65
Palmer	E	D	C	B	A	A	B	C	D	E
Class of Teeth	M	M	C	LI	CI	CI	LI	C	M	M
Palmer	E	D	C	B	A	A	B	C	D	E
FDI	85	84	83	82	81	71	72	73	74	75
Universal	T	S	R	Q	P	O	N	M	L	K
			RIGHT					LEFT		

Mandibular Teeth

Q 12. What are the functions of teeth?

Ans. Functions of Teeth (*May 2009, Nov. 2010*)

- The primary function of teeth is to prepare food for swallowing and to facilitate digestion.
- Different types of teeth with their respective forms are adapted to incise, shear and grind food.

- The teeth with their proper form and alignment protect the supporting periodontal tissues against trauma during mastication, facilitate jaw movement, speech, and enhance esthetic appearance of face by supporting lips and cheeks.
- In deciduous dentition the primary teeth maintain space in the dental arch for the development and eruption of permanent teeth.
- They function in the development of speech.
- Ability to use teeth for pronunciation is acquired entirely with the aid of primary dentition. Early and accidental loss of primary anterior teeth may lead to difficulty in pronouncing the sounds f, v, s, z, th.

Q 13. What are line angles and point angles? *(SAQ, Nov. 2015)*

Ans. Line Angles

A line angle is formed by the junction of two surfaces and derives its name from the combination of the two surfaces that join (Fig. 1.10).

The 'al' of the first term is changed to 'o'. *For example,* on the anterior tooth the junction of the mesial and labial surface is termed "mesiolabial".

Line angles of anterior teeth are 6	*Line angles of posterior teeth are 8*
1. Mesiolabial	Mesiobuccal
2. Mesiolingual	Mesiolingual
3. Distolabial	Mesioocclusal
4. Distolingual	Distobuccal
5. Labioincisal	Distolingual
6. Linguoincisal	Distoocclusal
Because the mesioincisal and distoincisal angles are rounded they are usually considered nonexistent and spoken as mesial incisal and distal incisal angle.	Buccoocclusal Linguoocclusal

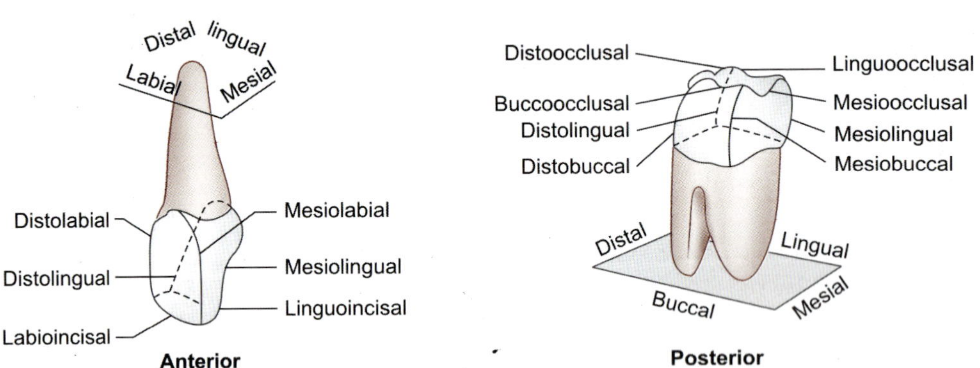

Fig. 1.10: Line angles

Point Angles

A point angle is formed by the junction of three surfaces. A point angle also derives its name from the combination of three surfaces (Figs 1.11A and B).

Point angles of both anterior and posterior teeth are four.

Anterior teeth [4]	*Posterior teeth [4]*
1. Mesiolabioincisal	Mesiobuccoocclusal
2. Mesiolinguoincisal	Mesiolinguoocclusal
3. Distolabioincisal	Distobuccoocclusal
4. Distolinguoincisal	Distolinguoocclusal

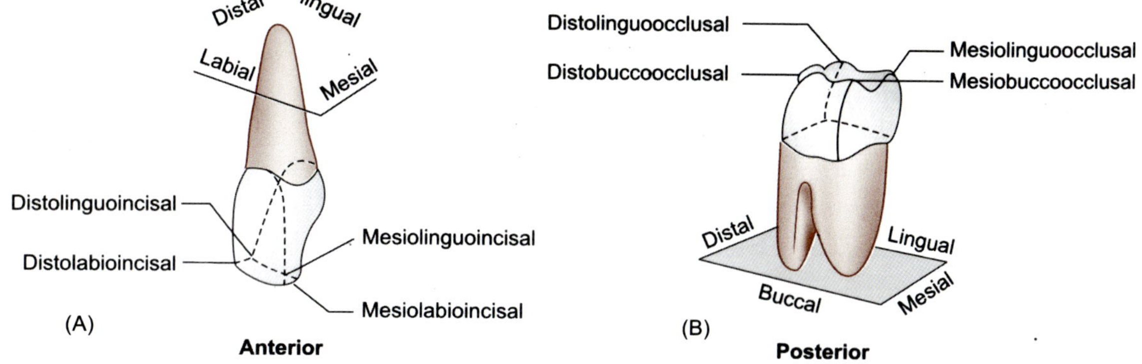

Figs 1.11A and B: Point angles

Q 14. What are embrasures? *(Oct. 2002, June 2006, May 2011, 2013)*

Ans. Embrasures

When the teeth in the same arch contact each other, there are four continuous spaces surrounding the contact area, these triangular shaped spaces or V-shaped spillway spaces adjacent to the contact area are called **embrasures** (Figs 1.12A and B).

They are named according to their location, which depends on the aspect from which the teeth are viewed.

When viewing the teeth from facial or lingual aspect, the two embrasures are incisal/occlusal and gingival/cervical.

The cervical embrasure corresponds to interproximal space and is normally larger in area than the incisal embrasure.

When viewing the teeth from the incisal/occlusal aspect the two embrasures which are visible are the facial and palatal embrasure.

Ideally if an imaginary line is drawn to bisect the embrasure space, the two portions would be symmetrical.

Embrasures have two physiologic purposes.

a. To serve as spillway for food during mastication.
b. To serve as an integral part of the self-cleansing process of the teeth.

Some general rules regarding normal embrasure form:

1. From facial and lingual aspect
   Incisal embrasure increases in size from anterior to posterior.
   Cervical embrasure decreases in size from anterior to posterior.
2. From incisal aspect, the labial and lingual embrasures are nearly equal in size in anterior teeth.

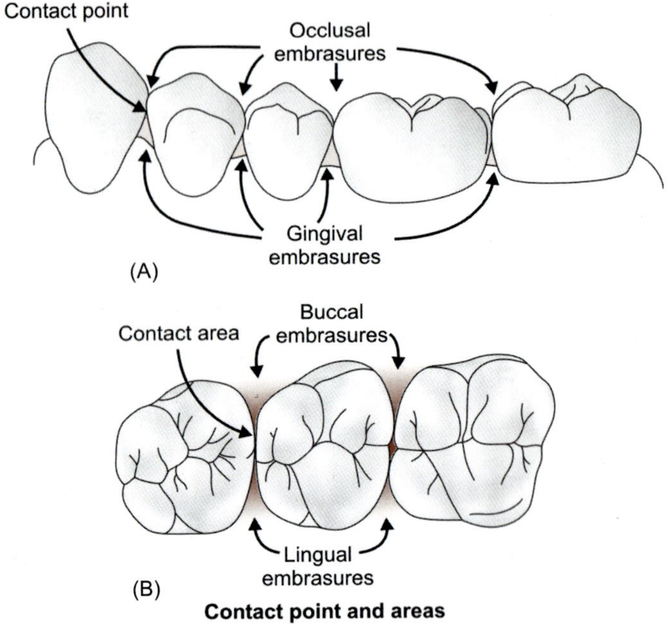

Figs 1.12A and B: Embrasures

3. From occlusal aspect, the lingual embrasure is normally larger than the buccal embrasure in the posterior teeth.
4. One side of the embrasure has a certain contour, the other side of the embrasure will normally have a similar contour.

It should now be easy to recognize the interrelationship between contact areas and embrasure form.

For example as the contact area becomes more cervically placed from anterior to posterior, the relative size of the incisal embrasure increases in size.

MULTIPLE CHOICE QUESTIONS (MCQs)

1. The information written about both maxillary and mandibular teeth of one side only is known as:
a. Dental formula
b. Palmer notation
c. FDI system
d. Universal system

2. A trait that distinguishes the characteristics between the same class of teeth is:
a. A set trait b. Arch trait
c. Class trait d. Type trait

3. A trait that distinguishes the features between the maxillary and the mandibular teeth is the
a. Class trait b. Type trait
c. Arch trait d. Dentition trait

4. A trait that distinguishes the features between the permanent and the primary teeth is the
a. Set trait b. Dentition trait
c. Class trait d. a and b

5. The part of a tooth which has enamel as the outer surface is
a. Anatomic crown
b. Anatomic root
c. Clinical crown
d. Clinical root

6. The part of a tooth which has cementum as the outer surface is
a. Clinical crown
b. Clinical root
c. Anatomic crown
d. Anatomic root

7. The part of a tooth that is visible in the oral cavity is
a. Anatomic crown b. Anatomic root
c. Clinical crown d. Clinical root

8. A line that separates the anatomic crown from the anatomic root is the
a. Gum line
b. Cervical line
c. Cemento-enamel junction
d. Both b and c

9. The relationship between the following does not change over a patient's life time
a. Clinical crown and anatomic crown
b. Clinical root and anatomic root
c. Anatomic crown and anatomic root
d. Clinical crown and clinical root

10. The hard, white, shiny, protective outer covering of the anatomic crown is
a. Dentin b. Cementum
c. Enamel d. Pulp

11. The dull yellow external surface of the anatomic root is
a. Enamel b. Dentin
c. Pulp d. Cementum

12. The inner surface of cementum lining the root is
a. The cementoenamel junction
b. The cementodentinal junction
c. The dentinoenamel junction
d. The dentinopulpal junction

13. The surface of the tooth which is next to face is
a. The labial surface
b. The buccal surface
c. The facial surface
d. All of the above

14. The surface of the tooth which is next to the adjacent tooth is the
a. Proximal surface
b. Mesial surface
c. Distal surface
d. All of the above

1-a, 2-d, 3-c, 4-d, 5-a, 6-d, 7-c, 8-d, 9-c, 10-c, 11-d, 12-b, 13-d, 14-d

15. An elevation on the chewing surface of a molar or a premolar and on the incisal edge of the canine is known as

a. Tubercle b. Cingulum
c. Cusp d. Ridge

16. A longitudinal convexity or any linear elevation on the surface of a tooth is known as

a. A groove b. A ridge
c. Tubercle d. Cingulum

17. A rounded protuberance in the cervical third of the lingual surface of the anterior teeth is

a. Cusp b. Tubercle
c. Ridge d. Cingulum

18. The numbering system in which the permanent teeth in each quadrant are numbered 1 to 8 and the deciduous teeth are numbered 1 to 5 or A to E is

a. Palmer notation
b. FDI system
c. Universal system
d. Both a and b

19. The numbering system which uses two digits where the first digit denotes arch, dentition and side and the second digit denotes the tooth number is

a. Universal NS
b. Zsigmondy's NS
c. FDI NS
d. All of the above.

20. The primary centres of tooth development or primary anatomic divisions of tooth are known as

a. Lobes b. Ridges
c. Pits d. Grooves

21. The sloping areas found between the two cusp ridges are known as inclined planes, the number of inclined planes for each cusp are

a. 2 b. 6
c. 4 d. 8

22. A shallow, narrow, linear depression formed during tooth development and separating lobes is known as

a. Fissure
b. Developmental groove
c. Supplemental groove
d. Sulcus

23. An irregular depression or concavity found on the surface of the tooth, bounded by ridges is known as

a. Sulcus
b. Groove
c. Fossa
d. None of the above

24. The central fossa is found on the following surface of the tooth

a. Lingual surface of the anterior teeth
b. Occlusal surface of all the posterior teeth
c. Occlusal surface of all molars
d. Occlusal surface of y-shaped mandibular second premolar
e. Both c and d

25. The convex bulge or curvature on the crown of a tooth, that determines the direction of food as it is pushed cervically over the tooth surface during mastication is the

a. Height of contour
b. Crest of curvature
c. Both a and b
d. None of the above

26. The height of contour on the facial surface of all the crowns of tooth (as seen from mesial and dental aspect) is in the

a. Incisal third b. Middle third
c. Cervical third d. All of the above

27. The crest of curvature on the lingual surface of all the anterior teeth is in the

a. Incisal third
b. Middle third
c. Entire lingual surface
d. Cervical third

15-c, 16-b, 17-d, 18-d, 19-c, 20-a, 21-c, 22-b, 23-c, 24-e, 25-c, 26-c, 27-d

28. The crest of curvature on the lingual/palatal surface of the posterior teeth is in the

a. Middle third b. Incisal third
c. Cervical third d. Entire surface

29. Crest of curvature on the proximal surfaces of the crowns of the teeth, where the adjacent teeth in the same arch touch each other are known as

a. Contact point b. Contact area
c. Both a and b d. None of the above

30. Contact areas are located in

a. Incisal third
b. Middle third
c. In the cervical third
d. Both a and b

31. The continuous triangular spaces surrounding the contact area between the two adjacent teeth in contact with each other is known as

a. Incisal embrasure
b. Cervical embrasure
c. Labial embrasure
d. Lingual embrasure
e. All of the above

32. The relative position of contact area in the facial view of teeth is demonstrated

a. Cervicoocclusally
b. Buccolingually
c. Both of the above
d. None of the above

33. In teeth, embrasures are

a. Wider facially than lingually
b. Wider lingually than facially
c. Same facially and lingually
d. None of the above

34. Although there are two dentitions, the primary and the secondary, the 'dentition periods' that occur during a patients lifetime are

a. One b. Two
c. Three d. Four

35. Teeth may have one or more roots, but all the roots of both the dentitions have common traits which are

a. Widest at CEJ and taper towards the apex
b. Taper facial to lingual
c. Bulbous uniformly
d. Both a and b

36. The occlusal view demonstrates the relative position of contact area

a. Faciolingually
b. Cervicoocclusally
c. Both of the above
d. None of the above

37. The only tooth other than maxillary third molar which has only one antagonist is

a. Mandibular CI
b. Mandibular LI
c. Mandibular second PM
d. Mandibular third molar

38. The largest embrasure in the dental arch is

a. Between maxillary canine and maxillary first PM
b. Between maxillary LI and maxillary canine
c. Between maxillary CI and maxillary LI
d. None of the above.

39. The height of epithelial attachment is dependent on

a. Height of contact area
b. Curvature of cervical line
c. Height of alveolar bone
d. All of the above

40. Midline foramina of incisive canal is called

a. Foramen of Scarpa
b. Foramen of Larschak
c. Foramen of Stenson
d. Foramen rotundum.

28-a, 29-c, 30-d, 31-e, 32-a, 33-b, 34-c, 35-d, 36-a, 37-a, 38-a, 39-c, 40-a

41. The number of line angles in the crowns of mandibular first molar are

a. 4 b. 6
c. 8 d. 10

42. Human dentition has different classes of teeth incisors, canines, premolars, and molars such a condition where more than one type of teeth are present is called

a. Homodont b. Heterodont
c. Haplodont d. None of the above

43. The last succedaneous tooth to erupt is

a. Maxillary canine
b. Maxillary first premolar
c. Mandibular canine
d. Mandibular first premolar

44. The palatal cusp of upper first premolar develop from

a. One lingual lobe
b. Lingual lobe and distal lobe
c. Lingual lobe and mesial lobe
d. Distal and mesial lobe

45. Which of the premolars develop from five lobes?

a. Upper first premolar
b. Upper second premolar
c. Lower first premolar
d. Lower second premolar

46. Main function of proximal contact area

a. Stabilizes the dental arch
b. Helps prevent food impaction
c. Distribution of occlusal forces
d. All of the above

47. The line angle which does not exist in any tooth

a. Mesiobuccal
b. Mesiolingual
c. Mesiodistal
d. Distolingual

48. The mesial contact is at the junction of incisal and middle third and distal contact is at the centre of middle third in

a. Maxillary central and lateral inciser
b. Maxillary lateral incisor and canine
c. Maxillary canine and first premolar
d. Maxillary first and second premolar

49. In maxillary arch posterior embrasures are larger on the lingual side in all teeth except between

a. First and second premolar
b. Second premolar and first molar
c. First premolar and canine
d. First and second molar

50. In posterior teeth, wider lingual embrasure and shallow occlusal embrasure are due to the position of contact

a. Buccoocclusally
b. Buccogingivally
c. Linguogingivally
d. Linguoocclusally

51. The largest occlusal embrasure is found between maxillary

a. Second and third molars
b. Canine and first premolar
c. First premolar and second premolar
d. First and second molar

52. The widest incisal embrasure is found between

a. Maxillary central incisors
b. Maxillary central and lateral incisor
c. Maxillary lateral incisor and canine
d. Mandibular central incisors

53. Which of the following does not contribute to arch stability

a. Embrasure
b. Contact areas
c. Root form
d. Periodontal fibres

41-c, 42-b, 43-a, 44-a, 45-d, 46-d, 47-c, 48-b, 49-b, 50-a, 51-b, 52-c, 53-a

54. The part of the tooth outlined by its developmental grooves is called as
a. Fissure b. Lobes
c. Sulci d. Cusps

55. In the intercuspal position, which of the following anterior teeth contact one anterior and one posterior antagonists
a. Maxillary canine
b. Mandibular canine
c. Maxillary lateral incisor
d. Mandibular lateral incisor

56. Wilson curve in mandibular arch is
a. Concave
b. Convex
c. Concave-convex
d. Convexo-concave

57. Mesial contact area is found in incisal third of the crown surface of
a. Maxillary central incisor
b. Mandibular central incisor
c. Mandibular lateral incisor
d. Mandibular canine
e. All of the above

58. Contact area present at the junction of incisal and middle third of the crown surface are at
a. Distal surface of maxillary CI
b. Mesial surface of maxillary LI
c. Mesial surface of maxillary canine
d. Distal surface of mandibular canine
e. All of the above

59. The distal contact point is in the middle of the middle third of the distal surface of the crown of
a. Maxillary LI b. Maxillary canine
c. Both a and b d. None of the above

60. What is the term used for the division of the root into 3 segments
a. Furcation b. Bifurcation
c. Trifurcation d. All of the above

61. The height of the clinical root is determined by the position of the
a. CEJ b. Gingival margin
c. Alveolar bone d. Both a and b

62. All are hard tissues of tooth *except*
a. Pulp b. Cementum
c. Dentin d. Enamel

63. Tissues of tooth which develop from mesodermal structure are
a. Enamel b. Dentin
c. Pulp d. Both b and c

64. The fibres which attach or anchor the teeth to the alveolus are
a. PDL fibres b. Gingival fibres
c. Both a and b d. None of the above

65. The opening present at the apex of the tooth is termed
a. Apical foramen
b. Accessory foramen
c. Both a and b
d. None of the above

66. Compared to incisal embrasure between maxillary central and lateral incisor, the incisal embrasure between the maxillary central incisors is
a. Larger b. Smaller
c. The same size d. None of the above

67. The first succedaneous tooth to erupt is a
a. Maxillary central incisor
b. Maxillary lateral incisor
c. Mandibular central incisor
d. Mandibular first molar

68. The following groove separates cusp ridges from marginal ridges
a. Supplemental
b. Developmental
c. Mesiomarginal developmental
d. Marginal ridge developmental

54-b, 55-a, 56-a, 57-e, 58-e, 59-c, 60-c, 61-b, 62-a, 63-d, 64-a, 65-a, 66-b, 67-c, 68-b

69. Mamelons are present on
a. Newly erupted deciduous incisors
b. Newly erupted permanent incisors
c. Newly erupted canines
d. All newly erupted anteriors

70. In reptiles the mandible consists of
a. Dentary b. Quadrate
c. Articulare d. All of the above

71. Out of the three bones found in reptile mandible the bone retained in human mandible is
a. Dentary b. Quadrate
c. Articulare d. None of the above

72. The proper contact relation between neighbouring teeth in each arch is important
a. To prevent food lodgement
b. Stabilize the dental arches
c. Protect interdental papilla
d. All the above

73. The last molars are prevented from drifting distally
a. By the angulation of their occlusal surface with their roots
b. By the angle of the direction of the occlusal forces in their favour
c. Both a and b
d. None of the above

74. The interproximal space is affected by or depends on
a. Form of teeth
b. Relative position of contact areas
c. Both a and b
d. None of the above

75. All aspects of each tooth crown except the incisal or occlusal aspect may be outlined schematically within geometric figures
a. A triangle b. Trapezoid
c. Rhomboid d. All of the above

76. The crown and root are separated by
a. Cervical line
b. Dentinoenamel junction
c. Cementoenamel junction
d. Both a and c

77. Occlusal and incisal surface are together termed as
a. Proximal surfaces
b. Facial surfaces
c. Masticatory surfaces
d. Both a and b

78. The angle formed by junction of 3 surfaces is
a. Point angle b. Line angle
c. None d. Both

79. Fossa is
a. A shallow depression seen between the primary parts of a tooth
b. An irregular depression on the surface of a tooth
c. It is a linear depression separating the cusps
d. All the above

80. According to the Universal notation system 'E' denotes
a. Primary second molar
b. Primary right central incisor
c. Primary first molar
d. Primary left central incisor

81. In the universal notation system, maxillary permanent right central incisor and maxillary left canine are designated as
a. 1 and 3 b. Number 8 and 11
c. 11 and 23 d. 9 and 12

82. The numbering system accepted by World Health Organisation is
a. The universal notation system
b. The palmer notation
c. The FDI system
d. All the above

69-b, 70-d, 71-a, 72-d, 73-c, 74-c, 75-d, 76-d, 77-c, 78-a, 79-b, 80-b, 81-b, 82-c

83. The numbering system acceptable to computer language is
a. FDI
b. Palmer notation
c. The universal system
d. Both a and c

84. A two digit system for numbering is
a. FDI
b. The universal system
c. None of the above
d. Palmer notation

85. According to FDI system, the permanent maxillary right first molar and the primary maxillary left canine are designated as
a. 16 and 63 b. 6 and c
c. 46 and 73 d. 3 and H

86. Calcification and eruption of both deciduous and permanent teeth was given by
a. Nolla
b. Anderson
c. Logan and Kronfeld
d. Mccall and Schour

87. The number of centers for formation of each tooth are
a. One b. Two
c. Three d. Four or more

88. Mesial surface of one tooth contacts the distal surface of its neighbour except for the distal surfaces of
a. Distal surfaces of third molars of permanent teeth
b. Distal surfaces of second molars of deciduous teeth
c. Both a and b
d. None of the above

89. The teeth which have their mesial surfaces contacting each other are
a. Maxillary central incisors
b. Mandibular central incisors
c. Both are correct
d. Both are wrong

90. Cusps and mamelons represent
a. Tubercule b. Ridge
c. Lobe d. None

91. The longest uneven side of each of the trapezoid outlines of the facial and lingual aspects of all teeth forms the
a. Occlusal line b. Cervical line
c. Buccal line d. Lingual line

92. The longest uneven side of the trapezoid outline of the mesial and distal aspect of maxillary posterior represents the
a. Occlusal line
b. Buccal line
c. Lingual line
d. Base of the crown (cervical line)

93. Cervical portion of a posterior tooth is smaller than that of occlusal portion when viewed from
a. Mesial or distal
b. Buccal or lingual aspect
c. Both
d. None of the above

94. When the posterior tooth is viewed from mesial or distal aspect the occlusal portion is
a. Smaller than cervical
b. Larger than cervical
c. Equal to cervical
d. None of the above

95. With increasing age
a. Anatomical crown > clinical crown
b. Anatomical crown < clinical crown
c. Anatomical crown = clinical crown
d. Any of the above

96. Which tooth occupies the centre of the fully developed adult jaw?
a. First premolar
b. Second premolar
c. Second molar
d. First molar

83-d, 84-a, 85-a, 86-c, 87-d, 88-c, 89-c, 90-c, 91-a, 92-d, 93-b, 94-a, 95-b, 96-d

97. Deepest position in tooth is
a. Pit b. Fossa
c. Groove d. Marginal ridge

98. Transverse ridge is formed by
a. The junction of the buccogingival ridge with marginal ridge
b. Joining of buccal and lingual triangular ridges
c. Junction of two marginal ridge with cingulum
d. The buccal ridge of distolingual cusp with the lingual ridge of mesiolingual cusp.

99. The nature has provided sufficient overlap of maxillary and mandibular teeth in buccal segment. This is to
a. Increase chewing efficiency
b. Add to esthetic value
c. Prevent soft tissue from cheek bite
d. None

100. Main function of proximal contact area is
a. To guide the food over occlusal table
b. For distribution of occlusal stresses
c. To prevent impaction of food in inter-proximal areas
d. All

101. The tooth anatomy common to anterior teeth only is
a. Cingulum b. Fossa
c. Pits d. Marginal ridges

102. Any union of two triangular ridges produces a single ridge which is
a. Cusp ridge
b. Transverse ridge
c. Marginal ridge
d. Proximal ridge

103. The surfaces of the following teeth have a triangular outline
a. Mesial and distal of anterior teeth
b. Mesial and distal of posterior teeth
c. Labial of anterior teeth
d. Lingual of anterior teeth

104. The surfaces of the following teeth have a trapezoid outline
a. Lingual and labial of posterior teeth
b. Lingual and facial of all teeth
c. Lingual and labial of anterior only
d. Proximal of anterior teeth only

105. The divergence of two proximal surfaces from the area of contact facially, lingually, occlusally and gingivally create a space called
a. A contact area
b. An occlusal curvature
c. A gingival space
d. An embrasure

106. Cemento-enamel junction of teeth curves in the following two directions
a. Towards the apex on the facial and lingual surfaces
b. Away from the apex on the facial and lingual surfaces
c. Away from the apex on the mesial and distal surfaces
d. Towards the apex on the mesial and distal surfaces
e. Both a and c

107. The two ridges which are present on all teeth are
a. Triangular ridge
b. Mesial and distal cusp ridge
c. Oblique ridge
d. Mesial and distal marginal ridge

108. A primary centre of growth or calcification on a tooth is called
a. Lobe b. Ridge
c. Cingulum d. Groove

109. The arrangement of natural teeth was first described by
a. GV Black b. Bolton
c. Wilson d. Graf Von Spee

97-a, 98-b, 99-c, 100-d, 101-a, 102-b, 103-a, 104-b, 105-d, 106-e, 107-d, 108-a, 109-d

110. Anisognathus refers to

a. Unequal teeth
b. Unequal jaws
c. Unequal cusps
d. Nonuniform teeth

111. The tooth in the closest relation to the zygomatic buttress is

a. Maxillary second PM
b. Maxillary first M
c. Maxillary second M
d. Maxillary third M

112. Humans have two sets of dentition, one primary and the other permanent, such a condition where two sets of teeth are present is called

a. Polyphyodonty
b. Diphyodonty
c. Monophyodonty
d. None of the above

113. The embrasures that increae in size from anterior toposteror are

a. Occlusal
b. Lingual
c. Labial
d. Gingival
e. a and b

110-b, 111-b, 112-b, 113-e

Chapter 2

The Permanent Incisors

SAQs (3 Marks)

Q 1. Describe type traits of maxillary incisors. *(May 2008, Nov. 2015)*

What are differences between maxillary central and lateral incisor? *(May 2009)*

Ans. Incisors are anterior teeth. They are 8 in number, 4 in each arch. Their functions is incising, esthetics, and phonetics.

Type Traits of Maxillary Incisors

Central incisor (CI)	*Lateral incisor (LI)*
Labial aspect (La)	
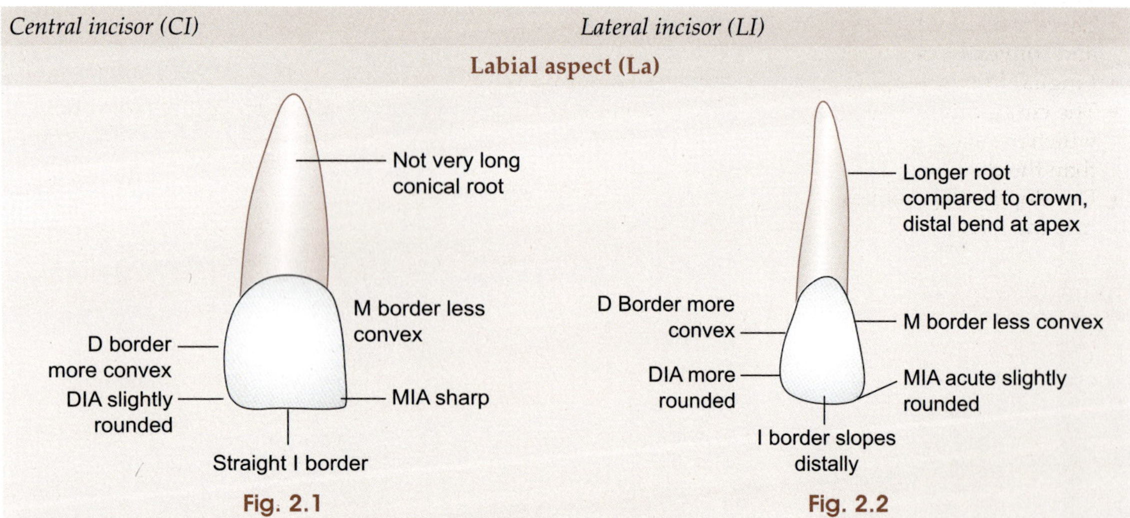 Fig. 2.1	Fig. 2.2
• Crown has more square or rectangular appearance and smooth surface. It is wider and longer.	• Crown is **oblong,** narrower, shorter and has more curvature.
• The mesial (M) border is less convex distal (D) border is more convex.	• Same as CI.
• Mesioincisal angle (MIA) is sharp and disto-incisal angle (DIA) is rounded.	• Both mesioincisal and distoincisal angles are rounded, where distoincisal angle is more rounded.

(Contd.)

Central incisor (CI)	*Lateral incisor (LI) (Contd.)*
• Mesiodistally the incisal ridge is almost straight.	• Incisal ridge is rounded. Mesial half in relatively straight and distal half is more rounded curving (sloping) towards the cervical line to join the distal border.
• Root is cone-shaped with blunt apex.	
• In proportion to crown, root is not much longer.	• In proportion to crown, the root is much longer and has a distal bend.

Lingual view (Li)

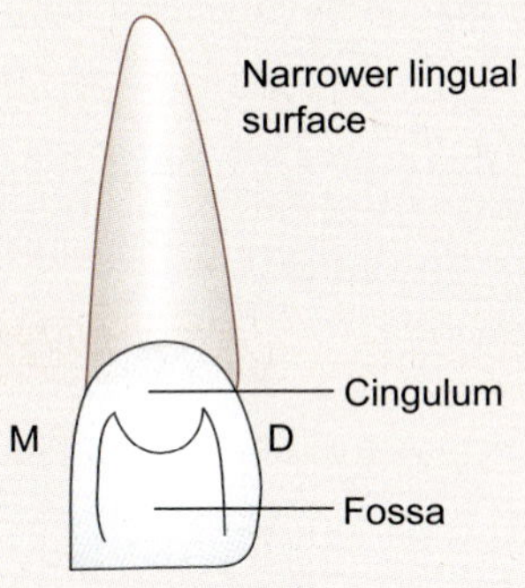

Fig. 2.3

Fig. 2.4

Central incisor (CI)	Lateral incisor (LI)
• The crown and root are narrower towards lingual and marginal ridges are less prominent.	• The crown and root are narrow towards lingual and marginal ridges are prominent.
• The surface is not smooth.	• Same as CI.
• There is concavity, fossa in the incisal two-thirds and convexity, cingulum in cervical third.	• Same as CI.
• Lingual fossa has shallow concavity.	• Lingual fossa has more concavity.
• The **cingulum** is **off-centered to distal** due to which mesial marginal ridge (MMR) is longer than the distal marginal ridge (DMR).	• The **cingulum** is **centered** but still the MMR is longer than the DMR due to the slope of the incisal ridge from M to D.
• Developmental grooves extend from cingulum into the fossa.	• More often a **deep developmental groove** is present at the distal side of the cingulum which may extend up onto the root.

Proximal view

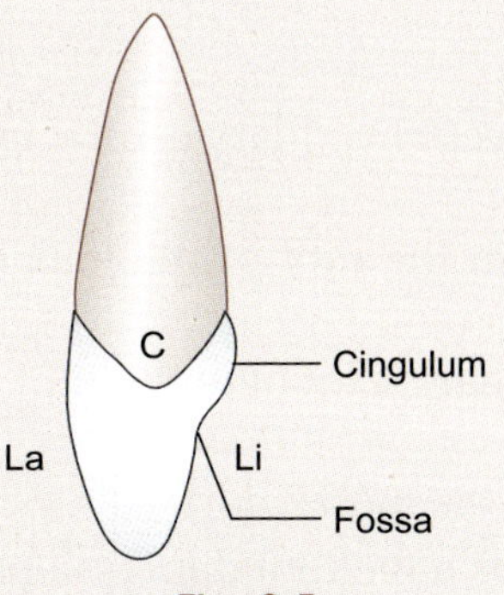

Fig. 2.5

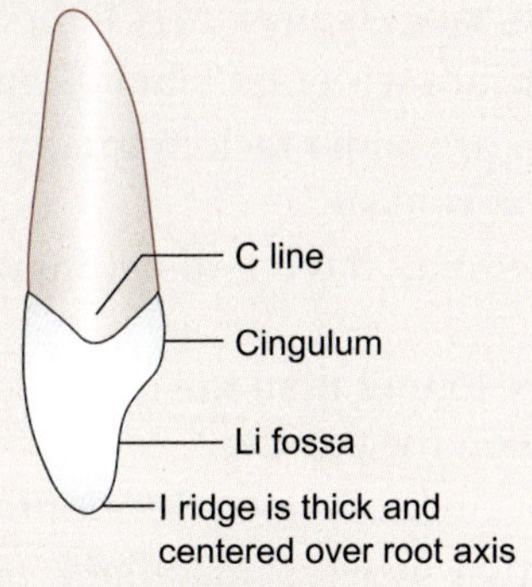

Fig. 2.6

(Contd.)

Central incisor (CI)	Lateral incisor (LI) (Contd.)
• The outline of the crown is triangular. • The crown is larger in size. • Incisal ridge centered over root axis. • The crest of curvature on both labial and lingual surfaces in the cervical third of the crown. • Crown from this aspect appears thicker in the incisal third due to distolingual slope of the labial surface.	• The outline of crown is also triangular. • The crown is **shorter.** • The incisal ridge is centered over root axis. • The crest of curvature on both labial and lingual surfaces is in cervical third of the crown. • Crown from this aspect appears thicker because of the more rounded distoincisal angle.
• The cervical line curvature on mesial aspect is more than that on the distal aspect. The cervical curvature is greater on the mesial surface of this tooth than on any other tooth in the mouth.	• The cervical line curvature on mesial aspect is more than that on the distal aspect.
• Root from this aspect is conical and apex bluntly rounded.	• Root from this aspect is conical, **longer** and has a pointed apex.
Incisal aspect (I)	
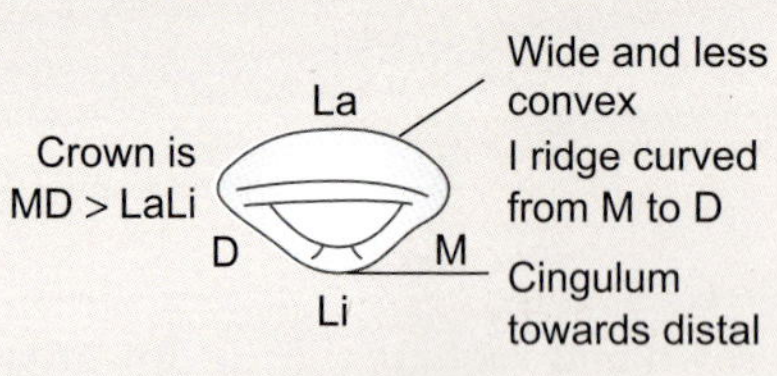 Fig. 2.7	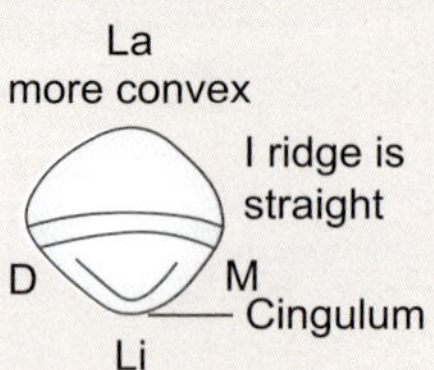 Fig. 2.8
• The crown outline is **triangular** • Crown is wider mesiodistally than labiolingually.	• The crown outline is **ovoid.** • The crown may be wider labiolingually than mesiodistally (MD).
• Labial outline is broad and flat **compared to lingual.** • The incisal ridge is slightly curved from mesial to distal.	• Labial and lingual outlines are more convex. • The incisal ridge is straight.

Q 2. Describe the roots of anterior teeth. *(June 2010)*

Ans.

- More often the anterior teeth have single roots.
- The roots taper from cervix to apex.
- The roots are wider on labial than on lingual.
- The roots are wider faciolingually than mesiodistally except maxillary central incisor where the root is conical.
- The roots may have a distal bend at the apex except in the root of the maxillary central incisor.
- Roots are longer than the crown except in case of maxillary CI where the root is not much longer than the crown.
- Maxillary incisors have developmental depressions on the mesial surface.
- Mandibular incisors, maxillary, and mandibular canines have root depressions on both M and D surfaces with distal depression being more distinct.
- Maxillary canine has the longest root of all the teeth.

Q 3. What are variations in permanent maxillary incisors? *(Nov. 2010)*

Ans. **Central Incisor**

- Hutchinson's incisors are found in congenital syphilis. They are screw-driver shaped with notched incisal edge.
- Central incisors may have very short root or very long root.
- Talon's cusp, fusion, gemination may be found.
- Shovel-shaped CI is one of the variations found in maxillary CI.

Lateral Incisor

- **Peg-shaped** is relatively common.
- The crown may be distorted.
- The tooth may be missing.
- The tooth may have a twisted root.
- Incisal side of cingulum may show a tubercle.
- Talon's cusp, an accessory cusp may be present on the lingual surface.
- Lingual surface may have a deep lingual pit.
- **Deep palatogingival groove** from cingulum to root may be present.

Q 4. Explain about type traits of permanent mandibular incisors.

Ans. Mandibular incisors are 4 in number.

They have uniform development and have narrowest of mesiodistal dimension.

Type Traits of Mandibular Incisors

Central incisor (CI)	*Lateral incisor (LI)*
Labial aspect (La)	

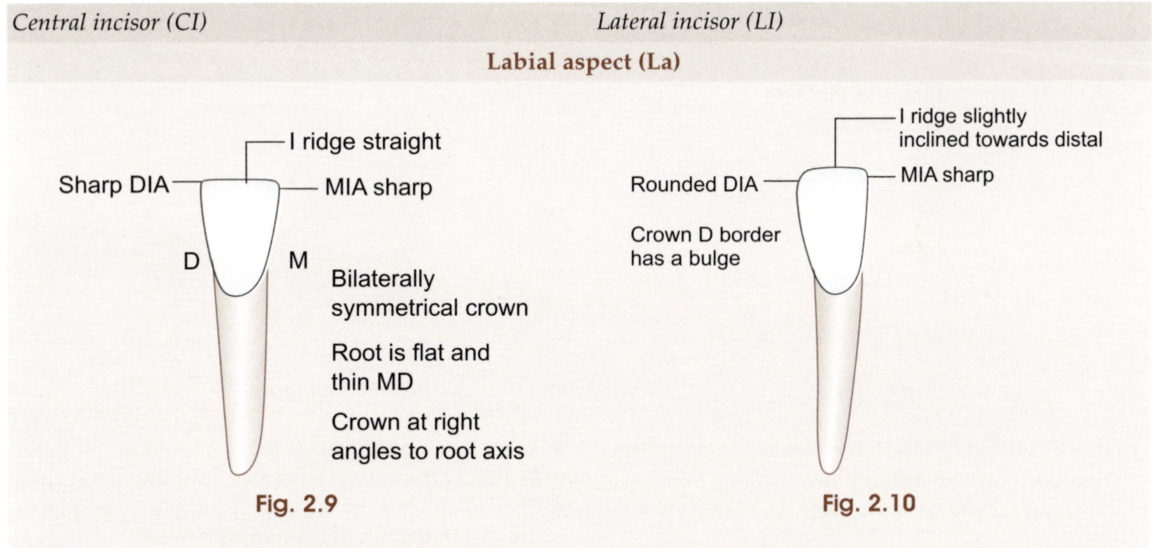

Fig. 2.9 Fig. 2.10

Central incisor (CI)	Lateral incisor (LI)
• The labial surface is regular and convex. • The crown is long and narrow and is bilaterally symmetrical. • Mesial and Distal incisal angles (MIA and DIA) are sharp (90°).	• Same as central incisor. • The crown is slightly wider and longer than that of central incisor and is not bilaterally symmetrical. • MIA is sharp whereas DIA is rounded. • DIA is rounded.

(Contd.)

Central incisor (CI)	*Lateral incisor (LI) (Contd.)*
• Incisal ridge (IR) is straight and at right angles to long axis.	• Incisal ridge is not straight.
• The root from this aspect is very thin mesiodistally.	• Same as that of CI.
• It may have a distal bend in the apical third.	• The root is longer and may have a distal bend.
Lingual aspect (Li)	
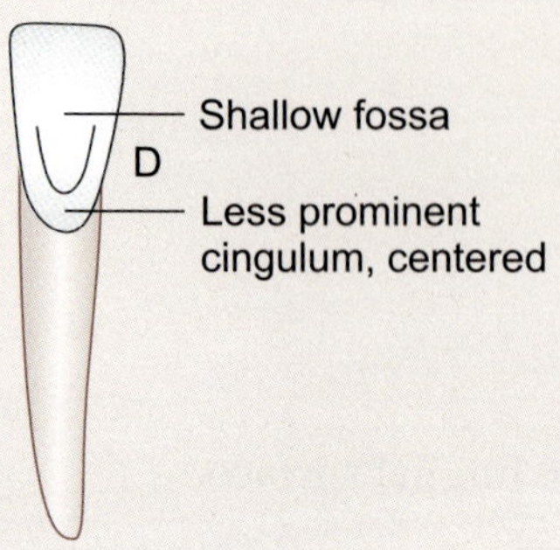 Fig. 2.11	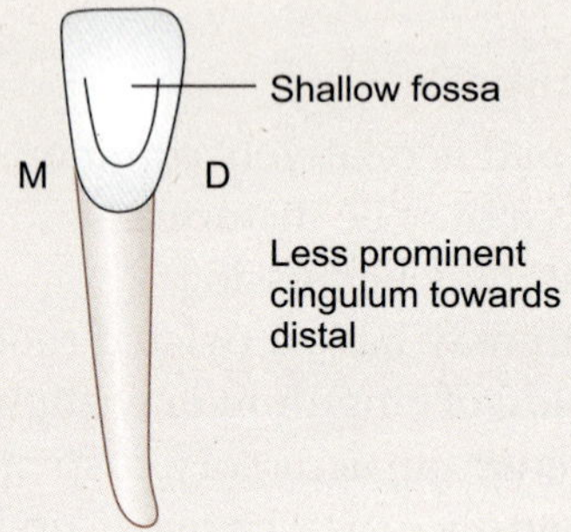 Fig. 2.12
• The lingual surface is smooth and shallow.	• Same as central incisor.
• The cingulum is small, convex, and centered.	• The cingulum is small, convex and off-centered to distal.
• No developmental grooves or pits.	• Same as central incisor.
• M and D developmental grooves on roots are visible from this aspect.	• Same as central incisor.
Proximal aspect	
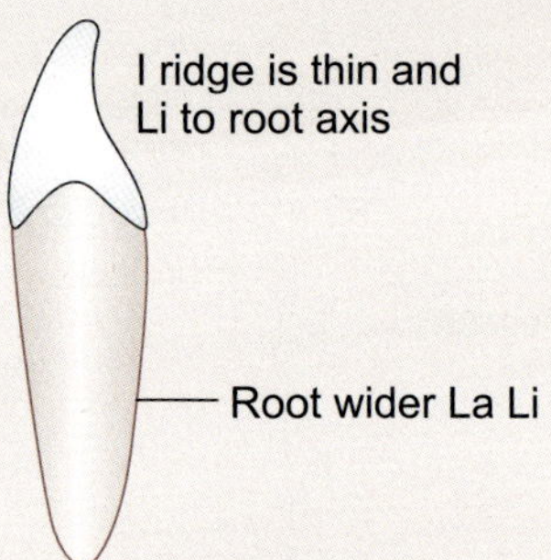 Fig. 2.13	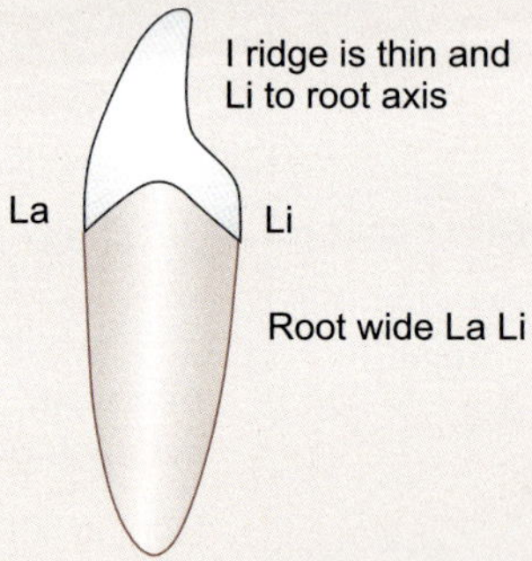 Fig. 2.14
• Mesial (M) and distal (D) surfaces are wedge-shaped.	• Same as central incisor.
• M and D surfaces are similar.	• M side of the crown is longer than the distal side.
• The incisal ridge is on or lingual to the root axis.	• The distoincisal twist of the incisal ridge places the distal portion of the incisal ridge more lingual than mesial portion.
• Crest of curvature on both labial and lingual surfaces is in the cervical third of the crown.	• Same as central incisor.
• The cervical line curvature on mesial is more than on distal surface.	• Same as central incisor.

(Contd.)

Central incisor (CI)	*Lateral incisor (LI) (Contd.)*
• The root from this aspect is wider labiolingually (LaLi) than mesiodistally (MD)	• Same as central incisor.
• Developmental depressions present on both M and D surface of the root.	• Same as central incisor.

Incisal aspect (I)

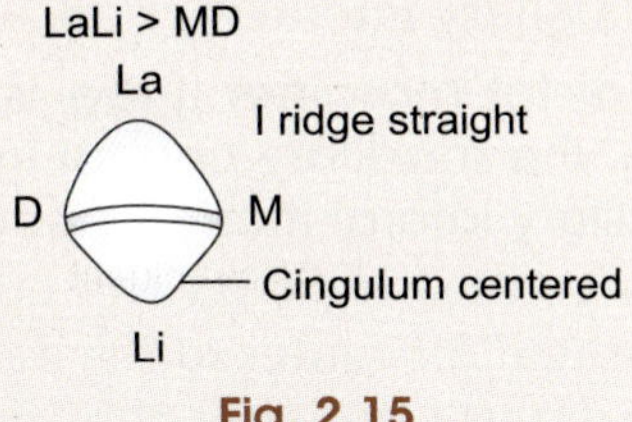

Fig. 2.15

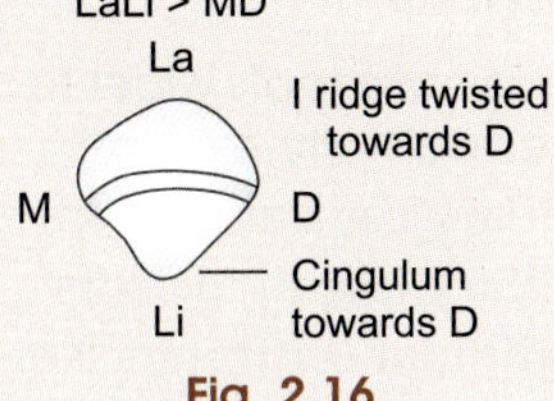

Fig. 2.16

Central incisor (CI)	*Lateral incisor (LI) (Contd.)*
• The tooth is bilaterally symmetrical. Mesial half is identical with the distal half.	• It is not bilaterally symmetrical.
• Incisal ridge is straight and at right angles to the line bisecting the cingulum.	• Incisal ridge not straight twisted towards distal. It follows the curvature of the mandibular arch.
• Labiolingually (LaLi) dimension > mesiodistally (MD) dimension.	• Same as central incisor.
• Labial (La) surface wider than lingual surface (Li).	• Same as central incisor.
• Cingulum is centered.	• Cingulum is toward distal.

MULTIPLE CHOICE QUESTIONS (MCQs)

1. The scallops found on the newly erupted teeth are known as
a. Perikymata
b. Mamelons
c. Imbrication lines
d. None of the above

2. All incisors have roots wider faciolingually than mesiodistally *except*
a. Maxillary central incisors
b. Maxillary lateral incisors
c. Mandibular central incisors
d. Mandibular lateral incisors

3. The incisal wear pattern on maxillary incisors is as
a. Incisal edge slopes cervically towards labial
b. Incisal edge slopes cervically towards lingual fossa
c. Incisal edge with no slope
d. None of the above

4. In mandibular incisors the incisal edge wear slopes
a. Cervically towards labial
b. Cervically towards lingual fossa
c. Neither labially nor lingually
d. None of the above

5. For all human teeth, contact areas are located
a. In incisal or occlusal thirds
b. At the junction of incisal and middle thirds
c. Cervical thirds
d. Both a and b

6. Maxillary central incisor is generally considered to be a poor abutment tooth when making a dental bridge because
a. Of its position
b. Root being short and conical
c. Due to size of the crown
d. None of the above

7. The mesial curvature of the cervical line is deepest on which of the following?
a. Mandibular central incisors
b. Maxillary canine
c. Maxillary central incisors
d. Maxillary lateral incisors.

8. The distal marginal ridge is shorter in both, the maxillary central Incisors and maxillary lateral Incisors because
a. In central incisors the cingulum is located off center to the distal side
b. In lateral incisors the incisal edge slopes cervically from mesial to distal
c. Both a and b
d. None of the above

9. A longitudinal depression is found on the middle of the mesial surface of the root of
a. Maxillary central incisors
b. Maxillary lateral incisors
c. Both
d. None of the above

10. The incisor more likely to have a bifurcated root is a variation found in
a. Maxillary lateral incisors
b. Mandibular central incisors
c. Mandibular lateral incisors
d. Maxillary central incisor

11. Shovel shaped incisors and a deep groove running cervicoincisally on the cingulum are associated with dentition in the following ethnic group
a. Caucasian b. Negro
c. Mongoloid d. None of the above

12. The only incisor that is symmetrical, having M and D contact points at the same level and is difficult to tell Right from Left is
a. Maxillary central incisors
b. Mandibular central incisors
c. Mandibular lateral incisors
d. Maxillary lateral incisor

1-b, 2-a, 3-b, 4-a, 5-d, 6-b, 7-c, 8-c, 9-c, 10-c, 11-c, 12-b

13. The labiolingual dimension is more than mesiodistal dimension in
a. Maxillary central incisors
b. Maxillary lateral incisors
c. Mandibular incisors
d. Both a and b

14. From proximal view, incisal edge is lingual to mid root axis, root is thin mesiodistally with inconspicuous marginal ridges and lingual fossa, is characteristic of
a. Maxillary incisors
b. Mandibular incisors
c. Maxillary canine
d. Mandibular canine

15. Longitudinal root depressions on both M and D root surface is characteristic of
a. Maxillary incisors
b. Mandibular incisors
c. Premolars
d. Molars

16. The cingulum is centred in
a. Maxillary central incisors and mandibular central incisors
b. Maxillary lateral incisors and mandibular lateral incisors
c. Maxillary lateral incisors and mandibular central incisors
d. Only maxillary central incisors

17. Palatal gingival groove, peg-shape, missing tooth are the variations found in
a. Maxillary lateral incisors
b. Mandibular lateral incisors
c. Mandibular canines
d. Maxillary central incisors

18. Crown bent distally on root, the bulge on the distal side of the crown and distal placement of the cingulum are characteristics of
a. Maxillary lateral incisors
b. Mandibular lateral incisors
c. Maxillary central incisors
d. Mandibular canine

19. In maxillary central incisors outline of the pulp chamber is
a. Round b. Oval
c. Triangular d. Square shaped

20. The distolingual twist of the incisal edge to the root axis is common to
a. Mandibular central incisors
b. Mandibular lateral incisors
c. Both a and b
d. None of the above

21. Most common incisors to show morphologic variation is
a. Permanent maxillary lateral incisors
b. Permanent mandibular central incisors
c. Deciduous maxillary central incisors
d. Permanent mandibular lateral incisor

22. The apex of the roots are generally tilted to
a. Buccal side b. Lingual side
c. Distal side d. Mesial side

23. The only root which is triangular in cross-section at cervix is of
a. Maxillary canine
b. Maxillary lateral incisor
c. Maxillary central incisor
d. Mandibular central incisor

24. The curve of the cervical line is deepest incisally on the mesial surface of
a. Maxillary central incisors
b. Maxillary lateral incisors
c. Mandibular central incisors
d. Mandibular lateral incisors

25. A deep lingual pit is usually found on the lingual surface of
a. Permanent maxillary central incisors
b. Permanent maxillary lateral incisors
c. Permanent maxillary canine
d. Permanent maxillary mandibular incisors

13-c, 14-b, 15-b, 16-c, 17-a, 18-b, 19-c, 20-b, 21-a, 22-c, 23-c, 24-a, 25-b

26. The tooth least likely to have a divided pulp canal is
a. Maxillary central incisor
b. Maxillary first PM
c. Mandibular central incisor
d. Mandibular first PM

27. The mesial contact area between the two maxillary and the two mandibular central incisors is present in the
a. Incisal third
b. Middle third
c. Cervical third
d. At the junction of middle and cervical third

28. The first evidence of calcification of permanent central incisors take place at
a. 3–4 months after birth
b. 3–4 months in intrauterine life
c. 6 months after birth
d. 8 months after birth

29. The first evidence of calcification of permanent maxillary LI takes place at
a. 8 months in intrauterine life
b. 8 months in after birth
c. 10 to 12 months after birth
d. At birth

30. Eruption of permanent maxillary CI takes place at the age of
a. 4–5 years b. 6–7 years
c. 7–8 years d. 9–10 years

31. Eruption of permanent maxillary LI takes place at the age of
a. 6–7 years b. 7–8 years
c. 8–9 years d. 9–10 years

32. The crown completion of permanent central incisors takes place at the age?
a. 4–5 years
b. 5–6 years
c. 6–7 years
d. 3–4 years

33. The first evidence of calcification of permanent mandibular LI takes place at the age of
a. 3–4 months after birth
b. 3–4 years after birth
c. 3–4 months in intrauterine life
d. 6–8 months in intrauterine life

34. In all the permanent incisors first evidence of calcification takes place at about 3ñ4 months after birth *except*
a. Maxillary central incisor
b. Maxillary lateral incisor
c. Mandibular central incisor
d. Mandibular lateral incisor.

35. An anatomic feature that is most likely to complicate root planing of a maxillary lateral incisor is
a. A root bifurcation
b. A mesial concavity
c. An enamel projection
d. A distolingual groove

36. The following structure calcifies first in an anterior tooth
a. Cingulum
b. Cervical ridge
c. Marginal ridge
d. Incisal ridge

37. The wear facets on the incisal edges of the mandibular lateral incisors are caused by occlusion with the
a. Maxillary central incisors only
b. Maxillary central and lateral incisors
c. Maxillary lateral incisors and canines
d. None of the above

38. Developmental depressions are not present on both mesial and distal surfaces of the roots of permanent.
a. Mandibular central incisors
b. Maxillary central incisors
c. Maxillary canine
d. None of the above

26-a, 27-a, 28-a, 29-c, 30-c, 31-c, 32-a, 33-a, 34-b, 35-d, 36-d, 37-b, 38-b

39. The maxillary permanent central incisor develops from

a. Two lobes and has two mamelons
b. Four lobes and has three mamelons
c. Three lobes and has three mamelons
d. Four lobes and has two mamelons

40. The permanent anterior tooth which may have a lingual groove extending from enamel to cementum of root

a. Maxillary canine
b. Maxillary lateral incisor
c. Maxillary central incisor
d. None of the above.

41. The permanent anterior tooth having developmental grooves extending from the cingulum into the lingual fossa is

a. Maxillary central incisor
b. Mandibular central incisor
c. Mandibular lateral incisor
d. Mandibular canine

42. The root of permanent tooth which is completed by 10 years is

a. Maxillary central incisors
b. Maxillary first molars
c. Mandibular first molars
d. None of the above

43. Depressions on the M and D aspect of the root is seen in

a. Mandibular central and lateral incisors
b. Maxillary canines
c. Maxillary central and lateral incisors
d. Maxillary first premolars

39-b, 40-b, 41-a, 42-a, 43-a

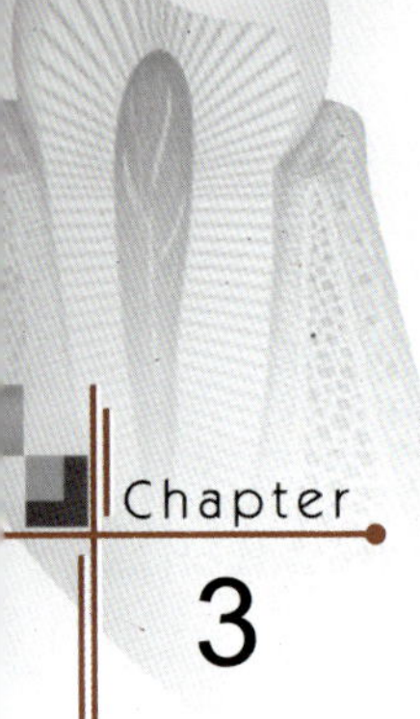

Chapter

3

The Permanent Canines

LAQ (10 Marks)

Q 1. Compare and contrast maxillary canine with mandibular canine in tabular form.
(June 2006)

Ans.

Maxillary canine

Introduction:
It is the third tooth from the midline in the maxillary arch.

Numbering system:

Palmer	3⌋	⌊3
Universal	Right-6	Left-11
F.D.I.	Right-13	Left-23

Chronological data:

First evidence of calcification	4–5 months
Enamel completion	6–7 years
Eruption	11–12 years
Root completion	13–15 years

Mandibular canine

Introduction:
It is the third tooth from the midline in the mandibular arch.

Numbering system:

Palmer	3⌉	⌈3
Universal	Right-27	Left-22
FDI	Right-43	Left-33

Chronological data:

First evidence of calcification	4–5 month
Enamel completion	6–7 years
Eruption	9–10 years
Root completion	12–14 years

Canine from each aspect

Labial aspect (La) (SAQ, Nov. 2015)

Maxillary canine	Mandibular canine
Crown: *Shape, size, and surface*: • It has trapezoid or pentagon shape due to 2 incisal ridges meeting at cusp tip which is pointed. • The length of the crown is short – (10 mm). It is 7.5 mm wide at contact area and 5.5 mm wide at cervix. • The labial ridge (LaR) is more prominent.	**Crown:** *Shape, size, and surface*: • It also has pentagon shape with two incisal ridges meeting at cusp tip which is not pointed. • The crown is **longer** (11 mm), and **narrower.** It is 7 mm wide at contact area and 5.5 mm wide at cervix. • The labial ridge is not prominent.

(*Contd.*)

Maxillary canine

Long conical root with distal bend
M and D borders of crown converge more at cervix
La R
MIA sharp
Short M cusp slope
DIA rounded
Longer D cusp slope
Both cusp slopes make acute angle at cusp tip

Fig. 3.1

Outlines:
- The mesial (M) and distal (D) outlines of the crown **converge towards the cervix**
- The M outline is convex from cervix to the contact point.
- D outline is concave near the cervix and convex at the contact point.
- Mesial cusp slope (MCS) is shorter than the distal cusp slope (DCS).
  Both the cusp slopes may have concavity before wear.
- M and D cusp slopes make an **acute angle** at the cusp tip which is centred over the root axis.
- The cusp slopes and the cusp make-up for the **incisal one-third** of the crown.
- The cervical line is convex towards the root apex.
- Mesioincisal angle (MIA) is sharp. Distoincisal angle (DIA) is rounded.

Contact point:
- Mesial contact point is at the **junction of incisal and middle third.**
- Distal contact point is in the middle third of the crown and is rounded.
- M and D contact areas are at different levels.

Root:
- The root is long, (17 mm), slender, and conical.
- The apex is bluntly pointed and may have a distal bend.

Mandibular canine (Contd.)

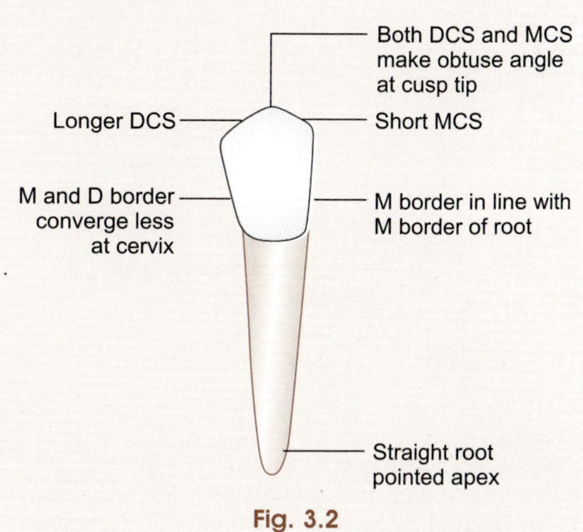

Fig. 3.2

Outlines:
- The mesial and distal outlines of the crown are **less converging,** they are more or less parallel.
- M outline of the crown is more or **less straight** in line with the mesial outline of the root.
- D outline is slightly concave in the cervical third.
- It is same as Maxillary Canine.
- M and D cusp slopes make an **obtuse angle** at the cusp tip which is centered over the root axis.
- The cusp slopes and the cusp make-up for the **incisal one-fifth** of the crown.
- The cervical line is convex towards the root apex.

Contact point:
- Mesial contact point is in the **incisal third** near the mesioincisal angle.
- Distal contact point is cervical to the mesial contact point.

Root:
- The root is 16 mm. It is **shorter** and **narrower** mesiodistally than that of maxillary canine.
- The apex is sharply pointed.

(Contd.)

Maxillary canine	*Mandibular canine (Contd.)*

Lingual aspect (Li)

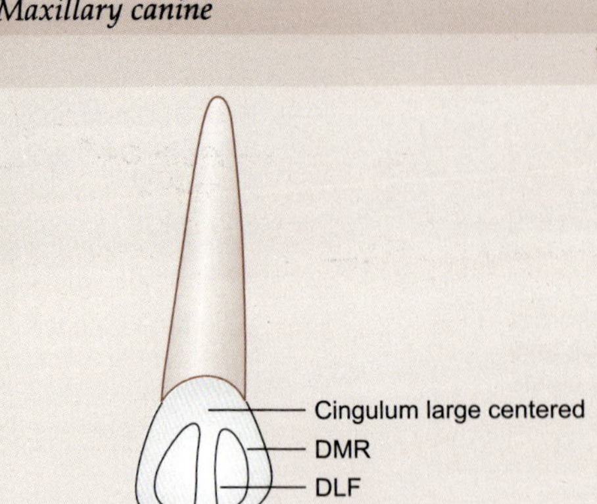

Fig. 3.3

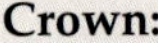

Crown:

Shape, size, and surface:

- The crown and root are narrower towards lingual.
- The **lingual ridge (LiR)** is prominent, runs from the cusp tip to the cingulum.
- The lingual surface is not **smooth.**
- The mesial and distal fossa (MLF and DLF) lie on either side of the lingual ridge and are usually shallow. Marginal ridges are strongly developed.
- The cingulum is large and centered and in some cases it is pointed like a small cusp or tubercle.

Outline:

- Outlines are similar to the labial surface.
- The mesial marginal ridge (MMR) is longer compared to the (DMR) because of the shorter mesial cusp slope.

Root:

- Root is narrow on the lingual side therefore it is possible to see the M and D surfaces of the root as well as the M and D developmental depressions.

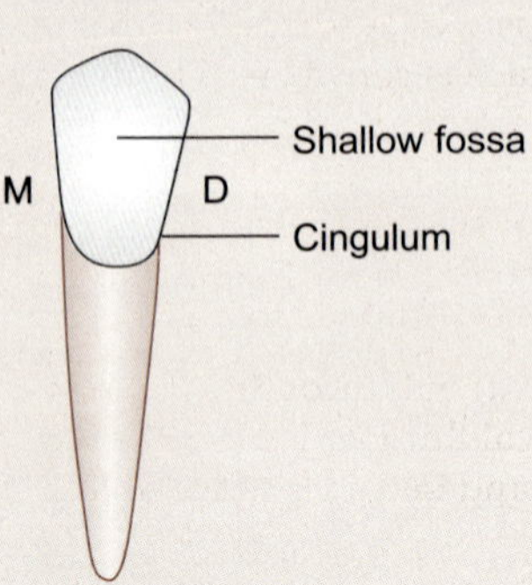

Fig. 3.4

Crown:

Shape, size, and surface:

- Same as maxillary canine.
- The lingual ridge is faint except at the cusp tip where it may be raised.
- The lingual surface is smooth regular and flatter.
- Fossa is less prominent. Marginal ridges are less distinct.
- The cingulum is smooth and poorly developed and off-centred distally or may be centered.

Outline:

- Outlines are similar to the labial surface.
- MMR is longer because of shorter mesial cusp slope as well as the cingulum being off-centred to distal.

- The lingual portion of the root is relatively narrower than that of the maxillary canine.

Proximal aspect

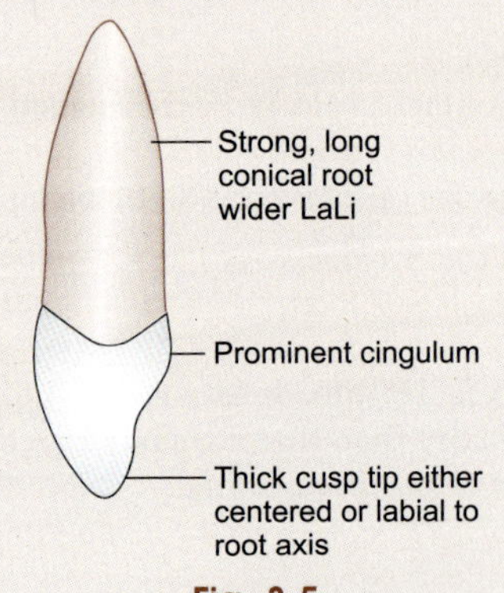

Fig. 3.5

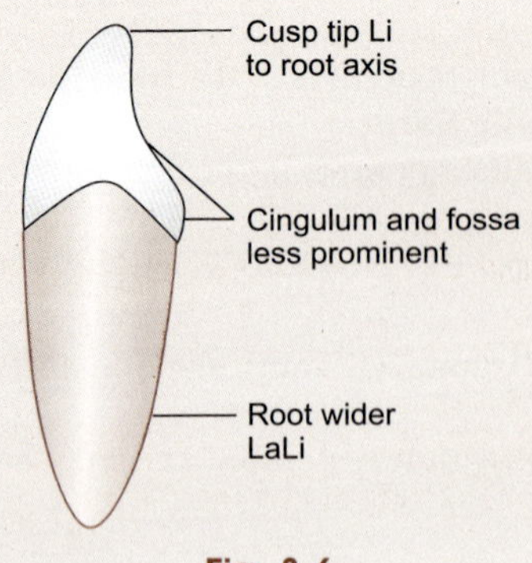

Fig. 3.6

(*Contd.*)

Maxillary canine	*Mandibular canine (Contd.)*
Crown: *Shape, size, and surface*: • The crown is wedge-shaped with smooth surface. • Mesial surface is convex except the area between the contact point and the cervical line which is slightly concave or flat. • On the distal surface there is more concavity in the area between the contact point and the cervical line.	**Crown:** *Shape, size, and surface*: • It is same as maxillary canine. • Mesial surface is not convex except at the contact point. • On the distal surface there is more concavity in the area between the contact point and the cervical line.
Outlines: • The labial (La) outline of the crown is more convex in the cervical third and is less convex in the incisal two-thirds and becomes more or less straight near the cusp.	*Outlines*: • The labial (La) outline has very less curvature, with very little curvature directly above the cervical line.
• The lingual (Li) outline is represented by a convex line describing the cingulum. In the middle third the outline is straight and becomes convex again in the incisal third.	• The lingual (Li) outline is very less convex. Cingulum is low and somewhat flattened. There is almost continuous crown-root outline.
• The crest of curvature on both labial and lingual surface is in the cervical third of the crown which shows **greater bulk labiolingually (LaLi)** than any other anterior tooth.	• The crest of curvature on both labial and lingual surfaces is in the cervical third but the bulk is much less and closer to the cervical line.
• The cusp tip is thicker labiolingually and is located either labial to root axis or centred over it.	• The cusp tip is thinner labiolingually and is located lingual to the root axis or may be centered over it.
• The cervical line curvature is towards incisal and more so on the mesial surface than on the distal surface.	• The cervical line curvature is more on the mandibular than on the maxillary canine and more so on the mesial surface than the distal surface.
• Distoincisal angle (DIA) is in line with the mesioincisal angle (MIA).	• Distoincisal angle is slightly more lingually placed than the cusp tip because of the distolingual twist of the crown, so much so that the lingual surface is visible from the mesial aspect.
Root: • Root is wide labiolingually in cervical third and middle third, it tapers at the apex. Labial outline is slightly convex while lingual outline is more convex. • Developmental depression on the distal surface is more pronounced whereas mesial depression is shallow.	**Root:** • Root from this aspect is very similar to that of maxillary canine except that the root tip is more pointed. • Both the M and D root depressions are more pronounced in the apical third.
Incisal aspect	
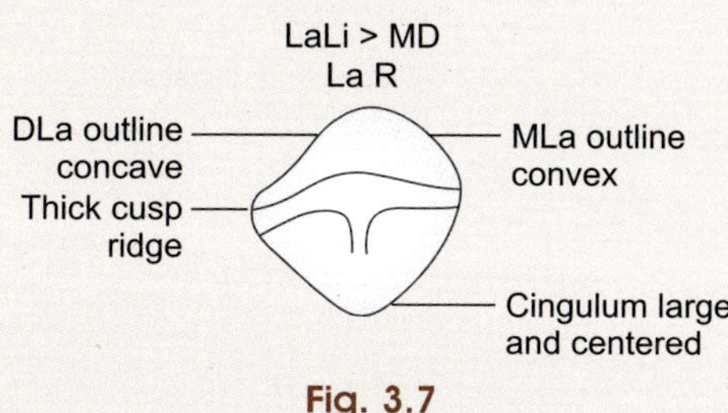 **Fig. 3.7**	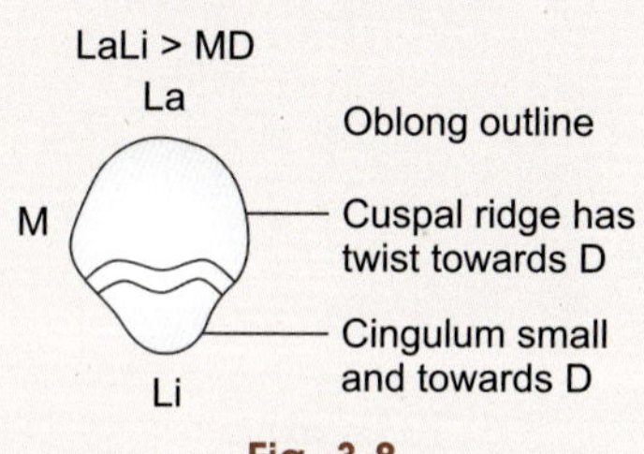 **Fig. 3.8**

(Contd.)

Maxillary canine	*Mandibular canine (Contd.)*
• The crown outline is not symmetrical.	• The crown outline is more symmetrical.
• Labiolingual dimension (Lali) is more than mesiodistal (MD) dimension.	• The labiolingual dimension is noticeably larger than mesiodistal dimension.
• Labial outline is convex due to prominent labial ridge.	• Oblong labiolingual outline is characteristic of mandibular canine.
• The mesial half of the labial surface (MLa) is very much convex while the distal half (DLa) is slightly concave giving it the appearance as if it is pinched or stretched to make contact with the first premolar.	• Mesiolabial outline is convex, distolabial outline flat or slightly concave.
• The **cingulum** is **large** and **centered** mesiodistally.	• The cingulum is **small** and **off-centred to distal.**
• The incisal ridge is straight mesiodistally.	• The incisal ridge is not straight it has a disto-lingual twist.
• The tip of the cusp is labial to the centre of the crown labiolingually and mesial to the centre mesiodistally.	

SAQ (3 Marks)

Q 1. What are class traits of canines? *(May 2014)*

Ans. **Class Traits of Canines**

- Canine is the longest tooth in the oral cavity.
- **Maxillary canine has a functional lingual surface.**
- It has a single pointed cusp. Incisal ridge of canine is divided into two inclines or slopes by a cusp as opposed to a straight ridge in the incisors, which gives the crown a pentagon shape. The mesial slope is shorter than the distal slope. Canine does not have mamelons but may have a notch on either of the cusp slope.
- It has a single, longest and strongest root of all the teeth providing best anchorage amongst all anterior teeth.
- **It is the only anterior tooth with a labial ridge.**
- Canines typically have mesial and distal contact areas at different levels cervicoincisally because of the mesial and distal contact with different classes of teeth.

MULTIPLE CHOICE QUESTIONS (MCQs)

1. The longest teeth in the mouth are
a. Canines b. Incisors
c. Premolars d. Molars

2. The feature that distinguishes maxillary canine from mandibular canine are
a. The pointed, acute angle at cusp tip and constriction of crown at the cervix
b. Asymmetrical outline from incisal view
c. Both a and b
d. Symmetrical outline from incisal view

3. Mesiodistal dimension of this tooth is less than labiolingual dimension
a. Permanent maxillary central incisor
b. Permanent maxillary canine
c. Permanent maxillary lateral incisor
d. None

4. The characteristic that differentiates maxillary canine from mandibular canine
a. Cusp tip labial to centre
b. Attrition on lingual surfaces
c. Cingulum is centred
d. All of the above

5. The tooth having mesial side of the crown in line with mesial side of the root is
a. Maxillary canine
b. Mandibular canine
c. Mandibular lateral incisor
d. Maxillary central incisor

6. The cingulum is off centred to distal in
a. Permanent maxillary central incisor
b. Mandibular lateral incisor
c. Mandibular canine
d. All the above

7. The canine eminence ridge on the anterior surface of maxilla, forms the following fossa anterior to it
a. Incisive fossa
b. Canine fossa
c. Triangular fossa
d. Central fossa

8. The anterior teeth most likely to have a bifurcated root is
a. Permanent maxillary canine
b. Permanent mandibular lateral incisor
c. Permanent mandibular canine
d. Permanent maxillary lateral incisor
e. Both b and c

9. The distinguishing features between maxillary right and left canine are
a. Shorter mesial cusp slope
b. Mesioincisal angle sharp, distoincisal rounded
c. Mesial cervical line is more convex
d. All the above

10. The surface of mandibular canine crown which is relatively straight and is in continuation with the same on the root is
a. Mesial b. Labial
c. Lingual d. Distal

11. The permanent tooth in the oral cavity having the longest crown length is
a. Maxillary canine
b. Mandibular lateral incisor
c. Maxillary 1st premolar
d. Mandibular canine

12. Anterior teeth having two roots, i.e. root divided into labial and lingual part is variation found in
a. Maxillary canine
b. Mandibular canine
c. Maxillary incisor
d. Mandibular incisor (lateral)
e. Both b and d

13. From incisal view distolingual twist of the crown is common to
a. Mandibular canine
b. Mandibular lateral incisor
c. Both a and b
d. Maxillary central incisor

1-a, 2-c, 3-b, 4-d, 5-b, 6-d, 7-a, 8-e, 9-d, 10-a, 11-d, 12-e, 13-c

14. From incisal aspect the labial outline of the crown appears to be pinched faciolingually on the distal half, this is the characteristic of
a. Maxillary canine
b. Mandibular canine
c. Both maxillary and mandibular canine
d. None of the above

15. From incisal view, compared to the axis of the root, the cusp tip of maxillary canine is placed
a. Labially and distally
b. Labially and mesially
c. Lingually and distally
d. Lingually and mesially

16. The largest labiolingual root dimension is of
a. Maxillary central incisor
b. Maxillary lateral incisor
c. Maxillary canine
d. Mandibular canine

17. On the lingual surface (in cingulum region) of permanent maxillary canine is a sharp cusp like eminence called
a. Lobe
b. Tubercle
c. Mamelon
d. Perikymata

18. The fossa above the roots of premolars, posterior to canine eminence on maxilla is
a. Canine fossa b. Incisive fossa
c. Linear fossa d. Central fossa

19. Of the four cusp ridges the longest cusp ridge of the permanent canines is
a. Labial ridge b. Lingual ridge
c. Mesial ridge d. Distal ridge

20. The permanent maxillary canine is most likely to occlude with mandibular
a. Lateral incisor and canine
b. Canine only
c. Canine and first premolar
d. First premolar only

21. The first evidence of calcification of permanent maxillary canine takes place at the age of
a. 4–5 months after birth
b. 4–5 years after birth
c. 6 months in intrauterine life
d. None of the above

22. The crown completion of permanent maxillary canine is at
a. 6–7 years b. 4–5 years
c. 7–8 years d. 8–9 years

23. When a permanent mandibular canine has more than one root, usually the position of the root is
a. Mesial and distal
b. Facial and lingual
c. Mesial and lingual
d. Distal and facial.

24. The distal contact point of maxillary canine is usually located at
a. Junction of middle and cervical third
b. Middle of cervical third
c. Middle third
d. Junction of incisal and middle third

25. In a maxillary canine, from proximal aspect the line bisecting the root apex will pass
a. Labial to the cusp tip
b. Lingual to the cusp tip
c. Through the cusp tip
d. None of the above

14-a, 15-b, 16-c, 17-b, 18-a, 19-a, 20-c, 21-a, 22-a, 23-b, 24-c, 25-b

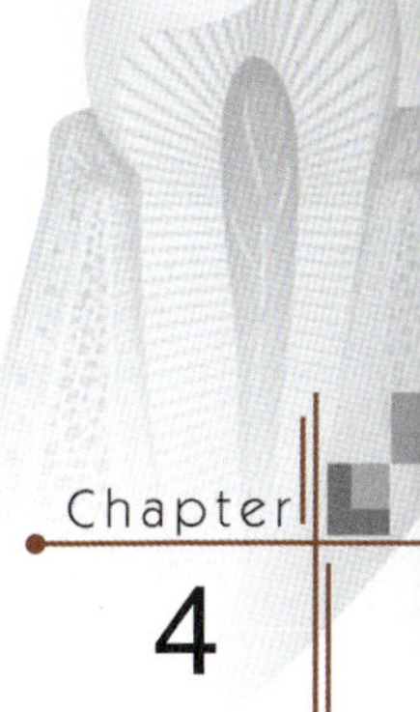

Chapter 4

Premolars

LAQs (10 Marks)

Q 1. Describe class and arch traits of premolars. Compare and contrast maxillary first and second premolars. (*June 2011*)

Ans. Class Traits of Premolars

- Premolars have a single buccal (B) cusp.
- They usually have two cusps, one buccal and one lingual and are called bicuspids but the term is misnomer because very often mandibular second premolar may have three cusps.
- They may have one or two roots.

Arch Traits of Premolars (*SAQ, Oct. 2003, Nov. 2010, 2014*)

- Maxillary first premolars are larger than the second premolars whereas mandibular first premolars are smaller than the second premolars.
- Maxillary first and second premolars are more similar to each other as compared to mandibular first and second premolars.
- Maxillary premolars usually erupt before the eruption of maxillary canines.
- Mandibular premolars usually erupt after the eruption of mandibular canines.
- From proximal view
  - Mandibular premolar crowns appear to be tilted lingual to the root axis.
  - In mandibular premolars the lingual cusps are much shorter than the buccal cusps as compared to those of maxillary premolars.
  - Mandibular premolars show rhomboid outline from this aspect due to the lingual tilt of the crown whereas maxillary premolars show trapezoid outline from this aspect.
- From occlusal view
  - The maxillary premolars have hexagonal or ovoid outline.
    The crown is wider buccolingually than mesiodistally.
  - The mandibular premolars have more or less square outline or rounded or ovoid.
  - Lingual cusp-tips are off-centered to the mesial most often on maxillary premolars and may be off-centered to mesial on mandibular first premolars and second premolars with two cusps.
  - Mandibular premolars exhibit more variation in occlusal form as compared to maxillary premolars.

Maxillary first premolar

Introduction:

- It is located fourth from the midline and contacts maxillary canine mesially and maxillary second premolar distally.
- It is larger than the second premolar.

Numbering system:

Palmer	4┘	└4
Universal	R # 5	L # 12
FDI	14	24

Chronological data:

First evidence of calcification	1½–13/4 yrs
Enamel completed	5–6 yrs
Eruption	10–11 yrs
Root completed	12–13 yrs

Maxillary second premolar

Introduction:

- It is located fifth from the midline and contacts maxillary first premolar mesially and maxillary first molar distally.
- It is smaller than the first premolar.

Numbering system:

Palmer	5┘	└5
Universal	R # 4	L # 13
FDI	15	25

Chronological data:

First evidence of calcification	2–21/4 yrs
Enamel completed	6–7 yrs
Eruption	10–12 yrs
Root completion	12–14 yrs

Buccal aspect (B)

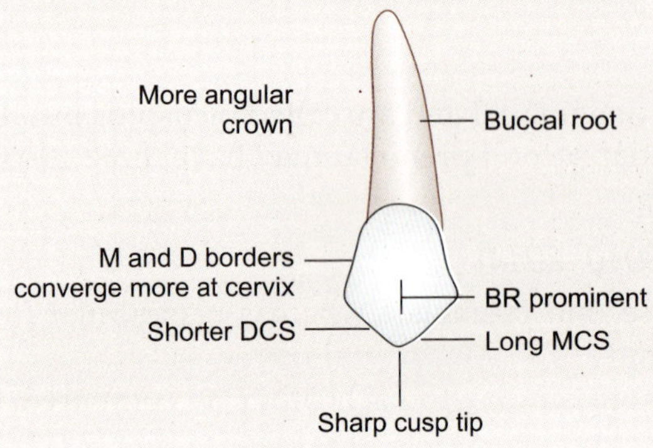

Fig. 4.1

Crown:

Shape, size, and surface:

- The crown has pentagon/trapezoid shape.
- The outlines are **more angular.**
- The crown is longer than that of the second premolar.
- Buccal surface (B) is convex with more **prominent buccal ridge (BR).**

Outlines:

- The mesial (M) and distal (D) outlines of the crown **converge** towards the cervix.
- Mesial outline is slightly concave from cervix to the contact point whereas distal outline is almost straight.
- The buccal cusp tip is long and pointed resembling canine but contact areas in this tooth near at same level.

Single root
Less angular crown
M and D border converge less
BR less prominent
Longer DCS
Short MCS
Blunt cusp tip

Fig. 4.2

Crown:

Shape, size, and surface:

- Same as that of first premolar.
- The outlines are **less angular.**
- The crown is not as long as that of first premolar.
- The buccal ridge is **less prominent.**

Outlines:

- The mesial and distal outlines **converge less** as compared to that of first premolar.
- Mesial outline is slightly convex whereas distal outline is more convex.
- The buccal cusp tip is short and blunt.

(Contd.)

Maxillary first premolar	*Maxillary second premolar (Contd.)*
• Location of buccal cusp tip is towards distal with a longer mesial cusp slope (MCS).	• Location of buccal cusp tip is **towards mesial with a shorter mesial cusp slope.**
• Mesial and distal cusp slopes (DCS) meet at right angles at the cusp tip.	• M and D cusp slopes meet at an obtuse angle at the cusp tip.
• Cervical line is convex towards the root apex.	• Same as that of first premolar.
• Mesial contact point lies at the junction of occlusal and middle third and it is narrower as compared to the distal contact point.	• Mesial contact point is at the junction of the occlusal and middle third.
• The distal contact point lies in the middle third of the crown and slightly cervical to the mesial contact point.	• Distal conact point same as that of first premolar.
	• Both the contact points are broader because the crown is in contact with posterior teeth.
Root:	**Root:**
• The root tapers from cervix to the apex	• Same as that of first premolar.
• Apex of the root may bend distally, mesially or may be straight.	• Same as that of first premolar.

Palatal aspect (P)

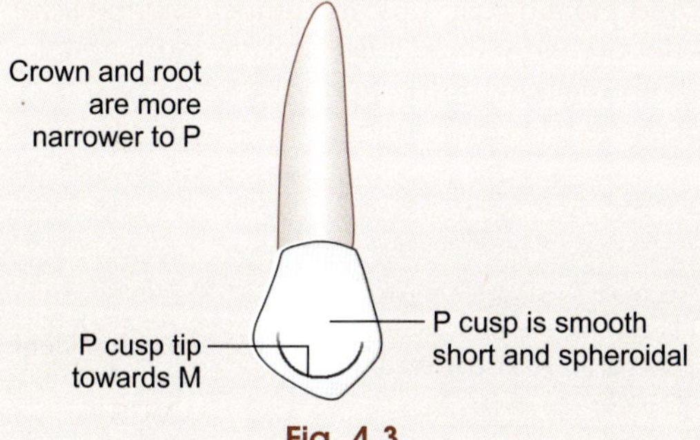

Fig. 4.3

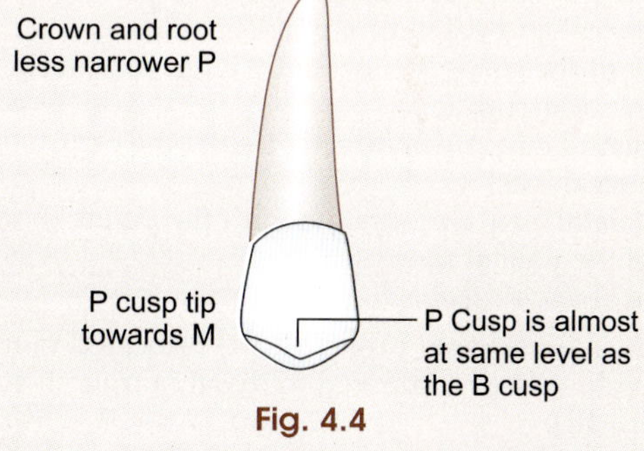

Fig. 4.4

Crown:	**Crown:**
• Crown is narrower on the palatal side.	• The crown is less narrower on the palatal side.
• Palatal (P) cusp is smooth, spheroidal and shorter than the buccal (B) cusp.	• Palatal cusp is almost of the same height as the buccal cusp.
• The tip of the unworn palatal cusp is placed mesially. The cusp tip is pointed.	• Same as that of first premolar.
• Because the palatal cusp is narrower and shorter than the buccal cusp, part of the M and D surfaces of the crown and root are seen from this aspect, and also the cusp tips and cusp slopes of both the buccal and palatal cusps are seen from this aspect.	• The palatal cusp is almost as long as the buccal cusp. The palatal cusp is slightly narrower than the buccal cusp.
• M and D outlines are convex and are continuous with the MCS and DCS.	
Root:	**Root:**
• The palatal root of the two rooted first premolar is smooth, convex, and shorter than the buccal roots.	• The single root is narrow towards the palatal aspect.
• The apex of the palatal root is blunt and may have a mesial or distal bend.	

(*Contd.*)

Maxillary first premolar | *Maxillary second premolar (Contd.)*

Proximal aspect

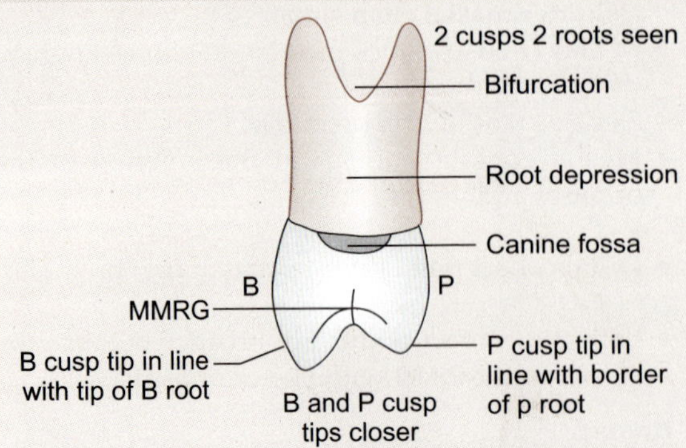

Fig. 4.5

Crown:

Shape, cusp tips, and cusps:

- Proximal surface has trapezoid shape.
- Two cusps are seen from this aspect. The buccal cusp is noticeably longer than the palatal cusp.
- Buccal and palatal cusp tips are closer.
- Both the cusps are located well in the confines of the root outline.
- Buccal cusp tip is directly below the centre of the buccal root.
- Palatal cusp tip is in line with the palatal border of the palatal root.

Outlines and surfaces:

- Mesial marginal ridge (MMR) is located more occlusally as compared to distal marginal ridge (DMR).
- Cervical line is convex towards the occlusal. It is more convex on the mesial surface.
- Crest of curvature on the buccal surface is in the cervical third.
- Crest of curvature on the palatal surface is in the middle third.

Mesial surface has distinguishing features:

- A prominent concavity, **the canine fossa (CF)** is **located at cervical to the mesial contact area.** (below the cervical line)
  It accommodates the rounded disto-incisal angle of the canine.
- This crown concavity is in continuation with the concavity on the root.
- A well defined developmental groove, the **mesial marginal ridge groove (MMRG)** crosses the mesial marginal ridge (MMR) immediately lingual to the mesial contact area.
  It is continuous with the central groove (CG) on he occlusal surface.

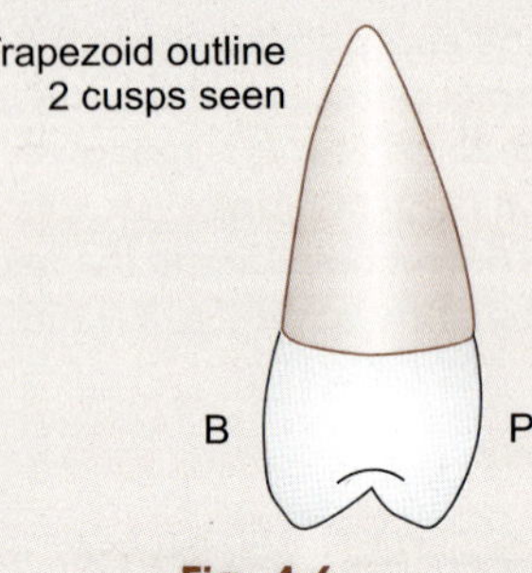

Fig. 4.6

Crown:

Shape, cusp tips, and cusps:

- The proximal surface has same shape.
- Two cusps are seen from this aspect. The buccal and palatal cusp tips are almost at same level.
- Buccal and palatal cusp tips are more apart.
- Same as that of first premolar.

Outlines and surfaces:

- Same as first premolar.
- Same as first premolar.
- Same as first premolar.
- Same as first premolar.

- There is **no concavity** on the mesial surface of the crown.
- The depression is present on the mesial surface of the root.
- There is no MMRG present.

(Contd.)

Maxillary first premolar	*Maxillary second premolar (Contd.)*
Root:	**Root:**
• The root is **bifurcated** in the apical third or half its length with **one buccal** and **one palatal** root.	• It has a **single root** which may be longer than the root of the first premolar.
• On the mesial surface of the root trunk there is a deep developmental depression which is in continuation with the canine fossa.	• On the mesial surface the depression is shallow.
• On the distal surface of the root trunk the depression is shallow.	• On the distal surface the depression is deeper.
Occlusal aspect	
Hexagonal outline MBDG MMRG DBDG DTF CG longer **Fig. 4.7**	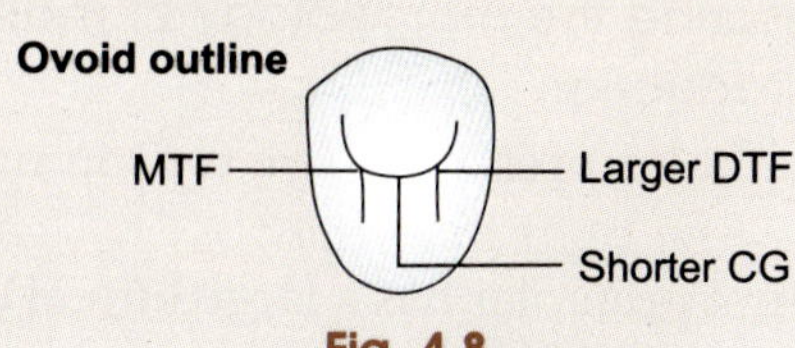 **Fig. 4.8**
Shape, surface, outline, and ridges:	*Shape, surface, outline, and ridges*:
• Occlusal surface has **hexagonal** outline.	• Occlusal surface has rounded or oval outline.
• The outline is asymmetrical.	• The outline is symmetrical.
• The six sides are the mesiobuccal (MB), mesial (M), mesiopalatal (MP), distobuccal (DB), distal (D), and distopalatal (DP).	
• The occlusal surface consists of B and P cusps, B and P triangular ridges, M and D marginal ridges, triangular fossa, pits, and central groove (CG).	• It is same as that of first premolar.
• The angle formed by the mesiobuccal cusp ridge and the MMR approaches a right angle.	• The angle formed by the mesiobuccal cusp ridge and MMR is an obtuse angle.
• The angle formed by the distobuccal cusp ridge and the DMR is an acute angle.	• The angle formed by the distobuccal cusp ridge and the DMR is not an acute angle.
• The MMR is shorter than the DMR.	• It is same as that of first premolar.
• Buccal triangular ridge (BTR) of the B cusp is prominent and arises near the centre of the CG and ends at the tip of the B cusp.	• Buccal triangular ridge (BTR) is less prominent.
• Lingual/palatal triangular ridge (PTR) extends from the P cusp tip to the CG.	• It is same as that of first premolar.
• BTR and PTR join to form a transverse ridge.	• It is same as that of first premolar.
Fossa:	*Fossa*:
• Mesial and distal triangular fossa (MTF and DTF) are triangular depressions closer to the marginal ridges.	• Mesial and distal triangular fossae are triangular depressions away from the marginal ridge.
Grooves and pits	*Grooves and pits*
• Occlusal surface of the first premolar **has fewer supplemental** grooves.	• Occlusal surface **has multiple supplemental grooves** radiating from the CG hence it appears **wrinkled.**
• A well-defined CG divides the occlusal surface evenly buccolingually.	• Same as in first premolar.
• The length of the **CG is longer** as compared to that of second premolar.	• The length of the **CG is shorter.**

(Contd.)

Maxillary first premolar	*Maxillary second premolar (Contd.)*
• The CG extends from distal pit to mesial pit where it joins the MMRG.	• The CG extends from mesial pit to distal pit.
• M and D pits are closer to the marginal ridges.	• M and D pits are farther from marginal ridges.
• Mesial pit is the point of union of three developmental grooves: (1) MMRG, (2) Mesiobuccal developmental groove (MBDG), (3) CG.	
• Distal pit is the point of union of two developmental groves: (1) distobuccal developmental groove (DBDG), (2) central groove (CG).	

Q 2. Describe the morphology of mandibular first premolar. *(May 2007)*

Ans. Introduction

- Mandibular premolars are four in number two on either side of the midline in the lower arch.
- The first premolar has a large buccal cusp, which is long and well-formed with a small non-functioning lingual cusp.
- It has many of the characteristics of a small canine.
- It is smaller than the second premolar.

Eruption

It erupts between the age of 10–12 years.

Numbering System

- Palmer 4 | 4 (below horizontal line)
- Universal R - # 28, L - # 21
- FDI R - # 44, L - # 34

Mandibular first premolar from all aspects

Buccal aspect

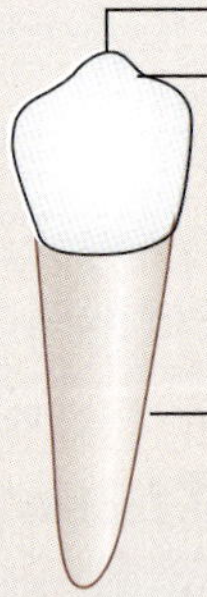

Fig. 4.9

Crown: *Shape, size, and surface:*	• From this aspect the form of the crown is nearly symmetrical bilaterally. • The crown is roughly trapezoid in shape. • The crown is long and narrow at cervix.

(Contd.)

	Mandibular first premolar from all aspects (Contd.)
	• The buccal surface is more convex than in maxillary premolars especially at cervical and middle-thirds. • The buccal ridge is prominent with developmental depressions on either side of the buccal ridge. • The crown tapers form contact area to the cervix.
Outlines and cusp tip:	• The mesial outline (M) is straight or slightly concave from cervical line to the mesial contact area. • The distal outline (D) is slightly concave from the cervical line to the distal contact area. • The mesial cusp slope **(MCS)** is shorter than the distal cusp slope (DCS). Both the cusp slopes form an acute angle at the cusp tip. • There is a shallow notch on the mesial cusp slope. • **Buccal cusp tip** is long and pointed and located a little mesial to the root axis. • Cervical line slightly convex towards the root.
Contact areas:	• Mesial contact area is more cervical than the distal contact area (This is an exception along with deciduous maxillary canine.)
Root	• It has a pointed apex and a distal bend in the apical third. • Some mandibular first premolars have slight distal tilt of the crown on the root.
	Lingual aspect
	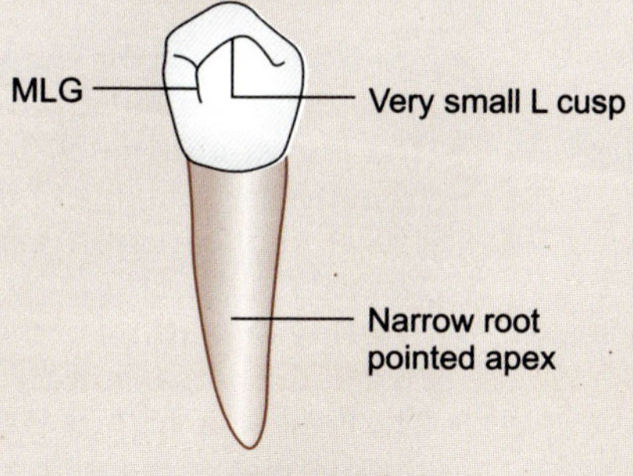 **Fig. 4.10**
Crown: *Shape, size, surface, and cusp*:	• The crown is narrower on the lingual aspect. • The major portion of the cown is made-up of the middle buccal lobe. • The cervical portion of the crown lingually is narrow, and convex with concavities between the cervical line and the contact areas on the lingual portion of the mesial and distal surfaces. • The contact areas and marginal ridges are pronounced and extend above the narrow cervical portion of crown. • **Lingual cusp** is very small, pointed and non-functional. • Lingual (L) cusp tip is in line with the buccal triangular ridge. • Because of the smaller lingual cusp much of the buccal profile and occlusal surface may be seen from this aspect. • Occlusal surface slopes sharply lingually in cervical direction, down to the short lingual cusp. Most of the occlusal surface of the tooth is therefore seen from this aspect.

(Contd.)

Mandibular first premolar from all aspects (Contd.)

- A characteristic of the lingual surface is the **mesiolingual developmental groove (MLG).**
- It separates the mesial marginal ridge (MMR) from the mesial slope of the lingual cusp.

Root:

- The root tapers from cervix to a pointed apex.
- The root is much narrower on the lingual side due to which the developmental depressions on the root are seen on the mesial and distal surfaces.
- Mesial surface of the root has a deep developmental groove present.

Proximal aspect (M)

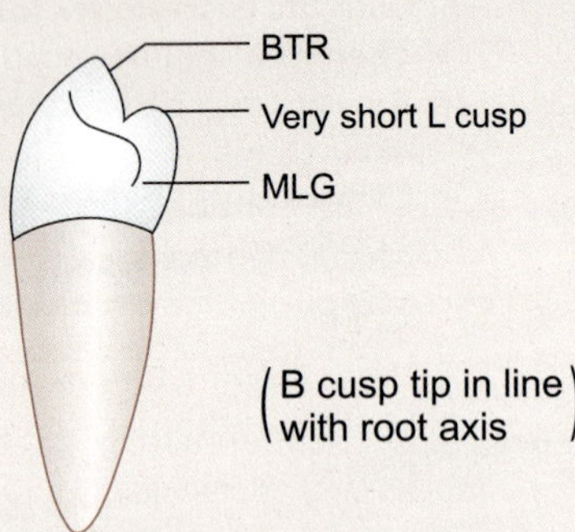

Fig. 4.11

Crown:

Shape and size:

- From this aspect, the **shape** of the crown is **rhomboid** which is characteristic of all the mandibular posterior teeth.

Outlines and the cusps:

- The **buccal outline** of the crown from this aspect is prominently curved from the cervical line to the tip of the buccal cusp.
  The crest of curvature is at the junction of cervical and middle third **more towards** middle third.
- The **lingual outline** of the crown is a curved outline of less convexity than that of the buccal surface.
- The crest of curvature is in the middle third of the crown, which is outside the confines of the root. The curvature ends at the tip of the lingual cusp.
- Cervical line curvature is more on the mesial surface than the distal surface.
- The **lingual tilt** of the crown over the root is more as compared to that of the crown of second premolar.
- Occlusal plane is tilted lingually.
- **Mesial marginal ridge (MMR)** is more cervical as compared to **distal marginal ridge (DMR)** because it inclines (slopes) at 45° towards the cervix and **is parallel to the long, prominent buccal triangular ridge (BTR).**
- Distal marginal ridge **(DMR) is horizontal** and more occlusal to the MMR and is confluent with the lingual cusp slope.
- The lingual triangular ridge (LTR) is short and horizontal.
- Mesiolingual developmental groove (MLG) is present between MMR and Mesial slope of the lingual cusp (from mesial aspect).
- The **buccal cusp tip** is in line with the root axis.
- The lingual cusp tip is in line with the lingual surface of the root.
- The lingual cusp is shorter than the buccal cusp by more than one-third of the total crown length.

(Contd.)

	Mandibular first premolar from all aspects (Contd.)
Contact area:	• Mesial contact area is in line with the buccal cusp tip. • Distal contact area is broader.
Root:	• The root tapers evenly from the cervix to a pointed apex which is in line with the buccal cusp tip. • Root depressions are present on both mesial and distal root surfaces.
	Occlusal aspect

Fig. 4.12

Shape, size, and surface:	• Both mandibular premolars exhibit more variations in form occlusally as compared to maxillary premolars. • Crown outline is roughly **diamond shaped** and similar to incisal aspect of mandibular canine and is asymmetrical. • Crown converges towards lingual.
Outlines:	• Mesial cusp slope is shorter than the distal cusp slope. • Mesial outline is flat or less curved. • Distal outline is more curved. • MMR is shorter and at an acute angle to the mesial cusp slope • Distal marginal ridge (DMR) is longer and at right angles to the distal cusp slope.
Contact areas:	• Mesial and distal contact areas are broad, distal being broader of the two.
Ridges:	• Middle lobe of the buccal cusp makes up for the major bulk of the crown. • **Buccal triangular ridge (BTR)** is more prominent, longer, and inclines **lingually from buccal** cusp tip to where it joins the short triangular ridge of the lingual cusp. • The two triangular ridges join to form a blunt transverse ridge, separating mesial and distal fossa.
Fossa:	• Mesial fossa (MF) is small, shallow, and linear with a mesial pit at its bottom. It contains mesio-buccal developmental groove (MBDG). • Distal fossa (DF) is large, deep and circular with a distal pit at its base.
Groove:	• Central groove is rarely present. • The mesiobuccal developmental groove (MBDG) runs buccolingually (BL) from mesial fossa and it is continuous with the mesiolingual developmental groove (MLG) as it passes over the mesiolingual surface. • A distal developmental groove (DDG) or a few supplemental grooves may extend from distal fossa.

Q 3. Define and enumerate different type traits. Write in detail maxillary first premolar with endodontic anatomy. *(Dec. 2005)*

Ans.

- A trait is a distinguishing characteristic.
- Type traits are the characteristics that differentiate the teeth within the same class, i.e. first premolars from second premolars.

Type Traits of Maxillary Premolars

First premolar	*Second premolar*
• Mesial cusp slope is longer than the distal cusp slope.	• Mesial cusp slope is shorter than the distal cusp slope.
• From proximal view the lingual cusp shorter than the buccal cusp and the cusp tips are closer.	• Both the cusps are almost of same height and the cusp tips are farther apart.
• Occlusal outline is sharp and hexagonal. Occlusal outline is asymmetrical.	• Occlusal outline is ovoid and is more symmetrical.
• On occlusal surface, the central groove is longer as compared to that on second premolar.	• Central groove is shorter.
• Occlusal surface is not wrinkled.	• Occlusal surface is wrinkled.
• More often it has two roots.	• It has a single root.
• Mesial crown and root depressions and mesial marginal ridge groove present.	• Mesial root depression only. • No MMRG.

Type Traits of Mandibular Premolars

First premolar	*Second premolar*
• The buccal cusp tip is more pointed.	• The buccal cusp tip is less pointed.
• The lingual cusp is very small and nonfunctional.	• In two cusp types the lingual cusp is longer as compared to that of first premolar and the lingual cusp tip is towards the mesial. • In three cusp types there are two lingual cusps the mesiolingual cusp is larger than the distolingual cusp.
• MMR is parallel to triangular ridge of buccal cusp. • The mesial marginal ridge (MMR) is more cervical as compared to distal marginal ridge (DMR).	• The MMR is horizontal and more occlusally placed. The DMR is more cervically placed.
• Root depressions present on both mesial and distal surfaces.	• Root depression present only on distal surface.
• From occlusal view the crown is diamond shaped.	• The crown has more of square or round shape.
• There is presence of mesiolingual groove, separating the mesial marginal ridge from the lingual cusp.	• Mesiolingual groove is absent.

(Detail description of maxillary first premolar is in Ans. 4)

- Endodontic anatomy of maxillary first premolar:
  Pulp chamber:
  - is narrow from buccal view and wider from proximal view.
  - Roof of the pulp chamber is coronal to the cervical line and floor is below the cervical line.
  - The pulp chamber does not constrict much near the cervical part as there are two separate roots and two canals.
  - One pulp horn is present under each cusp.
  - Buccal pulp horn is more prominent.
- Cross-section at the cervical level shows characteristic **kidney-shaped** outline because of indentation due to presence of mesial developmental groove.

Root and Root Canals

- The two well-formed roots divide in the middle third into buccal and lingual roots.
- A small percentage of teeth may have three roots.
- 40% of teeth have one root with two canals.
- There is possibility of roots having three canals, with one canal in the lingual root and two canals in the buccal root.
- Lingual canal is larger of the two canals.

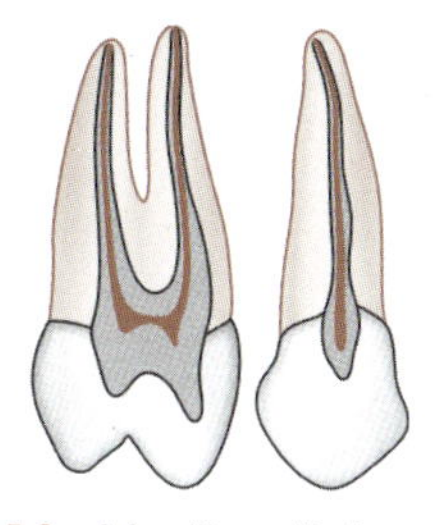

Fig. 4.13: Maxillary first premolar

Q 4. Describe morphology of maxillary first premolar and chronology.

(Dec. 2005, May 2009, 2014, 2015, June 2013)

Discuss chronology, odontometric data and morphology of maxillary first premolar in detail.

(Nov. 2015)

Ans. **Introduction**

- Premolars are eight in number. They succeed the deciduous molars.
- They are anterior to molars and present in permanent dentition only.
- They form a transition from anterior to posterior teeth.

Eruption

- It erupts between 10–11 years of age.

Numbering System

Palmer	4⌋
Universal	# 5
FDI	# 14

Chronological Data

Initiation of calcification	1½–1¾ years
Completion of enamel	5–6 years
Eruption	10–11 years
Completion of root	12–13 years

Odontometric data	
Length of crown	8.5 mm
Length of root	14.0 mm
Mesiodistal width of crown	7.0 mm
Mesiodistal width of crown at cervix	5.0 mm
Labiolingual width of crown	9.0 mm
Labiolingual width at cervix	8.0 mm
Curvature of cervical line on mesial	1.0 mm
On distal	0.0 mm

Maxillary first premolar from each aspect

Buccal aspect (B)

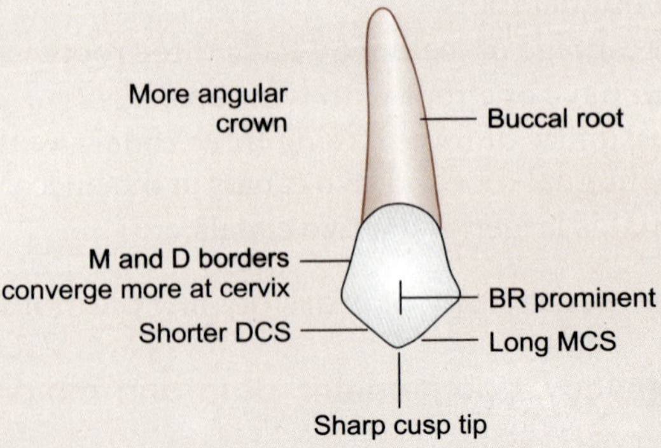

Fig. 4.14

Crown:

Shape, size, and surface:
- The crown has pentagon/trapezoid shape. It is more angular with buccal line angles more prominent. It has the widest crown of all the premolars.
- The crown is longer than that of the second premolar.
- Buccal surface is convex with a **prominent buccal ridge (BR).**
- Mesial and distal to the buccal ridge are the developmental depressions.

Outlines:
- The mesial (M) and distal (D) outlines of the crown converge towards the cervix.
- Mesial outline is slightly concave from the cervical line to the contact point whereas the distal outline is almost straight.
- The buccal cusp tip is long and pointed. The mesial and distal cusp slopes meet at right angles.
- Location of buccal cusp tip is towards distal to the vertical axis line with a longer mesial cusp slope and a shorter distal cusp slope.
- Cervical line is convex towards the apex.

Contact point:
- The mesial contact point lies at the junction of occlusal and middle third and it is narrower as compared to the distal contact point.
- The distal contact point lies in the middle third of the crown and slightly cervical to the mesial contact point.
- Even so, the contact areas are more nearly at same level than those found on anterior teeth.

Root:
- The root tapers from cervix to the apex.
- The apical end of the root bends distally or may be straight.

Palatal aspect (P)

Crown:

Size, shape, and cusp:
- On the palatal side the crown of the first premolar is more narrower than that of the second premolar.
- The tip of the unworn cusp is pointed and placed mesially.
- Palatal cusp is shorter, smooth, and spheroidal.
- Because the palatal cusp is narrower, part of mesial, and distal surfaces of crown and root are seen from this aspect.
- Because the palatal cusp is shorter the cusp tips and cusp slopes of both the cusps are seen from this aspect.

(Contd.)

Maxillary first premolar from each aspect (Contd.)

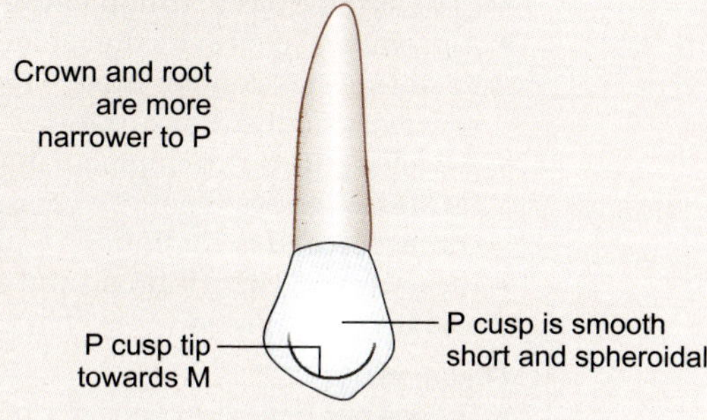

Fig. 4.15

Outlines:

- From this aspect the gross outline of the crown is reverse of the gross outline of the buccal aspect.
- Mesial and distal outline of the palatal cusp are convex and straighten at cervix, they continue with mesial and distal cusp slopes.

Root:

- The palatal root of two roots is smooth and convex.
- The apex of palatal root is more blunt compared to buccal root apex.

Proximal aspect

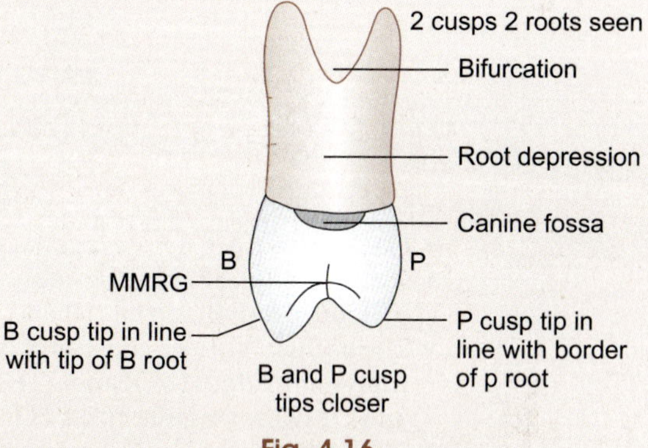

Fig. 4.16

Crown:

Shape, cusp tip, and cusps:

- Proximal surface has trapezoid shape. Longest uneven side towards cervical and shorter towards occlusal.
- 2 cusps are seen from this aspect. The buccal cusp is noticeably longer than the palatal cusp.
- Both the cusp tips are closer and located well in the confines of the root outline.
- Buccal cusp tip is directly below the centre of the buccal root.
- Palatal cusp tip is in line with the palatal border of the palatal root.

Outlines and surfaces:

- Mesial marginal ridge (MMR) is located more occlusally as compared to the distal marginal ridge (DMR).
- Cervical line is convex towards the occlusal outline. It is more convex on the mesial surface.
- Crest of curvature on the buccal surface is in the cervical third.
- Crest of curvature on the palatal surface is in the middle third.

(Contd.)

Maxillary first premolar from each aspect (Contd.)

	Mesial surface has distinguishing features: • A prominent concavity the canine fossa (CF) on the crown is located cervical to the mesial contact area. This concavity is in continuation with the concavity on the root surface. • A well-defined developmental groove, the mesial marginal ridge groove (MMRG) crosses the mesial marginal ridge immediately lingual to mesial contact area. It is continuous with the central groove on occlusal surface. • Mesial contact area is broad and at the junction of occlusal and middle third and buccally placed. **Distal surface:** • It does not have the concavity on the crown and the marginal groove. • Distal contact area is broader and more buccally placed.
Root:	• The root is bifurcated in the apical third with one buccal and one palatal root. • On the mesial surface of the root trunk is a deep depression which is in continuation with the canine fossa. • On the distal surface the depression is shallow.

Occlusal aspect

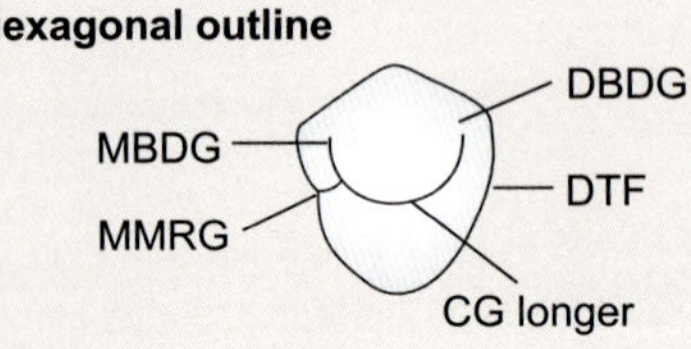

Fig. 4.17

Crown:	
Shape:	• Occlusal surface has hexagonal outline. • The six sides are the mesiobuccal (MB), mesial (M), mesiolingual (ML), distobuccal (DB), distal (D) and distolingual (DL).
Outline and surface:	• The occlusal surface consists of buccal and palatal cusps, buccal, and palatal triangular ridges (BTR and PTR), mesial, and distal marginal ridges (MMR and DMR), triangular fossa (TF), pit, and central groove (CG). • The angle formed by the mesiobuccal cusp ridge and mesial marginal ridge approaches a right angle. The angle formed by the distobuccal cusp ridge and the distal marginal ridge is an acute angle. The mesial marginal ridge is shorter than the distal marginal ridge. • Buccal triangular ridge of the buccal cusp is prominent and arises near the centre of the central groove and ends at the tip of the buccal cusp. • Palatal triangular ridge (PTR) extends from the palatal cusp tip to the central groove. • The buccal and palatal triangular ridges join to from a transverse ridge. • **Fossa:** Mesial and distal triangular fossa are triangular depressions closer to the marginal ridges. • **Grooves:** Occlusal surface of the first premolar has fewer supplemental grooves. A well-defined central developmental groove divides the occlusal surface evenly buccopalatally (BP). • The length of the central groove is longer as compared to that of the second premolar.

(Contd.)

Maxillary first premolar from each aspect (Contd.)

- The central groove extends from distal pit to mesial pit where it joins the mesial marginal ridge groove (MMRG).
- Two collateral developmental grooves join the CG inside the MMR and the DMR. These are the MBDG and the DBDG.
- Junction of these grooves is named as mesial and distal pits.
- **Pit:** Mesial and distal pits are closer to the marginal ridges. Mesial pit is the point of union of three primary developmental grooves.
  i. Mesial marginal ridge groove (MMRD)
  ii. Mesiobuccal developmental groove (MBDG), and
  iii. Central groove (CG).

The distal pit is the point of union of two developmental grooves.
  i. Distobuccal developmental groove (DBDG), and
  ii. Central groove (CG).

SAQs (3 Marks each)

Q 1. Describe arch traits of premolars. (Oct. 2003, Nov. 2014)

Mention morphological differences between maxillary and mandibular premolars. (Nov. 10)

Ans. Same as LAQ Q.1.

Q 2. What is Canine fossa on tooth surface? (June 2004)

Ans. **CANINE FOSSA (CF)**

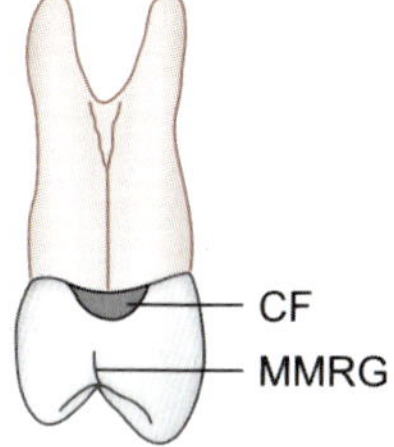

Fig. 4.18

- It is a small concavity present on the mesial surface of the crown of the maxillary first premolar just below the cervical line to accommodate the rounded distoincisal angle of the canine.
- It is a mesial developmental depression on the mesial surface of the maxillary first premolar where distal rounded surface of the canine rests. It is cervical to the mesial contact area.
- It is believed to be produced (formed) due to the pressure of the distal aspect of the maxillary canine as it develops earlier than the first premolar.

Q 3. Discuss about mesial aspect of maxillary first premolar. (May 2007)

Ans.

- Mesial surface of maxillary first premolar is trapezoid in shape.
- Mesial marginal ridge is more occlusal as compared to distal marginal ridge.
- Cervical line is more convex towards the occlusal as compared to the cervical line on the distal aspect.
- Crest of curvature on the buccal surface is in the cervical third.
- Crest of curvature on the lingual surface is in the middle third.
- A prominent concavity, the **canine fossa** is present on the crown just below the cervical line.
  This concavity is in continuation with the concavity on the mesial surface of the root trunk.
- A well-defined developmental groove, the mesial marginal ridge groove (MMRG) crosses the mesial marginal ridge immediately lingual to the mesial contact area.
  It is continuous with the central groove on the occlusal surface.

Q 4. Describe the type traits of mandibular premolars.

Ans.

Mandibular first premolar	*Mandibular second premolar*
• It is smaller in size than the second premolar.	• It is larger than the first premolar.
Buccal aspect	
• Crown is longer and narrower at cervix. • Cusp tip is pointed with steep cusp slopes. • Buccal ridge is more prominent.	• Crown is shorter and is wider at cervix. • Cusp tip less pointed and cusp slopes meet at an obtuse angle. • Buccal ridge is less prominent.
Lingual aspect	
• The lingual cusp is small and nonfunctional • One lingual cusp. • Mesiolingual developmental groove separates the mesial marginal ridge from the lingual cusp.	• The lingual cusp is longer and functional. • One or two lingual cusps. • Lingual groove separates the two unequal lingual cusps in 3-cusp type premolar. • No groove in two-cusp type premolar.
Proximal aspect	
• The lingual tilt of the crown is much more. • The mesial marginal ridge slopes cervically therefore it is at a lower level than the distal marginal ridge. • Depression present on both M and D surfaces of root.	• The lingual tilt is less. • The mesial marginal ridge is horizontal and more occlusally placed than the distal marginal ridge. • Depression present only on the distal surface of the root.
Occlusal aspect	
• Outline of the crown is diamond shaped.	• In two-cusp type the crown outline is rounded or ovoid. In three-cusp type crown outline is more or less square.

Q 5. Describe the occlusal surface of mandibular second premolar?

Ans.

- Mandibular second premolars are of two types.

  Two-cusp type, having one buccal and one lingual cusp.

  Three-cusp type, having one buccal and two lingual cusps.

- In **two-cusp** type the crown outline is more or less rounded or oval. The crown converges lingual to the mesiobuccal and distobuccal cusp ridges.

  The lingual cusp is smaller than the buccal cusp but larger than the lingual cusp on the first premolar.

- In the **three-cusp** type, the crown outline is more or less square lingual to the mesiobuccal and distobuccal cusp ridges due to the presence of two lingual cusps, which are uneven in size and smaller than the buccal cusp and are separated by a lingual groove. Mesiolingual cusp is longer and wider than the distolingual cusp.

Ridges, Grooves and Fossa

- **Two-cusp type.**
  - The triangular **ridge** of the buccal cusp is long and wide. It joins the not so prominent triangular ridge of the lingual cusp to form a transverse ridge.
  - The mesial **fossa** is small and circular. The distal fossa is large and circular.

  In two-cusp type more supplemental grooves present.

  In two-cusp type of mandibular second premolar, two types of groove pattern is seen.

U-type (Fig. 4.19A)

The central groove from mesial to distal pit is slightly curved towards lingual.

The central groove, along with the mesiobuccal developmental groove (MBDG) and the distobuccal developmental groove (DBDG) forms a U-shaped groove which is open and directed towards the buccal side.

H-type (Fig. 4.19B)

The central groove is straight and short from M to D pit. The CG along with the MBDG, MLDG, DBDG, DLDG forms the H-shaped groove pattern.

Three-Cusp Type (Fig. 4.19C)

- Each cusp has well-formed **triangular ridges** separated by deep developmental grooves. These grooves converge in a central pit (CP) and form a Y-shape, on the occlusal surface.
- There is no transverse ridge.
- The **central pit (CP)** located midway between the buccal cusp ridge and the lingual margin of the occlusal surface and slightly distal to the central point between the MMR and DMR.
- **Mesial fossa** is small and triangular. Distal fossa is smaller and also triangular.

  Distal fossa appears to be in the outer edge of the central fossa.

In the **three-cusp** type mandibular second premolar, the groove pattern is **Y-type.**

- There is no central groove.
- The longer mesial groove extends in MB direction from the central pit (CP) and ends in the mesial triangular fossa (MTF).
- The shorter distal groove continues from the central pit in DB direction and ends in Distal triangular fossa (DTF).
- A lingual groove also unique to the three-cusp type, begins in the CP and extends lingually between the ML and DL cusps and on to the lingual surface.
- The three grooves together form a Y-shaped groove pattern.

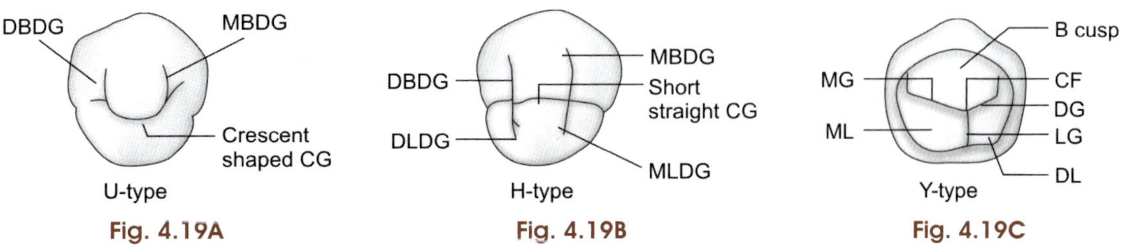

Fig. 4.19A **Fig. 4.19B** **Fig. 4.19C**

MULTIPLE CHOICE QUESTIONS (MCQs)

1. The term premolar is used to designate any tooth in the permanent dentition of mammals that succeeds
   a. A primary first molar
   b. A primary second molar
   c. Both a and b
   d. None of the above

2. The maxillary right and left first premolars can be identified by the universal numbering system as
   a. 4 and 11 b. 5 and 12
   c. 14 and 24 d. 13 and 22

3. The facial or buccal surface of all premolars develop from
   a. 2 facial lobes
   b. 3 facial lobes
   c. One lobe
   d. None of the above

4. The only premolar with buccal crest of curvature located as far cervically as in the anterior teeth is
   a. Maxillary first premolar
   b. Mandibular first premolar
   c. Mandibular second premolar
   d. Maxillary second premolar

5. Permanent canines and all premolars have the mesial slope of the buccal cusp shorter than the distal cusp slope except
   a. Mandibular first premolar
   b. Maxillary first premolar
   c. Maxillary second premolar
   d. Mandibular second premolar

6. Usually premolars have two cusps one buccal and one lingual except one premolar which has two lingual cusp; that is
   a. Maxillary second premolar
   b. Mandibular first premolar
   c. Mandibular second premolar
   d. Maxillary first premolar

7. Mesial marginal ridges are more occlusal than distal marginal ridges which are more cervical *except* in
   a. Mandibular first premolar
   b. Mandibular second premolar
   c. Maxillary first premolar
   d. Maxillary second premolar

8. From the occlusal view the shape of the maxillary premolar crown is
   a. Square b. Round
   c. Oblong d. Rectangular

9. From the occlusal view mandibular second premolar crown is
   a. Square b. Oblong
   c. Round d. Triangular
   e. Square or round

10. All premolar crowns are narrower on the lingual side than on the buccal side *except*
   a. Mandibular second premolar (Y-shaped)
   b. Mandibular first premolar
   c. Maxillary first premolar
   d. Maxillary second premolar

11. Lingual cusp tips are positioned off center to the mesial most often in
   a. Maxillary premolars
   b. Mandibular premolars
   c. Both a and b
   d. None of the above

12. The widest crown, buccal cusp long and pointed with M and D slopes meeting at right angles is common to
   a. Maxillary first premolar
   b. Maxillary second premolar
   c. Mandibular first premolar
   d. Mandibular second premolar

1-c, 2-b, 3-b, 4-b, 5-b, 6-c, 7-a, 8-c, 9-e, 10-a, 11-a, 12-a

13. The premolar commonly having two roots is
a. Maxillary first premolar
b. Maxillary second premolar
c. Mandibular first premolar
d. Mandibular second premolar

14. Cross-section of maxillary first premolar at cementoenamel junction is
a. Oval shaped
b. Round shaped
c. Kidney shaped
d. Triangular shaped

15. In maxillary first premolar, the pulp horn extends further occlusally under the
a. Buccal cusp b. Lingual cusp
c. None d. Both a and b

16. The lingual root of the two rooted maxillary first premolar is
a. Shorter than buccal root
b. Equal to buccal root
c. Longer than buccal root
d. None of the above

17. The mesial marginal ridge groove and mesial concavity is present in
a. Maxillary first premolar
b. Maxillary second premolar
c. Mandibular first premolar
d. Mandibular second premolar

18. The deepest mid root depression on the distal is common to
a. Maxillary first premolar
b. Maxillary second premolar
c. Mandibular second premolar
d. Mandibular first molar

19. The only premolar with an obvious concavity or depression on the mesial surface of the crown and this depression continues onto the root is
a. Mandibular first premolar
b. Maxillary first premolar
c. Maxillary second premolar
d. Mandibular second premolar

20. Pulp chamber floor in maxillary first premolar is at
a. Cervical level
b. Below cervical level
c. Above cervical level
d. None of the above

21. The only premolar having very small, pointed, nonfunctional lingual cusp is
a. Maxillary first premolar
b. Mandibular first premolar
c. Mandibular second premolar
d. Maxillary second premolar

22. The groove separating the mesial marginal ridge from the mesial slope of the small lingual cusp is the
a. Mesial marginal groove
b. Mesiolingual groove
c. Lingual groove
d. Distal marginal groove

23. Mesial marginal ridge is more cervical, mesial half of lingual surface is like a canine and distal half is like a molar this is a unique feature of
a. Mandibular first premolar
b. Maxillary first premolar
c. Maxillary second premolar
d. Mandibular second premolar

24. On the mandibular second premolar with two lingual cusps the mesiolingual and distolingual cusps are separated by
a. Mesiolingual groove
b. Distolingual groove
c. Lingual groove
d. None of the above

25. The tip of the buccal cusp is in line with the root axis in (Proximal view)
a. Mandibular first premolar
b. Second premolar
c. Maxillary first premolar
d. Maxillary second premolar

13-a, 14-c, 15-a, 16-a, 17-a, 18-b, 19-b, 20-b, 21-b, 22-b, 23-a, 24-c, 25-a

26. In cross-section of the tooth the classic indentation is present because of the mesial developmental groove in
a. Mandibular first premolar
b. Maxillary canine
c. Maxillary first premolar
d. Maxillary second premolar

27. The triangular ridge of the lingual cusp is in horizontal plane in
a. Mandibular second premolar with two lingual cusps
b. Mandibular second premolar with one lingual cusps
c. Mandibular first premolar
d. Maxillary first premolar

28. Because of the extreme lingual tilt of the crown of mandibular premolars, the tip of the lingual cusp
a. Is in line with the lingual surface of the root
b. Extends lingually beyond the lingual surface of the root
c. Placed buccally
d. Is in line with the root axis

29. Lingual tilt of the crowns is the characteristic of all the posterior teeth of
a. Maxillary arch
b. Mandibular arch
c. Both the arches
d. Neither arch

30. Premolars identified as #5 and #12 by universal numbering system are
a. Maxillary R and L first premolar
b. Maxillary R and L second premolar
c. Mandibular R and maxillary R second premolars
d. None of the above

31. By universal numbering system, maxillary R and L second premolar are
a. #4 and #13 b. #5 and #12
c. #28 and #21 d. #6 and #13

32. Buccolingual and mesiodistal dimension are more nearly equal and the occlusal surface more square in
a. Maxillary premolar
b. Mandibular premolar
c. Mandibular canine
d. Maxillary central incisor

33. The characteristic that differentiates maxillary first premolar from maxillary second premolar is
a. Mesial concavity cervical to contact area
b. Long buccal cusp
c. Mesial root depression, mesial marginal groove
d. All of above are correct

34. Premolar having canal that occasionally bifurcates at the apical third of the root is
a. Mandibular first premolar
b. Maxillary first premolar
c. Maxillary second premolar
d. Mandibular second premolar

35. Buccal and lingual pulpal projection or fins are present at the level of cemento-enamel junction and may show constriction at same level in
a. Maxillary first premolar
b. Maxillary second premolar
c. Mandibular first premolar
d. Mandibular second premolar

36. Wrinkled appearance of occlusal surface is common in
a. Maxillary 2nd premolar
b. Maxillary 1st premolar
c. Mandibular 1st premolar
d. Mandibular 2nd premolar

37. Maxillary first premolar erupts at the age of
a. 10–12 b. 9–11
c. 8–10 d. 7–9

26-c, 27-c, 28-a, 29-b, 30-a, 31-a, 32-b, 33-d, 34-c, 35-b, 36-a, 37-a

38. The first evidence of calcification of the maxillary first premolar takes place at the age of
a. 2–3 years after birth
b. 3–4 years after birth
c. 1½ to 1¾ years after birth
d. After birth

39. The tooth which shows kidney-shaped outline in the cervical cross-section is
a. Mandibular first premolar
b. Mandibular second premolar
c. Maxillary first premolar
d. Maxillary second premolar

40. A premolar having a well developed mesiolingual groove is
a. Maxillary first premolar
b. Mandibular first premolar
c. Maxillary second premolar
d. Mandibular second premolar

41. The mandibular second premolar resembles mandibular first premolar from
a. Buccal view b. Lingual view
c. Occlusal view d. All of the above

42. Maximum buccolingual dimension is found in
a. Maxillary first premolar
b. Mandibular first premolar
c. Mandibular second premolar
d. All of them have same dimension

43. Maximum mesiodistal dimension is present in which premolar?
a. Maxillary premolars
b. Mandibular first premolar
c. Mandibular second premolar
d. All of them have same dimension

44. The premolar which frequently has a central pit is
a. Maxillary first premolar
b. Maxillary 2nd premolar
c. Mandibular 1st premolar
d. Mandibular 2nd premolar

45. In a longitudinal section of a premolar crown, the enamel is thickest in the
a. Cervical third
b. Middle third
c. Occlusal third
d. Junction of cervical and middle third

46. In a mandibular arch, the greatest lingual inclination of the crown from its root is seen in
a. Canine b. First molar
c. First premolar d. Central incisor

47. The teeth that erupts at 10–12 years of age is
a. Permanent central incisor
b. Permanent first molar
c. Premolar
d. Permanent second molar

48. In the sequence of eruption of permanent dentition the maxillary canine usually follows
a. Maxillary lateral incisor
b. Mandibular first premolar
c. Mandibular second premolar
d. Mandibular canine

49. The three cusp form is seen in
a. Upper first premolar
b. Upper second premolars
c. Lower first premolar
d. Lower second premolar

50. The small and non-functional lingual cusp of mandibular first premolar is compared to
a. The cusp of Carabelli
b. Cingulum of canine
c. Distal cusp of molars
d. None of the above

51. Which of the following premolars frequently has only one pulp horn?
a. Maxillary first
b. Mandibular first
c. Maxillary second
d. Mandibular second

38-c, 39-c, 40-b, 41-a, 42-a, 43-d, 44-d, 45-c, 46-c, 47-c, 48-c, 49-d, 50-b, 51-b

52. In the mandibular arch the M and D contact points are at approximately same level in all teeth except the mandibular

a. Canine
b. First molar
c. First premolar
d. Lateral incisor

53. Lingual cusp is mesial in which maxillary premolars?

a. First premolar only
b. Second premolar only
c. Both first and second
d. Neither first or second

52-a, 53-c

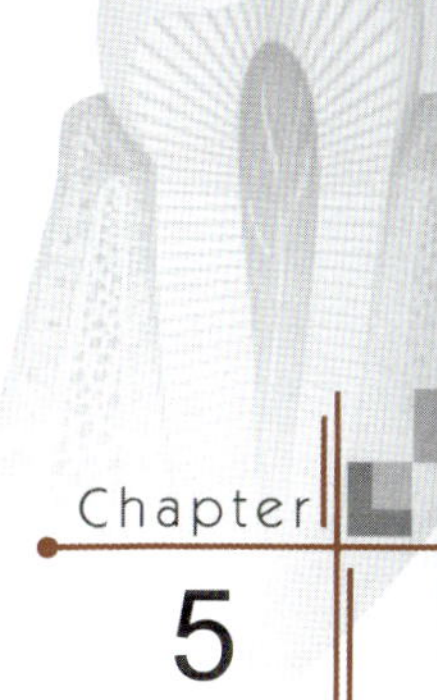

Chapter 5

The Permanent Molars

LAQs (10 Marks)

Q 1. Describe morphology of maxillary first molar. *(June 2004)*

Write class and arch traits of molars. Describe in detail the morphology of maxillary first molar. *(Second BDS) (Nov. 2010)*

Ans. Class and arch traits of molars refer page 76.

Morphology of Maxillary First Molar

Introduction

- The maxillary first molar is the largest tooth in the maxillary arch.
- It has four well-developed functioning cusps and one supplemental cusp of little practical use, the cusp of Carabelli.
- It has three well-developed and well separated roots.
- The crown of the tooth is wider buccopalatally (BP) than mesiodistally (MD).

Eruption

It erupts at around 6 years of age.

Numbering System

Palmer:	6┘
Universal:	# 3
FDI:	16

Maxillary first molar from each aspect

Buccal aspect

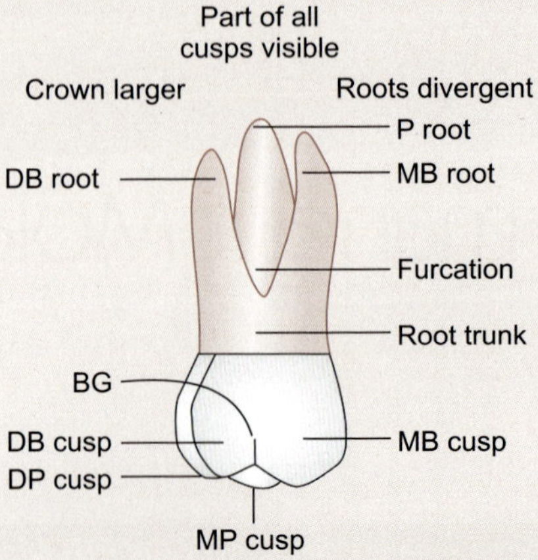

Part of all cusps visible
Crown larger
Roots divergent
P root
DB root
MB root
Furcation
Root trunk
BG
DB cusp
MB cusp
DP cusp
MP cusp

Fig. 5.1

Crown:

Shape, size, surface, cusps, and outlines:

- The crown is roughly trapezoidal with shorter cervical and longer occlusal sides representing the uneven sides. The crown is **wider mesiodistally (MD) than cervicoocclusally.**
- Crown is shorter from mesial (M) to distal (D).
- The crown tapers from contact area to the cervix.
- Mesial outline is straight from cervix to the contact point.
- Distal outline is convex.
- The cervical line has slight convexity towards the root.
- **The two buccal cusps** are separated by a **buccal groove (BG).**
- It has four functional cusps. **All four** cusps mesiobuccal (MB), distobuccal (DB) and part of mesiopalatal (MP) and distopalatal (DP) are **seen from this aspect.** This is possible because of the obtuse character of the disto-buccal line angle. This is possible because the two palatal cusps are offset to the distal in relation to the buccal cusps.
- The mesiobuccal cusp is wider than the distobuccal cusp. The distobuccal cusp is more pointed.

Contact area:

- Mesial contact area is at the junction of occlusal and middle third.
- Distal contact area is in the middle of the middle third.

Root:

- All the **three divergent** roots are seen from this aspect. The three roots are palatal root, which is longest, the mesiobuccal root and the distobuccal root.
- Root trunk is shorter (4 mm).
- Roots are about twice as long as the crown.
- The **palatal** root is longer than the mesiobuccal (MB) root. It is visible between the two buccal roots from this aspect, and the apex is located almost in line with the buccal groove (BG).
- Both mesiobuccal (MB) and distobuccal (DB) roots are nearly same length, both taper apically, mesiobuccal root apex is blunt and is in line with the tip of the MB cusp.
- The spread of the middle thirds of the two buccal roots is nearly as wide as the crown.

(Contd.)

Maxillary first molar from each aspect (Contd.)

- MB and DB roots bend in such a way that they look like handles on a pair of pliers.
- Often the MB and DB roots curve distally.
- A deep developmental groove is present on the root trunk from furcation area to the cervical 1ine.

Palatal/lingual aspect

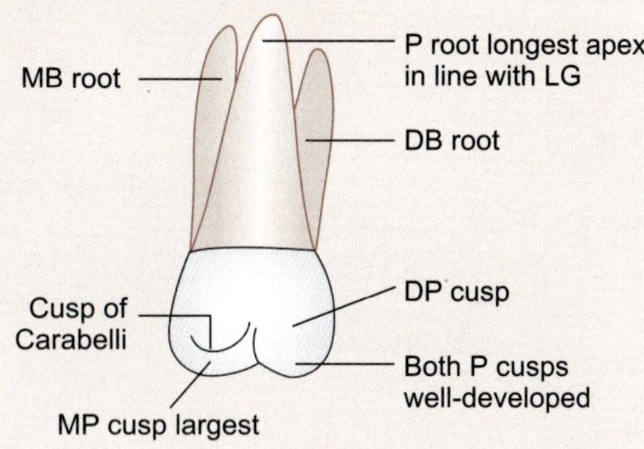

Fig. 5.2

Crown:

Shape, size, and surface:

- The shape is trapezoidal.
- The palatal surface is more convex.
- It is narrower in the cervical third.
- The M and D outline are similar except that distal outline is shorter and semicircular.
- The palatal developmental groove starts approximately in the centre of palatal surface mesiodistally, curves sharply to the distal as it extends between the two palatal cusps on to the occlusal surface.
- On the palatal surface of the mesiopalatal cusp a **fifth cusp, the cusp of carabelli** is present. It is mini cusp or tubercle. It is non-functioning. It is 2 mm short of mesiopalatal cusp tip. A groove normally separates the cusp of Carabelli from the cusp ridges of mesopalatal cusp.
- From this aspect only 2 palatal cusps visible.
- **Mesiopalatal** cusp is much **larger,** and before the occlusal wear it is always the longest cusp. Its mesiodistal width is about three-fifths of the MD crown diameter. Distopalatal cusp making the remaining two-fifths.
- Mesiopalatal cusp slopes make an obtuse angle.
- Distopalatal cusp is spheroidal.

Root:

- All three roots are visible from this aspect.
- The **palatal root** is longest, conical and tapers in blunt round apex which is in line with the palatal groove.
- The palatal portion of the palatal trunk is continuous with the entire cervical portion of the crown palatally.
- Longitudinal depression is present on the palatal aspect of the root.
- The wide mesiodistal spread of the buccal roots is visible from this aspect.

(Contd.)

Maxillary first molar from each aspect (Contd.)

Proximal aspect

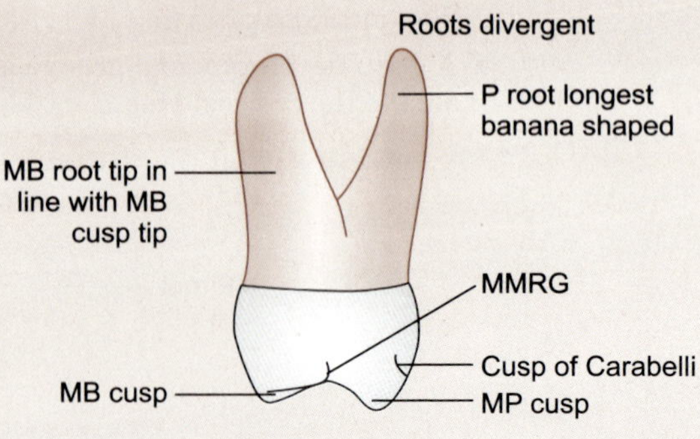

Fig. 5.3

Crown: *Shape, size, and surface:*	*Mesial aspect:* • Shape is trapezoidal, wider at cervical and narrow at occlusal. • Crown is shorter and wide buccopalatally.
Outline:	• The height of contour on the buccal surface is in the cervical one-third and on the palatal surface it is in the middle of the crown. • Cervical line is slightly convex above the contact area. • Mesial marginal ridge is confluent with the cusp ridges of MB and ML cusps. It is concave, longer and more occlusally placed as compared to distal marginal ridge.
Cusps:	• From this aspect two cusps **mesiobuccal** and **mesiopalatal** are seen and **the fifth cusp, the cusp of carabelli 2–3 mm** below the tip of the mesio-palatal cusp is also seen.
Contact area:	• Mesial contact area is at the junction of middle and occlusal thirds and buccal to the centre of the crown buccopalatally.
Root:	• Roots are more divergent. • From mesial aspect two roots are seen the mesiobuccal and the palatal root, the distobuccal root is hidden by the broader mesiobuccal root. • **Mesiobuccal root** is broad **buccopalatally** and flattened on its mesial surface. It is shorter than the palatal root. • The apex of the MB root is in line with the tip of the MB cusp. • **MB root** has two **root canals.** • From the buccal outline to the point of bifurcation, the width of the root on root trunk is approx two-thirds of the crown measurement BL at the cervix. • The root trunk is 3 mm long. • **Palatal root is** the longest, it is **banana-shaped and extends beyond** the crown palatally.
Crown: *Shape, size, and surface:*	*Distal aspect:* • Crown is narrower towards the distal and because of the rhomboid shape much of the buccal surface of the crown is seen from this aspect. • Distal marginal ridge is more cervical compared to MMR. Cervical line is almost straight. • **Tip of MB and MP cusps** are seen from this aspect.

(Contd.)

Maxillary first molar from each aspect (Contd.)

Root:

- **Distobuccal root** is shorter, narrower, and pointed therefore **mesiobuccal root is visible** from this aspect
- The root trunk is 5 mm long.
- (The length of the root trunk, from the cervical line to the point of bifurcation: on the mesial aspect is 3 mm, on the buccal aspect is 4 mm, and on the distal aspect is 5 mm.)

Occlusal aspect

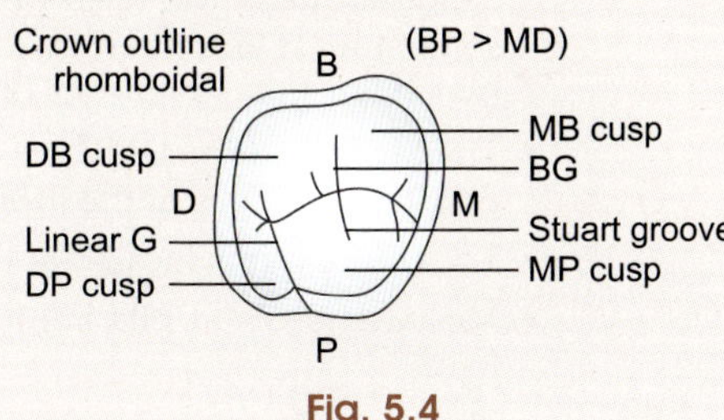

Fig. 5.4

Crown:

Shape, outline, and cusps:

- From this aspect it has somewhat rhomboidal outline following the four major cusp ridges and the marginal ridges.
- Buccopalatal (BP) dimension is more than mesiodistal (MD) dimension.
- Crown tapers from mesial to distal.
- In maxillary first molar (only molar) where the palatal side may be wider as compared to the buccal.
- The four major cusps and one minor cusp present.
- The **mesiopalatal cusp** is the largest with a rounded cusp tip.
- **Distopalatal cusp** is the smallest and most variable.
- Mesiobuccal cusp is second largest with sharp cusp tip and slightly larger than the distobuccal cusp.
- The distobuccal cusp is the third largest with sharpest cusp tip.

Fossa:

- There are two major fossae and 2 minor fossae.
- The major fossa is the central fossa (CF) which is roughly triangular and mesial to the oblique ridge and the distal fossa (cigar fossa) which is linear and distal to and parallel to the oblique ridge.
- The central fossa has connecting sulci within its boundries with developmental grooves at the deepest portion of these sulci (sulcate grooves).
- The two minor fossae are the mesial triangular fossa (MTF) and the distal triangular fossa (DTF) which are located just distal to and mesial to the MMR and the DMR.

Ridge:

- Each of the four cusps has at least one definite triangular ridge.
  The mesiopalatal (MP) cusp has two triangular ridges (few texts refer only one triangular ridge).
  The groove between the two triangular ridges of mesiopalatal cusp is called the **Stuart groove**.
  The mesial triangular ridge of mesiolingual/palatal cusp (MTRMP) joins the triangular ridge of mesiobuccal cusp (MB) to form a transverse ridge.

(Contd.)

Maxillary first molar from each aspect (Contd.)

The distal triangular ridge of mesiopalatal cusp (DTRMP) aligns with the triangular ridge of the distobuccal cusp (TRDB) to form a diagonal ridge called the **oblique ridge.** (OR)

Other texts refer to **DTRMP** by another name the distal cusp ridge of mesiopalatal cusp (DCRMP). Subsequently the OR is formed by the triangular ridge of distobuccal cusp and the **distal cusp ridge** of the mesiopalatal cusp (Refer page 399 Fig. 25.132).

- The oblique ridge is reduced in height in the centre of the occlusal surface being about at the level of the marginal ridges of the occlusal surfaces sometimes it is crossed by a developmental groove that partially joins the two major fossa by means of a shallow sulcate groove.
- The MMR and the DMR are irregular ridges confluent with the mesial and distal cusp ridges of the mesial and distal major cusps.

Pits:

- The central pit is located at the centre of the central fossa.
- Mesial and distal pits are located at the bottom of the mesial and distal fossa.

Grooves:

- There are **5 major developmental grooves.** Central groove **(CG)**, buccal groove (BG), distal oblique groove (DOG), palatal groove (PG), sometimes the **transverse groove of the oblique ridge,** and **the fifth cusp developmental groove (CDG).**
- **Central groove** extends in the mesial direction at an obtuse angle to buccal groove from the central pit (over the mesial transverse ridge) and ends in the mesial triangular fossa.
- A short developmental groove radiates from the central pit, extends distopalatally where it either crosses the oblique ridge and ends in the distal fossa or fades out before reaching the oblique ridge.

  This part of the CG which extends over the oblique ridge is called the **transverse groove of the oblique ridge,** it is a shallow developmental groove.
- **Buccal groove** extends from the central pit in buccal direction on to the buccal surface.
- **Distal oblique groove** or **linear groove** or **distopalatal groove** extends obliquely and traverses the distal linear fossa to join the palatal developmental groove between the mesiopalatal and distopalatal cusps. It shows several supplemental grooves.

  At distal pit it terminates into two branches which form the two sides of the distal triangular fossa (DTF).
- **Palatal developmental groove** (PG) separates the MP and DP cusps and extends on the palatal surface to terminate at the centre of the crown palatally below the palatal root.
- **Fifth cusp** groove outlines the fifth cusp (cusp of carabelli) it joins the palatal groove near its terminus.

The other grooves are:

- Distal marginal groove.
- Distobuccal triangular groove and distopalatal triangular groove.
- Mesial marginal groove.
- Mesiobuccal triangular groove and mesiopalatal triangular groove.

Q 2. Describe morphology of maxillary second molar. *(May 2002)*

Ans. Introduction

- The maxillary second molar is the second largest tooth in the maxillary arch.
- It is similar in form to the first molar, but is generally smaller, especially in the distopalatal arc.
- The buccopalatal dimension is almost the same as the first molar but mesiodistally it is noticeably narrower.

Eruption

- It erupts at around 12 years of age.

Numbering System

Palmer:	7┘	
Universal:	R # 2	L # 15
FDI:	17	L 27

Maxillary second molar from each aspect

Buccal aspect

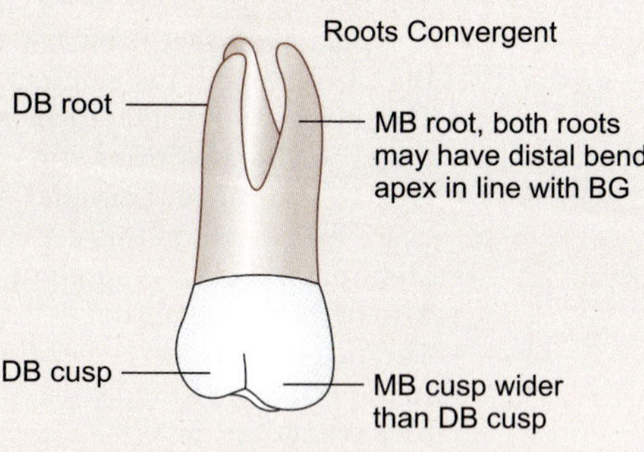

Fig. 5.5

Crown:	
Shape, size, and surface:	• The crown is roughly trapezoidal with shorter cervical and longer occlusal sides representing the parallel uneven sides. • The crown is narrower mesiodistally shorter cervicoocclusally than the maxillary first molar. • The crown tapers from contact area to cervix. • The larger and wider mesiobuccal cusp is separated from the smaller and sharper distobuccal cusp by a buccal groove. • Smaller DB cusp allows part of the distal marginal ridge and part of the DP cusp to be seen from this aspect.
Contact areas:	• Mesial contact area is at the junction of occlusal and middle third. • Distal contact area is little cervical to the mesial contact area.
Roots:	• The **three roots** are less divergent and are seen from this aspect.

(Contd.)

Maxillary second molar from each aspect (Contd.)

- The buccal roots are of the same length. These roots are more nearly parallel and are inclined distally more than those of the maxillary first molar so that the end of the distobuccal root is slightly distal to the distal extremity of the crown.
- The apex of the MB root is on a line with the buccal groove of the crown instead of the tip of the MB cusp.
- The root trunk is longer. The chances of fusion of roots is greater.

Palatal/lingual aspect

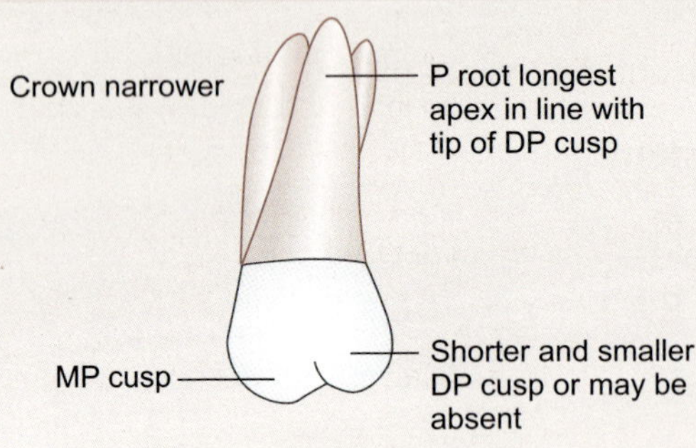

Fig. 5.6

Crown:

Shape, size, surface, and cusps:

- The shape is trapezoidal.
- The palatal surface is more convex.
- The palatal surface is narrower in the cervical third because of the taper of the crown to join the single palatal root.
- The mesial and distal outlines are same as on the buccal surface except that distal outline is shorter and semi-circular.
- Due to shorter and smaller distopalatal cusp or nonexistent distopalatal cusp, the crown on this aspect is less wide.
- **Distopalatal** cusp is small or absent.
- **The fifth** cusp is absent.
- The distobuccal cusp is seen through the sulcus between the MP and DP cusps.
- In the 4 cusp type of maxillary second molar, MP and DP cusps are separated by a palatal groove (PG).
- The **palatal root** is the longest and has a longitudinal depression on the palatal aspect.
- It tapers in blunt round apex.
- The palatal root apex is in line with the tip of the distopalatal cusp.
- **Buccal roots** are more parallel and have a distal bend.

Proximal aspect

Mesial aspect:

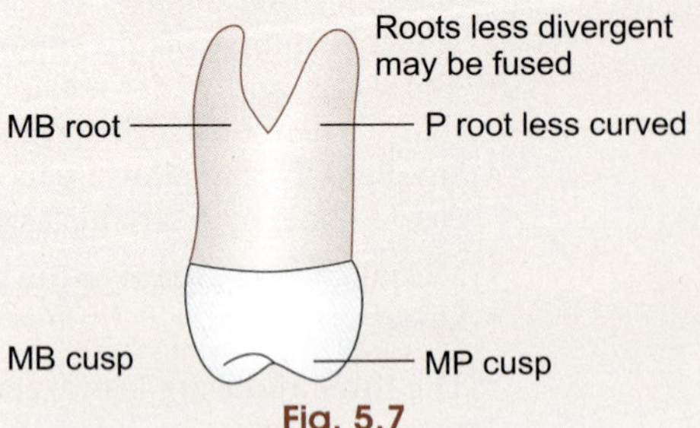

Fig. 5.7

(*Contd.*)

Maxillary second molar from each aspect (Contd.)

Crown :

Shape, size surface, and cusps:
- Shape is trapezoidal, wider at cervix and narrow towards occlusal.
- Crown is **shorter.**
- **Buccopalatally dimension** is same as that of first molar.
- From this aspect MB and MP cusps are seen **cusp of Carabelli is absent.**

Outline:
- The height of contour on the buccal surface is in cervical third and on palatal surface it is in the middle of the crown.
- The mesial marginal ridge (MMR) is concave, longer, and more occlusal.
- The mesial marginal ridge groove (MMRG) is less common.

Contact area:
- The mesial contact area is at the junction of middle occlusal third, and buccal to the centre of the crown buccopalatally.

Root:
- The roots are less spread being within the confines of the crown bucco-palatally.
- The roots are shorter and may be fused.
- Mesiobuccal root has a single canal.
- Palatal root is less curved or may be straight.

***Distal aspect*:**

Shape, size, and surface:
- Crown is narrower towards the distal, more of the buccal surface is seen.
- Distal marginal ridge is more cervical compared to MMR.
- Cervical line is almost straight.

Root :
- Distobuccal root is shorter and narrower therefore MB root visible from this aspect.
- The palatal root is less curved and the apex is in line with the tip of the DL cusp.

Occlusal aspect

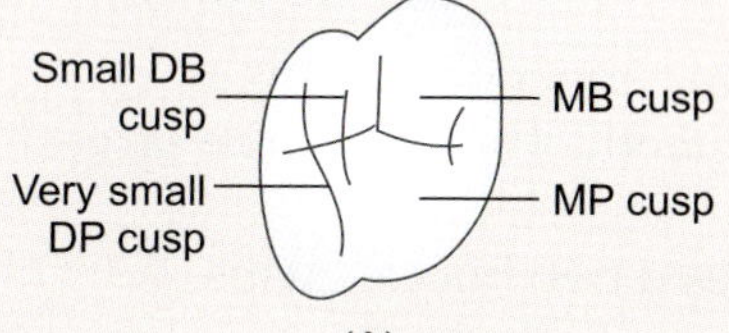

Figs 5.8A and B

Crown:

Shape, outlines, and cusps:
- There are two types of occlusal surfaces.
- The **rhomboid type** of second maxillary molar is more frequent.
- It has **four cusps.**
- It appears like a **twisted parallelogram** or **accentuated rhomboid,** rhomboid outline is more extreme with palatal portion twisted distally more acute angle on MB corner due to prominent MB cervical ridge.
- The **heart-shaped** type of second maxillary molar has **three-cusps.** The **disto-palatal cusp is absent.**
- The **occlusal surface** is narrower mesiodistally than the first molar.
- The crown tapers from mesial to distal.

(Contd.)

	Maxillary second molar from each aspect (Contd.)
	• There is more taper from buccal to palatal due to smaller DL cusp or due to absence of DP cusp. • The MB and DP acute line angles are smaller. • MP and DB obtuse line angles are wider. • MB and MP cusps are well-developed and as large as in first molar whereas DB and DP cusps are less developed. • MB cusp is much larger than the DB cusp. • MB cervical ridge is more prominent.
Fossa:	• In the **4-cusp type there** are 4 fossae. 2 major fossae, the central fossa, and the distal fossa. • 2 minor fossae, the mesial, and distal triangular fossae. • In the **3-cusp type,** there are 3 fossae. The distal fossa is absent.
Ridges:	• The **oblique ridge** is shorter and less prominent. • **MMR** is more occlusally placed than the DMR. • DMR which is more longer and more cervically placed. • In 3-cusp type there is no oblique ridge or may be faint.
Pits and grooves:	• There are 3 pits. • Central pit, mesial pit and distal pit. • **Central groove** extends from central pit to mesial triangular fossa. • The **buccal groove** extends from the central pit in the buccal direction between the MB and DB cusps onto the buccal surface. • Distal oblique groove, and palatal groove are absent in the 3-cusp type of second molar. • It 4-cusp type distal oblique groove, palatal groove present. • Groove pattern is similar to that of first molar, but is more variable and supplemental grooves are more numerous.

Q 3. What are arch and class traits of molars? *(Oct. 2002)*

- Describe the morphology of mandibular first molar. (May 2009)
- Write a note on its pulp cavity. (Nov. 2010, June 2012)

Ans. **Class Traits of Molars**

1. Molars are wider mesiodistally than cervicoocclusally.
2. They are the largest and strongest teeth. They have the largest occlusal surface of all the posterior teeth.
3. They are the only teeth having at least two buccal cusps.
4. They have 3–5 cusps and 2–3 roots.
5. Molars are not succedaneous teeth.

Arch Traits of Molars

Maxillary molar	*Mandibular molar*
1. Crowns of maxillary molars are wider bucco-palatally than mesiodistally.	1. Crowns are wider mesiodistally than bucco-palatally/lingually.
2. 3 roots are present in maxillary molars.	2. 2 roots are present in mandibular molars.
3. There is presence of oblique ridge on the occlusal surface.	3. There is no oblique ridge on the occlusal surface.
4. Maxillary molars are centred over their root axis.	4. Mandibular molars, from proximal aspect appear to be tilted lingually.
5. Root trunk is longer.	5. Root trunk is shorter.

MANDIBULAR FIRST MOLAR

Morphology of Mandibular First Molars

Introduction

- It is the largest tooth in the mandibular arch.
- It is located sixth from the midline.
- It has the widest mesiodistal dimension of all the teeth.
- It normally exhibits **five functional cusps and two well-developed roots,** one mesial and one-one distal which are very broad buccolingually.
- The crown is wider mesiodistally (MD) than buccolingually (BL).
- Flattened buccal cusps are typical of all mandibular molars.

Eruption

It erupts at around 6 years of age.

Numbering System

Palmer: 6 | 6 (lower)

Universal: # 30, 19

FDI: 46, 36

Mandibular first molar from each aspect

Buccal aspect

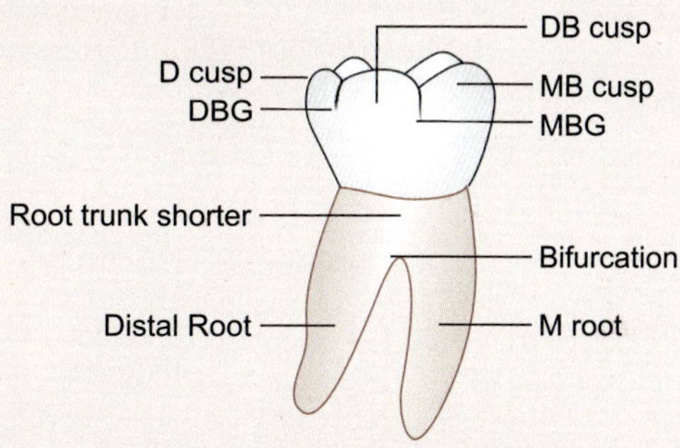

Fig. 5.9

Crown:

Shape, size, and surface:

- It has trapezoidal, shape with longer parallel side towards occlusal and shorter parallel side towards cervical.
- There is proportionately more taper from contact area to cervix because of the bulge of the distal cusp.
- The crown is wider mesiodistally than cervicoocclusally.
- The crown is shorter from mesial to distal.
- **It** has 5 cusps, 3 buccal cusps and 2 palatal cusps which are just visible from this aspect.
- Mesiobuccal cusp (MB) is the widest, next is distobuccal cusp (DB) and distal cusp (D) is smallest and more pointed than either of buccal cusp. MB and DB cusps are relatively flat.

(Contd.)

Mandibular first molar from each aspect (Contd.)

- The two buccal cusps make-up the major portion of the buccal surface of the crown.
- The distal cusp provides a very small part of the buccal surface because the major portion of the distal cusp makes up the distal portion of the crown providing the distal contact area on the centre of the distal surface of the distal cusp.
- The mesiobucccal and distobuccal cusps are separated by mesiobuccal groove (MBG) which is longer and terminates in a pit.
- The distobuccal and distal cusps are separated by a shorter distobuccal groove (DBG).

Outline:

- Mesial outline of the crown is concave from contact area to cervix.
- Distal outline of the crown is straight from contact area to cervix.
- At contact areas both outlines are convex.
- Cervical line is almost straight, dipping apically towards the root bifurcation.

Contact areas:

- Mesial contact area is more occlusal.
- It is close to the junction of occlusal and middle third.
- Distal contact area is cervical to the mesial contact area.

Root:

- The **root** is bifurcated near the cervical line.
- The **root trunk** is shorter (3 mm) and a depression is present.
- The **roots** are widely separated.
- The mesial root is longer, curved mesially from a point near the cervical line to the middle third then curves distally so that the tapered apex of the root is in line with the mesiobuccal groove.
- The distal root is shorter, straighter with pointed apex which extends beyond the distal of the crown.
- Both roots are wider mesiodistally at the buccal areas than they are lingually.
- The developmental depressions are present on the mesial and distal sides of both the roots.

Lingual aspect

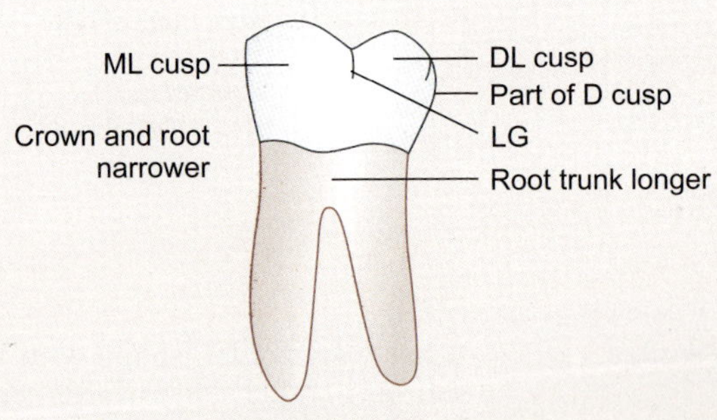

Fig. 5.10

Crown:

Shape, size, and surface:

- The crown is trapezoidal in shape. It is narrower from buccal to lingual.
- The **lingual cusps** are longer and sharper than the buccal cusps therefore from this aspect only mesiolingual and distolingual cusps and part of distal cusp is seen.
- The lingual groove (LG) separates the mesiolingual cusp from the disto-lingual cusp.

(*Contd.*)

Mandibular first molar from each aspect (Contd.)

- Mesiolingual cusp is slightly larger than the distolingual cusp.
- The tip of the mesiolingul cusp is somewhat higher than that of the disto-lingual tip.
- Cervical line is almost straight may dip cervically over the bifurcation.

Root:

- Roots are narrower on this aspect.
- Root trunk is longer on this aspect 4 mm because the cervical line is more occlusally placed.

Proximal aspect

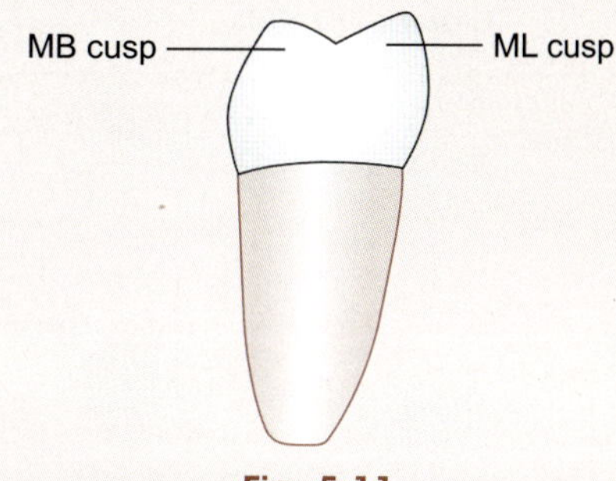

Fig. 5.11

Crown:

Shape, size, and surface:
- The proximal surface has **rhomboidal shape** due to the lingual tilt of the crown in relation to root axis.

Cusps and outline:
- The crown is shorter, narrower on distal aspect and the crown has a distal tilt therefore, more of occlusal surface and some part of each of the five cusps can be seen.

Distalaspect:
- And also more of buccal and lingual surface is seen from distal aspect.

Cusps and outline:
- Buccolingual dimension of the crown and root is greater on the mesial aspect than on the distal and because the mesial cusps are higher, from mesial aspect only mesiobuccal and mesiolingual cusps and mesial root are seen.

Mesial aspect:
- Mesial cervical line curves very slightly towards the occlusal.

Cervical line:
- Distal cervical line is almost straight.

Marginal ridge:
- Mesial marginal ridge (MMR) is longer, more occlusally placed and often crossed by mesial marginal groove.
- It is confluent with the mesial ridges of the MB and ML cusps.
- MMR is placed about 1 mm below the level of the cusp tips.
- There is a V-shaped notch at the mid-point of both the marginal ridges.
- The distal marginal ridge is short and more cervically placed.

Buccal and lingual outline:
- The buccal outline is more convex in the cervical third and in the occlusal two-thirds it becomes flatter.
- The MB cusp is located directly above the buccal third of the mesial root.
- The cervical ridge is less prominent.
- The lingual outline is straight from the cervix to the maximum convexity in the middle third, from this point it is curved towards the mesiolingual cusp tip. The tip of the mesiolingual cusp is in a position directly above the lingual third of the mesial root.

Contact areas:
- The mesial contact area is almost centred buccolingually and is placed at the junction of occlusal and middle third.

(Contd.)

Mandibular first molar from each aspect (Contd.)

- The distal contact area is placed just below the distal cusp ridge of the distal cusp at the middle of middle third.

Root:

- From mesial aspect only mesial root is seen which is wide buccolingually and has a deep depression on the mesial as well as inner surface. It has a blunt, wide apex.
- The distal root is narrower and shorter with a point apex.
- There is a shallow depression present on the distal surface of the distal root.

Occlusal aspect

Crown is MD > BL

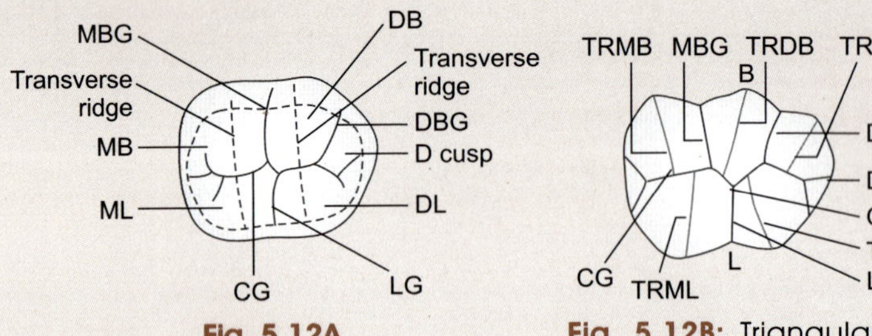

Fig. 5.12A

Fig. 5.12B: Triangular ridges and Grooves no transverse ridge

Shape and size:

- Occlusal surface is quadrilateral in form but due to the presence of buccal bulge of the distobuccal cusp and small distal cusp, it has a hexagonal shape.
- Mesiodistal (MD) dimension is 1 mm more than the buccolingual (BL) dimension.
- Crown tapers from mesial to distal therefore the crown is wider buccolingually on mesial half than on the distal half.
- Widest buccolingual (BL) dimension is in the middle third of the distobuccal cusp.
- Because of the lingual inclination of the crown more of the buccal surface is visible than the lingual surface.
- The crown narrows from buccal to lingual.
- Outline of the crown is convex on buccal, lingual, mesial, distal.
- The occlusal surface includes the cusps, the ridges, the fossae and the grooves.
- There are five **triangular ridges, 3 fossae, 3 pits and 4 developmental grooves.**

Cusps:

- Mesiobuccal cusp is larger than mesiolingual and distolingual cusps which are almost equal in size.
- Distobuccal is smaller than the mesiobuccal, mesiolingual, distolingual, and distal cusp is the smallest.

Ridges (Fig. 5.12B)

- Some texts refer that the occlusal surface of mandibular first molar has no transverse ridge.
- The triangular ridge of the mesiobuccal cusp (TRMB) extends lingually to end at the mesial portion of the central groove.
- The triangular ridge of the distobuccal (TRDB) cusp extends mesiolingual to the area of the central pit.
- The triangular ridge of the distal cusp (TRD) extends mesiolingual to the distal pit area.

(*Contd.*)

Mandibular first molar from each aspect (Contd.)	
	• The triangular ridge of the mesiolingual cusp (TRML) extends distobuccal to end at the mesial portion of the central groove. • The triangular ridge of the distolingual cusp (TRDL) extends mesiobuccally to end in the area of the junction of the distobuccal groove (DBG) and the distal portion of the central groove.
Ridges (Fig. 5.12A)	• Other texts refer that the occlusal surface of mandibular first molar has two transverse ridges. • The triangular ridges (TR) of the mesiobuccal and mesiolingual cusps (TRMB and TRML) meet to form a transverse ridge. • The triangular ridges of distobuccal and distolingual cusps (TRDB and TRDL) form a second transverse ridge. • Since the lingual cusps are higher, TR of lingual cusps of first molars are longer than the TR of buccal cusps.
Fossa:	• There is one major fossa and two minor fossae. • The major fossa is the central fossa. It is roughly circular and it is centrally placed on the occlusal surface between the buccal and lingual cusp ridges. • All of the developmental grooves converge in the centre of the central fossa at the central pit. • Mesial triangular fossa is smaller and distal triangular fossa is smallest.
Grooves:	• There are 4 developmental grooves. Central developmental groove (CG), mesiobuccal developmental groove (MBG), the distobuccal developmental groove (DBG) and the lingual developmental groove (LG). • Central groove (CG) extends from mesial pit to distal pit and has a zigzag course mesiodistally (MD). • Mesial portion of the central groove extends from central pit mesiobuccally for short distance, joins the mesiobuccal groove, then separates and continues mesially to the mesial pit. • Distal portion of CG extends from Central pit in distobuccal direction to a point, where it is joined by DBG. From this point, CG courses in distolingual direction terminating in the distal pit. • MBG extends mesiobuccally from the central pit for short distance to traverse on to the buccal surface passing between the MB and DB cusps. • LG extends lingually from the central pit between the mesiolingual and distolingual cusps but rarely extends on to the lingual surface.

PULP CAVITY OF MANDIBULAR FIRST MOLAR

Pulp Chamber (PC)

- Roof of pulp chamber is rectangular in cross-section.
- It has four pulp horns MB, DB, ML, DL.
- Floor of the PC is rhomboid in cross-section.
- It has 2 funnel-shaped openings of the mesial root canals and 1 opening of the distal canal.

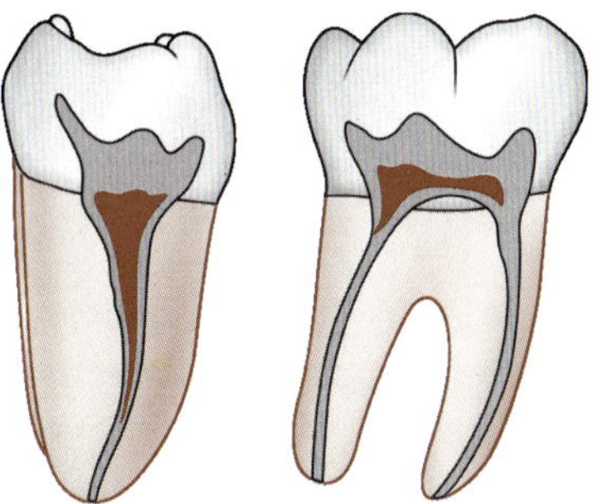

Fig. 5.12C: Mandibular first molar

Root Canals

- The molar has two separate and distinct roots :
- The mesial root has 2 distinct canals leaving the floor.
- It has a more complicated RC system because of presence of two root canals.

- The mesial canals may be severely curved or straight.
- The two canals may join each other and exit in a single foramen or may exit in separate foramen.
- The distal root has one large, straighter and shorter root canal, may have two canals.

Q 4. Describe morphology of mandibular second molar. *(May 2008)*

Ans. Introduction

- It is the second largest tooth in the mandibular arch.
- It is located seventh from the midline.
- It resembles the first molar in many respects, although it is more symmetrical and smaller in all dimensions.
- It has the least complicated occlusal design of any molar.
- Normally only four cusps present.

Eruption

It erupts at around twelve years of age.

Numbering System

Palmer:	7 | 7 (lower quadrants)	
Universal:	R # 31	L # 18
FDI:	R 47	L 37

Mandibular second molar from each aspect

Buccal aspect

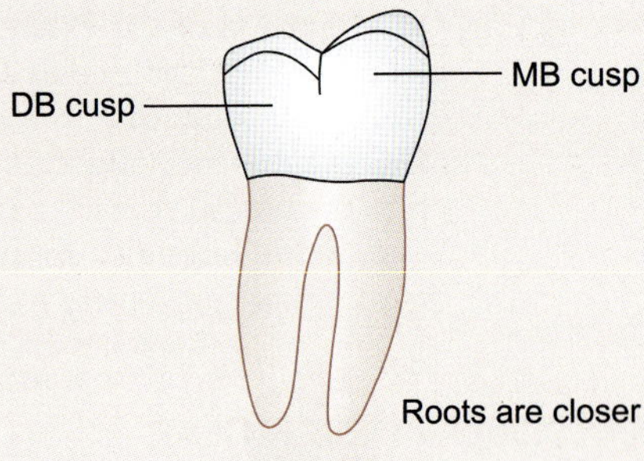

Fig. 5.13

Crown :	
Shape, size, surface:	• It has trapezoidal shape with longer parallel side towards the occlusal and shorter towards the cervical. • The crown tapers from contact area to the cervix. • The crown is shorter from mesial to distal. • It has four cusps, two buccal and two lingual which are just visible from the aspect. • Mesiobuccal (MB) cusp wider than distobuccal cusp. Two buccal cusps are separated by a buccal groove which terminates in a pit.
Outline:	• Mesial border of the crown is either straight or concave from contact area to cervix.

(Contd.)

Mandibular second molar from each aspect (Contd.)

- Distal border is either straight or convex from contact area to cervix.
- At contact area both outlines are convex.
- Cervical line is almost straight and points towards bifurcation.
- Occlusal border is flattened.

Contact area:

- Mesial contact area is more occlusal. It is close to the junction of occlusal and middle-third.
- Distal contact area is cervical to the mesial contact area.

Root:

- Two roots. Mesial root slightly longer than the distal root.
- Root bifurcation is near the cervical line.
- The root trunk is longer as compared to that of the first molar.
- Roots are more or less parallel, i.e. less separated.
- Either both the root apices are directed towards the centre line or both the roots curve distally.
- Both the roots taper apically in a pointed apex.

Lingual aspect

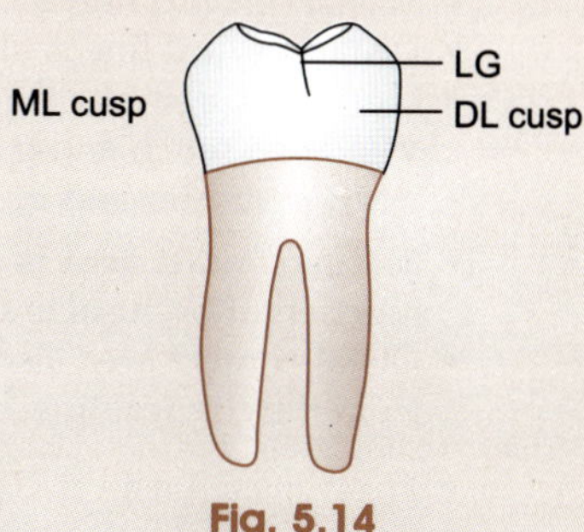

Fig. 5.14

Crown:

Shape, size, and surface:

- The crown is trapezoidal in shape.
- It is narrow from buccal to lingual.
- Since the lingual cusps are longer and sharper than the buccal cusps, from this aspect only ML and DL cusps are seen.
- Lingual groove separates the mesiolingual and the distolingual cusps.
- Cervical line is straight, may dip cervically over the bifurcation.

Root:

- Roots are narrower on this aspect.
- Root trunk appears longer because cervical line is more occlusal on lingual.

Proximal aspect

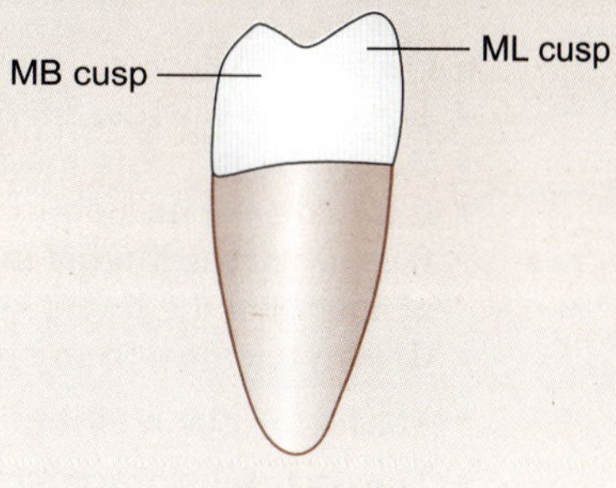

Fig. 5.15

(Contd.)

Mandibular second molar from each aspect (Contd.)

Crown:

Shape, size, and surface cusps:

- The proximal surface has rhomboid shape due to the lingual tilt of the crown in relation to root axis.

***Distal aspect*:**

- Due to the distal tilt of the crown and crown being shorter and narrower on this aspect, more of occlusal surface, part of MB and ML cusps are also seen behind the DB and DL cusps and also more of buccal and lingual surface is seen.

***Mesial aspect*:**

- Buccolingual dimension of the crown and root is more on the mesial aspect than on the distal and because the mesial cusps are longer, from this aspect only mesiobuccal and mesiolingual cusps and mesial root are seen.

Outline:

- Buccal outline is more convex in the cervical third and the lingual outline is more convex in the middle third.
- **The lingual cusp tips** more pointed than buccal cusp tips.
- The buccal cervical ridge is more prominent.
- Mesial cervical line is curved very slightly towards the occlusal.
- Distal cervical line is almost straight.
- Mesial marginal ridge is longer, more occlusally placed, has a sharp V-shaped notch and is crossed by mesial marginal ridge groove.
- DMR is shorter and more cervically placed.

Contact areas:

- Mesial contact area is almost centred buccopalatally and is placed at the junction of occlusal and middle third.
- Distal contact area also centered buccolingually and is placed equidistant from the cervical line and the marginal ridge.

Root:

- From mesial aspect compared to first molar the root is less wide bucco-lingually and narrower in the cervical third ending in a pointed apex.
- Deep depression on mesial surface of mesial root.
- Distal root is less wide, shorter with pointed apex.

Occlusal aspect

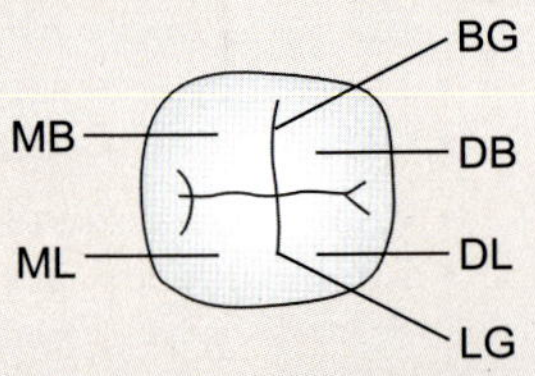

Fig. 5.16

Shape and size:

- Occlusal surface has a rectangular shape because of four cusps.
- The crown is wider mesiodistally than buccolingually.
- Crown tapers from mesial to distal.
- It is widest at mesiobuccal cusp because of prominent buccal cervical ridge.
- Because of the lingual inclination of the crown more of the buccal surface is visible than the lingual surface.
- Crown narrows from buccal to lingual.

Outline:

- Mesial outline is straight and longer, distal outline is convex and shorter.

Cusp:

- The occlusal surface includes cusps fossae, ridges and grooves.

(Contd.)

	Mandibular second molar from each aspect (Contd.)
	• The four cusps are more nearly equal even so MB is largest and DL is smallest. Palatal cusps are long and sharp.
Ridges:	There are four triangular ridges and two transverse ridges.
Groove:	Groove pattern is simple cross-type. Three major grooves present. • The central groove (CG), the buccal groove (BG), and the lingual groove (LG). MMRG and supplemental grooves also present. • The central groove extends from the central pit mesially and distally in a straight line. • Buccal and lingual grooves extend from central pit buccally and lingually onto the buccal and lingual surfaces to form a cross-pattern.
Fossa:	There are three fossae: • The major, large, circular central fossa and two minor mesial and distal triangular fossae.

SAQ (3 Marks)

Q 1. Describe arch traits of molars. *(2000, May 2007)*

Ans. Arch traits of molars and differences between maxillary and mandibular molars:

Maxillary molar	*Mandibular molar*
• The crowns of maxillary molars have three large cusps and one smaller cusp the distopalatal cusp. • Developmentally—three major cusps	• Mandibular molars have four relatively/large cusps, two buccal and two lingual. • Developmentally—four major cusps.
Buccal aspect	
• Buccal surface of the crown relatively vertical and flat.	• Buccal surface of the crown is convex.
• The crown does not appear to be tilted.	• First molar crown appears to tip distally relative the root axis due to increase taper from contact area to the cervical line.
• Buccal cusps not flattened	• Buccal cusps flattened.
• Two buccal cusps and one buccal groove	• In second molar, two buccal cusps and one buccal groove but in first M three buccal cusps and two buccal grooves.
Palatal aspect	
• Palatal cusps are unequal in size with MP cusp being largest and longest.	• Lingual cusps are almost equal in size.
• A fifth smaller cusp found on the palatal surface of the MP cusp of the Maxillary first molar.	• No cusp of carabelli present on the palatal/lingual surface.
Proximal aspect	
• Maxillary molars are centered over their roots.	• Mandibular molar crowns are tilted lingually.

(Contd.)

Maxillary molar	*Mandibular molar (Contd.)*
Occlusal aspect	
• From this aspect crown is wider bucco-palatally than mesiodistally.	• From this aspect crown are wider mesiodistally than buccolingually.
• The largest and longest MP cusp is connected to the DB cusp by an oblique ridge.	• There is no oblique ridge present.
• There is no palatal tilt, therefore buccal surface not seen.	• Since the crown is tilted lingually more of buccal surface is seen from this aspect.
• One transverse ridge from MB cusp to MP cusp.	• Two transverse ridges from MB to ML cusp and from DB to DL cusp.
• Four fossae.	• Three fossae.
• CG from central pit to mesial pit.	• CG from mesial pit to central pit to distal pit.
• Palatal groove/LG extends from distal pit and parallel to oblique ridge.	• LG extends from central fossa and at right angles to central groove.

Q 3. Describe type traits of maxillary molars. *(June 2006, 2011)*

Ans.

Maxillary first molar	*Maxillary second molar*
• It erupts at 6-year of age.	• It erupts at 12-year of age.
• It is the largest tooth in the arch.	• It is smaller than the first.
• It is least variable of all maxillary molars and it has rhomboid shape.	• Three cusps type is heart-shaped or four cusp type has accentuated rhomboid shape.
• Buccopalatally both molars are same in dimension.	• But mesiodistally second molar is narrower than the first molar.
• The crown is wider on palatal.	• Crown is narrower towards palatal.
• MB cusp longer and wider than DB cusp.	• MB cusp **much wider** than DB cusp.
• DP/DL cusp slightly smaller than MP.	• DP cusp is much smaller than MP cusp.
• Cusp of Carabelli present on palatal surface of MP cusp.	• No cusp of Carabelli.
• **The three roots** more divergent and are outside the confines of the crown.	• The three roots **less divergent** and are within the confines of the crown.
• MB and DB roots are curved like handle of pliers.	• MB and DB roots are more or less parallel.
• Palatal root is longest and has banana shape.	• Palatal root is straight.
• Less prominent MB cervical ridge.	• More prominent MB cervical ridge.
• More prominent oblique ridge (OR)	• Smaller and less prominent OR.
• Fewer supplemental grooves	• More supplemental grooves.

Q 4. What is Cope Osborn hypothesis? *(Nov. 2004)*

Ans. Cope Osborn Hypothesis

- The occlusal table of the maxillary first molar may be divided into two distinct components the trigon and the talon by an oblique ridge.
- The triangular shape is formed by the three major cusps mesiobuccal, distobuccal, mesiopalatal collectively known as "maxillary molar primary cusp triangle" or "Trigon" made by tracing the cusp outlines of these cusps, the MMR, and the oblique ridge and ridges of the occlusal surface.
- Developmentally only three major cusps may be considered as primary cusps the mesiopalatal cusp which is most primitive and two buccal cusps.
- The distopalatal cusp common to all maxillary molars and cusp of Carabelli on first molar maybe regarded as secondary cusps.

- Maxillary molar primary cusp triangle supposition follows "Cope Osborn hypothesis of tooth origin."
- There was a tritubercular stage in human tooth development when the molars had three cusps.
- The primary triangular design is also reflected in the outline of the root trunk when the tooth is sectioned in that area.
- One more observation that supports the explanation of maxillary molar having three major primary cusps is that distopalatal cusp becomes progressively smaller on second and third molars, often disappears as a major cusp.

Q 5. Draw, label occlusal surface of maxillary first molar.

(*June 2005, 2010, 2013, Nov. 2009*)

Ans.

Occlusal aspect

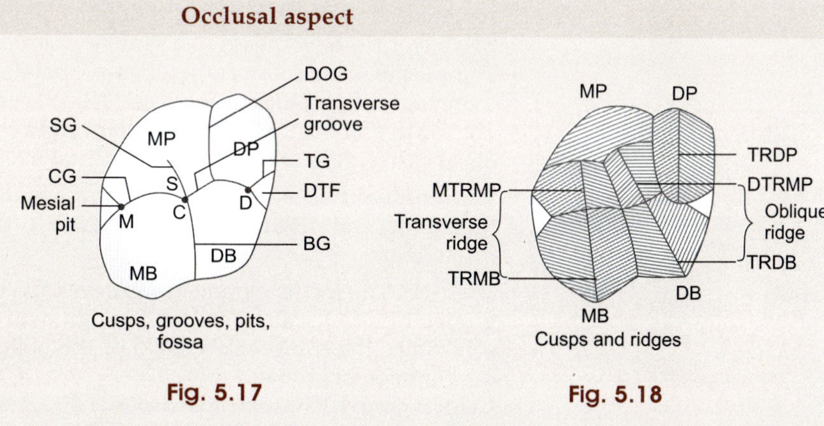

Fig. 5.17

Fig. 5.18

Crown:

Shape, outline, cusps:

- From this aspect it has somewhat rhomboid outline following the four major cusp ridges and the marginal ridges (MR).
- **Buccopalatal dimension** is more than mesiodistal dimension.
- Crown tapers from mesial to distal.
- In maxillary first molar the palatal side may be wider as compared to the buccal.
- The four major cusps and one minor cusp present.
- The mesiopalatal (MP) cusp is the largest with a rounded cusp tip.
- Distopalatal cusp (DP) is the smallest and most variable.
- Mesiobuccal (MB) cusp is second largest with sharp cusp tip and is slightly larger than the distobuccal cusp.
- The distobuccal cusp (DB) is the third largest with sharpest cusp tip.

Fossa:

- There are two major fossae and two minor fossae.
- The major fossa is the central fossa which is roughly triangular and mesial to the oblique ridge and the distal fossa (cigar fossa) which is linear and distal to and parallel to the oblique ridge (OR).
- The central fossa has connecting sulci within its boundaries with developmental grooves at the deepest portion of these sulci (sulcate grooves).
- The two minor fossae are the mesial triangular fossa (MTF) and the distal triangular fossa (DTF) which are located distal to and mesial to the MMR and the DMR.

(*Contd.*)

Occlusal aspect (*Contd.*)	
Ridges:	• The mesiopalatal cusp has two triangular ridges (TR). • The distopalatal cusp has a straight single triangular ridge. • The groove between the two triangular ridges of the mesiopalatal cusp is the "Stuart groove" (SG). • The distal triangular ridge of mesiopalatal cusp (DTRMP) and the triangular ridge of distobuccal cusp (TRDB) join to form a diagonal or oblique transverse ridge called "Oblique ridge" (OR). • Other texts refer to **DTRMP** by another name the **distal cusp ridge of mesiopalatal cusp (DCRMP):** Subsequently the OR is formed by union of triangular ridge of distobuccal cusp and distal cusp ridge of mesiopalatal cusp (Refer page 399 Fig. 25.132). • The oblique ridge is reduced in height in the centre of the occlusal surface being about on the level of the marginal ridges of the occlusal surface sometimes it is crossed by a developmental groove that partially joins the two major fossa by means of a shallow sulcate groove. • The mesial triangular ridge of mesiopalatal cusp (MTRMP) joins the triangular ridge of the mesiobuccal (TRMB) cusp to form a transverse ridge. • The MMR and the DMR are irregular ridges confluent with the mesial and distal cusp ridges of the mesial and distal major cusps.
Pits:	• The central pit (C) is located at the centre of the central fossa. • Mesial (M) and distal pits (D) are located at the bottom of the mesial and distal fossa.
Grooves:	• There are 5 major developmental grooves. CG the central groove, the buccal groove BG, DOG the distal oblique groove, PG the palatal groove, and sometimes the transverse groove of the oblique ridge and the fifth cusp developmental groove. • **Central groove (CG)** extends in mesial direction at an obtuse angle to buccal groove from the central pit (over the mesial transverse ridge) and ends in the mesial triangular fossa. A short developmental groove radiates from the central pit, extend disto-palatally where it other crosses the oblique ridge and ends in the distal fossa or fades out before reaching the OR. This part of the CG which extends over the oblique ridge is called the **transverse groove** of the oblique ridge, it is a shallow developmental groove. • **Buccal groove (BG)** extends from the central pit in buccal direction on to the buccal surface. • **Distal oblique groove (DOG)** or linear groove or distopalatal groove extends obliquely and traverses the distal linear fossa to join the palatal developmental groove between the mesiopalatal and distopalatal cusps. It shows several supplemental grooves. At distal pit it terminates into two branches (TG) which form the two sides of the distal triangular fossa (DTF). • **Palatal developmental groove (PG)** separates the MP and DP cusps and extends on the palatal surface to terminate at the centre of the crown palatally below the palatal root. • **Fifth cusp** groove outlines the fifth cusp (cusp of carabelli) it joins the palatal groove near its terminus. The other grooves are : • Distal marginal groove (DMG). • Distobuccal triangular groove and distopalatal triangular groove. • Mesial marginal groove. • Mesiobuccal triangular groove and mesiopalatal triangular groove.

Q 6. Describe the occlusal surface of mandibular first molar. *(Nov. 2009, May 2015)*

Ans.

Occlusal aspect	
	Crown is MD > BL

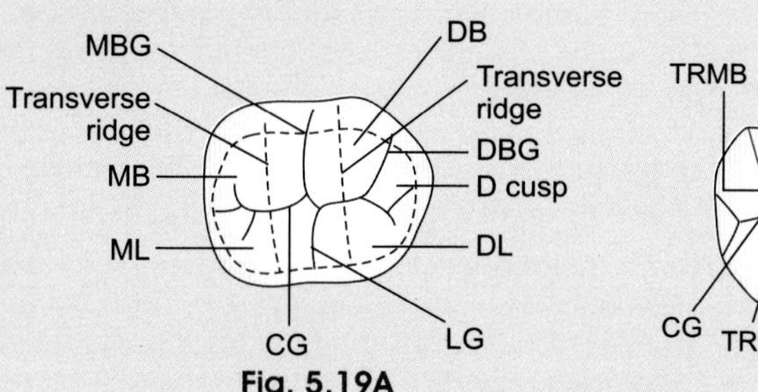

Fig. 5.19A Fig. 5.19B

Shape and size:	• Occlusal surface is quadrilateral in form but due to the presence of buccal bulge of the distobuccal cusp and small distal cusp, it has a pentagon shape. • Mesiodistal dimension is 1 mm more than the buccolingual dimension. • Crown tapers from mesial to distal therefore the crown is wider bucco-lingually on mesial half than on the distal half. • Widest buccolingual dimension is in the middle third of the distobuccal cusp. • Because of the lingual inclination of the crown more of the buccal surface is visible than the lingual surface. • The crown narrows from buccal to lingual. • Outline of the crown is convex on buccal, lingual, mesial, distal. • The occlusal surface includes the cusps, the ridges, the fossae and the grooves. • There are five triangular ridges, three fossae, three pits and four developmental grooves.
Cusps:	• Mesiobuccal cusp is larger than mesiolingual and distolingual cusps which are almost equal in size, distobuccal cusp is smaller than the mesiobuccal, mesiolingual, distolingual and distal cusps is the smallest.
Ridges: (Fig. 5.19B)	• Some texts refer that the occlusal surface of mandibular first molar has no transverse ridge. • The triangular ridge of the mesiobuccal cusp (TRMB) extends lingually to end at the mesial portion of the central groove. • The triangular ridge of the distobuccal cusp (TRDB) extends mesiolingual to the area of the central pit. • The triangular ridge of the distal cusp (TRD) extends mesiolingual to the distal pit area. • The triangular ridge of the mesiolingual cusp (TRML) extends distobuccal to end at the mesial portion of the central groove. • The triangular ridge of the distolingual cusp (TRDL) extends mesiobuccally to end in the area of the junction of the distobuccal groove (DBG) and the distal portion of the central groove.
Ridges: (Fig. 5.19A)	• Other texts refer that the occlusal surface of mandibular first molar has two transverse ridges. • The triangular ridges (TR) of the mesiobuccal and mesiolingual cusps (TRMB and TRML) meet to form a transverse ridge.

(Contd.)

Occlusal aspect (*Contd.*)	
	• The triangular ridges of distobuccal and distolingual cusps (TRDB and TRDL) form a second transverse ridge. • Since the lingual cusps are higher, TR of lingual cusps of first molars are longer than the TR of buccal cusps.
Fossa:	• There is one major fossa and two minor fossae. • The major fossa is the central fossa. It is roughly circular, and it is centrally placed on the occlusal surface between the buccal and palatal cusp ridges. • All of the developmental grooves converge in the centre of the central fossa at the central pit. • Mesial triangular fossa is smaller and distal triangular fosa is smallest.
Grooves:	• There are four developmental grooves. Central developmental groove (CG), mesiobuccal developmental groove (MBG), the distobuccal developmental groove (DBG) and the lingual developmental groove (LG). • Central groove (CG) extends from mesial pit to distal pit and has a zigzag course mesiodistally. • Mesial portion of the central groove extends from central pit mesiobuccally for short distance via mesiobuccal groove, then separates and continues mesially to the mesial pit. • Distal portion of the central groove extends from distal pit passes mesiobuccally to becomes confluent with the distobuccal groove (DBG). • MBG extends mesiobuccally from the central pit for short distance to traverse on to the buccal surface passing between the MB and DB cusps. • LG extends lingually from the central pit between the mesiolingual and distolingual cusps but rarely extends on to the lingual surface.

Q 7. What is endodontic anatomy of maxillary first molar? *(Nov. 2009)*

Ans. Endodontic Anatomy of Maxillary First Molar

Pulp Chamber (PC)

- It has large pulp chamber with four pulp horns mesiobuccal, distobuccal, mesiopalatal and distopalatal.
- Roof of the pulp chamber is rhomboid in cross-section whereas the floor of the PC is triangular in cross-section.
- The three orifices of the root canals are present at triangles of the floor.
- It an accessory mesiobuccal canal is present the 4th canal orifice may be present at its palatal end.
- Mesiobuccal orifice under the mesiobuccal cusp is long buccopalatally.
- Distobuccal orifice is slightly mesial and palatal to the mesiobuccal orifice.
- Palatal orifice is largest, is round or oval and is centered palatally.

Root and Root Canals

- It usually has three roots and three canals. Mesiobuccal root usually possesses an accessory canal.
- The mesiobuccal canal is often very small and curved but some may be wide.
- The palatal root canal is the largest.

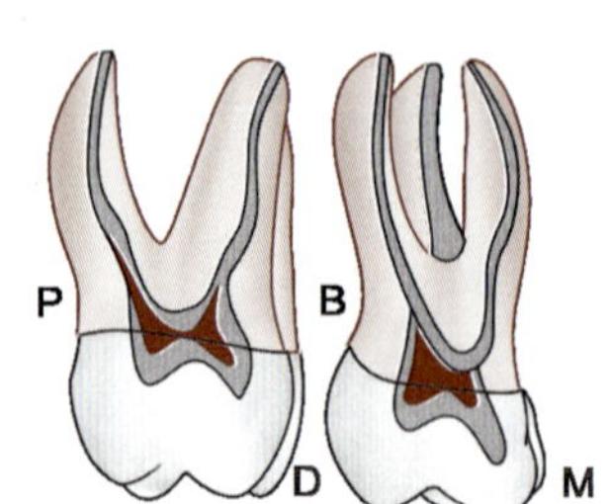

Fig. 5.20: Maxillary first molar

- The distobuccal root canal is straighter and smaller and centred.
- The entire removal of pulp is an impossibility in many maxillary first molars because of the compleixities of the root canal system.

Q 8. What is cusp of Carabelli?

Ans. Cusp of Carabelli

- It is a supplemental cusp palatal to mesiopalatal cusp which is largest of the well-developed cusps of the deciduous and permanent maxillary first molar.
- Usually a developmental groove is found.
- This morphological trait can take the form of a well-developed fifth cusp, or it can grade down to a series of grooves, depressions or pits on the mesial portion of the palatal surface.
- This trait has been used to distinguish populations.
- Fifth cusp or a developmental trace at its usual site serves to identify the maxillary first molar.

MULTIPLE CHOICE QUESTIONS (MCQs)

1. **The molar having the crown, wider bucco-palatally than mesiodistally is**
   a. Maxillary molars
   b. Mandibular molars
   c. Both
   d. None
2. **The cusp or tubercle of Carabelli is found in**
   a. Mandibular second molar
   b. Maxillary second molar
   c. Maxillary first molar
   d. Mandibualr first molar
3. **The largest cusp on the maxillary molars is**
   a. Mesiopalatal
   b. Mesiobuccal
   c. Distobuccal
   d. Distopalatal
4. **The three roots in maxillary molars are**
   a. Mesiopalatal, distopalatal, and buccal
   b. Mesiobuccal, mesiopalatal, and distal
   c. Mesiobuccal, distobuccal, and palatal
   d. None of the above
5. **The longest root in maxillary first molar is**
   a. Mesiobuccal
   b. Distobuccal
   c. Palatal
   d. None of the above
6. **In maxillary first molar, bifurcation is seen from**
   a. Buccal aspect b. Proximal aspect
   c. Both a and b d. Palatal aspect
7. **From the occlusal aspect the crown is rhomboid in shape, wider bucco-palatally than mesiodistally, is the characteristic of**
   a. Maxillary molars
   b. Mandibular molars
   c. Maxillary and mandibular molars
   d. Maxillary premolars
8. **The oblique ridge is formed by the union of triangular ridge of**
   a. Distobuccal cusp and distal ridge of mesiopalatal cusp
   b. Mesiobuccal cusp and distopalatal cusp
   c. Mesiopalatal and mesiobuccal cusp
   d. Distobuccal and distopalatal
9. **The developmental groove traversing from the linear distal fossa which connects with the palatal development groove is called the**
   a. Distal developmental groove
   b. Distopalatal groove
   c. Distal oblique groove
   d. Mesial development groove
10. **The crown with more extreme rhomboid outline, having buccal roots that are more nearly parallel is the characteristic of**
    a. Maxillary first molar
    b. Maxillary second molar
    c. Maxillary third molar
    d. Mandibular first molar
11. **The poor development of distopalatal cusp and heart shape form is common to**
    a. Maxillary first molar
    b. Maxillary second molar
    c. Maxillary second and third molar
    d. Mandibular second molar
12. **The apex of the palatal root of maxillary second molar is**
    a. In line with the palatal groove
    b. In line with the distopalatal cusp tip
    c. In line with mesiopalatal cusp tip
    d. In line with root axis
13. **The apex of palatal root of maxillary first molar is**
    a. In line with the palatal groove
    b. In line with the distopalatal cusp tip
    c. In line with mesiopalatal cusp tip
    d. In line with root axis

1-a, 2-c, 3-a, 4-c, 5-c, 6-c, 7-a, 8-a, 9-c, 10-b, 11-c, 12-b, 13-a

14. Crowns are wider mesiodistally than buccopalatally in
a. Maxillary molars
b. Mandibular molars
c. Both a and b
d. Mandibular second premolar

15. Taper of crown from B to L is more in
a. Maxillary first
b. Maxillary second
c. Maxillary third
d. None of the above

16. From proximal view the crown is tilted palatally at cervix in
a. Maxillary molars
b. Mandibular molars
c. Mandibular premolars
d. Both b and c

17. The longest pulpal horn in mandibular permanent first molar is
a. Distobuccal
b. Mesiobuccal
c. Distopalatal
d. Mesiopalatal

18. In maxillary first molar the root which is more often curved is
a. Mesiobuccal b. Distobuccal
c. Palatal d. Mesiopalatal

19. Molars having short root trunk and two roots M and D are
a. Maxillary molars
b. Mandibular molars
c. Both
d. None

20. The most common feature to differentiate between maxillary first, second, and third molars is
a. Position of distopalatal groove and size of DL cusp
b. Number of roots
c. Cusp of Carabelli
d. All the above

21. Flattened buccal cusps are typical of all
a. Maxillary first molars
b. Mandibular molars
c. All mandibular premolars
d. Maxillary second molar

22. The distal cusp of mandibular first molar is located
a. On distal surface of the teeth
b. Part of it on palatal surface and part of it on distal surface
c. Small portion on buccal and major portion on distal surface.
d. On buccal surface

23. In mandibular first molar the mesiobuccal developmental groove is shorter of the two grooves and is situated
a. Mesial to the root bifurcation
b. In line with the root bifurcation
c. Distal to the root bifurcation
d. None of the above

24. The mesial root and canal show considerable curvature, distal root is straighter and shorter than the curved mesial root is common to
a. Mandibular first molar
b. Mandiular second molar
c. Mandibular third molar
d. Maxillary first molar

25. No transverse ridge, zigzag groove pattern, two buccal grooves, is the characteristic of permanent
a. Maxillary first molar
b. Mandibular first molar
c. Mandibular second molar
d. Maxillary second molar

26. The widest mesiodistal dimension is found on permanent
a. Maxillary first molars
b. Maxillary central incisors
c. Mandibular first molars
d. None of the above

14-b, 15-c, 16-d, 17-b, 18-a, 19-b, 20-a, 21-b, 22-c, 23-a, 24-a, 25-b, 26-c

27. The size of the cusps from largest to smallest in mandibular first molar is

a. Mesiopalatal, mesiobuccal, distobuccal, distopalatal, distal
b. Mesiopalatal, distopalatal, mesiobuccal, distobuccal, distal
c. Mesiopalatal, mesiobuccal, distopalatal, distobuccal, distal
d. Distopalatal, distal, mesiopalatal, mesiobuccal, distobuccal

28. The size of the cusps in maxillary first molar from largest to smallest

a. Mesiopalatal, distopalatal, mesiobuccal, distobuccal, cusp of Carabelli
b. Mesiopalatal, mesiobuccal, distobuccal, distopalatal, fifth cusp.
c. Mesiopalatal, mesiobuccal, distopalatal, distobuccal, fifth cusp
d. Distopalatal, distobuccal, mesiobuccal, mesiopalatal

29. Irregular groove pattern, numerous supplemental groove bulbous (B and L convex) and short crown, distal tilt is characteristic of

a. Mandibular third molars
b. Mandibular second molars
c. Maxillary third molars
d. Maxillary second molars

30. The largest tooth in the maxillary arch is

a. Maxillary first molar
b. Mandibular second molar
c. Mandibular first molar
d. Maxillary second molar

31. Using occlusal morphology as a guide, the mandibular third molar is most similar to the

a. Permanent maxillary first molar
b. Permanent mandibular first molar
c. Permanent mandibular second molar
d. Deciduous mandibular second molar

32. The cusp of Carabelli is located on the

a. Maxillary permanent third molar
b. Maxillary permanent first molar
c. Maxillary permanent CI
d. Maxillary permanent second molar

33. Oblique ridge connects

a. Mesiobuccal cusp to distopalatal cusp
b. Mesiobuccal cusp to distobuccal cusp
c. Mesiopalatal cusp to distopalatal cusp
d. None of the above

34. The occlusal surface of permanent maxillary first molar is

a. Oval in shape
b. Trapezoid in shape
c. Rectangular in shape
d. Rhomboid in shape

35. Fourth canal in maxillary first molar is commonly located in

a. Mesiobuccal root
b. Distobuccal root
c. Palatal root
d. None of the above

36. Wrinkled occlusal surface is found in

a. Mandibular third molars
b. Mandibular second molars
c. Maxillary third molars
d. Maxillary second molars

37. The mandibular first molars having sixth cusp located on the distal marginal ridge between the distal cusp and distopalatal cusp is named

a. Tubercle of carabelli
b. Tuberculum sextum
c. Tuberculum intermedium
d. Tubercle genial

38. Sixth cusp on mandibular first molar when located between two palatal cusps is named

a. Cusp of Carabelli
b. Genial tubercle
c. Tuberculum sextum
d. Tuberculum intermedium

27-b, 28-b, 29-a, 30-a, 31-c, 32-b, 33-d, 34-d, 35-a, 36-a, 37-b, 38-d

39. Primary feature that distinguishes maxillary molars from mandibular molars is
a. Number of roots
b. Number of cusps
c. Number of Surfaces
d. All of the above

40. A developmental groove that partially joins the two major fossae of maxillary first molar is
a. Stuart groove
b. Sulcate groove/transverse groove
c. Central groove
d. Buccal groove

41. The most symmetrical permanent molar is
a. Maxillary first molar
b. Maxillary second molar
c. Mandibular first molar
d. Mandibular second molar

42. Occlusocervically, the height of the distal marginal ridge of a permanent maxillary first molar is the same height as the following:
a. Mesial marginal ridge of maxillary second molar
b. MMR of mandibular first molar
c. MMR of mandibular second molar
d. DMR of maxillary second molar

43. A fissured groove is most frequently found on
a. Facial of maxillary molar
b. Palatal of maxillary molar
c. Facial of mandibular molar
d. Palatal of mandibular molar

44. The tooth most often restored, extracted or replaced is
a. Maxillary first molar
b. Maxillary third molar
c. Mandibular first molar
d. Mandibular first premolar

45. Pits in the occlusal surface of molars and premolars are at the junction of
a. Marginal ridge and inclined planes
b. Inclined planes and cusp tips
c. Development grooves
d. Facial and mesial surfaces

46. In persmanent maxillary first molar, the level of the oblique ridge on the occlusal surface near the center is at a level with
a. Marginal ridges
b. Cusp of Carabelli
c. Tips of ML and DB cusps
d. Depth of cental and distal fossa

47. In maxillary first M from which aspect bifurcation is closer to cervical line
a. Buccal b. Mesial
c. Distal d. Palatal

48. Pulp horn most likely to be exposed accidentally during class II cavity preparation in a maxillary first molar are
a. ML and DL b. MB and ML
c. ML and DB d. MB and DB

49. Primates have conical cusps and are called
a. Bunodont
b. Haplodont
c. Diphyodont
d. Bilophodont

50. Human teeth like incisors, canines premolars, molars can be described as
a. Monophyodont
b. Homodont
c. Heterodont
d. None of the above

51. Simplest form of tooth with single cone is called as
a. Haplodont
b. Triconodont
c. Tritubercular
d. Quadritubercular

39-a, 40-b, 41-d, 42-a, 43-b, 44-c, 45-c, 46-a, 47-b, 48-b, 49-a, 50-c, 51-a

52. A transverse ridge in maxillary first molar is formed by

a. Triangular ridge of mesiobuccal cusp and the mesial triangular ridge of the mesiopalatal cusp
b. Triangular ridge of distobuccal cusp and triangular ridge of mesiopalatal cusp
c. Triangular ridge of mesiobuccal cusp and triangular ridge of distopalatal cusp
d. None of the above

53. A deep concavity on the mesial surface of the crown in cervical area is present in maxillary

a. First premolar
b. First molar
c. Second premolar
d. Second molar

54. A deep concavity on the distal surface of the crown in the cervical area is present in the maxillary

a. First molar b. Canine
c. Incisors d. First PM

55. The two major fossa of permanent maxillary first M as

a. M and D triangular fossa
b. Central fossa and distal fossa
c. Central fossa and mesial fossa
d. Mesial fossa and mesial triangular fossa

56. Which furcation of roots in permanent maxillary first molar is closer to cervical line?

a. Mesial b. Distal
c. Buccal d. Palatal

57. The tooth which has longest root trunk from buccal view is

a. Maxillary 1st molar
b. Maxillary 2nd molar
c. Mandibular 1st molar
d. Mandibular 2nd molar

58. Which of the following is most likely to show an anomaly in radicular morphology?

a. Maxillary canine
b. Maxillary third molar
c. Maxillary first molar
d. Mandibular first molar

59. The occlusal outline of a permanent mandibular first molar is usually

a. Square b. Parallelogram
c. Circle d. Trapezoid

60. The maxillary molar crown of early primates has trigon of three cusps namely

a. Mesiobuccal, mesiopalatal, distobuccal
b. Mesiobuccal, mesiopalatal, distopalatal
c. Distobuccal, distopalatal, mesiopalatal
d. None of the above

61. The crown formation of all permanent teeth except third molars is completed between

a. 2–3 years
b. Birth to 6 years
c. Birth to 8 years
d. Birth to 12 years

62. In carving an occlusal amalgam restoration in a permanent mandibular second molar, the shape of the groove pattern is

a. H b. +
c. U d. Y

63. In a molar, the root canals usually join the pulp chamber

a. At the level of the furcation
b. At varying levels, depending on age
c. Within the cervical third of the crown
d. Apical to the cementoenamel junction

64. The root of permanent maxillary first molar that is flattened mesiodistally and has depressions on both its mesial and distal surfaces is the

a. Palatal b. Distobuccal
c. Mesiobuccal d. Distopalatal

52-a, 53-a, 54-b, 55-b, 56-a, 57-c, 58-b, 59-d, 60-a, 61-c, 62-b, 63-d, 64-c

65. From occlusal aspect, the greatest bucco-palatal dimension of a permanent mandibular second molar crown is located in the

a. Mesial half b. Distal half
c. Middle d. None

66. Cross-section of the floor of the pulp chamber is triangular in

a. Permmanent maxillary molars
b. Permanent mandibular first molar
c. Permanent mandibular second molar
d. None

67. When a fourth root canal is present in a maxillary first molar it is most likely located in the

a. Palatal root
b. Mesiobuccal root
c. Distobuccal root
d. Distopalatal root

68. The smallest pulp horn in permanent mandibular first molar is

a. Distal b. Mesiobuccal
c. Distobuccal d. Distopalatal

69. The statement which is correct regarding permanent mandibular first molar is

a. It has four root canals
b. Mesial root has concavities on both mesial and distal surfaces
c. Distal root has concavities on both buccal and palatal sides
d. No concavities seen on any root.

70. The pulp horn most commonly exposed in cavity preparation on newly erupted permanent molar is

a. ML and MB b. DL and DB
c. DL and ML d. None of the above

71. The tooth having five pulp horns and three root canals is most likely to be

a. Maxillary first molar
b. Mandibular first molar
c. Mandibular second molar
d. Maxillary second molar

72. The three root canals of mandibular first molars are

a. MB, ML, and distal
b. Mesial, distal, and palatal
c. MB, DB, and palatal
d. DL, ML, and buccal

73. The occlusal outlines of the permanent posterior teeth is correctly matched in the following:

a. Mandibular second premolar—square
b. Mandibular first molar—trapezoid
c. Maxillary first molar—rhomboidal
d. All of the above

74. The statement not true about the molars is

a. Mandibular molar crowns are tilted palatally
b. Palatal cusp on mandibular molars are almost equal in size.
c. Mandibular molars are wider mesio-distally
d. Maxillary molar crowns are titled palatally.

75. The most constant feature that differentiates maxillary first, second, and third molars is

a. The size of the DL cusp
b. Number of roots
c. Cusp of Carabelli
d. The shape of the crown

76. Maxillary molar can be differentiated from mandibular molar by all of the following except

a. Number of roots
b. Number of cusps
c. Arrangement of roots
d. All of the above

77. The statement not true about the occlusal morphology of mandibular first molars is

a. Buccal cusps are functional
b. Palatal cusps are non-functional
c. MB cusp is the widest
d. Presence of oblique ridge

65-a, 66-a, 67-b, 68-a, 69-b, 70-a, 71-b, 72-a, 73-d, 74-d, 75-a, 76-d, 77-d

78. The permanent molar having similar occlusal morphology to mandibular third molar is

a. Mandibular first
b. Maxillary first
c. Mandibular second
d. Maxillary second

79. The two major fossa, of maxillary first molar are

a. M and D triangular fossa
b. Central and distal fossa
c. Central and mesial fossa
d. Mesial and mesial triangular fossa

80. The permanent tooth with occlusal surface characterized by five cusps, three primary and two secondary; two major and two minor fossa, four triangular ridges and one oblique ridge is

a. Maxillary first molar
b. Maxillary second molar
c. Mandibular second
d. Mandibular second

81. The permanent tooth with occlusal surface characterized by five cusps, one major and two minor fossa and five triangular ridges is

a. Mandibular first molar
b. Mandibular second molar
c. Maxillary first molar
d. Maxillary second molar

82. The furcation in permanent maxillary first molar is closest to cervical line on

a. Mesial
b. Distal
c. Buccal
d. Palatal

83. The longest root trunk from buccal aspect is seen in

a. Maxillary first molar
b. Maxillary second molar
c. Mandibular first molar
d. Mandibular second molar

78-c, 79-b, 80-a, 81-a, 82-a, 83-a

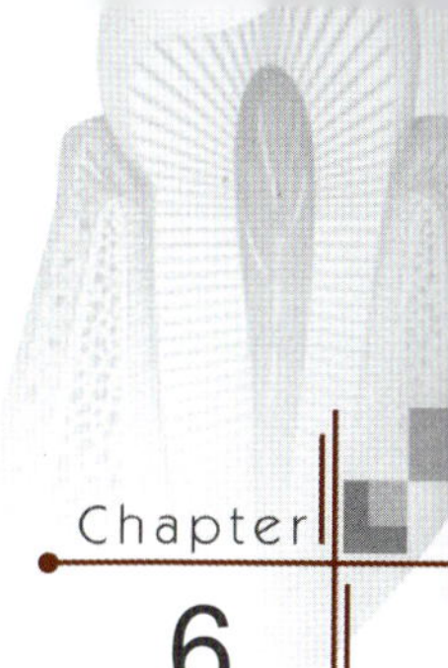

Differences between Deciduous and Permanent Dentition

LAQs (10 Marks)

Q 1. Differences between deciduous and permanent dentition. *(Oct. 2003, June 2010)*

Ans. Differences are macroscopic and microscopic or histological:

Macroscopic (SAQ 2000, 2001, Nov. 2014)		
	Deciduous dentition	*Permanent dentition*
I. General features		
1. Number and size of teeth 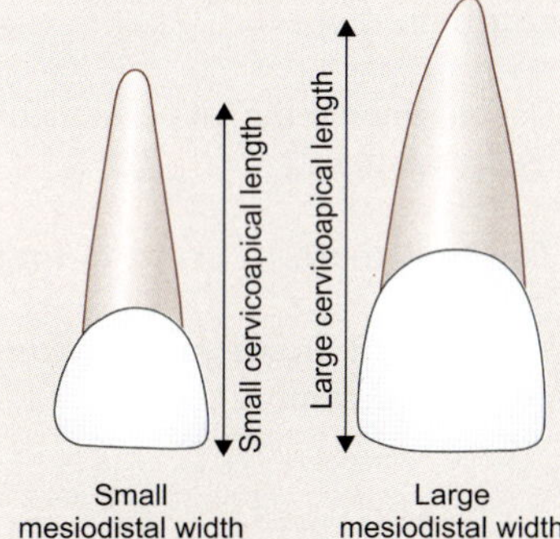	• The jaws are smaller in size and number of teeth are less. A total of 20 teeth, 10 in each jaw. • Teeth are smaller in size. • Crown of second molar is larger than crown of first molar.	• The jaws are larger. The number of teeth are 32 with 16 teeth in each jaw. • Teeth are larger in size than the deciduous teeth. • Crown of first molar is larger than that of the second and third molar.
2. Classes of teeth and dental formula	• There are 3 classes of teeth. Incisors, canines and molars. Premolars and third molars are not present. • Molars are distal to canines. Dental formula is: $I\frac{2}{2}, C\frac{1}{1}, M\frac{2}{2}$ • Total of 10 teeth, 5 in upper and 5 in lower jaw. Dental Formula is written for one side of the mouth.	• There are 4 classes of teeth. Incisors, canines, premolars, and molars. • Molars are distal to premolars. Dental formula is: $I\frac{2}{2}, C\frac{1}{1}, P\frac{2}{2}, M\frac{3}{3}$ • Total of 16 teeth, 8 in upper and 8 in lower jaw. Dental formula is written for one side of the mouth only.

(Contd.)

Macroscopic (SAQ 2000, 2001, Nov. 2014) (*Contd.*)		
	Deciduous dentition	*Permanent dentition*
3. Colour	• Teeth are lighter in colour. They appear bluish white (milky white) and are also called as **milk-teeth.** Their refractive index is comparable to that of milk. The enamel is opaque and less mineralized.	• Teeth are darker in colour. They appear yellowish white or grayish white. Enamel is highly mineralized and translucent therefore reflects the yellowish white colour of the underlying dentin.
4. Placement in the jaw	• Teeth are arranged perpendicular to the jaw.	• Teeth are not perpendicular to the jaw, but are labially inclined which allows to accommodate the larger permanent teeth.
5. Interdental spacing	• Interdental spacing is present which is physiological or developmental spacing.	• No spacing present. If present it is due to decay or loss of tooth.
6. Duration of dentition and period of eruption	• Deciduous dentition period lasts from 6 months to 6 years. Six years to 12 years is mixed dentition period. • Total period of eruption is from 6 months to 2.5–3 years. • Root completion is 1 year after eruption.	• Permanent dentition period is from 12 years onwards. • Period of eruption is between 6 years to 12 years except for third molars which erupt between 18–25 years. • Root completion is 2–3 years after eruption.
7. Development time	• Development time for deciduous teeth is shorter.	• Development time for permanent teeth is longer.
8. Sequence of eruption	• The first tooth to erupt is mandibular central incisor. • Deciduous teeth erupt from anterior to posterior except first molar which erupts before canine. • $\frac{\text{A B D C E}}{\text{A B D C E}}$	• The first tooth to erupt is first molar. • Permanent teeth erupt from posterior to anterior. • $\frac{6\,1\,2\,4\,5\,3\,7\,8}{6\,1\,2\,3\,4\,5\,7\,8}$
9. Shedding	• Shedding is physiological. • Teeth start exfoliating from about 7–10 years due to physiologic resorption of roots.	• Shedding or loss of teeth is due to some pathology.
10. Mineralization	• The teeth are less mineralized therefore, wear out faster.	• Teeth are highly mineralized.

(*Contd.*)

Macroscopic (SAQ 2000, 2001, Nov. 2014) (*Contd.*)		
	Deciduous dentition	*Permanent dentition*
II. Crown morphology **11. Shape and cervical constriction** 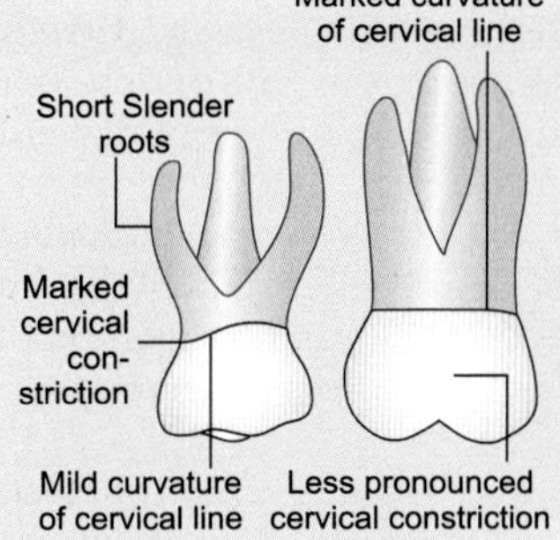 	• **Incisors** – Width of the crown is more than the length. – More constriction at the cervix. • **Molar** Molars have more bulbous shape due to more constriction at the cervix.	• The length of the crown is more than the width. • Less constriction at the cervix. • Do not have bulbous shape.
Clinical significance	• Cervical constriction has to be kept in mind while forming gingival floor during class II cavity preparation.	• Crowns of permanent teeth are not so constricted at the cervix.
12. Surface and cingulum and cervical ridge 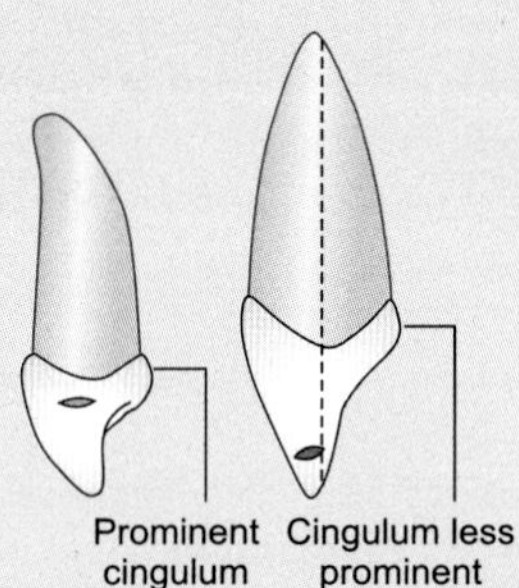 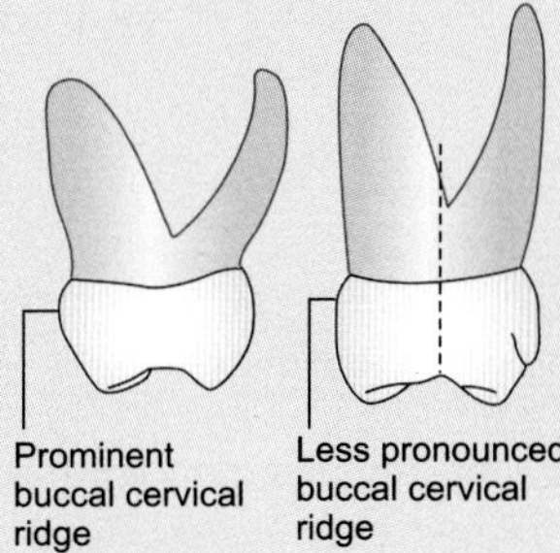 	**Incisors** • In incisors the surface is flat above the cervical ridge. • There are no developmental depressions on the labial surface. • Cervical ridge on labial surface of anterior teeth is very prominent. • Cingulum is more prominent. **Molars** • In molars also the surface is flat above the cervical ridge up to the occlusal. • Cervical ridge on the buccal surface of molar is very prominent, especially on buccal surface of first molars. If overdeveloped, it is referred to as "tubercle of zuckerkandl" or buccal cingulum.	• In incisors, the surface above the height of contour is slightly convex. • Transient developmental grooves separating the mamelons are present on the labial surface. • No prominent cervical ridge • Comparatively cingulum is less prominent. • In molars the surfaces are convex above the cervical ridge up to the occlusal. • Cervical ridges are not prominent except in mandibular second molars.
13. Mamelons	• No mamelons in newly erupted incisors.	• Mamelons are present on the incisal ridge of the newly erupted incisors.
14. Cervical line	• Cervical line is less curved.	• It is more curved.

(*Contd.*)

Macroscopic (SAQ 2000, 2001, Nov. 2014) (*Contd.*)		
	Deciduous dentition	*Permanent dentition*
15. Contact areas Clinical significance 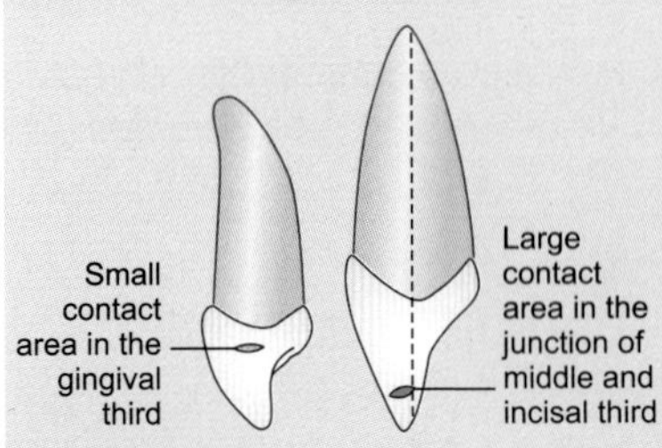	• Contacts areas between teeth are flatter, broader and situated gingivally. • While preparing class II cavity, buccal and lingual walls should be made divergent.	• Contact areas between permanent teeth are narrower and situated either in the middle third or at the junction of incisal and middle third.
16. Molar		
	• Upper first molar has 3–4 cusps, it resembles a premolar.	• Upper first molar has four cusps and accessory cusp the cusp of Carabelli.
	• Upper second molar has four cusps and one accessory cusp, the cusp of Carabelli. It resembles permanent upper first molar.	• Upper second molar has four cusps or three cusps.
	• Lower first molar has four cusps (it does not resemble any permanent tooth).	• Lower first molar has five cusps.
	• Lower second molar has five-cusps (it resembles permanent lower first molar.)	• Lower second molar has four cusps.
Relation between distal planes of last molars	• Mesiodistal relation between distal surfaces of upper and lower second molars is called the **terminal plane.**	
	• Distal surfaces of upper and lower second molars are in one vertical plane due to a greater mesiodistal width of lower second molar and is called **Flush-terminal plane** or end-on-occlusion which is necessary for normal eruption and occlusion of permanent first molar.	• There is no such distal plane relation in permanent molar.
Cusps	• The cusps are short and sharp but may become flat due to wear.	• The cusps are less sharp.
Occlusal surface	• Since the cusps are short and the fossae and ridges are less prominent the occlusal surface is shallow.	• Due to longer cusps and more prominent fossae and ridges the occlusal surface is deeper and has curved contour.
Grooves	• More supplemental grooves due to which more prone to caries. To prevent caries, pit and fissure sealants are advisable.	• Fewer supplemental grooves.

(*Contd.*)

Macroscopic (SAQ 2000, 2001, Nov. 2014) (*Contd.*)		
	Deciduous dentition	*Permanent dentition*
Occlusal table area 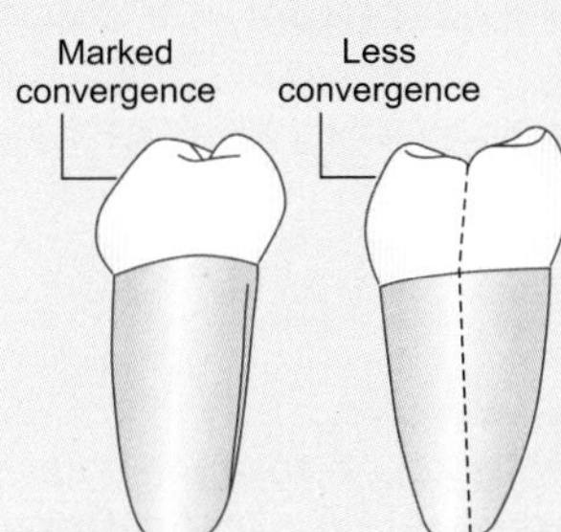	• Buccal and lingual surfaces converge sharply occlusally, thus forming a narrow occlusal table area buccolingually. • Deciduous molars are functionally adapted to withstand less occlusal load.	• There is less convergence of buccal and lingual surface towards occlusal thus occlusal table appears wider buccolingually.
Clinical significance	• Occlusal cavity preparation should be kept narrow buccolingually.	
III. Root morphology		
17. Length and width	• Roots of deciduous teeth are shorter and slender and they are narrower mesiodistally.	• Roots are longer and stronger and they are broader mesiodistally.
18. Crown root ratio	• In deciduous teeth, the roots are longer in proportion to the crown size.	• Roots are not as long in proportion to the crown size.
19. Inclination of the root 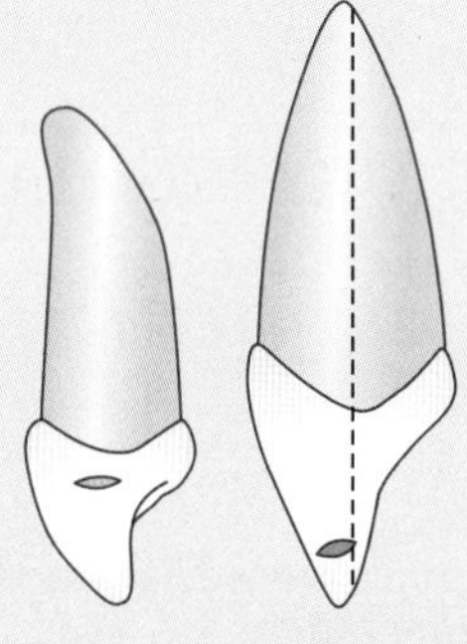	• The roots of the anterior teeth have a slight labial inclination of about 10° in the apical third to accommodate the developing permanent anterior teeth.	• The roots do not show any labial inclination.
20. Root trunk and furcation 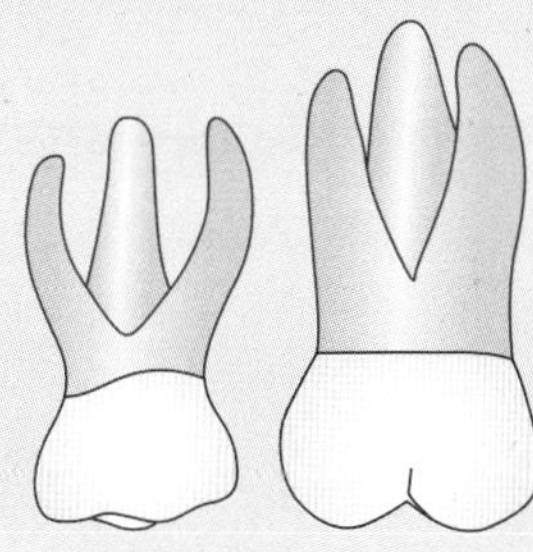	• The furcation of the roots of molars is near the cervical line so that the root trunk is almost absent.	• The furcation of the root is more apically placed, thus the root trunk is longer.

(*Contd.*)

Macroscopic (SAQ 2000, 2001, Nov. 2014) (*Contd.*)		
	Deciduous dentition	*Permanent dentition*
21. Flaring of roots in molars	• Roots of deciduous molars flare out markedly to accommodate the developing premolars.	• Roots of permanent molars do not flare markedly.
Clinical significance	• Thin, slender and flared roots with absence of root trunk may cause fracture during extraction.	
22. Apical foramen and resorption	• The apical foramen is larger. • Roots undergo physiologic resorption. Pathoogical resorption is less common.	• It is narrower. • Physiologic resorption is absent. Pathological resorption is commonly seen.
IV. Pulp morphology		
23. Pulp chamber	• Pulp chamber is larger as compared to the crown size.	• Pulp chamber is smaller as compared to the crown size.
24. Pulp horns 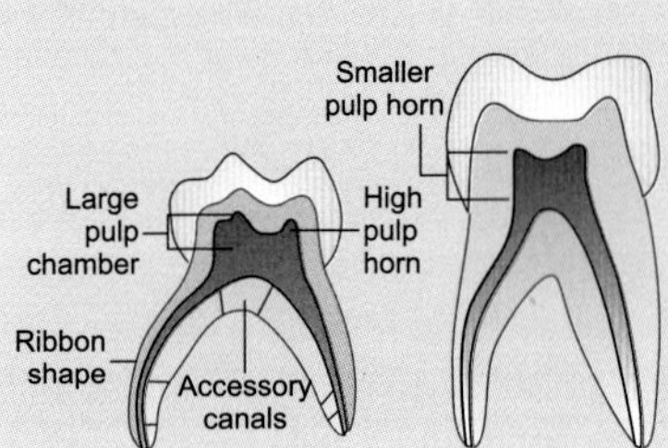 	• Pulp horns of molars (especially, mesial horns) are higher and close to the outer surface than that of permanent molars.	• Pulp horns are lower and away from the outer surface.
Clinical significance	• Pulp horns more longer and pointed than cusps would indicate. • Care should be taken during cavity preparation to prevent pulp exposure.	
25. Pulp canals	• Root canals are flat, ribbon shaped, more tortuous and branching which makes complete debridement impossible.	• Root canals are well-defined and less branching.
26. Accessory canals	• Accessory pulp canals are more in number and found in furcation area. • Floor of the pulp chamber is more porous due to which the inflammation can directly reach periodontium.	• Accessory canals are found near the apex of the root.

Q 2. Explain histologic/microscopic differences. *(Nov. 2004)*

Ans.

	Deciduous dentition	*Permanent dentition*
1. Enamel		
Thickness	• Enamel is thinner but of uniform thickness. (1 mm) decay progresses faster to the pulp.	• Enamel is thick (2–3 mm) and not uniform in thickness.
Clinical significance	• Depth of the cavity should be less and less pressure required during cavity preparation.	
Mineralization	• Enamel is less mineralized thus wears out faster. It is more permeable.	• Enamel is more mineralized.
Clinical significance	• Greater permeability facilitates better uptake of fluoride in caries preventive measures.	
Direction of enamel rods	• In the cervical region the enamel rods are directed occlusally from DEJ to the enamel surface.	• In the cervical region the enamel rods are directed gingivally.
Incremental lines	• Incremental lines of Retzius are less common.	• Lines of Retzius are more common.
Neonatal line	• Neonatal line is present in all deciduous teeth.	• Neonatal line is present in first molar only.
2. Dentin		
Thickness	• Dentin is thin and of variable thickness, increased thickness near occlusal fossa area.	• Dentin is thick and is of more uniform thickness.
Dentinal tubules	• Dentinal tubules are less regular.	• Dentinal tubules more regular.
Secondary dentin	• Less deposition of secondary dentin.	• Greater deposition of secondary dentin.
Interglobular dentin	• Interglobular dentin is absent.	• Interglobular dentin is present beneath the well-calcified mantle dentin.
Neonatal line	• Neonatal line is present in all deciduous teeth.	• Neonatal line present only in first molar.
Mineralization	• It is less mineralized and softer.	• It is more mineralized and harder.
DEJ	• Dentinoenamel junction is not scalloped.	• Dentinoenamel junction is scalloped.
3. Cementum		
Thickness	• Cementum is relatively thin and made-up of only primary cementum. Anchorage is less firm.	• Cementum is relatively thick. Both cellular and acellular cementum present. Cellular cementum being thicker in the apical region.

(*Contd.*)

	Deciduous dentition	Permanent dentition (Contd.)
CDJ	• Cementodentinal junction is scalloped.	• Cementodentinal junction is not scalloped.
4. Pulp		
Pulp chamber	• Pulp chamber is proportionately larger.	• Pulp chamber is smaller in proportion to the crown size.
Pulp horns	• Pulp horns are pointed and at a higher level especially the mesial pulp horns. • Hence care should be taken during cavity preparation to prevent pulp exposure.	• Pulp horns are lower and not as pointed.
Accessory canals	• Accessory canals are present in furcation area.	• Accessory canals are more near the apex of the root.
Apical foramen	• Apical foramen larger, thus abundant blood supply and exhibit a more typical inflammatory response. • Poor localization of infection and inflammation.	• Apical foramen is narrower.
Root canals	• Root canals flatter.	• Root canals are round or oval or triangular.
Nerves	• Pulp is less innervated thus primary teeth are less sensitive to operative procedure.	• Pulp is densely innervated.
5. PDL	• Periodontal space is wider.	• Periodontal space is narrower.

SAQs (3 Marks)

Q 1. Describe functions of deciduous teeth. *(July 2008)*

Ans.

1. The deciduous teeth are useful for mechanical preparation of child's food for digestion and assimilation during one of the most active periods of growth and development.
2. They maintain space in the dental arch for the permanent teeth to erupt.
3. They stimulate the growth of jaws through mastication especially in the development of the height of the dental arches.
4. They function in the development of speech.

   Ability to use the teeth for pronunciation is acquired entirely with the aid of primary teeth.

   Early and accidental loss of primary anterior teeth may lead to difficulty in pronouncing the sounds f, v, s, z, th.
5. The normal facial appearance and smile of the child is maintained due to support provided by the teeth to cheeks and lips.

Q 2. Differentiate type traits of deciduous maxillary molars. (*Nov. 2004*)

Ans.

Maxillary first molar	*Maxillary second molar*
• It is most atypical of all molars.	• It resembles the permanent first molar that erupts distal to it.
• It resembles the maxillary first premolar that replaces it.	
• It is mesial to the deciduous second molar.	
• It is the smallest deciduous molar	• It is larger than the first molar.
• Occlusal outline is relatively flat with no definite cusp form.	• Occlusal outline is formed by the tips of MB and DB cusps.
• Two buccal cusps are unequal in size and MB cusp is wider, longer and less sharp.	• Two buccal cusps are more equal in size.
• There is no cusp of Carabelli.	• Cusp of Carabelli is present.
• Distolingual cusp is inconspicious.	• DL cusp is smallest but well-developed.
From occlusal aspect	
• It generally has four cusp giving it quadrilateral occlusal form.	• It generally has four major cusps and one minor cusp of Carabelli.
• Two larger cusps MB and ML show premolar like form.	• Occlusal form is rhomboidal.
• Two smaller cusps DB and DL which may be absent giving triangular occlusal form.	
• Oblique ridge is less prominent.	• Oblique ridge is well-defined prominent and straighter.
• There are three fossae.	• There are four fossae.
• The central fossa, the mesial fossa is larger and smaller distal triangular fossa.	• The central fossa, the mesial triangular fossa.
	• The distal fossa located distal to oblique ridge and less distinct distal triangular fossa.
• The central groove runs mesiodistally from mesial pit to distal pit.	• The central groove runs from mesial pit to the central pit.
• The buccal developmental groove separates MB and DB cusps and may extend onto buccal surface.	• The buccal developmental groove separates MB and DB cusps and may extend onto buccal surface.
• The distal developmental groove separates the two lingual cusps and may or may not extend onto lingual surface.	• The distal developmental groove separates the two lingual cusps and extends onto the lingual surface as the lingual developmental groove.
• Three roots are thin, slender, divergenent, and visible from both buccal and lingual aspects.	• Three roots are thin, slender and divergenent and visible from both buccal and lingual aspects.

Q 3. Describe importance of primary teeth. (*Nov. 2010, June 2011*)

Ans.

- Care of primary dentition is very much essential for the normal growth and development of the jaws and establishment of the normal occlusion of permanent dentition.
- Neuromuscular coordination required for masticatory process is established at primary dentition stage.
- With the establishment of primary occlusion, child learns to masticate food efficiently.
- Functional occlusion of primary teeth helps to maintain a proper diet and good nutrition.
- A well-cared set of primary teeth helps to maintain normal facial appearance which in turn helps normal psychological development of the child.

- The primary teeth, especially the anteriors are necessary for normal pronunciation of consonants and for development of clear speech.
- The proper care of primary teeth is important to avoid infection and spread of infection.
- The primary teeth maintain the normal eruption schedule of permanent successors.
- The primary teeth help in maintaining the space for eruption of permanent successor.
- The premature loss of primary teeth due to caries or trauma causes migration of adjacent teeth into the available space leading to decrease in arch length. This causes lack of space for the erupting permanent tooth resulting in development of malocclusion.

Q 4. What is buccal cingulum/tuberculum of Zukerkandl? *(Dec. 2005, May 2007)*

Ans.

- The cervical ridge running mesiodistally in the cervical third of the buccal surface of the primary first molars is sometimes called **buccal cingulum.** It is present in both maxillary and mandibular first molars.
- It is more prominent in the cervical third of the mesiobuccal cusp of the primary maxillary first molar and is referred to as Tuberculum of Zukerkandl. When viewed from mesial aspect, the buccal outline of the molar shows pronounced convexity of the cervical enamel ridge in the cervical third and then the buccal outline is straight line converging in an occlusal direction. This makes the occlusal table narrower buccolingually compared to that of the permanent molars.

MULTIPLE CHOICE QUESTIONS (MCQs)

1. Divergent roots with very short root trunk is present in
a. Permanent maxillary molars
b. Permanent mandibular molars
c. Primary molars
d. All posterior teeth

2. The teeth not included in primary set are
a. Canines b. Third molars
c. Premolars d. Both b and c

3. The predecessor of permanent molars are
a. Primary first molar
b. Primary second molar
c. Primary canine
d. None of the above

4. Mixed dentition is present from
a. 1–5 years b. 3–8 years
c. 6–12 years d. 8–16 years

5. The number of teeth present in the oral cavity at the age of 8 years are
a. 20 b. 32
c. 24 d. 48

6. Primary maxillary second molars most closely resemble
a. Primary maxillary first molar
b. Permanent maxillary first molar
c. Permanent maxillary second molar
d. Primary maxillary second molar

7. The highest and sharpest cusp on a primary mandibular first molar is
a. Mesiolingual b. Distolingual
c. Mesiobuccal d. Distobuccal

8. Primary mandibular second molars resemble
a. Primary mandibular first molar
b. Permanent mandibular second molar
c. Permanent mandibular first molar
d. None of the above

9. Man has two sets of dentition, one primary, the other permanent, this can be correctly described as
a. Polyphyodont
b. Monophyodont
c. Diphyodont
d. Homodont

10. Which tooth does not exist in primary dentition?
a. Incisors b. Canines
c. Premolars d. Molars

11. Primary first molars are
a. Larger in size than primary second molars
b. Much smaller in size than primary second molars
c. Same as primary second molars
d. None of the above

12. The primary teeth having strange and primitive appearance is
a. Maxillary 1st molar
b. Maxillary 2nd molar
c. Mandibular 1st molar
d. Mandibular 2nd molar

13. Primary teeth when in occlusion, each teeth occludes with two teeth of the opposing jaw *except*
a. Mandibular central incisors
b. Maxillary central incisors
c. Maxillary second molar
d. Both a and c

14. Primary teeth are worn off rapidly on incisal edges and occlusal surfaces because
a. Of food habits
b. Of brittle teeth
c. Teeth do not hold their relative positions for long-time
d. All the above

1-c, 2-d, 3-d, 4-c, 5-c, 6-b, 7-a, 8-c, 9-c, 10-c, 11-b, 12-c, 13-d, 14-c

15. The human dentition is referred to as
a. Omnivorous dentition
b. Carnivorous dentition
c. Herbivorous dentition
d. All the above

16. The groove that separates the gumpads from the palate and floor of the mouth is
a. Gingival groove
b. Dental groove
c. Transverse groove
d. Mesiogingival groove

17. Even though upper and lower gumpads are almost similar to each other the upper gum pad is
a. Wider and longer than the lower
b. Narrower and shorter than the lower
c. Wider and shorter than the mandibular gum pad
d. Narrower and longer than lower

18. When upper and lower gum pads are approximated
a. There is complete over jet all around
b. Contact occurs only at first molar region
c. Space exists between them in anterior region
d. Infantile open bite is normal and helps suckling
e. All of above

19. The spaces between the deciduous teeth are called
a. Normal and physiological spaces or developmental spaces
b. Abnormal spaces
c. Diastema
d. Leeway space

20. The location and relationship of the first permanent molar depends much upon
a. Mesial surface relationship between upper and lower first deciduous molars
b. Distal surface relationship between upper and lower second deciduous molars
c. Both a and b
d. None of the above

21. Leeway space of Nance is the difference between the combined MD width of
a. C, D, E and 3, 4, 5
b. C, D, E and 4, 5, 6
c. A, B, C and 1, 2, 3
d. C, D, E and 5, 6, 7

22. The Leeway space on each side of the maxillary and mandibular arch is
a. 1.8 mm and 3.4 mm
b. 0.9 mm and 1.7 mm
c. 0.5 mm and 0.9 mm
d. 0.2 mm and 0.5 mm

23. When thickness of dentin in primary teeth is compared with that of permanent teeth the dentin in primary teeth is about
a. One-fourth of the thickness of permanent teeth
b. Half of the thickness of the permanent teeth
c. Two-thirds of the thickness of the permanent teeth
d. One-sixth of the thickness of the permanent teeth

24. The pulp horn which is more likely to be exposed during cavity preparation on deciduous molars is
a. Mesiobuccal of first molar
b. Distobuccal of first molar
c. Mesiobuccal of second molar
d. Distobuccal of second molar

25. In general, first deciduous tooth to erupt in oral cavity is
a. Mandibular central incisor
b. Maxillary central incisor
c. Mandibular first molar
d. Maxillary second molar

15-a, 16-a, 17-a, 18-e, 19-a, 20-b, 21-a, 22-b, 23-b, 24-a, 25-a

26. Mixed dentition period in an average child is between
a. 10 years to 15 years of age
b. 6 years to 13 years of age
c. 4 years to 13 years of age
d. 15 years to 17 years of age

27. Generally the sequence of eruption of permanent teeth in maxilla is
a. 1 – 6 – 2 – 3 – 4 – 7 – 5 – 8
b. 6 – 1 – 2 – 4 – 3 – 5 – 7 – 8
c. 6 – 1 – 2 – 3 – 4 – 5 – 7 – 8
d. 1 – 2 – 3 – 4 – 5 – 6 – 7 – 8

28. In deciduous dentition, the tooth which is more wider mesiodistally is
a. Maxillary first molar
b. Mandibular first molar
c. Maxillary second molar
d. Mandibular second molar

29. Generally the sequence of eruption of permanent teeth in lower jaw is
a. 1 – 6 – 2 – 3 – 5 – 4 – 7 – 8
b. 6 – 1 – 2 – 4 – 5 – 3 – 7 – 8
c. 6 – 1 – 2 – 3 – 4 – 5 – 7 – 8
d. 1 – 7 – 6 – 5 – 4 – 3 – 2 – 8

30. The permanent tooth which succeeds the deciduous first molar is
a. First premolar
b. First molar
c. Second premolar
d. Second molar

31. Abscess from a primary tooth can cause dark spot on the underneath permanent developing tooth is called
a. White spot b. Black spot
c. Turner's spot d. None of the above

32. Calcification of the primary teeth begins *in utero*
a. 18–20 weeks
b. 15–18 weeks
c. 13 and 16 weeks
d. 6–10 weeks

33. The general order of eruption of primary dentition is
a. A – B – C – D – E
b. D – A – B – C – E
c. A – B – D – C – E
d. B – A – C – D – E

34. The process of exfoliation of the primary teeth takes place during
a. 5th and 10th year
b. 6th and 14th year
c. 7th and 12th year
d. 8th and 11th year

35. The primary teeth remain in normal alignment and occlusion for
a. 6 years b. 5 years
c. 4 years d. 3 years

36. In primary dentition, the canine which has its mesial cusp slope longer than the distal cusp slope is
a. Primary maxillary canine
b. Primary mandibular canine
c. Both the above
d. None of the above

37. Which of the following is not a succedaneous tooth
a. Permanent first molar
b. Permanent third molar
c. Permanent second molar
d. All of the above

38. Zukerkandl tubercle is present on
a. Deciduous first molar
b. Deciduous second molar
c. Deciduous canine
d. Deciduous incisors

39. The primary molar having a prominent transverse ridge that unites the mesiofacial and mesiolingual cusps is
a. First mandibular molar
b. Second mandibular molar
c. First maxillary molar
d. Second maxillary molar

26-b, 27-b, 28-d, 29-c, 30-a, 31-c, 32-c, 33-c, 34-c, 35-c, 36-a, 37-d, 38-a, 39-a

40. Primary maxillary canine exfoliates at the age of

a. 6–7 years b. 7–8 years
c. 9–10 years d. 10–11 years

41. Resorption of roots of primary molars begins at the age of

a. 5 years b. 4 years
c. 3 years d. 2 years

42. The last succedaneous tooth to erupt in mouth is

a. Maxillary second molar
b. Maxillary first molar
c. Maxillary canine
d. Maxillary first premolar

43. Generally permanent maxillary central incisors has

a. Three mamelons and two developmental lobes
b. Two mamelons and two developmental lobes
c. Three mamelons and four developmental lobes
d. Three mamelons and three developmental lobes

44. An approximation of the curvature of the circles of a 4-inch equilateral triangle was given by

a. Von Spee b. Monson
c. Bolton d. Bonwill

45. Under normal condition the presence of mamelons in a 14-year-old patient is indicative of

a. Malnutrition b. Flurosis
c. Malocclusion d. Malformation

46. A transverse ridge is prominently present on the following primary molar

a. Maxillary first molar
b. Maxillary second molar
c. Mandibular first molar
d. Mandibular second molar

47. Calcification of the roots of primary teeth is normally completed between

a. 1–2 years b. 3–4 years
c. 5–6 years d. 7–8 years

48. The primary molar in which the mesial portion of the occlusal table is separated from the remainder by a transverse ridge is

a. Maxillary first molar
b. Mandibular first molar
c. Mandibular second molar
d. None

49. The dentition of a normally developed 6½-year old child usually consists of

a. 8 primary and 8 permanent teeth
b. 10 primary and 10 permanent teeth
c. 18 primary and 6 permanent teeth
d. 20 primary teeth

50. A one-year old child is expected to have the following maxillary and mandibular teeth

a. Incisors and canines
b. Incisors and first molars
c. Central incisors and canines
d. Mandibular central and lateral incisors

51. The highest and sharpest cusp on the deciduous mandibular first molar

a. Mesiobuccal b. Distobuccal
c. Mesiolingual d. Distolingual

52. The primary teeth that present the most outstanding morphological deviation from permanent teeth are

a. Central incisors
b. Lateral incisors
c. Canines
d. First molars

53. The primary mandibular second molars have

a. 2 cusps b. 3 cusps
c. 4 cusps d. 5 cusps

40-d, 41-b, 42-c, 43-c, 44-d, 45-c, 46-c, 47-b, 48-b, 49-c, 50-b, 51-c, 52-d, 53-d

54. The lingual surface of primary maxillary central incisors closely resembles that of
a. Mandibular lateral incisor
b. Maxillary canine
c. Mandibular lateral incisor
d. Mandibular central incisor

55. Initial calcification of primary teeth occurs before birth in the following
a. Incisors
b. Canines
c. Molars
d. All of the above

56. Hypoplasia of primary teeth limited to incisal or occlusal one-third indicates
a. Flouridated water
b. Tetracycline medication
c. Metabolic disturbance
d. Dentinogenesis imperfecta

57. The deciduous molar which has greatest resemblance to a premolar is
a. Maxillary first molar
b. Maxillary second molar
c. Mandibular first molar
d. Mandibular second molar

58. The developmental space or primate space in mandibular arch is present between
a. Canine and first molar
b. First and second molar
c. Lateral incisor and canine
d. Central and lateral incisor

59. The occlusal outline of the primary mandibular first molar
a. Rhomboidal
b. Trapezoidal
c. Diamond shaped
d. Rectangular

60. Number of grooves present on the occlusal surface of primary mandibular first molar are
a. 4 b. 6
c. 3 d. 8

61. The outline of the labial surface of deciduous maxillary canine
a. Diamond shaped
b. Rhomboidal
c. Angular
d. Both a and c

62. Occlusal outline seen in deciduous maxillary first molar
a. Two-cusp type
b. Three-cusp type
c. Four-cusp type
d. Both b and c

63. The primary mandibular left canine according to universal numbering system is written as
a. R b. M
c. 73 d. 83

64. Cusp of Carebelli is seen in the
a. Deciduous maxillary first molar
b. Deciduous maxillary second molar
c. Permanent maxillary first molar
d. Both b and c

65. The number of teeth in deciduous dentition and permanent dentition are
a. 31 and 20
b. 20 and 32
c. 52 and 20
d. 20 and 52

66. The deciduous teeth are white in colour because
a. Enamel is less mineralized
b. Enamel does not reflect the colour of the underlying dentin
c. Enamel is opaque
d. All of the above

67. The degree of labial bend in the apical third of the roots of the deciduous anterior teeth is
a. 20° b. 12°
c. 10° d. 8°

54-b, 55-d, 56-c, 57-a, 58-a, 59-a, 60-a, 61-d, 62-d, 63-b, 64-d, 65-b, 66-d, 67-c

68. The level of furcation of the roots of the deciduous teeth is

a. 4 mm from cervix
b. 3 mm from cervix
c. Near the cervix
d. Both a and c

69. In deciduous teeth the accessory pulp canals are situated at the

a. Apical region
b. Furcation
c. Middle third
d. All

70. Initial calcification of which of the primary teeth occurs before birth

a. Incisors b. Canines
c. Molars d. All of the above

71. In the sequence of eruption of permanent dentition, the maxillary canine usually follows

a. Maxillary LI
b. Mandibular 1st PM
c. Mandibular 2nd PM
d. Mandibular canine

72. The crown formation of all the permanent teeth except third molars is completed between

a. 2–3 years
b. Birth to 6 years
c. Birth to 8 years
d. Birth to 12 years

73. Root development of permanent dentition except third molar is completed by

a. 12 years
b. 14 years
c. 16 years
d. 18 years

74. The lingual surface of primary maxillary CI closely resembles that of

a. Maxillary lateral incisor
b. Maxillary canines
c. Mandibular LI
d. Mandibular CI

75. The primary second molars have

a. 2 cusps b. 3 cusps
c. 4 cusps d. 5 cusps

68-c, 69-b, 70-d, 71-c, 72-c, 73-c, 74-b, 75-d

Chapter 7

Occlusion

LAQ (10 Marks)

Q 1. Define occlusion. Describe factors governing occlusion. *(Nov. 2004, 2014, June 2016)*
Ans. Occlusion is derived from the Latin word *Occlude* meaning "to close".

Definition

- It is defined as the contact relationship of the teeth in function and parafunction.
- In addition to the contact at an occlusal interface, occlusion is also concerned with other factors associated with the development and stability of the masticatory system and with the use of teeth in oral motor behavior.

Factors influencing occlusion

1. Development of the dentition.
2. Dental arch form.
3. Curvatures of occlusal planes.
4. Inclination and angulation of the roots of the teeth.
5. Functional form of the teeth at incisal and occlusal thirds.
6. Facial and lingual relations of each tooth in one arch to its antagonists in the opposing arch in centric occlusion (overlap of the teeth).
7. Occlusal contacts and intercuspal relations between arches.
8. Occlusal contact relations and intercuspal relations of the teeth.
9. Neurobehavioral aspects of occlusion.

1. DEVELOPMENT OF THE DENTITION

The different periods of dentition are pre-dentition period, deciduous dentition period, mixed dentition period, and permanent dentition.

Pre-dentition Period (Figs 7.1 and 7.2)

- This period is the time from birth to 6 months (till the first deciduous tooth erupts).
- The dental arches during this period are referred to as gum pads. These are pink, firm and covered by a dense layer of fibrous periosteum.

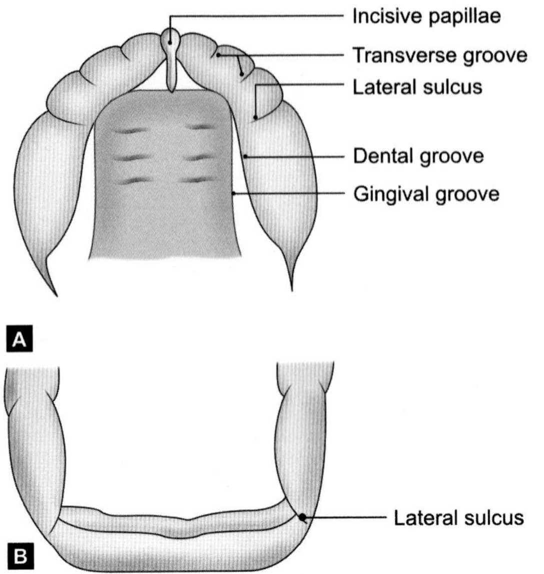

Figs 7.1A and B: (A) Upper gum pad; (B) Lower gum pad

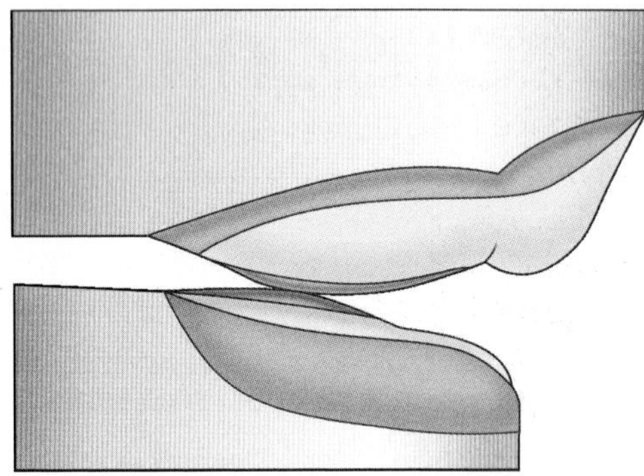

Fig. 7.2: Gum pads in occlusion

- The upper gum pads are wider than the lower gum pads.
- Upper and the lower gum pads are U-shaped.
- The contact between the gum pads occur in the first molar region with absence of contact at the anterior region of the jaws. This spacing is physiologic and aids the infant in suckling.
- This period ends when first deciduous tooth erupts and period of deciduous dentition begins.

Clinical Implications

Natal and neonatal teeth: These refer to the teeth that erupt prematurely before their normal eruption time. Natal teeth are those which erupt before 30 days of birth and neonatal teeth are referred to those teeth that erupt between 30 days to 6 months. The natal and neonatal teeth are usually present in the mandibular region and interfere with suckling and hence have to be managed appropriately.

Deciduous Primary Dentition

- This period extends from 6 months of age when the deciduous mandibular incisors erupt till 6 years of age when permanent first molar erupts.
- The primary teeth are arranged in the form of two arches; maxillary and mandibular and outline is roughly elliptical when following the labial and buccal surface which is wider in the maxillary arch than the mandibular arch.
- Time taken for eruption of deciduous teeth: 6 months to 2 and half-year and root formation is completed by 3 years of age.
- Sequence of eruption: A B D C E.
- ***Interdental spacing***: (Fig. 7.3)
  - After the deciduous teeth are fully formed and occupy their respective position, rapid development of the jaws results in interdental spacing between the teeth. These spaces between the teeth are referred to as **physiological spaces** or **developmental spaces** and

are necessary to accommodate the permanent teeth which have a larger mesiodistal dimension than the primary teeth.

- **Simian space or primate space or anthropoid space:** The physiological spaces occurring mesial to maxillary canine or distal to mandibular canine are referred to as primate spaces.

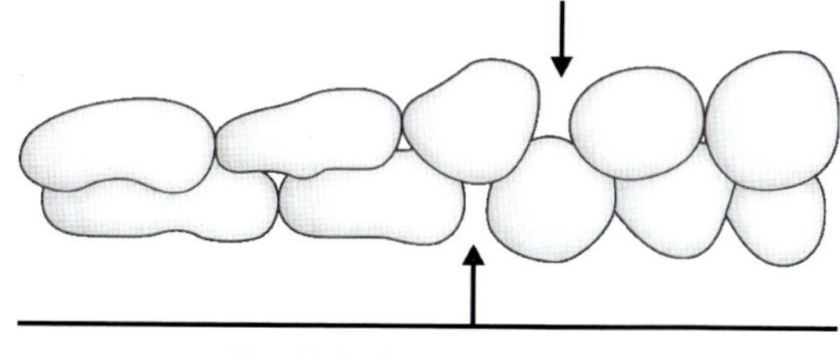

Fig. 7.3: Primate space

- The absence or presence of these spaces serves as an indicator of future sufficiency of space in the dental arches for the permanent teeth.

- ***Primary molar relationships*:** (Fig. 7.4)
  - *Described in three ways*: Flush terminal plane, mesial step and distal step based on the relationship of the distal surface of second primary molar.
  - *Flush terminal plane***:** Distal surface of primary mandibular second molar and maxillary second molar are in the same plane. This is also referred to as end to end molar relationship.
  - *Mesial step*: The distal surface of primary mandibular second molar is mesially located to the distal surface of the primary maxillary second molar.
  - *Distal step*: Distal surface of the primary mandibular second molar is distally located to the distal surface of the primary maxillary second molar.
- ***Effects of terminal plane relationship*:** The effects of these relationships have a bearing on the relationship of permanent molars.
  - It is considered that a flush terminal plane in deciduous dentition may lead to either an end on molar relation, a class I or a class II molar relation in permanent dentition.
  - Distal step in primary dentition may lead to class II permanent molar relation.
  - Mesial step in primary dentition may lead to either a class I relation or class III molar relation.

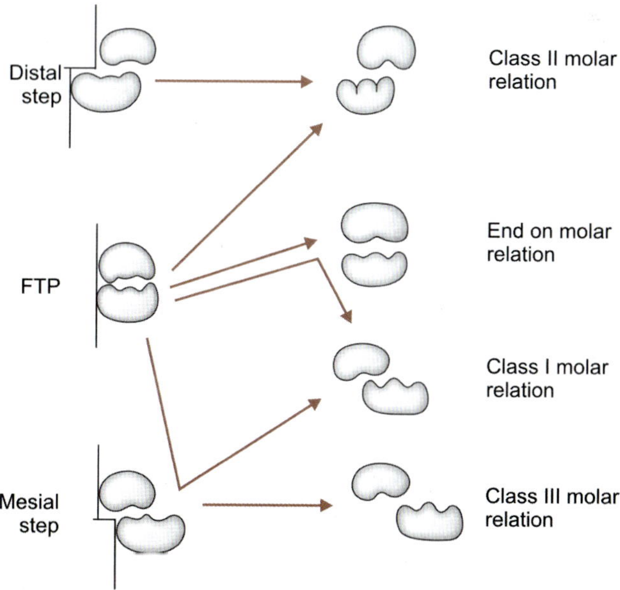

Fig. 7.4: Primary molar relationship

  - Other factors which have an influence on molar relationships include differential growth of the jaws, forward growth of the mandible and sufficient Leeway space to accommodate a mesial drift of the permanent molars.
- The deciduous dentition period ends with the eruption of the permanent first molars and the mixed dentition or transition period starts from then.

Mixed (Transitional) Dentition

- This period which indicates the transition from primary to permanent dentition begins about **6 years of age with the emergence of permanent molars.**
- As the permanent teeth in general have a greater mesiodistal dimension than the primary teeth, they are accommodated by the space provided by the growth of the jaws. In addition, the erupting permanent teeth utilize the physiological spaces available in the deciduous dentition.
- ***Leeway space of Nance*:** (Fig. 7.5)
  - This space is defined as the difference in the combined mesiodistal width of C, D, and E (deciduous canine, first molar, and second molar) and mesiodistal width of 3, 4, and 5 (permanent canine, first premolar, and second premolar).
  - The space is 1.8 mm in maxilla (0.9 mm in each quadrant) and 3.4 mm in mandible (1.7 mm in each quadrant).
  - *Significance:* This space allows the mesial movement of mandibular molar thereby guiding them into proper occlusion.
- Permanent molars are initially in an end-on relationship. Later this is converted into a class I molar relationship by the following factors:
  - Mesial drifting of mandibular molar utilising the physiological space and Leeway space of Nance.
  - Differential forward growth of the mandible.

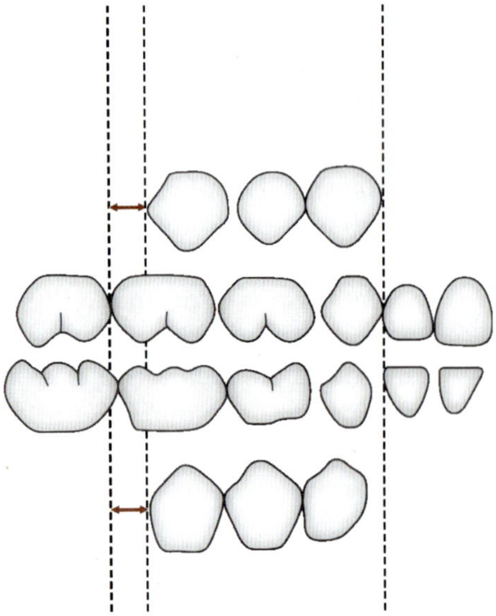

Fig. 7.5: Leeway space of Nance

- ***Incisal liability*:** Because of the discrepancy in mesiodistal crown dimensions between the primary and permanent incisors, some degree of transient crowding may occur at around 8 to 9 years of age until the emergence of canine when the space for the teeth may again be adequate. This is referred to as incisal liability.
- ***Ugly duckling stage*:** Around 8–10 years of age, while the permanent maxillary canines are erupting; they exert pressure on the roots of the maxillary lateral incisors. This causes flaring of the crowns of permanent maxillary central and lateral incisors in distal direction resulting in spacing between the teeth. This is known as ugly duckling stage and disappears as soon as the canines erupt. They do not possess much clinical significance except for the appearance (Fig. 7.6).
- The permanent molar relationship is categorized as follows:
  - *Class I*: When the mesiobuccal cusp of the maxillary first molar aligns with the buccal groove of the mandibular first molar.
  - *Class II*: When the buccal groove of the mandibular first molar is distally positioned when in occlusion with the mesiobuccal cusp of the maxillary molar.

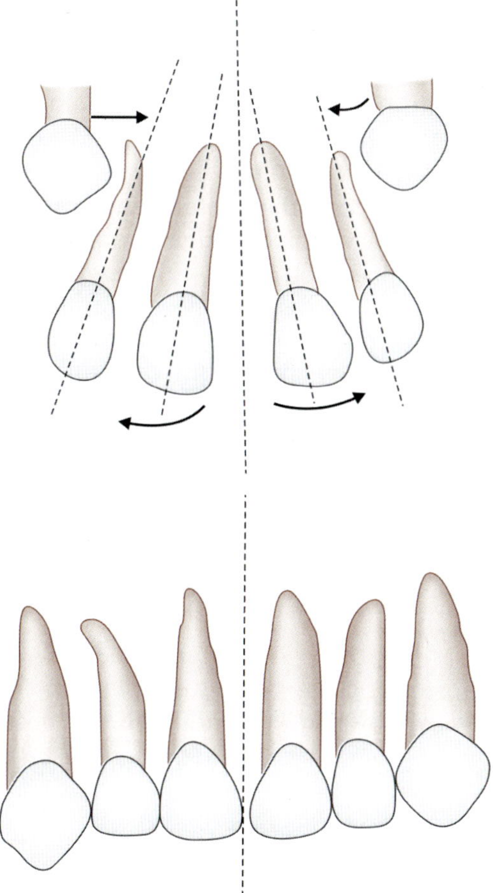

Fig. 7.6: Ugly duckling stage

- *Class III*: When the buccal groove of mandibular first molar is mesially placed in relation to the mesiobuccal cusp of the maxillary first molar when the teeth are in occlusion.

Permanent Dentition

***Sequence of eruption*:**

- Maxilla: 6-1-2-4-3-5-7-8 or 6-1-2-4-5-3-7-8
- Mandible: 6-1-2-3-4-5-7-8

2. DENTAL ARCH FORM

a. The teeth are positioned on the maxilla and mandible in such a way to produce a curved arch when viewed from the occlusal aspect. This arch form is largely determined by the shape of the underlying basal bone.

b. In general, the alignment of the teeth in both the arches follows a parabolic curve. Variations of the arch form are U-shaped (square form), ellipsoid, rotund or tapered. The tapered arch form (V-shaped) generally occurs in the maxillary arch where there is narrowing of the anterior maxilla secondary to thumb sucking habit.

c. The tooth alignment in the arches is divided into three segments—anterior, middle, and posterior. The anterior segment is described by a curved line and includes anterior teeth up to the labial ridge of canine. The middle segment is described by a straight line which includes distal portion of canine, premolars, and mesiobuccal cusp of first molar. The posterior segment is again a straight line from distobuccal cusp of first molar and includes the buccal surface of second and third molar.

d. Under resting conditions, the teeth, and the dental arches are in space referred to as **Neutral space** which is balanced by two set of forces. The lips and cheeks generate muscular forces externally which are balanced by the internal muscular forces arising from the tongue thereby maintaining the dental arches and the teeth in normal alignment. Any imbalance of these forces may result in malocclusion or abnormal alignment of arches. **Examples** of such forces are tongue thrusting which generates greater outward forces from the tongue against the teeth leading to its protrusion. In mouth breathing, pressure of the lips on the teeth is more than the outward pressure of the tongue.

3. CURVATURES OF OCCLUSAL PLANES

a. The occlusal surfaces of the dental arches do not generally conform to a flat plane. The mandibular arch conforms generally to one or more curved planes which appear concave while the curvature at the opposing maxillary arch appears convex.

b. Some of the curves are:
   i. Curve of Spee (anteroposterior curve of occlusal plane).
   ii. Curve of Wilson (side to side curve)
   iii. Curve of Monson

- ***Curve of Spee*:** (Fig. 7.7)
  - This is an anteroposterior curve of the occlusal surfaces and is viewed from buccal surface.
  - The curve of Spee begins at the tip of the lower cuspid and touches the buccal cusp tips of all the mandibular posterior teeth and continues to the anterior border of the ramus. An ideal curve of Spee is aligned so that a continuation of this arc would extend through the condyles. The curvature of this arc would relate, on average, to part of a circle with a 4-inch radius.

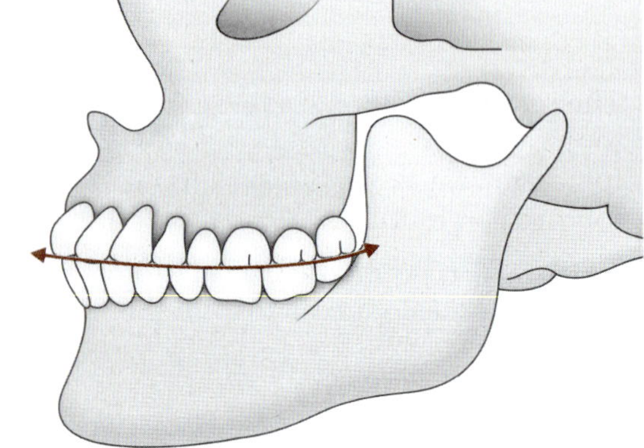

Fig. 7.7: Curve of Spee

  - *Function*: Allows for the normal functional protrusive movements of the mandible.

- ***Curve of Wilson*:** (Fig. 7.8)
  - This is a mediolateral curve and is viewed from the anterior aspect with the mouth slightly open.
  - The curve of Wilson contacts the buccal and lingual cusp tips of each side of the arch. It results from the inward inclination of the lower posterior teeth, making the lingual cusps lower than the buccal cups on the mandibular arch; the buccal cusps are higher than the lingual cusps on the maxillary arch because of the outward inclination of the upper posterior teeth.

- *Functions*: Allows for those requisite movements that are used in chewing functions. The lingual inclination of the lower posterior teeth positions the lingual cusps lower than the buccal cusps. This design permits easy access to the occlusal table. As the tongue lays the food on the occlusal surfaces, it is stopped from going past the chewing position by the taller buccal cusps.

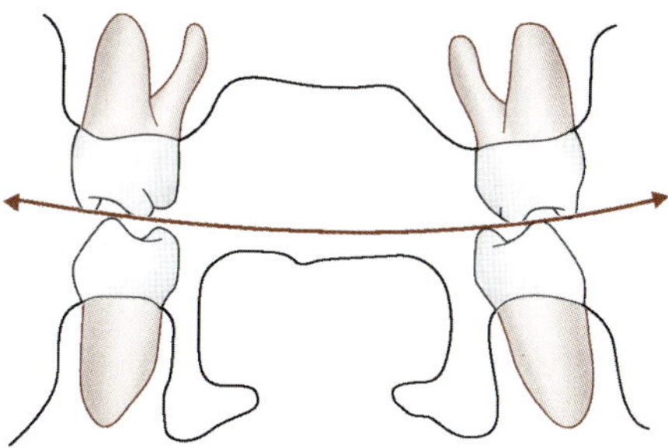

Fig. 7.8: Curve of Wilson

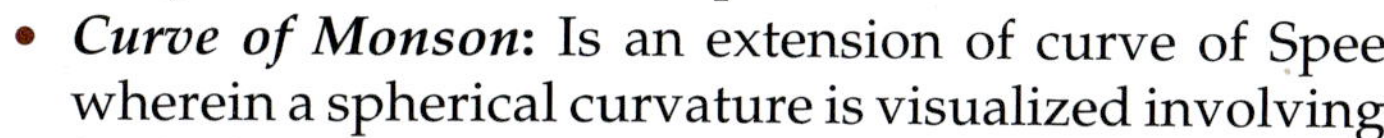

- ***Curve of Monson*:** Is an extension of curve of Spee wherein a spherical curvature is visualized involving both the right and left bicuspid and molar cusps and the right and left condyles. It was supposed that the centre of a sphere with an eight inch diameter was the vector for converging lines of masticatory forces passing through the center of the teeth and that the occlusal surfaces of the molar teeth were congruent with the surface of the sphere of some dimension.
- ***Bennett movement*:** The movement of the mandible to the right or left during mastication is referred to as Bennett movement.

Relationship of teeth:

Centric relation: It is the most posterior position of the mandible relative to the maxilla at a given vertical dimension.

Centric occlusion: Refers to the relationship of the mandible to the maxilla when the teeth are in maximum occlusal contact, irrespective of the position or alignment of the condyle-disk assemblies.

4. INCLINATION AND ANGULATION OF THE ROOTS OF THE TEETH

The inclination of axes of the maxillary and mandibular teeth to each other varies with each tooth group. The importance of the relative root angles helps relate the direction of occlusal forces in restorations along the long axis of teeth, guides the control of orthodontic forces for proper tooth angulation, aids in using templates for implant placement and also in visualization how the X-ray beam must be directed. The angle at which the tooth is placed depends on its function and lines of forces brought about during function. The mesiodistal and faciolingual inclincations are described in terms of angle between the long axis of a tooth and a line drawn perpendicular to a horizontal or median plane. The maximum faciolingual inclination of teeth is seen with maxillary central incisors which has an inclination of 28° while the least is with maxillary premolars at 4–5°. The mesiodistal angulation of the mandibular molars is highest between 10–14° while mandibular lateral incisors do not show any angulation.

5. FUNCTIONAL FORM OF THE TEETH AT INCISAL AND OCCLUSAL THIRDS

The incisal or occlusal thirds of the tooth crowns present convex or concave tooth surface at all contacting tooth areas. When the teeth of one jaw comes in contact with the occlusal surface of the antagonist teeth, these curved surfaces come in contact with each other. The lingual surface of maxillary incisors present some concave surfaces which come in contact with the convex portions present in the incisal ridges of mandibular incisors. In the posterior teeth, the depressions in the depth of sulci and developmental grooves contact with the curved portion of the cusp and marginal ridges.

Escapement Spaces/Spillway Spaces (Fig. 7.9)

Although the teeth in centric occlusion seem to intercuspate closely, escapement spaces have been provided between the teeth which are needed for efficient occlusion during mastication. Escapement space is provided in the teeth by the form of cusp and ridges, the sulci and development grooves and the interdental spaces or embrasures when the teeth come together in occlusion. The escapement spaces are reduced with increase in occlusal contact and vice-versa.

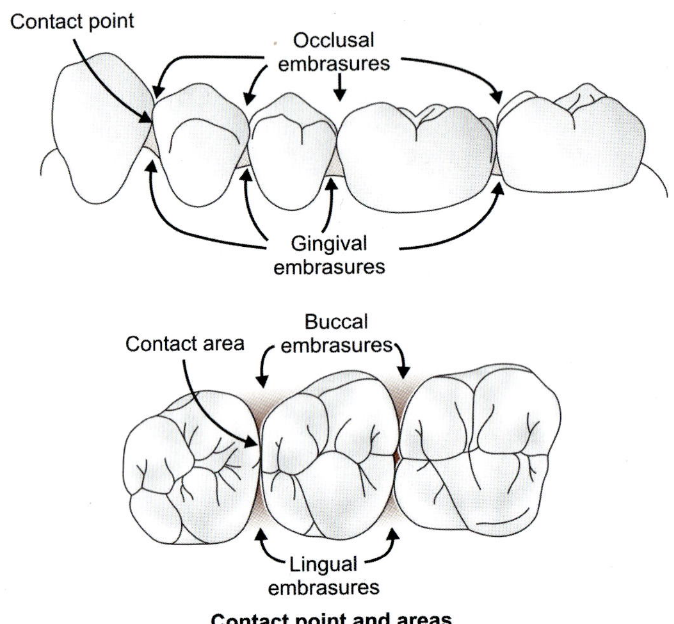

Fig. 7.9: Escapement spaces/spillway spaces

6. FACIAL AND LINGUAL RELATIONS OF EACH TOOTH IN ONE ARCH TO ITS ANTAGONISTS IN THE OPPOSING ARCH IN CENTRIC OCCLUSION (OVERLAP OF THE TEETH)

a. The arch form of the maxilla tends to be larger than that of the mandible. This results in the maxillary teeth overhanging the mandibular teeth when the teeth are in centric occlusion.
b. Under normal circumstances of maximal intercuspation the maxillary anterior teeth overlap the mandibular teeth. The overlap could be horizontal (overjet) or vertical (overbite).
c. **Overbite** (Fig. 7.10): Overbite is defined as the vertical overlap of the maxillary and mandibular anterior teeth, where the maxillary anterior teeth extend below the incisal edges of the mandibular anterior teeth.
d. **Overjet** (Fig. 7.11): Overjet is defined as the horizontal overlap of the maxillary and mandibular anterior teeth, where the maxillary anterior teeth are labial to incisal edges of the mandibular anterior teeth.

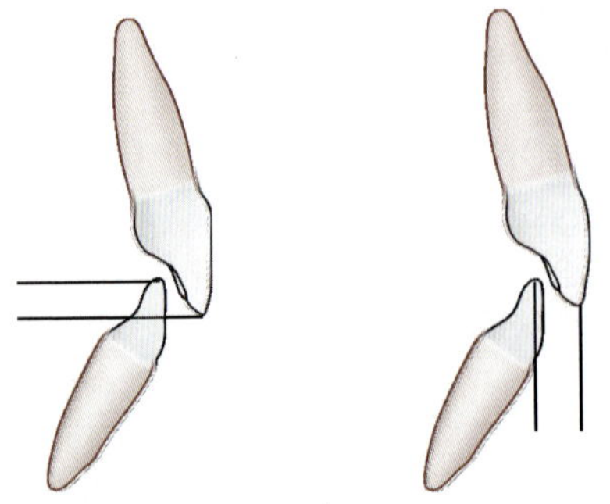

Fig. 7.10: Overbite **Fig. 7.11:** Overjet

e. Ideally overjet and overbite is in the range of 2–4 mm.
f. **Clinical significance:**
   i. Overlapping of the maxillary teeth over the mandibular teeth protects the cheeks, lips and tongue during the opening and closing movements of the jaws. Insufficient horizontal overlap of the molars may result in cheek biting.
   ii. There should be sufficient vertical overlap to enable the disocclusion of the posterior teeth in function.
g. Excessive vertical overlap of the anterior teeth may result in tissue impingement and is referred to as **impinging overbite**.
h. **Incisal guidance:** Is a measure of the amount of movement and angle at which the lower incisors and mandible must move from the overlapping position (centric occlusion) to an edge to edge relationship with maxillary incisor.

7. OCCLUSAL CONTACT RELATIONS AND INTERCUSPAL RELATIONS BETWEEN THE ARCHES

- ***Supporting cusps*:** The lingual cusps of the maxillary posterior teeth and the buccal cusps of the mandibular posterior teeth that make contact with the opposing teeth are referred to as supporting cusps.
- ***Centric stops*:** The areas of occlusal contact that a supporting cusp makes contact with opposing teeth in centric occlusion are centric stops. These contribute to occlusal stability.
- ***Guiding cusps*:** The upper buccal cusps and the lower lingual cusps make contact on their occlusal sides only when the mandible makes gliding movements. Since these cusps provide guidance for the mandibular movement, they are known as guiding cusps.

8. OCCLUSAL CONTACT RELATIONS AND INTERCUSPAL RELATIONS OF THE TEETH

- ***Eccentric movements*:** Occlusal contact relations away from the intercuspal position involve all possible movements of the mandible within the envelope of border movements. These movements are referred to as lateral, protrusive and retrusive movements. Lateral movements may be either to the right or left.
- ***Lateral movements*:** When the mandibular teeth make their initial contact with the maxillary teeth in right or left lateral occlusion, they bear a right or left lateral position to centric occlusion. During the right lateral movement, the mandible is depressed and the dental arches are separated, the jaw moves to the right and brings the teeth together at points right of the intercuspal position in right working position. On the left side, the teeth may or may not make contact. In respect to lateral movements, the side towards which the mandible moves is the working side and the opposite side is the non-working side (known as balancing side in complete dentures).
  - *Working side/working occlusion*: During lateral movements, when the teeth are brought together with the mandible to one side, the condyle of the same side (working side) remains in the posterior position and the condyle of the opposing side (non-working side) have been moved forward in the glenoid fossa. This type of closure is referred to as working position and the sliding action of the mandible from working position back to centric occlusion is working occlusion.
  - *Balancing side/Balanced occlusion*: The opposite side of working side in lateral movements is referred to as non-working side or balancing side. The teeth on this side may or may not make contact. The function of this side during all types of mandibular movement is

to balance the mandible against the maxilla. When all the teeth in both the arches occlude perfectly in all positions and excursions of the mandible, they are said to be in balanced occlusion. Balanced occlusion is seen only in complete dentures and is rarely seen in natural dentition.

- ***Protrusive occlusion*:** When the teeth are closed with the protruded mandible so that both the condyles are equally forward in the glenoid fossa and the incisors are edge to edge, while at the same time the mandibular posterior teeth contact the maxillary posterior teeth, the closure is called protrusive position. As the mandible is retracted from the protrusive position to centric occlusion, the relationship of upper and lower teeth changes in such a manner that the incisal edges of the mandibular anterior teeth slide along the sulci and cross the marginal ridge of the opposing teeth at the same time. This sliding action is called as **protrusive occlusion** and is used mostly in the act of cutting of food when it is too large to be taken wholly into the mouth.
- ***Retrusive movements*:** A retrusive movement normally follows a protrusive movement back to the intercuspal position (centric occlusion). Retrusive movement from centric occlusion to the retruded contact position where the condyles are in the rearmost, uppermost position seems to occur in bruxism but infrequently in mastication and swallowing.

9. NEUROBEHAVIORAL ASPECTS OF OCCLUSION

The neurobehavioral aspect of occlusion relates to the function and parafunction action of stomatognathic system. Functions include a variety of actions such as chewing, sucking, swallowing, speech and respiration while parafunctional habits refer to habits like bruxism. The stability of the occlusion and the maintainance of tooth position are dependent on all the forces that act on the teeth. Occlusal forces, eruptive forces, lip, and cheek pressure, periodontal support and tongue pressure are all involved in maintaining the position of teeth. This requires a very intricate control system involving a number of guiding influences from teeth and their supporting structures along with the involvement of higher centers in the central nervous system.

SAQs (3 Marks)

Q 1. What are curvatures of occlusal planes?

(Dec. 2005, June 2006, May 2007, 2011, Nov. 2010, 2011)

Ans. The occlusal surfaces of the dental arches do not generally conform to a flat plane. The mandibular arch conforms generally to one or more curved planes which appear concave while the curvature of the opposing maxillary arch appears convex.

Some of the curves are:

1 Curve of Spee
2. Curve of Wilson
3. Curve of Monson
4. Bonwill's equilateral triangle.

1. CURVE OF SPEE (May 2011)

- Concept of this curve was introduced by F. Graf Von Spee in 1890.
- This is an anteroposterior curve of the occlusal surface and is viewed from buccal surface.

- This curvature is within sagittal plane only.
- The curve of Spee begins at the tip of the lower cuspid and touches the buccal cusps of all the mandibular teeth and continues to the anterior border of the ramus.
- An ideal curve of Spee is aligned so that a continuation of this arc would extent through the condyles.

  The curvature of this arc would relate, on an average, to part of a circle with 4-inch radius.

Significance

- It has clinical significance in relation to tooth guidance—that is canine and/or incisal guidance as applied in orthodontics and restorative dentistry.
- Curve of Spee allows for the normal functional protrusive movements of the mandible.

2. CURVE OF WILSON

- This is a mediolateral curve viewed from anterior aspect with the mouth slightly open.
- The cusp tips of posterior teeth follow a gradual curve from left side to right side. This is curve of Wilson.
- The curve of maxillary arch is convex and the curve of mandibular arch is concave.
- Thus, the lingual cusps of the posterior teeth are aligned at a lower level than the buccal cusps on both sides and in both the arches.

Significance

It allows for those requisite movements that are used in chewing functions.

3. CURVE OF MONSON

- It is a three-dimensional combination of curves of Spee and Wilson.
- The concept was introduced by G. S. Monson in 1920.
- According to Monson, all cusps and incisal edges in a natural dentition are tangent to a surface of a sphere, approximately 4-inches in radius with center in the area of glabella.

4. BONWILL'S EQUILATERAL TRIANGLE (May 2007) (Fig. 7.12)

Taking the point between two mandibular central incisors and mid-point of condyles, an equilateral triangle is formed with the sides approximately 4-inches in measurement known as **Bonwill's equilateral triangle.**

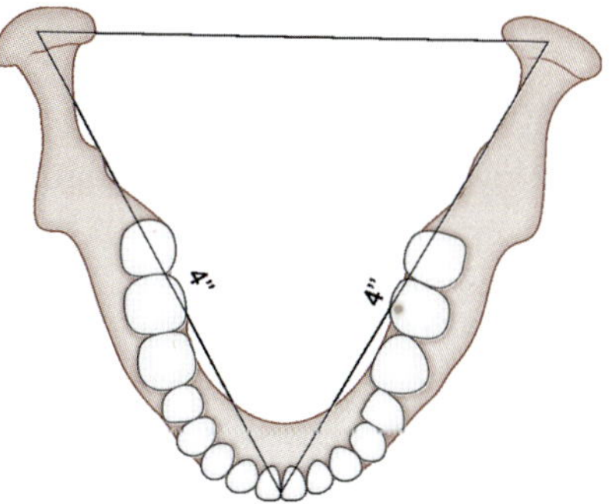

Fig. 7.12: Bonwill's triangle

Q 2. Describe compensating curvatures. (June 2005, Nov. 2015)

Ans. Compensating curvatures

- All surfaces of dental arch conform to the curvatures.
- When viewed from occlusal aspect each dental arch is U-shaped.
- The buccal cusp tips follow a curved line around the outer edge of the dental arch.
- The lingual cusp tips follow a curved line nearly parallel to the buccal cusp tip curved line.
- Between the buccal and lingual cusps is the sulcular groove which runs anteroposteriorly throughout the length of the posterior teeth. The curvature of the mandibular arch is concave and the maxillary arch is convex. As mandibular teeth appear in advance of maxillary teeth, the mandibular teeth are the ones which establish compensating curvatures. The maxillary teeth have to adapt themselves to the mandibular teeth. The curve of one arch is compensated by another arch hence they are called 'compensating curvatures'.

***Importance of compensating curvatures*:** Compensatory curves are developed to compensate for the paths of the condyle as the mandible moves from centric to eccentric position.

Although the maxillary and mandibular curvatures are opposite, they are complimentary and thereby may help achieve occlusal balance during mastication by encouraging simultaneous contact in more than one area of the dental arches.

Q 3. Define overjet. (May 2002, 2012, Nov. 2010)

Overjet and overbite

Ans. Overjet

- The arch form of the maxilla tends to be larger than that of the mandible. As a result the maxillary teeth overhang the mandibular teeth when the teeth are in centric occlusion (the position of maximal intercuspation).
  The lateral or anteroposterior aspect of this overhang is called 'overjet'.
- Overjet is defined as the horizontal overlap of the maxillary and mandibular anterior teeth where the maxillary anterior teeth are labial to incisal edges of the mandibular anterior teeth.
- Ideally overjet is in the range of 2–4 mm.

Significance

- Overjet protects the cheeks, lips and tongue during the opening and closing movements of the jaws.
- Insufficient horizontal overlap of the molars may result in cheek biting.

Overbite

It is defined as the vertical overlap of the maxillary and mandibular anterior teeth, where the maxillary anterior teeth extend below the incisal edges of the mandibular anterior teeth.

Ideally, the overbite is in the range of 2–4 mm.

Significance

- There should be sufficient overlap to enable the disocclusion of the posterior teeth in function.
- Excessive vertical overlap of the anterior teeth may result in tissue impingement and is referred to as "impinging overbite."

Q 4. Define freeway space. (Oct. 2003)

Ans.

- Freeway space is the normal 2–6 mm space between occluding surfaces of the maxillary and mandibular teeth when mandible is in physiologic resting position or
- The amount of separation between the occlusal surfaces of maxillary and mandibular teeth when mandible is in its rest position.
- ***Synonyms***: Interocclusal clearance, interocclusal distance, interocclusal gap interocclusal rest space.

Q 5. Describe Bennett shift (movement). (Oct. 2003)

Ans.

- The movement of the mandible to the right or left during mastication is referred to as 'Bennett movement'. It is the lateral movement of mandible produced when the mandibular condyles slide along mandibular fossae during sideway jaw movement.
- It is the bodily side shift of the mandible toward the side in function and occurs to some extent in most patients during lateral functional movements.
- It may significantly influence the movement of the mandibular cusp tips, thereby determining the proper inclination, direction and contour of the facial and lingual grooves in posterior teeth.

Q 6. What is ugly duckling stage? (July 2005)

Ans.

- The ugly duckling stage was first described by B H Broadbent in 1937.
- It is a mixed dentition stage also called as 'Broadbent phenomenon'.
- It is a transient or self-correcting malocclusion seen in the maxillary incisor region between the age of 8–10 years during the eruption of permanent maxillary canines.
- It is a stage of dental development preceding the eruption of permanent canines which exert pressure on the roots of maxillary lateral incisors causing flaring of crowns of maxillary central and lateral incisors in distal direction resulting in spacing between the teeth.

  It is called ugly duckling stage because dentition in children at this stage looks ugly due to spacing between the teeth. It disappears as soon as canines erupt (around 11–12 years).

Q 7. What is dental arch form? (Nov. 2010)

Ans. Dental Arch Form

- The teeth are positioned on the maxilla and mandible in such a way as to produce a curved arch when viewed from the occlusal aspect. This arch form is largely determined by the shape of the underlying basal bone.
- In general, the alignment of the teeth in both the arches follows a parabolic curve. Variations of the arch form are U-shaped (square form), ellipsoid, round or tapered. The tapered arch form (V-shaped) generally occurs in the maxillary arch where there is narrowing of the anterior maxilla secondary to thumb-sucking habit.
- The tooth alignment in the arches is divided into three segments, anterior, middle, and posterior. The anterior segment is described by a curved line and includes anterior teeth up to the labial ridge of canine. The middle segment is described by a straight line which includes distal portion of canine, premolars and mesiobuccal cusp of first molar. The posterior segment is again a straight line from distobuccal cusp of first molar and includes

the buccal surface of second and third molars. The concept of arch segment allows the arches to overlap slightly so that canines and first molars are cooperating in more than one segment indicating that canines and molars function as anchor supports for both arches.

- Under resting conditions, the teeth and the dental arches are in space referred to as **Neutral space** which is balanced by two set of forces. The lips and cheeks generate muscular forces externally which are balanced by the internal muscular forces arising from the tongue thereby maintaining the dental arches and the teeth in normal alignment. Any imbalance of these forces may result in malocclusion or abnormal alignment of arches. Examples of such forces are tongue thrusting which generates greater outward forces from the tongue against the teeth leading to its protrusion.
- In mouth breathing, pressure of the lips on the teeth is more than the outward pressure of the tongue.

Overlap of the Teeth

- The maxillary arch form of the maxilla tends to be larger than that of the mandible. This results in the maxillary teeth overhanging the mandibular teeth when the teeth are in centric occlusion.
- The mandibular arch is narrower in width than the maxillary arch. This relation is caused by the difference in MD width between mandibular and maxillary anterior teeth and by the lingual projection of the crowns of the mandibular posterior teeth. This relationship is reflected by the overjet and overbite characteristics of teeth.
- Mandibular arch is smaller compared to maxillary arch hence all the teeth of this arch are forwarded to midline.
- Under normal circumstances of maximal intercuspation the maxillary anterior teeth overlaps the mandibular teeth. The overlap could be horizontal (overjet) or vertical (overbite).
- ***Overbite*:** It is defined as the vertical overlap of the maxillary and mandibular anterior teeth where the maxillary anterior teeth extend below the incisal edges of the mandibular anterior teeth.
- ***Overjet*:** It is defined as the horizontal overlap of the maxillary and mandibular anterior teeth where the maxillary anterior teeth are labial to incisal edges of the mandibular anterior teeth.
- Ideally overjet and overbite is in the range of 2–4 mm.

Clinical Significance

- Overlapping of the maxillary teeth over the mandibular teeth protects the cheeks, lips, and tongue during the opening and closing movements of the jaws. Insufficient horizontal overlap of the molars may result in cheek biting.
- There should be sufficient vertical overlap enable the disocclusion of the posterior teeth in function.
- Excessive vertical overlap of the anterior teeth may result in tissue impingement and is referred to as **impinging overbite.**

Q 8. What is Leeway space of Nance?

Ans. Leeway Space of Nance

- Leeway Space of Nance is defined as the difference between combined mesiodistal width of primary canine and molars, i.e. deciduous canine, first molar, second molar, and mesiodistal width of permanent canine and both premolars.

- Usually, the sum of mesiodistal width of C, D, E, is larger than the sum of mesiodistal width of 3, 4, 5.
  This difference, i.e. the Leeway Space in maxilla is 1.8 mm (0.9 mm in each quadrant) and in mandible it is 3.4 mm (1.7 mm in each quadrant).

Significance

It is partly used for alignment of permanent incisors and partly for normal permanent molar relationship.

Q 9. Define occlusion in deciduous dentition. *(May 2013)*

Ans.

- Deciduous dentition stage starts with eruption of mandibular central incisors at around 6 months of age and ends with the eruption of first permanent molar at around 6 years of age.
- The eruption of all primary teeth is completed by the age of 2½–3 years of age. With the eruption of second primary molar.
- Each tooth in the arch occludes with two teeth in the opposing jaw except for mandibular central incisor and the maxillary second molar.
- ***Features of normal primary dentition*:**
  1. Spaced anteriors
  2. Primate spaces
  3. Deep overbite and increased overjet
  4. Straight terminal plane
  5. Sallow cuspal interdigitation
  6. Almost vertical inclination of anterior teeth
  7. Ovoid arch form
  8. Flat occlusal plane or almost no curve of Spee.
- ***Sequence of eruption*:**

$$\frac{\text{AB} \qquad \text{D} \qquad \text{C} \qquad \text{E}}{\text{A} \qquad \text{B} \qquad \text{D} \qquad \text{C} \qquad \text{E}}$$

- ***Characteristics of occlusion in deciduous dentition*:**
  1. Interdental spacing
  2. Incisor relationship
  3. Molar relationship
  1. **Interdental spacing:** Generalized spacing is very common in deciduous dentition. These spaces are called **physiological or developmental spaces.**
     These spaces are necessary to accommodate the permanent teeth which have a larger mesiodistal dimension than the primary teeth.
     This space is about 4 mm in the maxillary arch and 3 mm in mandibular arch.
     Primate/Simian/Anthropoid/Baume space.
     The physiological space seen mesial to maxillary canine and distal to mandibular canine is called 'primate space'. These spaces are similar to the dentition of the primates.
     These spaces are utilized during early mesial shift of molars from end-on to Class I relation.

2. **Incisor relationship:** There is increased overbite and overjet in the initial phase of deciduous dentition.
   Gradually, it gets corrected due to attrition of anteriors, eruption of posterior teeth and due to growth of mandible.
3. **Primary molar relationship:** In deciduous dentition the mesiodistal relation between the upper and lower second molar is called 'terminal plane'.
   - In flush terminal plane distal surface of deciduous lower second molar and upper second molar are in the same vertical plane. It is also referred to as end-on molar relationship 37%.
   - In mesial step, the distal surface of deciduous lower second molar is mesial to the distal surface of deciduous upper second molar 49%.
   - In distal step, the distal surface of deciduous lower second molar is distal to the distal surface of upper second molar.

Q 10. What are escapement spaces/spillway spaces?

Ans.

- Although the teeth in centric occlusion seem to intercuspate closely, escapement spaces have been provided between the teeth which are needed for efficient occlusion during mastication.
- Escapement space is provided in the teeth by the form of cusp and ridges, the sulci and developmental groove and the interdental spaces or embrasures. When the teeth come together in occlusion.
- The escapement spaces are reduced with increased in occlusal contact or vice-versa.
- When two adjacent teeth in the same arch are in contact with each other there are four triangular continuous spaces adjacent to the contact areas. These are embrasures.
- They are named according to their location which depends on the aspect from which the teeth are viewed.
- From facial and lingual aspect—incisal and cervical embrasures are seen.
- From occlusal aspect—facial and lingual embrasures are seen.
- It is significance that it provides a Spillway for food during mastication and makes teeth self-cleansing, prevents food from impinging on gingiva.

Q 11. Explain theories of occlusion. *(Oct. 2002)*

Ans.

1. ***Theory of equilateral triangle*:** This theory was proposed by Bonwill which states that an equilateral triangle is formed with the three corners of the triangle being right condyle, left condyle, and a point between the two mandibular central incisors. The distance between the two points (or one side of he triangle) is 4 inches or 10 cm. The theory postulates that the teeth move in relation to each other as guided by the condyle control and the incisal point.
2. **Conical theory of occlusion:** This theory postullates that lower teeth move over the surface of the upper teeth as over the surface of a cone with a generating angle of 45°. The central axis of the cone is tipped at an angle of 45° to the occlusal plane. In case of posterior teeth, the cusps of teeth have 45° and each cusp behaves like a separate cone. The cusps of the lower posterior teeth incline over the cusps of the maxillary teeth similar to that of the anterior teeth.

3. ***Spherical theory of occlusion*:** This theory was proposed by G.S. Monson in 1918. According to the theory, the lower teeth move over the surface of the upper teeth as over the surface of a sphere. This sphere has a diameter of 8 inches or 20 cm with its center near the glabella. The surface of the sphere passes through the glemoid fossa along the articular eminence. This theory postulated that teeth are positioned in such a way that the anteroposterior and mesiodistal inclinations of the teeth are in harmony with the spherical surface.
4. ***Theory of organic occlusion*:** The theory was proposed by Stuart and Stallard in 1947. They proposed that teeth are in harmony with muscles and joints in function; the latter determining the mandibular position of occlusion throughout tooth guidance. Organic occlusion has the following features teeth are passive to the paths of mandibular movements, cusp fossa contact relationship are developed when jaws are in centric relation, posterior teeth protect anteriors during centric occlusion, separation of posterior teeth on both sides of the arch when jaw moves away from the centric occlusion, vertical overlap of maxillary central incisors is sufficient to provide separation of posterior teeth when the incisor are at an end to end relation and during lateral movement of the mandible, the canines cause disclusion of all the other teeth.

MULTIPLE CHOICE QUESTIONS (MCQs)

1. All teeth have two antagonists in the opposing jaw *except*
   a. Mandibular central incisor
   b. Maxillary third molar
   c. Both a and b
   d. Mandibular third molar

2. In centric occlusion, the massive and pointed mesiolingual cusp portion of maxillary first molar fits into
   a. Distal fossa of lower first molars
   b. Mesial fossa of lower first molars
   c. Major/central fossa of lower first molars
   d. Mesial fossa of upper first molar

3. The distolingual cusp of maxillary first molars are in apposition
   a. To the distal triangular fossa and marginal ridge of mandibular first molars
   b. To the mesial marginal ridge of the molar distal to the mandibular first molar
   c. Both a and b
   d. None of the above

4. In centric occlusion, lingual cusp of mandibular first premolar
   a. Contacts with distal marginal ridge of maxillary canine
   b. Contacts with cingulum of maxillary canine
   c. Does not contact with any teeth
   d. Contacts with mesial marginal ridge of maxillary canine

5. In physiologic rest position of mandible
   a. There is slight contact
   b. There is maximum contact
   c. There is no contact
   d. The contact depends on the size of the cusp

6. Usually the canine erupts before premolar in
   a. Maxillary arch
   b. Mandibular arch
   c. Both a and b
   d. None of the above

7. Dentition in girls erupts earlier than in boys by about
   a. 5 months
   b. 3 months
   c. 2 months
   d. 1 months

8. In Angle's class I molar relationship mesiolingual cusp of maxillary first molar occludes into the
   a. Mesial triangular fossa
   b. Distal triangular fossa
   c. Central fossa
   d. None of the above

9. In normal occlusion, the buccal cusps of maxillary teeth occlude
   a. With the lingual surface of mandibular teeth
   b. With the buccal surface of mandibular teeth
   c. In the central sulci of mandibular teeth
   d. Distal surface of permanent mandibular first molar

10. In normal occlusion mesiobuccal cusp of permanent maxillary first molar occludes with
   a. Mesiobuccal groove of permanent mandibular first molar
   b. Distobuccal groove of permanent mandibular first molar
   c. Mesial surface of permanent mandibular first molar
   d. Distal surface of permanent mandibular first molar.

1-c, 2-c, 3-c, 4-c, 5-c, 6-b, 7-a, 8-c, 9-b, 10-a

11. If a permanent first molar is lost, the permanent second molar drifts to the

a. Distal side
b. Mesial side
c. Buccal side
d. Lingual side

12. 'Leeway space' is

a. Physiologic spacing between deciduous teeth
b. The difference in labiolingual width between deciduous molars and premolars
c. The difference in mesiodistal width of deciduous molars and permanent molars
d. The difference in combined mesiodistal width of deciduous canine and molars and of permanent canines and premolars

13. The interocclusal freeway space in normal circumstances should be

a. 0–1 mm b. 1–2 mm
c. 2–4 mm d. 3–5 mm

14. In Primary dentition the physiologic space mesial to maxillary canine and distal to mandibular canine is called

a. Primate/Simian space
b. Leeway space
c. Freeway space
d. Diastema

15. Curve which runs in anteroposterior direction is

a. Curve of Spee
b. Curve of Wilson
c. Monson's curve
d. None of the above

16. Freeway space is maximum at

a. Incisor region
b. Canine region
c. Premolar region
d. Molar region

17. In the unworn dental arch all the following occlusal contacts are there *except*

a. Point to point b. Point to area
c. Edge to edge d. Edge to area
e. Area to area

18. The cusp of the maxillary molar that serves as a reference point in identifying Angleís Class I, Class II, Class III occlusion is

a. Distobuccal cusp
b. Mesiobuccal
c. Mesiolingual
d. Distolingual

19. When the mandible is in its physiologic rest or postural position, contact of teeth is

a. Maximum b. Premature
c. Slight d. Not present

20. When posterior teeth are in normal ideal relationship, the following cusps are considered supporting cusps

a. Maxillary lingual
b. Maxillary facial
c. Mandibular lingual
d. Mandibular facial
e. Both a and d

21. The following cusps are referred to as 'stamp cusps'

a. Maxillary lingual cusps
b. Maxillary buccal
c. Mandibular buccal
d. Mandibular lingual
e. Both a and c

22. In the intercuspal position distobuccal cusp of permanent mandibular first molar occludes into

a. The interproximal marginal ridge area between maxillary second premolar and first molar
b. Central fossa of maxillary first molar
c. Central fossa of maxillary second molar
d. Interproximal marginal ridge area between maxillary first molar and second molar

11-b, 12-d, 13-c, 14-a, 15-a, 16-a, 17-e, 18-b, 19-d, 20-e, 21-e, 22-b

23. Cusptip articulating with a marginal ridge area is called as
   a. Normal cusp
   b. Plunger cusp
   c. Non-working cusp
   d. Deflected cusps

24. Forces of occlusion are mainly sustained by
   a. Tough enamel
   b. Resilience of dentin
   c. Supporting cancellous bone
   d. PDL

25. Maximum mesiodistal inclination with respect to mid-sagittal plane is found in
   a. Maxillary canine
   b. Mandibular lateral incisor
   c. Mandibular canines
   d. Maxillary molar

26. From proximal view, the tooth which has least labiolingual inclination is
   a. Maxillary canine
   b. Maxillary central incisor
   c. Maxillary lateral incisor
   d. Mandibular central incisor

27. The teeth which have only one antagonist in the opposite arch are
   a. Mandibular third molar and maxillary lateral incisor
   b. Mandibular central incisors and maxillary third molars
   c. Maxillary and mandibular third molars
   d. Maxillary and mandibular central incisor

28. Opening of mandible is initiated by
   a. Cortical center
   b. Bulbay center
   c. Pre-central gyrus
   d. Post-central gyrus

29. The position of the jaw that is exclusively determined by the behavior of the mandibular musculature is
   a. Postural b. Terminal
   c. Intercuspal d. None of the above

30. During nonmasticatory swallowing teeth are usually
   a. Protruded
   b. In a working arrangement
   c. In contact in intercuspal position
   d. None of the above

31. Spacing between anterior teeth in the primary dentition is most frequently caused by
   a. Thumb sucking
   b. Tongue thrusting
   c. The growth of the dental arches
   d. The pressure from the succedaneous teeth

32. The lingual cusps of the mandibular first molar must be restored to accomodate
   a. Centric relation
   b. Working movement
   c. Non-working movement
   d. Maximum intercuspation

33. The smallest vertical dimenson measurement will be present in one of the following position
   a. Edge-to-edge
   b. Retruded contact
   c. Maximum intercuspation
   d. Retruded contact

34. When the mandible slides in a protrusive contacting movement, the mandibular teeth that make contact with maxillary lateral incisors are
   a. Central and lateral incisors
   b. Central incisors and canines
   c. Lateral incisors and canines
   d. All of the above

23-b, 24-d, 25-a, 26-a, 27-b, 28-c, 29-a, 30-c, 31-c, 32-b, 33-c, 34-c

35. Moving the mandible from a maximum intercuspal position to a retruded contact position usually results in

a. Increased occlusal vertical dimension
b. Decreased vertical overlap
c. Increased horizontal overlap
d. All of the above

36. In an ideal permanent tooth relationship, the tip of a mandibular canine in lateral excursion passes

a. Distal to the tip of maxillary canine cusp
b. Mesial to the tip of maxillary canine cusp
c. Directly in line with the maxillary canine cusp tip
d. Through the embrasure between the maxillary canine and first premolar

37. The wear facets on the incisal edges of the mandibular lateral incisors are caused by occlusion with the

a. Maxillary central incisors only
b. Maxillary central and lateral incisors
c. Maxillary lateral incisors and canines
d. None of the above

38. The non-working pathway of the maxillary cusps on the mandibular posterior teeth is towards the

a. Distobuccal
b. Mesiobuccal
c. Distolingual
d. Mesiolingual

39. The Bennett movement is best described as the

a. Medial shift of the working condyle
b. Lateral movement of the non-working condyle
c. Bodily shift of the mandible in the direction of the working condyle
d. Bodily shift of the mandible in the direction of the non-working condyle

40. In canine guided occlusion contact between posterior teeth occurs in

a. Centric occlusion only
b. Eccentric movement only
c. Protrusive movement only
d. Retrusive movement only

41. In protrusion mandibular right central incisor occludes with maxillary

a. Right lateral incisor only
b. Right central incisor only
c. Right and left central incisors only
d. Right central and lateral incisor

42. In protrusion maxillary right central incisor contacts with mandibular

a. Right and left mandibular central incisors
b. Right central and lateral incisors
c. Right central incisors only
d. Left central incisor only

43. In centric occlusion the cusp tip of maxillary canine opposes

a. Distal marginal ridge of mandibular canine
b. Facial embrasure between lower canine and premolar
c. Mesial marginal ridge of lower lateral incisors
d. Interproximal space between lower lateral and canine

44. The teeth in occlusion have

a. Surface contact
b. Cusp to cusp contact
c. Cusp to fossa contact
d. Marginal contact

45. Wilson curve in mandibular arch is

a. Concave
b. Convex
c. Concavoconvex
d. Convexoconcave

35-d, 36-b, 37-b, 38-a, 39-c, 40-a, 41-b, 42-b, 43-a, 44-d, 45-a

46. In ideal occlusion with class I molar and canine relationship, mesial cusp ridge of mandibular canine opposes maxillary
   a. Lateral incisor on distal side
   b. Canine on mesial side
   c. Lateral incisor on mesial slide
   d. Canine on distal side

47. In an ideal occlusion mesial marginal ridge of maxillary canine
   a. Opposes mesiobuccal cuspal ridge of mandibular first premolar
   b. Opposes distal marginal ridge of mandibular canine
   c. Is in line with mesial marginal ridge of mandibular canine
   d. Opposes mandibular lateral incisor

48. In centric occlusion, cusp of mandibular canine will oppose
   a. Marginal ridge of upper canine and first premolar
   b. Marginal ridge of upper canine and lateral incisors
   c. Cingulum of maxillary canine
   d. Distal ridge of maxillary first premolar

49. In physiologic rest position of mandible there is
   a. Slight contact
   b. No contacts
   c. Maximum contacts
   d. None of the above

50. The movements of mandible during chewing can be described as
   a. Being vertical and tear-drop in shape
   b. Being horizontal and rhomboidal in shape
   c. Occurring only on working side
   d. Occurring only on non-working side

51. Direct lateral shift of condyle occurs
   a. On working side
   b. On balancing side
   c. Both on working side and non-working side
   d. Laterla shift never occurs

52. During lateral movements the balancing side of condyle moves
   a. Forward, downwards, mesially
   b. Forward, downwards, laterally
   c. Forward, upwards, mesially
   d. Backwards, downwards and mesially

53. The effect of benett shift will be on mesio-distal positioning of
   a. Lingual cusps of all teeth
   b. Buccal cusps of all teeth
   c. Both buccal and lingual cusps
   d. No effect on cusps

54. Which is the active component in masticatory apparatus
   a. TMJ
   b. Muscles of mastication
   c. Molar teeth
   d. All of the above

55. Free way space is maximum at
   a. Incisor region
   b. Canine region
   c. Premolar region
   d. Molar region

56. Longest stage of deglutition is
   a. Stage I   b. Stage II
   c. Stage III   d. All stages are equal

57. The smallest permanent tooth in the mouth is
   a. Maxillary central incisor
   b. Mandibular canine
   c. Mandibular central incisor
   d. Maxillary lateral incisor

46-a, 47-b, 48-b, 49-b, 50-a, 51-b, 52-a, 53-b, 54-a, 55-d, 56-c, 57-c

Chapter 8

Blood and Nerve Supply to Teeth and Tongue

SAQs (3 Marks)

Q 1. Describe blood and nerve supply to tongue. *(May 2007)*

Ans. Blood and Nerve Supply to Tongue

- The tongue and floor of the mouth are supplied by lingual artery.
- The lingual artery is a branch of external carotid artery.
- Its dorsal lingual branch supplies the base of the tongue.
- The deep lingual branch supplies the body and apex of the tongue.
- One of its terminal branches communicates with the deep lingual artery of the opposite side and is called the 'arcus raninus'.
- Venous drainage of tongue is quite peculiar and is from two different routes for two different parts of tongue. The dorsal surface and side of the tongue drains into lingual vein, ventral surface drains into deep lingual veins.
- Venous blood from lingual vein drains into facial vein and later into internal jugular veins.

Nerve Supply

- The tongue is developed from the contribution of different arches which is reflected in the nerve supply.
- Mucous membrane of anterior two-thirds of the tongue is supplied by mandibular branch of trigeminal nerve.
- Posterior one-third of the tongue is supplied by glossopharyngeal nerve, the ninth cranial nerve which carries the taste sensation from the posterior part.
- The hypoglossal nerve, the 12th cranial nerve supplies the voluntary muscles.
- Lingual branch of the mandibular branch of trigeminal nerve supplies the anterior two-thirds of the tongue for general sensation of pain, temperature, touch, etc.
- Chorda tympanic branch of the 7th cranial nerve supplies the anterior two-thirds for special sensation of taste.
- Posterior one-third is supplied by 9th cranial nerve, the glossopharyngeal nerve.

Q 2. Write about blood and nerve supply to teeth.

Ans. Blood Supply

- Mandibular teeth and supporting structures are supplied by inferior alveolar artery which is a branch of maxillary artery.
- Interior alveolar artery passes through the mandibular foramen to enter into the mandibular canal and terminate as mental and incisive arteries.
- Maxillary teeth receive arterial supply from two different sources: Posterior superior alveolar artery supplies the molars and premolars while anterior superior alveolar artery supplies the anterior teeth.
- The veins drain into either facial vein or pterygoid plexus of veins.
- The lymph vessels from teeth run directly into the submandibular nodes on the same side. Lymph from lower incisors may drain into submental nodes. Sometimes molars may drain directly into jugulodigastric gray of nodes.

Nerve Supply

The pulp and periodontal membrane have the same nerve supply which is different from that of the overlying gingiva.

- Mandibular incisors are innervated by incisive nerve premolar and molars are innervated by inferior alveolar nerve.
- Maxillary anterior teeth are innervated by anterior superior alveolar nerve.
  Premolars and mesiobuccal root of first molar are innervated by middle superior alveolar nerve. Molars are innervated by posterior superior alveolar nerve.

MULTIPLE CHOICE QUESTIONS (MCQs)

1. The mental foramen on each side lies near the apex of the

a. Mandibular canine
b. Mandibular first premolar
c. Mandibular second premolar
d. In between mandibular first and second premolar

2. The mental foramen in most humans is located superior to the inferior border of the mandible at a distance of

a. 10–12 mm b. 8–10 mm
c. 13–15 mm d. 6–8 mm

3. The single, bilaterally symmetrical, movable, bone of the skull is

a. Maxilla b. Temporal
c. Mandible d. Occipital

4. The carotid artery that supplies the mouth

a. External carotid
b. Internal carotid
c. Both a and b
d. Middle carotid

5. The blood supply to maxillary and mandibular teeth is by

a. Mandibular part of maxillary artery
b. Anterior tympanic
c. Middle meningeal
d. Laryngeal

6. The inferior alveolar artery supplies

a. Maxillary molars
b. Mandibular molars and premolars
c. Both a and b
d. Maxillary central incisor

7. The symphyseal cartilage ossifies

a. Before birth
b. At birth
c. One year after birth
d. At 21 years of age

8. Lymph from mandibular posterior teeth is drained into

a. Submental lymph nodes
b. Submandibular lymph nodes
c. Submental and submandibular lymph nodes
d. Cervical lymph nodes

9. Branches of maxillary artery that supply the temporomandibular Joint are

a. Anterior tympanic
b. Masseteric
c. Middle meningeal
d. All the above

10. The facial nerve is

a. Sensory nerve
b. Motor nerve
c. Mixed nerve
d. None of the above

11. Mandibular torus is found on the

a. Labial side of the mandible
b. Lingual side of the mandible
c. Angle of the mandible
d. Lower border of the mandible.

12. Mandible is a following type of bone

a. Intracartilagenous
b. Intracartilagenous and intramembranous
c. Intramembranous
d. None of the above

13. The sections of the teeth clearly seen on standard radiographs are

a. The labial and buccal longitudinal sections
b. The mesial and distal aspect of longitudinal sections
c. Both
d. None of the above

1-c, 2-c, 3-c, 4-a, 5-a, 6-b, 7-c, 8-b, 9-d, 10-c, 11-b, 12-b, 13-a

14. The lingual plate is paper thin over the lingual alveolus of the
a. Maxillary first molar
b. Maxillary premolar
c. Maxillary second and third molars
d. Mandibular molars

15. Mandibular anterior teeth have sensory nerve supply from
a. Superior alveolar nerve
b. Inferior alveolar nerve
c. Lingual nerve
d. Buccal nerve

16. Lower lip gets sensory nerve supply from
a. Buccal branch of facial nerve
b. Mandibular branch of facial nerve
c. Buccal branch of mandibular nerve
d. Mental nerve

17. Buccinator muscle receives its motor nerve supply from
a. Zygomatic branch of facial nerve
b. Buccal branch of trigeminal nerve
c. Buccal branch of facial nerve
d. Mandibular branch of facial nerve.

18. Hypoglossal nerve is motor nerve for all the muscles of tongue *except*
a. Superior longitudinal muscle
b. Inferior longitudinal muscle
c. Genioglossus
d. Palatoglossus

19. The line of posterior alveoli of mandibular teeth are inclined
a. Labially
b. Lingually
c. Not inclined, are straight
d. Mesially

20. The mandibular anterior teeth have alveoli tipped
a. Labially
b. Lingually
c. Not tipped
d. Mesially

21. The bone buccal to last two molars in mandible is
a. Very heavy and thick
b. Very thin
c. Moderately thick
d. Moderately thin

22. Mandible is formed by
a. Endochondral ossification method only
b. Intramembranous ossification
c. Both endochondral and intramembranous ossification
d. None of the above

23. The sutural junction where frontal and parietal bones unite is termed
a. Nasion
b. Bregma
c. Lamboid
d. Frontion

24. Lingula is the projection of bone on the following part of the mandible
a. Medial aspect of vertical ramus of mandible
b. Inner aspect of mandible at midline
c. Outer aspect of mandible near mental foramen
d. None of the above

25. Genial tubercles are the tiny projections of the bone present in
a. Inner aspect of mandible near mylohyoid ridge
b. External surface of mandible near symphysis menti
c. Inner aspect of mandible at midline
d. The lingula

26. Lingual foramen is present on
a. Inner aspect of vertical ramus
b. Outer aspect of mandible near premolar region
c. Inner aspect of mandible near midline
d. The symphysis menti

27. Lymph drainage from all the following structures go to submandibular lymph nodes, *except*
a. Mandibular teeth
b. Occipital part
c. Tongue
d. Maxillary teeth

14-a, 15-b, 16-d, 17-c, 18-d, 19-b, 20-a, 21-a, 22-c, 23-b, 24-a, 25-c, 26-c, 27-b

Chapter 9

Muscles of Mastication

SAQs (3 Marks)

Q 1. Enumerate and describe muscles of mastication. (*Oct. 2002, 2003, June 2005, 2006*)

Ans. Muscles of Mastication

- The masticatory muscles surrounding the joint are group of muscles that contract and relax in harmony so that the jaws function properly.
- There are four pairs of muscles of mastication, masseter, temporalis, medial pterygoid, and lateral pterygoid.

Masseter

- It is the principal and strongest muscle of mastication, which stems from the temporal bone and extends down the outside of the mandible to its lower angle. It consists of two overlapping heads:
- ***Origin:*** Zygomatic arch.
- ***Insertion:*** Lateral surface of ramus, angle and border of mandible.
- ***Nerve supply:*** Masseter nerve.
- ***Function:*** To close the jaw and apply power in crushing food.

Temporalis Muscle

- It is a fan-shaped muscle and the largest masticatory muscle that fills the temporal fossa.
- ***Origin:*** Temporal fossa and the overlying temporal fascia.
- ***Insertion:*** Coronoid process of mandible, anterior border of ramus and temporal crest of mandible via one common tendon.
- ***Nerve supply:*** Temporal branch of mandibular nerve.
- ***Function:*** Its anterior fibers help in elevation of mandible. Its posterior fibers help in retracting the protruded mandible.

Medial Pterygoid Muscle

- It runs parallel to the masseter muscle but on the inside of the jaw.
- ***Origin:*** From the medial surface of the lateral pterygoid plate.
- ***Insertion:*** On the medial surface of mandible in the triangular region just above the angle.

- ***Nerve supply:*** The nerve to the medial pterygoid, a branch of main trunk of mandibular teeth.
- ***Function:*** Elevation and protrusion of mandible.

Lateral Pterygoid Muscle

- It is a short conical muscle and has upper and lower heads.
- ***Origin:*** Sphenoid bone.
- ***Insertion:*** Into the neck of condyle.
- ***Nerve supply:*** Branch of anterior division of mandibular nerve.
- ***Function:*** In opening of the jaw, in protrusion and lateral movements of mandible.

Q 2. What is Mastication? *(July 2005)*

Ans. Mastication

- It is a complex rhythmical activity that requires coordination of the neuromusculature. It is the cutting down of food substances in small particles and grinding them into a small bolus.
- Mastication is a repititive sequence of jaw opening and closing with a profile in the vertical plane called the 'chewing cycle'.
- Mastication consists of number of chewing cycles opening phase, closing phase, occlusal or intercuspal phase.
- Each chewing cycle lasts approximately for .8 to 1.0 sec.
- During normal function 7 to 15 kg force occurs during swallowing and chewing.
- The act of mastication begins with "setting the system" by sight, tactile sense and smell to receive the food.
- When food is taken into mouth, the lips, tongue and periodontium function to estimate size, hardness, etc. of food.
- This information sets the chewing program in pattern.
- Chewing is highly complex.
- The duration of chewing cycle varies between 1 to 6 sec, depending on the type of food.
- Speed, duration and form of the chewing cycle vary with the type of occlusion, kind of food, and presence of dysfunction.

MULTIPLE CHOICE QUESTIONS (MCQs)

1. Retraction results from the bilateral contraction of the
a. Medial pterygoid
b. Lateral pterygoid
c. Posterior fibers of the temporalis muscle
d. Masseter

2. Protraction results from the simultaneous contraction of
a. Right and left medial pterygoid
b. Right and left lateral pterygoid
c. Temporalis
d. Buccinator

3. Sideway movement of mandible results from the contraction of
a. One lateral pterygoid muscle on opposite side
b. One medial pterygoid muscle on opposite side
c. Pterygoid muscle
d. Temporalis

4. In the opening of the mouth, all of the following muscles take part, *except*
a. Temporalis
b. Platysma
c. Digastric
d. Lateral pterygoid

5. Muscle attached to articular disc is
a. Lateral pterygoid
b. Medial pterygoid
c. Masseter
d. Temporalis

6. The muscle which moves the disc of the TMJ forward is
a. Lateral pterygoid
b. Medial pterygoid
c. Temporalis
d. Masseter

7. Contraction of posterior fibres of temporalis muscle results in
a. Retrusion b. Protrusion
c. Opening d. Closing

8. The position in which there is relative muscular equilibrium is
a. Retruded contact position
b. Postural position
c. Protruded contact position
d. None of the above

9. Except one pair all the following are jaw elevators
a. Masseter
b. Temporalis
c. Medial pterygoid
d. Lateral pterygoid

10. All the following muscles are elevators of mandible *except*
a. Masseter b. Digastric
c. Temporalis d. Medial pterygoid

11. Medial pterygoid takes its origin on
a. Medial surface of lateral pterygoid plate (sphenoid bone)
b. External pterygoid plate
c. Styloid process
d. Zygoma

12. Buccinator muscle receives its motor nerve supply from
a. Zygomatic branch of facial nerve
b. Buccal branch of trigeminal nerve
c. Buccal branch of facial nerve
d. Mandibular branch of facial nerve

13. The following muscles take their origin on medial surface of mandible *except*
a. Medial pterygoid muscle
b. Mylohyoid muscle
c. Genioglossus muscle
d. Superior constrictor

1-c, 2-b, 3-a, 4-a, 5-a, 6-a, 7-a, 8-b, 9-d, 10-b, 11-a, 12-c, 13-d

14. The combined pull of two lateral pterygoid muscles along with the anterior bellies of the two digastric and the other suprahyoid muscles will result in

a. Protrusion
b. Retrusion
c. Closing
d. Opening of mandible

15. The fan shaped large and flat muscle is

a. Buccinator
b. Temporalis
c. Masseter
d. Medial pterygoid

16. Out of the four pairs of muscles of mastication the only pair of muscle which is oriented horizontally is

a. Medial pterygoid
b. Lateral pterygoid
c. Masseter
d. Temporalis

17. Closing of the mouth (elevation) results from the bilateral contraction of

a. Right and left temporalis
b. R and L masseter
c. R and L medial pterygoid
d. All of the above

18. Opening of mouth (depression) results from the bilateral contraction of

a. Both lateral pterygoid
b. Masseter
c. Medial pterygoid
d. Buccinator

19. During the opening of mouth there is

a. Only translation movement
b. Only hinge movement
c. First hinge and then translation movement
d. Sliding movement

20. Temporalis muscle performs the function of

a. Elevation b. Retraction
c. Clenching d. All of the above

21. The most superficial bulky and powerful muscle of mastication is

a. Temporalis
b. Masseter
c. Medial pterygoid
d. Lateral pterygoid

22. The muscle which is not antigravity muscle is

a. Masseter
b. Temporalis
c. Medial pterygoid
d. Lateral peterygoid

14-d, 15-b, 16-b, 17-d, 18-a, 19-c, 20-d, 21-b, 22-d

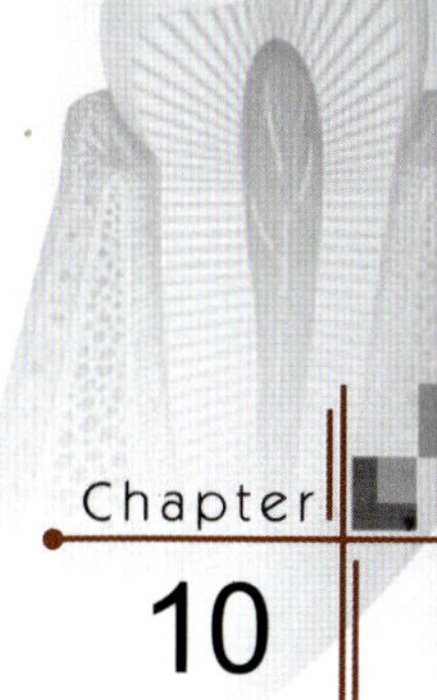

Chapter

10

Deglutition

SAQs (3 Marks)

Q 1. Define deglutition. *(Oct. 2004, July 2005, June 2007, May 2009, 2013)*

Ans. Swallowing of food is known as deglutition:

Deglutition occurs in 3 stages, namely.

1. Oral stage—when food enters from mouth into pharynx.
2. Pharyngeal stage—when food enters esophagus from pharynx.
3. Esophageal stage—when food enters stomach from esophagus.

- ***Oral stage***: It is preceded by mastication. The passage of food through oral cavity into the pharynx occurs in this stage. This is a voluntary stage.
- ***Pharyngeal or second stage***: In this stage, the bolus is pushed from pharynx into the esophagus. It is an involuntary stage.

  The pharynx is a common passage for food and air.

  It divides into larynx and esophagus.

  Larynx lies anteriorly and continues as respiratory passage. Esophagus lies behind the larynx and continues as GIT.

  During this stage of swallowing, the bolus can enter 4 ways into the pharnyx, which are:

  a. Back into mouth
  b. Upward into nasopharynx
  c. Forward into larynx
  d. Downward into the esophagus.

  The various movements are coordinated so that the bolus enters only the esophagus.

  The entrance of bolus through other outlets is prevented as follows:

  a. Back into mouth is prevented by position of the tongue and the high intraoral pressure created by the movement of the tongue.
  b. Upward into nasopharynx is prevented by elevation of soft palate.
  c. Forward into larynx is prevented by:
     - Approximation of vocal cords.
     - Forward and upward movement of larynx.

- Backward movement of epiglottis to close the larynx and by temporary arrest of breathing.
- This occurs during second stage of swallowing and apnea during deglutition is called "deglutition apnea", or "swallowing apnea".

d. Entrance of bolus into esophagus.

As the other three paths are closed for the Bolus, it has to only pass through the esophagus.

This occurs by the combined effects of various factors:

- Upward movement of the larynx.
- Relaxation of upper 3–4 cm of esophagus.
- Peristaltic contraction in the pharynx.
- Lifting away of glottis from the food passage due to elevation of larynx.

The whole process takes place within 1–2 sec and this process is purely involuntary.

- ***Esophageal or third stage*:** This is also an involuntary stage.

  The function of esophagus is to transport the food from pharynx to the stomach.

  The movements of esophagus are specifically organized for this function and these movements are called "peristaltic waves", which propel the bolus into the stomach.

Q 2. What is speech regulatory center? *(June 2007)*

Ans. Speech Regulatory Center

- Speech is one of the functions of the upper aerodigestive tract and is an activity that involves nerves, muscles, and mechanical factors such as movement of air and hearing.
- Speech is produced and modified in the vocal tracts.
- The term language center refers to the area of the brain which serves a particular function for speech processing and production. *For example,* Broca's area and Wernicke's area.
- Most areas of speech processing develop in second year of life in the dominant half (hemisphere) of the brain, which corresponds to the opposite of dominant hand. Nenety eight percent of right handed people are left hemisphere dominant and majority of left hand people as well.
- Broca's area is located in left inferior frontal cortex (left cerebral hemisphere in the inferior frontal gyrus of the frontal lobe).
- Wernicke's area is located in the superior temporal gyrus of the temporal lobe.
- Broca's area is an speech production center with motor functions.
- Wernicke's area is a language center with motor comprehension center which is next to primary auditory cortex. It controls meaningful or logical speech.
- The cranial nerves involved in speech production are V, VII, X, XII.

MULTIPLE CHOICE QUESTIONS (MCQs)

1. **The process of preventing entry of food bolus into the respiratory tract in the pharyngeal stage is known as**
   a. Respiration of swallowing
   b. Deglutition apnea
   c. Both
   d. None
2. **Muscle that closes nasopharynx during deglutition is**
   a. Levator palate
   b. Tensor palate
   c. both a and b
   d. Palato glossus
3. **The number of times swallowing takes place per day in an individual is approximately**
   a. 600 times b. 60 times
   c. 6000 times d. 1600 times
4. **The stage of deglutition which is voluntary is**
   a. Pharyngeal b. Esophageal
   c. Oral d. Both a and b
5. **Respiration stops for a while in the following phase of swallowing**
   a. Esophageal b. Oral
   c. Pharyngeal d. Both b and c
6. **Newborn and infants feed by a process called**
   a. Suckling b. Sucking
   c. Mastication d. All of the above
7. **Irritation or noxious stimulation of the posterior of the oral cavity results in the following reflex**
   a. Swallowing b. Masticatory
   c. Suckling d. Vomiting

1-b, 2-c, 3-a, 4-c, 5-d, 6-a, 7-d

Chapter

11

Temporomandibular Joint

SAQs (3 Marks)

Q 1. Describe ligaments of temporomandibular joint.

(June 2004, Nov. 2010, 2014, 2015, May 2012, Oct. 2015)

Ans. Ligaments of Temporomandibular Joint

- The TMJ has one major and three minor ligaments.
- The temporomandibular ligament is the major ligament.
- The sphenomandibular ligament, the stylomandibular ligament and pterygomandibular raphae are minor ligaments.
- **The temporomandibular ligament** (lateral ligament) strengthens the joint capsule. It is infact the thickened lateral portion of the capsule.
- The function of this ligament is to provide the main support to the joint and to resist dislocation during functional movements.
- **Sphenomandibular ligament** is a flat, thin band which is attached to the spine of the sphenoid above and to the lingula of the mandible below.
  The function of this ligament is to limit distension of the mandible in an inferior direction.
- **Stylomandibular ligament:** This ligament is a specialized band or the free border of the cervical fascia which extends from the apex of the styloid process of the temporal bone to the posterior border of the angle of the mandible, between the masseter and internal pterygoid.
  This ligament along with the sphenomandibular ligament, limits excessive opening of the mandible.
- **Pterygomandibular raphae:** It is a tendinous band of the buccopharyngeal fascia attached by one extremity to the hamulus of the medial pterygoid plate and by the other extremity to the posterior end of the mylohyoid line of the mandible.

Q 2. What is synovial membrane? *(Oct. 2004)*

Ans. Synovial Membrane

- The synovial membrane is a thin and flexible layer lining the inner surface of the capsule. It covers all the intraarticular surfaces except pressure-bearing fibrocartilage.
- The synovial membrane consists of two layers.
  The cellular intima layer and the vascular sub-intima layer.
- Function of synovial membrane is to produce fluid which helps in lubricating the joint, repairing the wear.

MULTIPLE CHOICE QUESTIONS (MCQs)

1. During the opening of mouth there is
a. Only translation movement
b. Only hinge movement
c. First hinge and then translation movement
d. Sliding movement

2. Temporomandibular joint is found in
a. Only mammals
b. Reptiles
c. Amphibians
d. Mammals and reptiles

3. Synovial membrane is present in
a. Temporomandibular joint
b. Knee joint
c. Wrist joint
d. All of the above

4. Capsule of TMJ is weakest
a. Anteriorly
b. Laterally
c. Medially
d. Posteriorly

5. The only ligament that gives direct support to the capsule of the TMJ is
a. Sphenomandibular ligament
b. Stylomandibular ligament
c. Temporomandibular ligament
d. None of the above

6. The amount of synovial fluid
a. Increases with age
b. Decreases with age
c. Does not depend on age
d. None of the above

7. The articular surface of TMJ in made-up of
a. Vascular fibrous tissue
b. Calcific tissue
c. Hyaline tissue
d. None of the above

8. Meniscus of TMJ in older person is
a. Synovial
b. Cartilagenous
c. Fibrocartilagenous
d. Fibrous

9. Muscle attached to articular disc is
a. Lateral pterygoid
b. Medial pterygoid
c. Massetor
d. Temporalis

10. The muscle which moves the disc of TMJ forward is
a. Lateral pterygoid
b. Medial pterygoid
c. Temporalis
d. Masseter

11. The articulation between the movable mandible and the stationary skull is known as
a. Temporomandibular joint
b. Craniomandibular joint
c. Both a and b
d. Gomiohosis

12. The mandible functions as which type of lever
a. Class I b. Class II
c. Class III d. Class IV

13. Medially and laterally, the articular disc is attached to
a. Lateral pterygoid
b. Squamotympanic fissure
c. Condylar neck
d. Joint capsule

14. Glenoid fossa is
a. Central fossa of mandibular first molar
b. Articulating surface of mandibular condyle
c. Depression in maxilla distal to canine fossa
d. None of the above

1-c, 2-a, 3-d, 4-c, 5-c, 6-b, 7-c, 8-d, 9-a, 10-a, 11-c, 12-c, 13-d, 14-b

15. TMJ is capable of performing full opening movements and slight gliding movements and this type of joint can be described as

a. Ball and socket joint
b. Hinge joint
c. Pivot joint
d. Condylar joint

16. Contraction of lateral ptyerygoid causes meniscus to move forwards and this results

a. Posterior movement of condyles in the glenoid fossa
b. Forward and downward movement of the condyles
c. Forceful closure of the mandible
d. None of the above

17. Which of the following protects TMJ in function?

a. Synovial fluid
b. Ligaments of the capsule
c. Muscles of mastication
d. All of the above

18. When mandible is brought forward to make edge to edge contacts there is both hinge and gliding movements. The condyles contacts there is both hinge and gliding movements. The condyles in the glenoid fossa moves.

a. Forward only
b. Backward only
c. Forwards and downwards
d. Forwards and upward.

19. The movement that occurs during opening of mandible from retruded contact position is

a. Hinge movement only
b. Sliding movement
c. Hinge followed by sliding
d. Sliding followed by hinge

20. The stylomandibular ligament of TMJ is attached

a. Above to the lateral surface of the styloid process
b. Below to the angle and posterior border of the ramus of the mandible
c. Both a and b
d. None of the above

21. TMJ gets its blood supply from

a. Branches from superficial temporal and maxillary arteries
b. Branches from mandibular arteries
c. External carotid artery
d. Mental artery

22. TMJ gets its nerve supply/TMJ is innervated by

a. Auriculotemporal nerve
b. Masseter nerve
c. Both a and b
d. None of the above

15-b, 16-b, 17-d, 18-c, 19-c, 20-c, 21-a, 22-c

Chapter 12

Maxillary Sinus

SAQ (3 Marks)

Q 1. Describe maxillary sinus. *(June 2008)*

Ans.

- It is also called "maxillary antrum", and the "antrum of Highmore".
- It is the pneumatic space that is lodged inside the body of the maxilla and it communicates with the environment by way of the middle nasal meatus and the nasal vestibule.
- It is large, four-sided, pyramid-shaped cavity. Its size is 25 × 30 × 30 mm. Capacity of 15 ml or about 1 tablespoon.
- The sinus cavity floor extends inferiorly into the base or top of the alveolar process where many projections of the apical ends of the molar roots and sometimes, premolar roots are found.
- ***Histology of maxillary sinus*:**
  - Microscopically three layers surround the maxillary sinus space—the epithelial layer, basal lamina, and subepithelial layer including periosteum.
  - The epithelium is pseudostratified, columnar and ciliated. The most numerous cellular type is columnar ciliated epithelial cell.
  - In addition basal cells, columnar nonciliated cells, and Goblet cells are also seen.
  - A **ciliated** cell has nucleus and cytoplasm with numerous mitochondria and enzyme containing organelles. The cilia are typically composed of 9+1 pairs of microtubules and they provide the motile apparatus to the sinus epithelium. By way of ciliary beating the mucous blanket lining the epithelial surface moves from sinus toward nasal cavity.
  - The **Goblet cell** displays all of the characteristic features of a secretary cell. In the basal segment of the cell is the nucleus, rough, and smooth endoplasmic reticulum and golgi apparatus. All of which are involved in the synthesis of secretory mucosubstances. From the golgi apparatus the zymogenic granules transport the mucopolysaccharides toward the cellular apex and finally release this material onto the epithelial surface by exocytosis.
  - In addition to the epithelial secretion, the surface of the sinus is provided with a mixed secretory product from the subepithelial glands. These are located in the subepithelial layer of the sinus and reach the sinus lumen by way of excretory ducts. Acini of subepithelial glands has varying proportions of serous and mucous cells.

- ***Functions***:
  - Lighten the skull, give resonance to voice, warm the air we breathe, moisten the nasal cavity.
  - It enhances faciocranial resistance to mechanical shock.
- ***Clinical considerations***:
  - Agenesis, aplasia or hypoplasia of the maxillary sinus occurs either alone or in association with other anomalies, e.g. cleft palate, high palate, and septal deformity.
  - Since upper first molar is very close to the floor of maxillary sinus, surgical manipulation on this tooth breaks the bony lamina and creates an oroantral fistula.

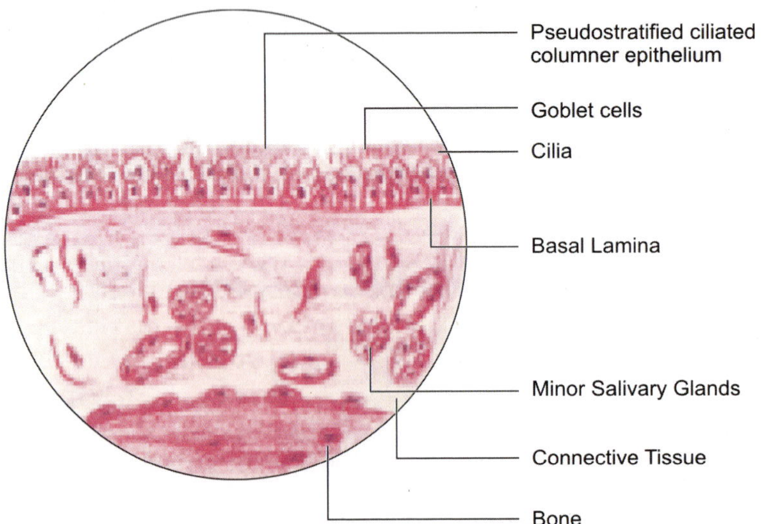

Fig. 12.1: Maxillary sinus

MULTIPLE CHOICE QUESTIONS (MCQs)

1. Opening of maxillary sinus is situated in
a. Superior meatus
b. Middle concha
c. Inferior meatus
d. Hiatus semilunaris

2. Maxillary sinus is lined with
a. Squamous cell epithelium
b. Columnar epithelium
c. Pseudostratified ciliated columnar epithelium
d. Stratified squamous epithelium

3. The largest sinus is
a. Maxillary
b. Frontal
c. Ethmoid
d. Sphenoid

4. The first formed sinus is
a. Maxillary b. Frontal
c. Ethmoid d. Sphenoid

5. The paranasal sinus which is not paired is
a. Maxillary b. Frontal
c. Ethmoid d. Sphenoid

6. The maxillary sinus communicates with the environment by
a. Superior nasal meatus
b. Middle nasal meatus
c. Middle nasal meatus and nasal vestibule
d. Inferior nasal meatus

7. The secretary cells present in the sub-epithelial glands of maxillary sinus are
a. Mucous cells
b. Serous cells
c. Both of the above
d. None of the above

8. The functions of maxillary sinus are
a. Protect the internal structures against exposure to cold air
b. Contribute resonance to voice
c. Mastication
d. Both a and b

9. The maxillary sinus is also called as
a. Antrum of maxilla
b. Antrum of mandible
c. Antrum of highmore
d. Antrum of lowmore

1-d, 2-c, 3-a, 4-a, 5-d, 6-c, 7-c, 8-d, 9-c

Section

II

Dental Histology

13. Development of Tooth and Face
14. Enamel
15. Dentin
16. Pulp
17. Cementum
18. Periodontal Ligament
19. Bone
20. Oral Mucous Membrane
21. Salivary Glands
22. Tooth Eruption
23. Shedding of Deciduous Teeth
24. Preparation of Specimen for Histologic Study

Chapter 13

Development of Tooth and Face

LAQs (10 Marks)

Q 1. Enumerate various stages of tooth development. Describe in detail early bell stage.

(Nov. 2000, May 2015)

Ans. Introduction

- The primitive oral cavity, *stomodeum* is lined by ectoderm. Deep to oral epithelium is the ectomesenchyme which is thought to instruct the overlying ectoderm to start tooth development.
- Oral epithelium gives rise to two horseshoe-shaped bands of tissues at the surface of stomodeum, one for each jaw. These are called as *primary epithelial bands.*
- At about 7th week, primary epithelial band divides into *dental lamina* and *vestibular lamina.*
- At certain points along the dental lamina, little outgrowths from the dental lamina grow into the underlying mesenchyme, these are known as *enamel organs.*
- As cell proliferation continues, each enamel organ increases in size and changes its shape. Based on the shape of enamel organ, *morphologic stages* of tooth development are described as:

  1. Bud stage 3a. Early bell stage
  2. Cap stage 3b. Advanced bell stage

  On the basis of *histophysiological process,* development of tooth can be described as:

  1. Initiation
  2. Proliferation
  3. Histodifferentiation
  4. Morphodifferentiation
  5. Apposition

Early Bell Stage (Fig. 13.1)

Features of tooth germ at early bell stage are:

- By the 14th week, further proliferation of the tooth germ leads to bell stage. As the under surface of the cap deepens, the enamel organ takes the shape of a bell.
- In this stage, the crown of the tooth gets its final shape (morphodifferentiation) and cells that form the hard tissues of the crown (the ameloblasts that form the enamel and

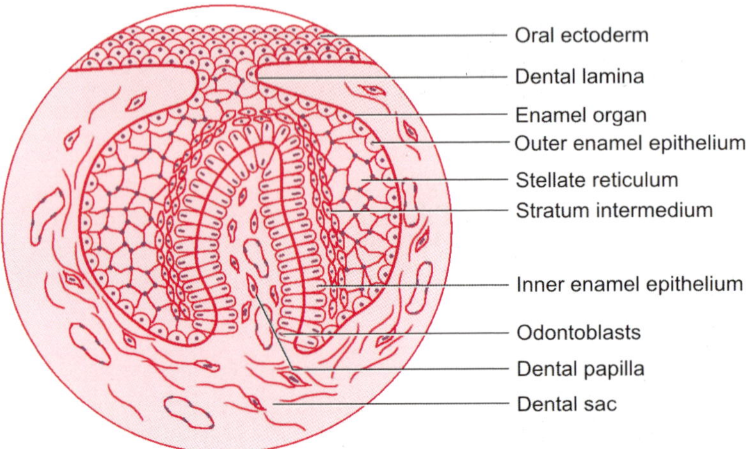

Fig. 13.1: Early bell stage of tooth development

odontoblasts that form the dentin) acquire histodifferentiation. The inner enamel epithelial cells at the future cusp tip or incisal region, stop dividing and begin to differentiate. Cell differentiation proceeds gradually cervically.

- During this stage, dental lamina joining the enamel organ to the oral epithelium, breaks up into discrete islands of **cell rests of Serres.**
- At this stage, developing tooth germ shows enamel organ, dental papilla and denta sac.

Enamel Organ

At bell stage, four different layers of cells can be distinguished in enamel organ, outer enamel epithelium, inner enamel epithelium, stellate reticulum, and stratum intermedium.

1. Inner Enamel Epithelium (IEE)

- IEE consists of a single layer of cells that differentiate prior to amelogenesis into tall columnar cells called *ameloblasts.* These cells are 4–5 nm in diameter and 40 nm high.
- The cells of IEE are separated from dental papilla by a basement membrane. They are attached to one another by junctional complexes laterally and to the cells of the stratum intermedium by desmosomes.
- At the regions associated with the future cusp tips or incisal regions the IEE cells become elongated and this differentiation gradually reaches cervically.
- The basement membrane that separates the enamel organ and dental papilla just prior to dentin formation is called the **membrana preformativa.**
- The folding of inner enamel epithelium causes different crown shapes due to difference in the rate of mitosis and differences in cell differentiation time.
- Inner enamel epithelium meets the outer enamel epithelium at the rim of the enamel organ. This junctional zone is known as **cervical loop.**
- ***Functions*:** Cells differentiate prior to amelogenesis into tall columnar cells called preameloblasts which later form enamel. These cells exert an organizing influence on peripheral cells of dental papilla so that they differentiate into *odontoblasts.*
  The folding of IEE causes different crown shapes.

2. Stratum Intermedium

- It first appears at early bell stage and consists of 2–3 layers of squamous cells lying between inner enamel epithelium and the stellate reticulum.
- It is absent in the root portion of the tooth germ.
- The cells are connected to one another and to the cells of inner enamel epithelium and stellate reticulum by desmosomes and gap junctions.
- These cells contain alkaline phosphatase and are rich in glycogen.
- ***Function***: It is concerned with the synthesis of enamel proteins and transport of nutrients to the ameloblasts. It is essential for enamel formation.

3. Stellate Reticulum (SR)

- SR is most fully developed at bell stage. It expands further mainly by increase in the amount of intercellular fluid. The cells are star shaped with bodies containing conspicuous nucleus and many branching processes.
- Desmosomal junctions are observed between the cells of stellate reticulum, stratum intermedium and outer enamel epithelium.
- ***Functions***: These serve to protect the delicate enamel forming cells, inner enamel epithelial cells, by acting as a shock absorber.
  Before enamel formation begins, the stellate reticulum collapses reducing the distance between the ameloblasts and the nutrient capillaries near the outer enamel epithelium.

4. Outer Enamel Epithelium

- Cells are flat to low cuboidal in shape, separated from the surrounding ectomesenchyme cells by a basement membrane.
- The cytoplasm consists of few organelles, free ribosomes, few rough endoplasmic reticulum, some mitochondria, and scattered tonofilaments. Adjacent cells are joined by junctional complexes.
- At the end of the bell stage, the smooth surface of the OEE is laid in folds. Between the folds, the adjacent mesenchyme of the dental sac forms papillae that contain capillary loops, thus providing nutritional supply to the enamel organ.
- ***Functions***: It maintains shape of the enamel organ.
  It helps in exchange of nutrients between the enamel organ and the dental sac.

Dental Papilla (DP)

- It is enclosed in the invaginated portion of the enamel organ. It consists of closely packed mesenchymal cells with only a few delicate extracellular fibrils.
- ***Function***: Before the cells of inner enamel epithelium begin to produce enamel, the peripheral cells of dental papilla differentiate into odontoblasts under the organizing influence of inner enamel epithelium and form dentin. The dental papilla ultimately gives rise to dental pulp once dentin formation starts.
- The basement membrane that separates the enamel organ and dental papilla just prior to dentin formation is called the *membrana preformativa.*

Dental Sac (DS)

- Before formation of dental tissues begins, dental sac shows a circular arrangement of its fibers and resembles a capsular structure.

- ***Function***: It serves as a primordium for formation of cementum, alveolar bone, and periodontal ligament.

Q 2. Name the stages of tooth development. Describe in detail the advanced bell stage.

(SAQ, July 2005, May 2009, 2015)

Ans. Introduction

- The primitive oral cavity or *stomodeum* is lined by ectoderm. Deep to oral epithelium is the ectomesenchyme which is thought to instruct the overlying ectoderm to start tooth development.
- Oral epithelium gives rise to two horseshoe-shaped bands of tissues at the surface of stomodeum, one for each jaw. These are called as *primary epithelial bands.*
- At about 7th week, primary epithelial band divides into *dental lamina* and *vestibular lamina.*
- At certain points along the dental lamina, little outgrowths from the dental lamina grow into the underlying mesenchyme, these are known as *Enamel organs.*
- As cell proliferation continues, each enamel organ increases in size and changes its shape. Based on the shape of enamel organ, *morphologic stages* of tooth development are described as:
  1. Bud stage
  2. Cap stage
  3a. Early bell
  3b. Advanced bell stage
- On the basis of *histophysiological process,* development of tooth can be described as:
  1. Initiation
  2. Proliferation
  3. Histodifferentiation
  4. Morphodifferentiation
  5. Apposition

ADVANCED BELL STAGE/LATE BELL STAGE (Hard tissue formation stage/crown stage/appositional stage) (Fig. 13.2)

- This stage commences at about 18th week.

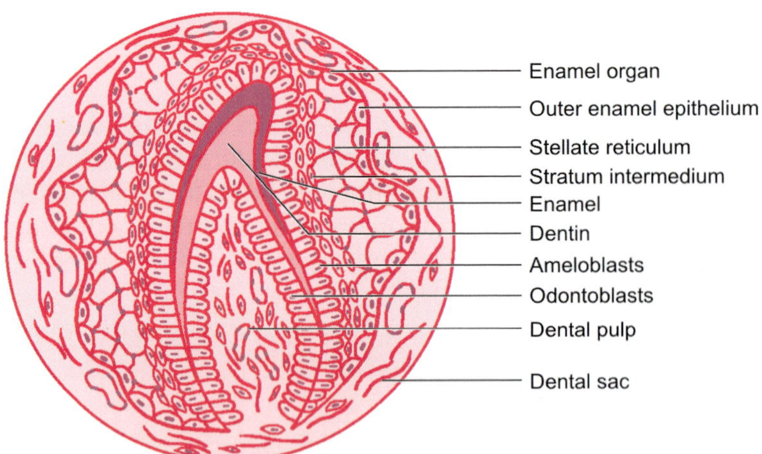

Fig. 13.2: Advanced bell stage of tooth development

Features of tooth germ at advanced bell stage are:

Enamel Organ

- It is characterized by formation of two principal hard tissues, enamel and dentin, and root formation. Formation of dentin always precedes enamel formation.
- Four different types of epithelial cells can be distinguished in enamel organ at advanced bell stage.

1. Inner Enamel Epithelium (IEE)

- At the site of future cusp tips and incisal areas where dentin will first be formed, the cells of inner enamel epithelium become tall columnar and their nuclei become aligned at the proximal end of the cells adjacent to the stratum intermedium. This is *reversal of polarity.*
- There is migration of cellular organelles responsible for enamel protein formation from proximal end to the distal end of the ameloblast.
- This reversal of polarity is in preparation to formation of enamel matrix.
- The cells of IEE exert an organizing influence on the underlying mesenchymal cells of dental papilla, which later differentiate into odontoblasts.
- After the first layer of dentin is formed only then the cells of the inner enamel epithelium differentiate further, assuming a secretory function and producing an organic matrix against the newly formed dentin surface. It immediately gets partially mineralized and becomes the enamel of the crown.
- Before the formation of first dentin, enamel organ and in particular the cells of the inner enamel epithelium receive nutrition from blood vessels located in the dental papilla and those situated along the periphery of the outer enamel epithelium.
- After the first layer of dentin is formed, blood supply from dental papilla to the enamel organ is cut-off. Enamel organ then gets nutrition from dental sac.
- The enamel formation then proceeds coronally and cervically, in all regions from the dentinoenamel junction towards the surface.

2. Stratum Intermedium

- It first appears at early bell stage and consists of 2–3 layers of squamous cells lying over inner enamel epithelium.
- The cells are connected to one another and to the cells of inner enamel epithelium and stellate reticulum by desmosomes and gap junctions.
- These cells contain alkaline phosphatase.
- ***Function*:** It has been suggested that stratum intermedium is concerned with the synthesis of enamel proteins and transport of nutrients to the ameloblasts. It is essential for enamel formation.
- It is absent in the part of the tooth germ that outlines the root portion of the tooth which does not form enamel.

3. Stellate Reticulum

- At early bell stage, stellate reticulum collapses so that the ameloblasts are approximated to the blood vessels lying outside the outer enamel epithelium and their demand of nutrition is satisfied.

4. Outer Enamel Epithelium

- In the late bell stage, preparatory to and during the formation of enamel, the formerly smooth surface of outer enamel epithelium is laid in folds. Between the folds, the adjacent mesenchyme of the dental sac forms papillae that contain capillary loops and thus provide a rich nutritional supply for the intense metabolic activity of the avascular enamel organ.

Dental Papilla

- The undifferentiated mesenchymal cells of dental papilla increase rapidly in size and ultimately differentiate into odontoblasts, the dentin forming cells. This differentiation is initiated by an organizing influence of inner enamel epithelium on dental papilla.
- The increase in size of the papillary cells to become odontoblasts eliminates the acellular zone between dental papilla and inner enamel epithelium.
- Odontoblasts contain increasing amount of rough endoplasmic reticulum and golgi complexes. They have highly polarized nuclei which are positioned away from inner enamel epithelium.
- Enamel formation cannot begin until some dentin has been formed. This interdependency between the two tissues is an example of epithelial-mesenchymal interaction.
- Odontoblasts as they differentiate, begin to elaborate organic matrix of the dentin, which gets ultimately mineralized.
- Formation of dentin occurs first as a layer along the future dentinoenamel junction in the region of future cusps and proceeds pulpally and apically. After the first layer of dentin is formed, the newly differentiated ameloblasts lay down enamel over the dentin.
- Cervical portion of the enamel organ gives rise to the epithelial root sheath of Hertwig. *Hertwig's epithelial root sheath* outlines the future root and is responsible for the shape, length, size, and number of roots.

Dental Sac

- Before the formation of dental tissues begins, dental sac shows a circular arrangement of its fibers and resembles a capsular structure.
- ***Function***: It serves as a primordium for formation of cementum, alveolar bone, and periodontal ligament.
- With the development of the root, fibers of the dental sac differentiate into periodontal fibers that become embedded in the developing cementum and alveolar bone.

Q 3. Enumerate various stages of tooth development. Describe in detail bell stage.

(July 2006, May 2008)

Ans. Describe early and advance bell stage from Q 1 and Q 2.

SAQs (3 Marks)

Q 1. Describe cap stage. *(June 2011, 2013)*

Ans.

- Based on the shape of enamel organ, morphologic stages of tooth development are described as bud stage, cap stage, early bell, and advanced bell stage.
- During tooth development, the enamel organ grows into cap shape due to unequal growth in different parts of tooth bud which leads to a shallow invagination on the deep surface of the bud.

1. Enamel Organ

- As the tooth bud continues to proliferate, it does not expand uniformly into a larger sphere. Unequal growth in different parts of the enamel organ into the underlying ectomesenchyme leads to cap stage (Fig. 13.3).
- The ectomesenchyme adjacent to the cap shaped enamel organ gets condensed. The condensed ectomesenchyme near the shallow invaginated (concave) portion of the enamel organ is called dental papilla. The ectomesenchyme surrounding the enamel organ and dental papilla is dental sac.
- The enamel organ at this stage has distinct cell layers, the outer enamel epithelium, the inner enamel epithelium and stellate reticulum.

Outer Enamel Epithelium (OEE)

- These are peripheral cuboidal cells that cover the convexity of the cap and are separated from dental sac by a delicate basement membrane and is anchored to it by hemidesmosomes.
- The cells contain a large centrally placed nucleus and small amount of cytoplasmic organelles.
- ***Function:*** Outer enamel epithelium cells are involved in maintaining the shape of enamel organ and in the exchange of substances between the enamel organ and the surrounding tissue.

Inner Enamel Epithelium (IEE)

- These are columnar cells that lie on the concavity (invagination) of the cap and are separated from the dental papilla by a delicate basement membrane and are anchored to it by hemidesmosomes.
- During bell stage, IEE cells differentiate into ameloblasts, enamel forming cells.

Stellate Reticulum

- These are polygonal cells located in the center of the enamel organ, between the OEE and IEE. They begin to separate due to water being drawn into the enamel organ from the surrounding dental papilla as a result of osmotic force exerted by glycosaminoglycans contained in the ground substance.
- As a result the polygonal cells begin to separate and become star shaped but maintain contact with each other by their cytoplasmic processes.
- As these star shaped cells form a cellular network, they are called the **stellate reticulum.** This gives the stellate reticulum a cushion-like consistency and acts as a shock absorber that may support and protect the delicate enamel forming cells.
- ***Transient structures*:** In enamel organ at cap stage, some transient structures appear which act as a reservoir of dividing cells for the growing enamel organ. These are **Enamel knot, enamel cord** and **enamel septum.** Enamel knot also plays an important role in determining the shape of the tooth.

2. Dental Papilla

- Under the organizing influence of the proliferating epithelium of the enamel organ, the ectomesenchyme (neural crest cells), that is partially enclosed by the invaginated portion of the IEE, proliferates.
- It condenses to form the dental papilla, which is the formative organ of the dentin and the primordium of the pulp.

- Dental pupilla shows active budding of capillaries and its peripheral cells adjacent to IEE later differentiate into odontoblasts.

3. Dental Sac/Dental Follicle

- Concomitant with the development of enamel organ and dental papilla, there is a marginal condensation in the ectomesenchyme surrounding the enamel organ to form dental sac.
- Dental sac gives rise to the supporting tissues of tooth, i.e. cementum, periodontal ligament and alveolar bone.

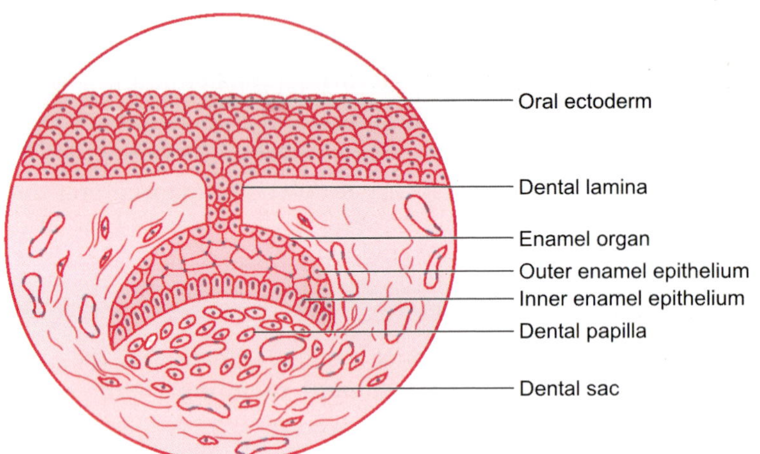

Fig. 13.3: Cap stage of tooth development

Q 2. Define transient structures.

Ans. In enamel organ during cap stage and early bell stage, before enamel formation begins, some transient structures appear which act as a reservoir of dividing cells for the growing enamel organ. These are **enamel knot, enamel cord** and **enamel septum.** These are temporary structures that disappear before enamel formation begins.

1. Enamel Knot

- It is a localized mass of cells in the center of the enamel organ which are densely packed. Characteristically it forms a bulge into the dental papilla at the center of the enamel organ, which is bordered by the labial and lingual enamel grooves.
- ***Function*:** It acts as a reservoir of dividing cells for the growing enamel organ. It may represent an important signalling center during tooth development and play an important role in determining the shape of the tooth. It plays prime role in controlling the growth as well as designing of tooth cusps.

2. Enamel Cord and Septum

- Enamel cord is vertical extension of the enamel knot. It is a strand of cells running from the knot towards outer enamel epithelium (OEE).
- When the enamel cord extends to meet the outer enamel epithelium, it is termed as *enamel septum*, as it divides the stellate reticulum into two parts.

- The point on OEE, where the enamel cord meets OEE, shows a small depression which is termed *enamel navel,* as it resembles the umbilicus.

Significance

Transient structures act as reservoir of dividing cells for the growing enamel organ.

Q 3. Write about stellate reticulum/enamel pulp. *(June 2002, 2004)*

Ans. Introduction

Stellate reticulum is a layer of cells present beween outer and inner enamel epithelia in enamel organ during development of tooth.

Structure (Refer Fig. 13.3)

- Stellate reticulum, also called **enamel pulp**, consists of the polygonal cells in the center of enamel organ.
- These cells begin to separate due to water being drawn into the enamel organ from the surrounding dental papilla as a result of osmotic force exerted by glycosaminoglycans contained in the ground substance.
- As a result, the polygonal cells become star shaped but maintain contact with each other by their cytoplasmic processes.
- These cells are star shaped with bodies containing conspicuous nucleus and many branching processes. As these star shaped cells form a cellular network, they are called as stellate reticulum.
- Stellate reticulum is fully developed at bell stage.
- Desmosomal junctions are observed between the cells of stellate reticulum, stratum intermedium, and outer enamel epithelium.

Functions

- Stellate reticulum has cushion like consistancy.
- It acts as a shock absorber that may support and protect the delicate enamel forming cells.
- In late bell stage just before enamel formation begins, stellate reticulum collapses reducing the distance between ameloblasts and the nutrient capillaries near the OEE.
- Its cells are then hardly distinguished from those of the stratum intermedium. This change begins at the height of the cusp and progresses cervically. This collapsed enamel organ along with stellate reticulum is called as *reduced enamel epithelium* and it serves to protect the newly formed enamel till eruption.

Q 4. Write about outer enamel epithelium. *(Oct. 2002)*

Ans.

- Enamel organ during development of tooth has distinct cell layers, outer enamel epithelium, inner enamel epithelium, stellate reticulum and stratum intermedium.
- Outer enamel epithelium (OEE) has cuboidal cells that cover the convexity of the enamel organ and are separated from the dental sac by a delicate basement membrane and are anchored to it by hemidesmosomes.
- The cells contain a large, centrally placed nucleus and the cytoplasm consists of few organelles, free ribosomes, few rough endoplasmic reticulum, some mitochondria and scattered tonofilaments. Adjacent cells are joined by junctional complexes.
- At bell stage the cells of OEE flatten to a low cuboidal form.

- ***Functions*:**
  1. OEE cells are involved in maintaining the shape of enamel organ and in the exchange of substances between enamel organ and surrounding tissue/dental follicle.
  2. In the late bell stage preparatory to and during formation of enamel, formerly smooth surface of outer enamel epithelium is laid in folds. Between the folds adjacent mesenchyme of the dental sac forms papillae that contain capillary loops which provide a rich nutritional supply for the intense metabolic activity of the avascular enamel organ.

Q 5. Explain root formation. Or write about Hertwing's Epithelia Root Sheath (HERS).

Ans.

- Development of root begins after enamel and dentin formation has reached the future cementoenamel junction. Enamel organ plays an important role in the formation of root by forming *Hertwig's Epithelial Root Sheath (HERS)* from the cervical loop.
- Cervical portion of the enamel organ at bell stage gives rise to HERS. It consists of inner enamel epithelium and outer enamel epithelium. It does not include stratum intermedium and stellate reticulum.
- HERS plays an important role in the determination of the shape, length, size, and number of roots. In addition, it initiates radicular dentin formation.
- The inner cells of the HERS induce differentiation of radicular dental papilla cells into odontoblasts. After the first layer of root dentin is laid down by these cells, HERS lose its structural continuity and breaks its remnants persist as epithelial network of strands which are found in PDL of erupted teeth and are called **cell rests of Malassez.**
- The cells of dental follicle surrounding the HERS, proliferate and come in contact with the outer surface of newly laid dentin and differentiate into cementoblasts that deposit a layer of cementum onto the surface of root dentin.
- At the proliferating end HERS bend into a horizontal plane. This area is termed as *epithelial diaphragm*. The epithelial diaphragm encircles the apical opening of the dental papilla.
- As the odontoblasts differentiate along the pulpal boundary, root dentinogenesis proceeds and the root lengthens. Dentinogenesis and cementogenesis continues until the appropriate root length is developed. The root then thickens till the apical opening is 1–3 mm which is sufficient to allow vascular and neural communication between the pulp and periodontal ligament.
- With the increase in root length, the tooth begins its eruptive movement which provides further space for further lengthening of the root. This is how a single root is formed.
- ***Root formation in multirooted teeth*:** Differential growth of the epithelial diaphragm causes the root trunk of multirooted tooth to divide into 2–3 roots. During the general growth of the enamel organ in a multirooted tooth, the expansion of its cervical opening occurs in such a way that long tongue like epithelial extensions of the horizontal diaphragm develop. Two or three such extensions can be present in multirooted teeth, depending on the number of roots to be formed.
- The single cervical opening of the coronal enamel organ is then divided into 2–3 openings by the horizontal extensions. On the pulpal surface of these horizontal bridges, dentin formation starts after the induction of odontoblasts. Root development then proceeds in the same way as single root formation.
- ***Significance*:** If cells of HERS remain adherent to the dentin surface, they may differentiate into ameloblasts and produce enamel. Such droplets of enamel, called **enamel pearls** are found in furcation area of roots of permanent molars.

  If continuity of HERS is broken or is not established prior to dentin formation a defect in dentinal wall of pulp ensures which accounts for the development of accessory root canals.

Q 6. Write about cell rests of Malassez. *(2000, Oct. 2003, May 2007)*

Ans.

- During development of tooth, root development begins after enamel and dentin formation has reached the future cementoenamel junction. Enamel organ plays an important role in the formation of root by forming *Hertwig's Epithelial Root Sheath (HERS)* from its cervical portion.
- The inner cells of the HERS induce differentiation of radicular dental papilla cells into odontoblasts. After the first layer of root dentin is laid down by these cells, HERS loses its structural continuity and breaks. Its remnants persist as epithelial network of strands which are found in periodontal ligament of erupted teeth and are called **cell rests of Malassez** (Figs 13.4A and B).
- ***Significance*:** They are inactive but can become active, proliferate to form odontogenic cysts, and tumors or may also undergo calcification to become cementicles.

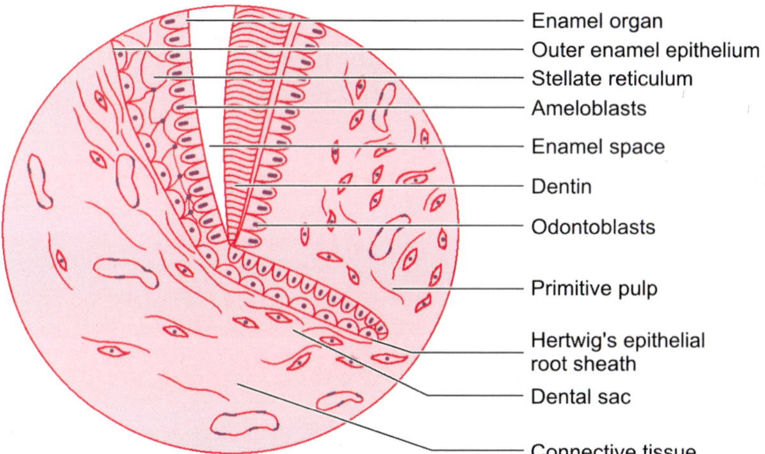

Fig. 13.4A: Root formation/Hertwig's epithelial root sheath

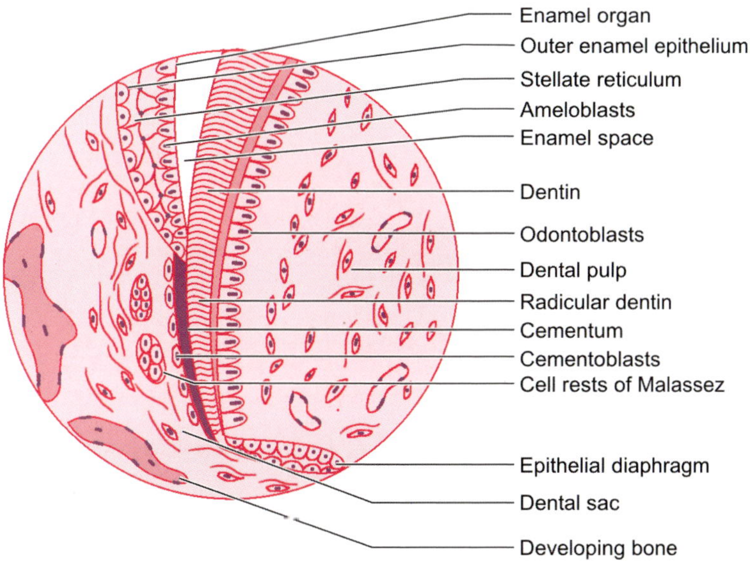

Fig. 13.4B: Root formation/Cell rests of Malassez

Q 7. Write about dental lamina and its fate. (2000, 2001, Nov. 2010)

Ans. Dental Lamina (Fig. 13.5)

- The primitive oral cavity, *or stomodeum,* is lined by oral ectoderm.
- At around 7th week of intrauterine life, due to proliferation of basal cells of the oral ectoderm there is formation of a continuous band of epithelium called as *Primary epithelial band.* It invades the underlying ectomesenchyme along each of the horseshoe-shaped future dental arches. At about 7th week the *primary epithelial band* devides into two subdivisions, *vestibular lamina* and *dental lamina.*
- Within dental lamina, continued localized proliferation leads to formation of a series of epithelial ingrowths into ectomesenchyme at sites corresponding to the position of future deciduous teeth.
- ***Functions*:**
  1. Dental lamina serves as the primordium for the ectodermal portion of deciduous teeth.
  2. Later during development of the jaws, permanent molars arise directly from a distal extension of the dental lamina.
  3. The lingual extension of the free end of the dental lamina, called as *successional lamina* gives rise to succedenous teeth.
- ***Fate of dental lamina*:**
  - It is evident that total activity of dental lamina extends over a period of at least 5 years.
  - As the teeth continue to develop, they lose their connection with the dental lamina. It then breaks up by the mesenchymal invasion.
- ***Significance*:** Remnants of the dental lamina persist as *epithelial pearls* or *islands* within the jaws as well as in the gingiva. These are referred to as **cell rests of Serres**. However, dental lamina may remain active in the third molar region. It may give rise to odontogenic cysts and tumors.

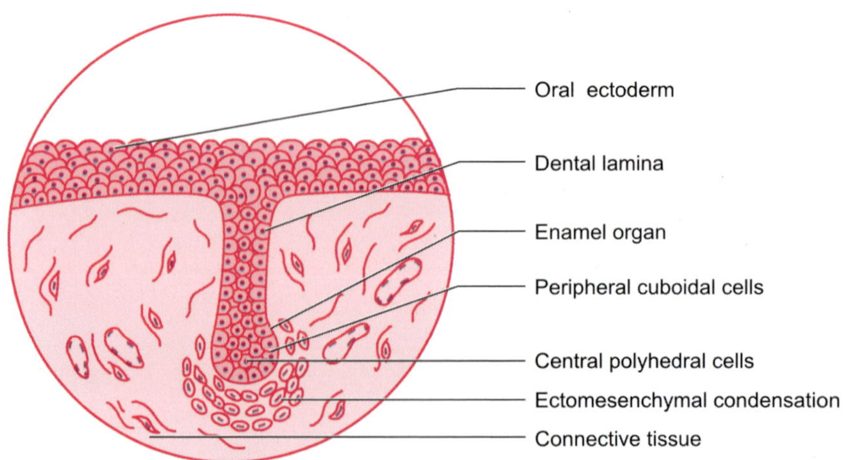

Fig. 13.5: Bud stage/Dental lamina

Q 8. Enumerate histophysiological stages of tooth development.

(Dec. 2005, July 2006)

Ans. Various physiologic growth processes participate in the progressive development of the teeth. On the basis of these histophysiological processes, the development of tooth can be studied under following headings:

1. Initiation
2. Proliferation
3. Histodifferentiation
4. Morphodifferentiation
5. Apposition

1. Initiation

- Initiation of tooth development depends on the epithelial-ectomesenchymal interaction. Dental lamina, a part of oral epithelium, has the ability to form enamel organs of the deciduous and permanent teeth, when instructed by underlying ectomesenchyme.

2. Proliferation

- Enamel organ formed due to initiation, undergoes proliferation to give the crown of the tooth its final size shape, and results successively in the bud, cap, and bell stage.
- Proliferative growth causes changes in the size and proportions of the growing tooth germ.

3. Histodifferentiation

- As the cells continue to proliferate, they undergo definite morphologic and functional changes and give up their capacity to multiply and prepare themselves to carry out their specific function, for example deposition of organic matrix. This is termed histo-differentiation.
- In the bell stage, the inner enamel epithelium influences adjacent cells of the dental papilla to differentiate into odontoblasts which form the dentin matrix. This constitutes histodifferentiation of odontoblasts. With the formation of dentin, the inner enamel epithelial cells differentiate into ameloblasts which form the enamel matrix. This constitutes histodifferentiation of the ameloblasts.
- Dentin formation precedes and is essential to enamel formation.

4. Morphodifferentiation

- The morphologic pattern, or basic form and relative size of the tooth, is determined by morphodifferentiation or differential growth.
- The dentinoenamel and dentinocemental junctions, which are different in characteristic for each type of tooth, acts as a blue print pattern and determines the form and size of the tooth.

5. Apposition

- It is the deposition of the matrix of the hard dental structures.
- Appositional growth of enamel and dentin is the layer like deposition of the extracellular matrix of dental hard tissues, characterized by alternate periods of activity and rest. It is this regular and rhythmic appositional growth that gives the tooth its final shape.

Clinical Significance

- Lack of initiation results in absence of teeth, known as *anodontia.*
- Abnormal initiation can result in development of supernumerary teeth.
- Improper histodifferentiation can result in failure of ameloblasts to differentiate as can occur in vitamin A deficiency.
- Disturbance in morphodifferentiation can result in peg shaped permanent incisors.
- *Enamel hypoplasia* is disturbed synthesis and secretion of organic matrix of enamel.
- Enamel hypocalcification is defective mineralization of enamel.

Q 9. Explain histo and morphodifferentiation. *(Nov. 2009)*

Ans. On the basis of various physiologic growth processes taking place, the development of tooth can be studied under following headings:

1. Initiation
2. Proliferation
3. Histodifferentiation
4. Morphodifferentiation
5. Apposition

Histodifferentiation

As the cells continue to proliferate, they undergo definite morphologic and functional changes, and prepare themselves to carry out their function, for example, deposition of organic matrix. This is termed histodifferentiation.

- In the bell stage, the inner enamel epithelium influences the adjacent cells of the dental papilla to differentiate into odontoblasts which form the dentin matrix. This constitutes the histodifferentiation of odontoblasts.
- With the formation of dentin, the inner enamel epithelial cells differentiate into ameloblasts which form the enamel matrix. This constitutes histodifferentiation of the ameloblasts.
- Dentin formation precedes and is essential to enamel formation. While, differentiation of the epithelial cells precedes and is essential to the differentiation of the odontoblasts and the initiation of dentin formation.
- Thus, formation of enamel and dentin are dependent on one another, and this forms the basis of reciprocal induction.

Clinical Significance

- In vitamin A deficiency, ameloblasts fail to differentiate properly and hence their organising influence on the adjacent cells of dental papilla is disturbed. As a result, odontoblasts fail to differentiate properly and the dentin formed by these odontoblasts will be atypical and known as osteodentin.

Morphodifferentiation

- The dentinoenamel junction and the dentinocemental junction are established before formation of the hard tissues. These junctions are different and characteristic for each type of tooth and acts as a blue print pattern which determines the form and size of the tooth.
- In accordance with their shape, the formative cells deposit enamel, dentin and cementum, giving the tooth their characteristic form and size.

- Disturbances occuring during the morphodifferentiation can affect the morphology of the crown or root without impairing the function of the ameloblast or odontoblasts.

Clinical Significance

- Examples of morphodifferentiation disturbances involving the crown are formation of supernumerary cusp, loss of cusp, and peg shaped teeth. Formation of supernumerary root and dilaceration (abnormal curvature in the root caused due to trauma) are some examples of disturbances involving the morphology of root with enamel and dentin which may be normal in structure.
- An abnormality in shape may result in peg or malformed tooth. Peg shaped teeth (screw-driver shaped) with the permanent upper central incisor showing a notched incisal edge may be seen in individuals born with congenital syphilis. This condition is known as Hutchinson's incisor.

Q 10. Describe bud stage.

Ans.

- By the 8th to 10th week *in utero*, continued and localized proliferative activity within dental lamina leads to the formation of epithelial downgrowths into the underlying ectomesenchyme. These are the primordia of the enamel organ, the tooth buds.
- These round or ovoid epithelial downgrowths into the underlying ectomesenchyme form at the sites corresponding to the position of 10 maxillary and 10 mandibular deciduous teeth.
- Since main function of certain epithelial cells of these epithelial downgrowths is formation of tooth enamel, these epithelial swellings are called as **enamel organs.**
- The epithelium of the enamel organ is separated from the underlying ectomesenchyme by a basement membrane.
- As cell proliferation continues, each enamel organ increases in size, sinks deeper into the ectomesenchyme and due to differential growth changes its shape from bud to cap to bell.
- At bell stage, proliferation of tissues of enamel organ occurs. No structural changes occur in the cells of the enamel organ or ectomesenchyme as later occurs during differentiation and morphogenesis.
- In the bud stage, the enamel organ consists of peripherally located low columnar cells and centrally located polygonal cells (Refer Fig. 13.5).
- Many cells of the tooth bud and the surrounding ectomesenchyme undergo mitosis. As a result of increased mitotic activity and migration of neural crest cells into the area, the ectomesenchymal cells surrounding the tooth bud condense.
- The area of ectomesenchyme condensation immediately subjacent to the enamel organ is the **dental papilla.**
- The condensed ectomesenchyme cells surrounding the tooth bud and the dental papilla is the **dental sac** or **dental follicle.**
- Both the dental papilla and dental sac become more well-defined as the enamel organ grows into cap and bell shape.

Q 11. What is enamel pearl?

Ans.

- The cells of the Hertwig's epithelial root sheath may differentiate into fully functional ameloblasts and form enamel if they remain adherent to the radicular dentin without becoming removed by the invading cells of dental follicle.
- This may appear as a globule of enamel called enamel pearl and is sometimes seen at the furcation area of roots of permanent molars.

Q 12. Describe development of tongue.

Ans.

- Tongue develops in relation to the pharyngeal arches in the floor of the developing mouth.
- Pharyngeal arch arises as a mesodermal thickening in the lateral wall of the foregut and it grows ventrally to become continuous with the corresponding arch of the opposite side.
- During 4th week of intrauterine life, the medial-most parts of the first (mandibular) arches proliferate to form two lingual swellings. The lingual swellings are partially separated from each other by a median swelling, *tuberculum impar*, which appears in the midline.
- Anterior two-thirds of the tongue is formed by fusion of the tunberculum impar and the two lingual swellings. Thus, anterior two-thirds of the tongue is derived from the mandibular arch.
- Immediately behind the tuberculum impar, the epithelium proliferates to form a downgrowth, thyroglossal duct, from which the thyroid gland develops.
- The site of this epithelial downgrowth is marked by a depression called *foramen caecum*.
- Posterior one-third of the tongue is formed by third arch mesoderm. The posterior-most part of tongue is derived from the fourth arch.
- Formation of posterior third of tongue is indicated by a midline swelling, hypobranchial eminence which is seen in relation to the medial ends of the second, third, and fourth pharyngeal arches. This eminence shows a subdivision into a cranial part (copula), and a caudal part.
- The posterior one-third of the tongue is formed from the cranial part of the hypobranchial eminence (copula).
- Anterior two-thirds of the tongue is covered by ectoderm and posterior one-third by endoderm.
- The connective tissue components of the anterior two-thirds of the tongue are derived from first arch mesenchyme while that of posteior one-third from third arch mesenchyme.
- The intrinsic musculature of the tongue is derived from the pharyngeal arch mesenchyme while the extrinsic muscles arise from the occipital myotomes and are supplied by the hypoglossal nerve.
- ***Formation of taste buds and papillae of the tongue***: Epithelium of the tongue is at first made-up of a single layer of cells. Later it becomes stratified and papillae become evident.
- The most common lingual papillae, filiform papillae, develop at around 10th to 11th weeks. The vallate and foliate papillae appear close to terminal branches of the glossopharyngeal nerve. The fungiform papillae appear later near the termination of the chorda tympani, branch of the facial nerve.
- Taste buds are formed in relation to the terminal branches of the innervating nerve fibers during 11th to 13th weeks by inductive interaction between the epithelial cells of the tongue and gustatory nerve cells from the chorda tympani, glossopharyungeal and vagus nerve.

Anomalies of Tongue

1. Macroglossia—too large tongue, or aglossia—tongue may be absent, bifid tongue due to non-function of the two lingual swellings, fissured tongue, are the developmental anomalies of tongue.
2. Ankyloglossia is tongue tie.
3. Remnants of thyroglossal duct may form cysts at the base of the tongue.

Q 13. Decribe development of maxilla/palate.

Ans.

- The face is developed by the fusion and merging of frontonasal process, a pair of maxillary process and a pair of mandibular processes.
- Palate consists of two parts, primitive (premaxilla) and permanent (secondary) palate. The primitive palate is formed from the frontonasal process while the secondary palate develops from the fusion of the palatine processes of maxillary prominences.
- The frontonasal process gets divided into a median nasal process and two lateral nasal processes by the ingrowth of a pair of olfactory pits. The primitive palate is formed by the fusion of the maxillary processes and the globular part of the median nasal processs.
- During the 6th week of intrauterine life a shelf like projection, the palatine process grows medially from the inner surface of each maxillary process.
- During 7th week, the mandibular arches grow more ventrally and caudally producing the prominence of the chin which causes necessary depression and ventral shifting of the tongue. As a result the palatine process assumes horizontal position, meet and fuse with each other, and form the permanent palate.
- The definitive palate is formed by the fusion of three parts as:
  a. The two palatal processes fuse with each other in the midline. Their fusion begins anteriorly and proceeds backwards.
  b. Each palatal process fuses with the posterior margin of the primitive palate in a "y" shaped manner. Each limb of "y" passes between the lateral incisor and canine.
- The primitive palate (premaxilla) is wedge shaped and carries four incisor teeth.
- Later, the mesoderm in the ventral three-fourths of the permanent palate undergoes ossification to form the hard palate.
- Ossification of the palate starts at 8th week of intrauterine life by intramembranous ossification of mesoderm.
- However, ossification does not extend into the most posterior portion which remains as the soft palate.
- The fusion of the palatine process with each other and with the primitive palate is completed at about ninth week of intrauterine life. Median palatine raphe indicates the line of fusion of the lateral palatine processes.

Clinical Considerations

- Defective fusion of the various compartments of the palate gives rise to clefts in the palate which results in communications between the mouth and the nose which can be unilateral or bilateral.

Q 14. Describe development of mandible.

Ans.

- A part of the mandibular arches forms the lower lip, lower jaw, and the integument covering the mandible.
- First or mandibular arch has a dorsal maxillary process, and a ventral mandibular part.
- The cartilaginous bar of the mandibular part is known as the *Meckel's cartilage* which extends dorsally up to the cartilaginous ear capsule. The dorsal part of the cartilage gets ossified to form the malleus and the incus, which are the two ossicles of the middle ear.
- The succeeding part of the cartilage regresses but its fibrous envelop persists as the anterior ligament of the malleus and the sphenomandibular ligament. The fibrous membrane of the ventral part of the Meckle's cartilage gets ossified to form the body of the mandible. This occurs at around 6th week of intrauterine life. The cartilage cells then disappear.
- The lingula of the mandibular foramen and the mental ossicles of the symphysis mentis are the ossified remnants of the cartilage and are incorporated with the body of the mandible.
- Between 10th and 14th week of intrauterine life, secondary cartilage develops which include the condylar cartilage, the coronoid and the symphyseal secondary cartilage. The condylar cartilage gives rise to condyle while secondary cartilage of coronoid forms coronoid.
- The two halves of mandible get united at midline by 4th–12th months postnatally.
- Major part of the mandible is formed by intramembranous ossification.

Clinical Considerations

- Mandibulofacial dysostosis—entire first arch may remain underdeveloped resulting in retrognathic mandible.

MULTIPLE CHOICE QUESTIONS (MCQs)

1. The basement membrane that separates the enamel organ and the dental papilla just prior to dentin formation is called the
a. Nasmyth's membrane
b. Enamel cuticle
c. Membrana preformativa
d. Dentinoenamel membrane

2. Enamel formation is influenced by
a. Stratum intermedium
b. Stratum reticulum
c. Membrane preformativa
d. All of the above

3. Stratum intermedium is present in
a. Bud stage
b. Bell stage
c. Cap stage
d. All of the above

4. The nucleus of the preameloblasts in the advanced bell stage is
a. In the basal region of the cell
b. In the distal end of the cell
c. In the middle of the cell
d. In the mesial region of the cell

5. The total activity of dental lamina extends over a period of
a. 2 years b. 4 years
c. 5 years d. 8 years

6. The dental lamina forms when the embryo is
a. 3 weeks old b. 4 weeks old
c. 6 weeks old d. 7 weeks old

7. Hertwig's epithelial root sheath consists of
a. Outer enamel epithelium (OEE) and inner enamel epithelium (IEE)
b. OEE, stellate reticulum and IEE
c. OEE, stratum intermedium and IEE
d. OEE and stratum intermedium only

8. The cells of dental follicle differentiate to form
a. Dentin and pulp
b. Pulp and cementum
c. PDL and cementum
d. Enamel

9. Initiation of tooth formation occurs at
a. First week of intrauterine life
b. Second week of intrauterine life
c. Sixth week of intrauterine life
d. Sixth month of intrauterine life

10. The cells of dental papilla differentiate to form
a. Enamel
b. Dentin and pulp
c. Pulp and cementum
d. Cementum and PDL

11. The buccopharyngeal membrane ruptures at approximately
a. 20th day of gestation
b. 25th day of gestation
c. 26th day of gestation
d. 27th day of gestation

12. The shape of the cells of stratum intermedium is
a. Squamous b. Columnar
c. Star shaped d. Cuboidal

13. The densely packed stellate reticulum cells in the center of the enamel organ in the cap stage is called
a. Enamel niche b. Enamel cord
c. Enamel knot d. Enamel tuft

14. The advanced bell stage marks the stage of
a. Histodifferentiation
b. Morphodifferentiation
c. Proliferation
d. Both a and b

1-c, 2-a, 3-b, 4-b, 5-c, 6-c, 7-a, 8-c, 9-c, 10-b, 11-d, 12-a, 13-c, 14-d

15. The following structures have influence in the initiation of enamel formation
a. Stratum intermedium
b. Membrana preformativa
c. Cervical loop
d. Stellate reticulum

16. If the organic matrix is normal but its mineralization is defective the condition is called
a. Hypoplasia
b. Hypocalcification or hypomineralization
c. Both a and b
d. None of the above

17. Both hypoplasia and hypocalcification can occur due to disturbance (insult) to the cells during
a. Proliferative stage
b. Histodifferentiation stage
c. Morphodifferentiation stage
d. Apposition stage

18. Disturbance in morphodifferentiation affects the
a. Form and size of the tooth
b. Matrix formation
c. Mineralization
d. All of the above

19. In vitamin A deficiency ameloblasts fail to differentiate properly due to which of the formation
a. Atypical enamel
b. Osteodentin
c. Hypoplastic dentin
d. Both a and b

20. All of the following structures are essential for tooth formation, *except*
a. Dental lamina
b. Membrana performativa
c. Dental papilla
d. Vestibular lamina

21. Stomodeum is lined by
a. Ectoderm b. Endoderm
c. Mesoderm d. Ectomesenchyme

22. The stellatet reticulum collapses
a. To facilitate the enamel formation
b. To facilitate the supply of nutrients to the IEE cells
c. To facilitate the supply of nutrients to the OEE cells
d. To facilitate the supply of nutrients to odontoblasts

23. The cells of stratum intermedium are closely attached by
a. Desmosomal junctions
b. Tight junctions
c. Gap junctions
d. Desmosomal and gap junctions

24. The time of initiation of first permanent molar is
a. Fourth month of intrauterine life
b. Sixth month of intrauterine life
c. Ninth month of intrauterine life
d. Sixth month after birth

25. The first evidence of calcification of the permanent first molars occurs approximately at
a. Six weeks of intrauterine life
b. At birth
c. Three years
d. Six years

26. The anatomical form of the roots of teeth is determined by
a. Dental lamina
b. Periodontal ligament
c. Epithelial attachment
d. Hertwig's epithelial root sheath

27. Stratum intermedium first appears during
a. Bud stage
b. Cap stage
c. Bell stage
d. None of the above

15-a, 16-b, 17-d, 18-a, 19-b, 20-d, 21-a, 22-b, 23-d, 24-a, 25-b, 26-d, 27-c

28. The permanent teeth are initiated by
a. Dental lamina
b. New tooth bud
c. Successional lamina
d. Enamel organ

29. The disturbance in the normal synthesis and secretion of the organic matrix leads to a condition called
a. Hypoplasia
b. Hypocalcification
c. Both a and b
d. None of the above

30. Morphologic outline of crown of tooth is determined by
a. Dentinoenamel membrane
b. Membrana preformativa
c. Dental papilla
d. Cervical loop

31. Lip furrow band is the
a. Dental lamina proper
b. Lateral dental lamina
c. Vestibular lamina
d. None of the above

32. The first hard tissue that is formed in the tooth is
a. Enamel
b. Dentin
c. Cementum
d. Alveolar bone

33. The successors of deciduous teeth develop from the
a. Distal extension of dental lamina
b. Lingual extension of dental lamina
c. Vestibular extension
d. None of the above

34. A cell active in secretory function usually shows
a. Decreased number of mitochondria
b. Increased rough endoplasmic reticulum
c. Increased number of lysosomes
d. Increase in size of nucleus

35. Remnants of dental lamina persist as
a. Enamel pearls
b. Epithelial pearls
c. Enamel cord
d. Cell rests of Malassez

36. The name for the lingual extension of dental lamina is
a. Vestibular lamina
b. Distal lamina
c. Successional lamina
d. All of the above

37. Tooth germ is made-up of
a. Dental organ
b. Dental papilla
c. Dental follicle
d. All of the above

38. Tomes' processes are
a. Conical processes of odontoblasts
b. Conical processes of ameloblasts
c. Conical processes of cementoblasts
d. Processes of osteoblast

39. Mulberry molars and peg laterals are formed as a result of disturbances in
a. Initiation
b. Histodifferentiation
c. Morphodifferentiation
d. Mineralisation

40. Hertwig's epithelial root sheath is formed by
a. Enamel organ
b. Dental lamina
c. Oral epithelium
d. None of the above

41. An enzyme present in stratum intermedium is
a. Acid phosphatase
b. Alkaline phosphatase
c. Esterase
d. Lysosomal sulfatase

28-c, 29-a, 30-b, 31-c, 32-b, 33-b, 34-b, 35-b, 36-c, 37-d, 38-b, 39-c, 40-a, 41-b

42. Enamel pulp is same as
a. Dental papilla
b. Stellate reticulum
c. Outer enamel epithelium
d. Inner enamel epithelium

43. Dental papilla becomes the pulp when
a. Cementum is laid down around dentin
b. Dentin is laid down around pulp
c. First layer of enamel is formed over it
d. None of the above.

44. The following is not a part of tooth bud
a. Dental papilla
b. Dental follicle
c. Vestibular lamina
d. Enamel organ

45. The permanent molars arise from the following extension of dental lamina
a. Lingual
b. Buccal
c. Distal
d. Mesial

46. The space between the jaws into which the teeth erupt is provided by growth at the
a. Alveolar process
b. Mandibular condyles
c. Intermaxillary sutures and mental symphysis
d. None of the above

47. A narrow developmental pit is most likely to be found on the lingual surface of
a. Maxillary canine
b. Maxillary central incisor
c. Maxillary lateral incisor
d. Mandibular central incisor

48. In a developing tooth, alkaline phosphate in present in
a. OEE
b. IEE
c. Stellate reticulum
d. Stratum intermedium

49. The number of visceral arches in humans are
a. 2 b. 4
c. 5 d. 6

50. The name of the first visceral arch is
a. Hyoid b. Maxillary
c. Mandibular d. None of the above

51. The second visceral arch is
a. Hyoid b. Mandibular
c. Maxillary d. None of the above

52. Which of the following statement is true?
a. Foramen caecum is present at the junction of anterior two-thirds and posterior one-third of the tongue
b. Anterior two-third of the tongue is covered by ectoderm and posterior one-thirds is covered by endoderm
c. The epithelial components of the salivary glands are derived from oral ectoderm
d. All of the above

53. Median rhomboid glossitis is
a. Caused by persistence of tuberculum impar
b. Red and rhomboidal smooth zone of the tongue
c. Found in midline in front of the foramen caecum
d. All of the above

54. Membrane preformativa is seen during
a. Bell stage
b. Cap stage
c. Bud stage
d. Advanced bell stage

55. Life of successional lamina is from the
a. 5th month *in utero* to the 10th month of age
b. Third month *in utero* to the 10th month of age
c. 5th month *in utero* to the 10th month *in utero*
d. 6 weeks of embryo to the 10th month *in utero*

42-b, 43-b, 44-c, 45-c, 46-b, 47-c, 48-d, 49-d, 50-c, 51-a, 52-d, 53-a, 54-a, 55-a

56. Epithelial pearls are found
a. Within the jaw
b. In the gingiva
c. None of the above
d. Both a and b

57. Retarded eruption of teeth occurs in persons with
a. Hypopituitarism and hypothyroidism
b. Hyperpituitarism
c. Hyperthyroidism
d. None of the above

58. The layer of enamel organ which has Cushioning effect is
a. Inner enamel epithelium
b. Stellate reticulum
c. Stratum intermedium
d. Outer enamel epithelium

59. The component that is absent in enamel organ is
a. Dental sac
b. Stellate reticulum
c. Stratum intermedium
d. Outer enamel epithelium

60. One of the following is not true about dental lamina
a. The total activity lasts for approximately 5 years
b. It persists as epithelial pearls
c. It is derived from ectoderm
d. Derived from mesoderm

61. The calcified tissue which has the largest hydroxyapatite crystals is
a. Enamel
b. Dentin
c. Cementum
d. Bone

62. Periodontal ligament develops from
a. Enamel organ
b. Dental papilla
c. Perifollicular mesenchyme
d. None of the above

63. In the bell stage, the cells in the center of enamel organ continue to synthesize and secrete
a. Glycogen
b. Glycosaminoglycans
c. Alkaline phosphatase
d. Proteins

64. The branchial arches are separated from each other by
a. The stomodeum
b. Prosencephalon
c. The neural groove
d. Ectodermal to endodermal groove

65. The process which does not play any role in the development of face is
a. Maxillary process
b. Mandibular
c. Frontonasal
d. Ethmoidal

66. Each maxillary process forms a horizontal extension termed as
a. The lateral nasal process
b. The internal nares
c. The median nasal septum
d. The palatal process

67. The anterior two-thirds of the tongue develops from the
a. The first arch mesenchyme
b. The copula
c. The hypobranchial eminence
d. The tuberculum impar and adjacent tissue

68. The salivary glands develop from
a. Ectodermal germ layer
b. Endodermal germ layer
c. Ectodermal and endodermal germ layers
d. Oral mesenchyme

56-d, 57-a, 58-b, 59-a, 60-d, 61-a, 62-c, 63-a, 64-d, 65-d, 66-a, 67-a, 68-a

69. The developing mandible grows back (not surrounding Meckel's Cartilage) to form

a. The malleus
b. Otic capsule
c. The hyoid cartilage
d. The coronoid process

70. When a tooth erupts, the percentage of root formation completed is

a. 20%
b. 30%
c. 50%
d. 80%

71. The embryonic connective tissue under the oral ectoderm is termed ecto-mesenchyme because

a. It has both ectodermal and mesenchymal cells
b. It has migrated neural crest cells in it
c. It has characteristics similar to ectodermal cells
d. None of the above

72. The primary epithelial band is

a. Same as dental lamina
b. It is the structure that gives rise to dental lamina and vestibular lamina
c. Same as lip furrow band
d. None of the above

73. The cell rests of Malassez in the periodontal ligament are derived from

a. Dental pulp
b. Lamina propria
c. Odontogenic epithelium
d. Vestibular lamina

74. The precise expression of growth and transcription factors associated with future cusp formation takes place in the

a. Enamel cord
b. Enamel knot
c. Inner enamel epithelium
d. None of the above

75. Reciprocal induction is seen between the

a. Cementoblast and odontoblast
b. Cementoblast and osteoblast
c. Ameloblast and odontoblast
d. None of the above

76. Hypoplasia is

a. Disturbance in matrix formation
b. Disturbance in calcification
c. Disturbance in maturation
d. All of the above

77. The correct sequence of dental tissues from softest to hardest is

a. Dentin, cementum, enamel
b. Cementum, dentin, enamel
c. Dentin, enamel, cementum
d. Cementum, enamel dentin

69-a, 70-c, 71-b, 72-b, 73-c, 74-b, 75-c, 76-a, 77-b

Chapter

14

Enamel

LAQ (10 Marks)

Q 1. Describe different stages in the life cycle of ameloblasts in detail.

(June 2006, 2009, 2011, 2014, Nov. 2015)

Ans. LIFE CYCLE OF AMELOBLASTS

Introduction

- During development of tooth, the inner enamel epithelial (IEE) cells of enamel organ differentiate into ameloblasts which produce enamel matrix and help in its mineralization.
- According to their function, the life cycle of ameloblasts can be divided into 6 stages.
  1. Morphogenic stage } pre-secretory stage
  2. Organizing stage } pre-secretory stage
  3. Formative stage/secretory stage
  4. Maturative stage/transitional or maturation proper
  5. Protective stage } post-maturation stage
  6. Desmolytic stage } post-maturation stage
- Differentiation of ameloblasts is most advanced in the region of incisal edge or cusp tip.

1. Morphogenic Stage

- During the bell stage of tooth development, the cells of the IEE interact with adjacent mesenchymal cells, determining the shape of the dentinoenamel junction and the crown.
- At this stage, the cells of the IEE are short and columnar with large oval nucleus that almost fills the cell body (Fig. 14.1A).
- The golgi apparatus are near the proximal (basal) portion of the cells (near the stratum intermedium) whereas the mitochondria and other cytoplasmic components, are scattered throughout the cytoplasm.

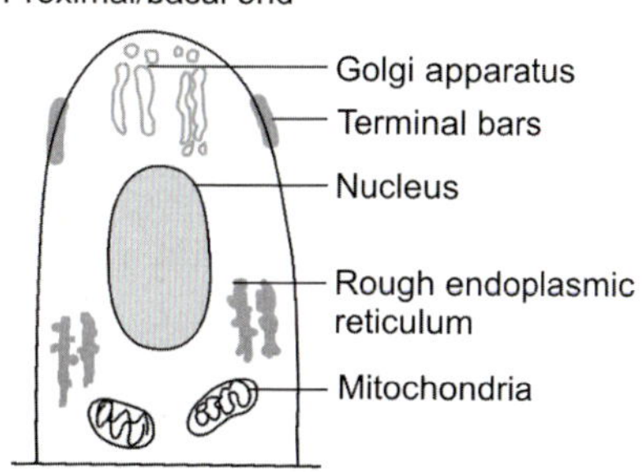

Fig. 14.1A: Morphogenic stage of ameloblast

- During ameloblast differentiation, terminal bars appear between the adjacent cells concomitantly along with migration of mitochondria to the basal region of the cells. Terminal bars represent areas of close contact between the cells.
- IEE is separated from the connective tissue of dental papilla by a delicate basal lamina.
- The adjacent pulpal layer is a cell-free zone.

2. Organizing Stage

- This stage is characterized by a change in the appearance of the IEE cells. They become elongated and the nucleus-free zone at the distal end becomes almost as long as the proximal part containing the nucleus.
- Majority of the cell organelles migrate from the proximal end of the cell to the distal end. This is called as **"reversal of functional polarity" (Fig. 14.1B).** Thus, ameloblast becomes a highly polarized cell for the functional need to secrete the enamel matrix from the distal end.

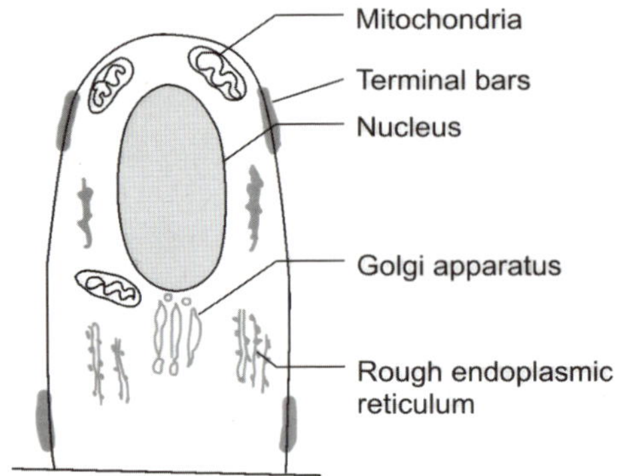

Fig. 14.1B: Organizing stage of ameloblast: Reversal of functional polarity

- Clear cell-free zone between IEE and dental papilla disappears as elongation of the cells of IEE occurs. This causes the epithelial cells to come in contact with the connective tissue cells of the dental papilla which differentiate into odontoblasts. This is a part of epithelial-mesenchymal interaction during tooth development.
- During the terminal phase of this stage, formation of dentin by odontoblasts begins.
- The first appearance of dentin seems to be a critical phase in the life cycle of the cells of IEE. As long as the IEE cells are in contact with the connective tissue cells of the dental papilla they receive nutrients from the blood vessels of the dental papilla. However, after deposition of first layer of dentin, the IEE cells are cut-off from their original source of nourishment and from then on they are supplied by the capillaries that surround outer enamel epithelium (OEE).
- This reversal of nutritional source is characterized by proliferation of capillaries of the dental sac and by reduction and gradual collapse of the stellate reticulum. Thus, the distance between the capillaries and stratum intermedium and ameloblasts is reduced.

3. Formative/Secretory Stage

- Ameloblasts enter the formative stage after the first layer of dentin is laid down (Fig. 14.1C).
- Presence of dentin seems to be necessary for the beginning of enamel matrix formation.
- Morphology of ameloblasts at this stage reveals their intense synthetic and secretory activity, so as to form enamel matrix.
- The earliest apparent change is the development of a blunt process on the ameloblast surface called the Tomes' process.
- Synthesis of enamel proteins occurs in the rough endoplasmic reticulum from where it is passed to golgi complex in which it is condensed and packaged into membrane bound secretory granules (Fig. 14.1D).
- Contents of secretory granules are released as enamel matrix against the newly formed mantle dentin.

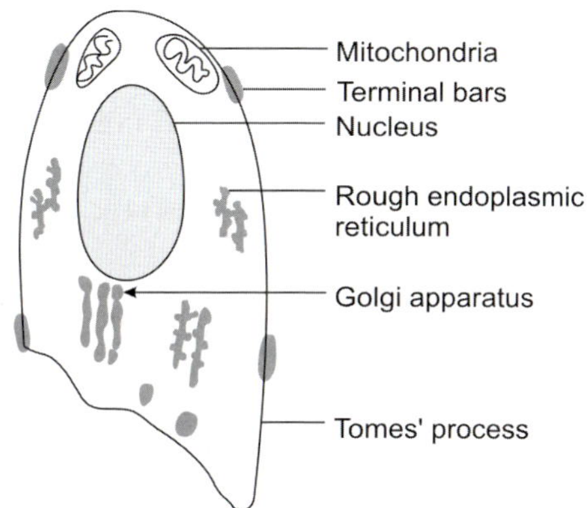

Fig. 14.1C: Formative/secretory stage of ameloblast

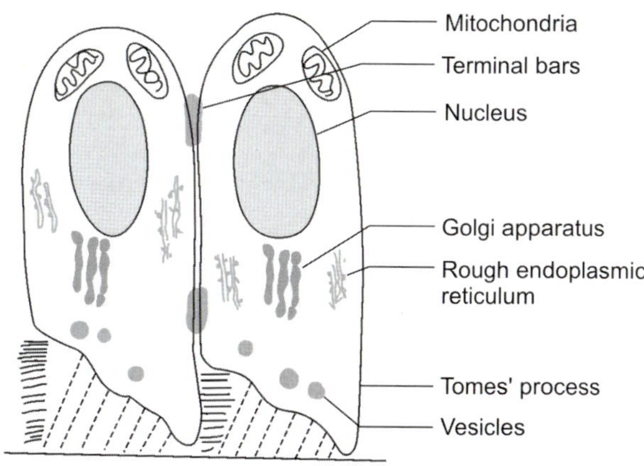

Fig. 14.1D: Synthesis of enamel proteins by Tomes' process

4. Maturative Stage

- Enamel maturation (full mineralization) occurs after most of the thickness of the enamel matrix has been formed in the occlusal or incisal area.
- During this stage there is reduction in the height of the ameloblasts and decrease in its volume and organelle content.
- Ameloblasts display microvilli at their distal extremities which indicate an absorptive function of these cells (Fig. 14.1E).
- This morphology alternates with that of smooth ended ameloblasts (Fig. 14.1E).

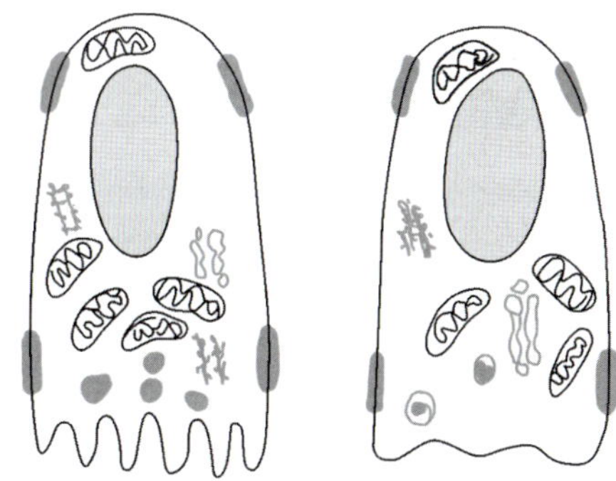

Fig. 14.1E: Maturative stage of ameloblast

- Ameloblasts with microvilli promote the calcium influx into the maturing enamel and smooth bordered ameloblasts promote the removal of proteins and water.
- Process of maturation starts from the height of the crown and progresses cervically.

5. Protective Stage/Post-maturation

- When the enamel has completely developed and has fully calcified, ameloblasts cease to be arranged in a well-defined layer.
- They are no longer differentiated from the cells of the stratum intermedium and outer enamel epithelium.
- These cell layers then form a stratified epithelial covering of the enamel which is known as **reduced enamel epithelium** (REE).
- Function of REE is to protect the mature enamel by separating it from the connective tissue until the tooth erupts (Fig. 14.1F).
- During this stage if the connective tissue comes in contact with the enamel, anomalies may develop. Under such conditions enamel may be either resorbed or covered by a layer of cementum.

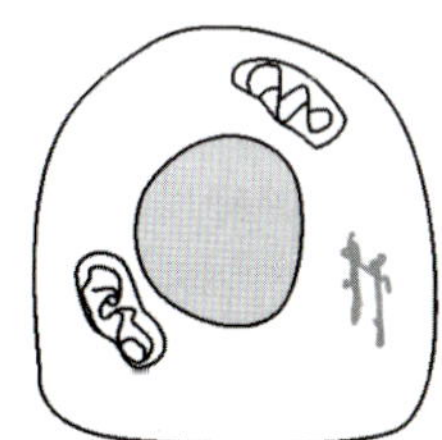

Fig. 14.1F: Protective stage of ameloblast

6. Desmolytic Stage

- REE proliferates and seems to induce atrophy of the connective tissue, which separates it from the oral epithelium, so that fusion of REE with oral epithelium can occur.
- The epithelial cells elaborate enzymes that are able to destroy connective tissue fibers by desmolysis.
- Premature degeneration of the REE may prevent eruption of tooth.

Clinical Significance

1. Ameloblasts are very sensitive cells. Infections, trauma, chemicals and metabolic changes involving calcium or phosphorus affect ameloblasts. As a result, they produce decreased thickness of enamel, called *enamel hypoplasia* or decreased mineralization, called *enamel hypomineralization.*
2. Fluorosis affects enamel. It is chemical intoxication of ameloblasts when drinking water has fluoride in excess of 1.5 parts per million.

SAQs (3 Marks)

Q 1. Describe physical and chemical properties of enamel. (*May 2002, Nov. 2009, 2010*)

Ans. PHYSICAL AND CHEMICAL PROPERTIES OF ENAMEL

Introduction

- Enamel is the hard mineralized tissue covering the anatomic crown of tooth. It is acellular and avascular.
- Highest content of mineral salts along with crystalline arrangement makes it hardest calcified tissue in the human body.

Physical Properties

- ***Thickness:*** Enamel forms a protective covering of variable thickness over different parts of the crown with a maximum of 2.5 mm at the cusp tips to less than 100 at the neck of the tooth.
- ***Density and hardness:*** High mineral content and crystalline arrangement of mineral salts makes enamel the hardest tissue in the human body. This hardness enables it to withstand the heavy masticatory forces. Density of enamel is 2.8–3. Knoop hardness number is 343.
- ***Brittleness:*** Enamel is brittle, having a low tensile strength due to its structure and the hardness.
- ***Colour:*** Enamel is translucent. Its colour varies from light yellow to grayish white. Colour is determined by difference in the translucency of enamel, which is influenced by the thickness of enamel. Thinner areas appear more yellowish as the underlying dentin is seen through the thin translucent enamel.
- ***Permeability:*** It is semipermeable.
- ***Temperature resistance:*** Enamel is an insulator at room temperature. It is a non-electrical conducive material.

Chemical Properties

- Enamel consists mainly of inorganic (96%) and only a small amount of organic substance (4%).
- ***Organic content:*** Organic part is present between and around the crystals. It consists of protein and water. It has two groups of proteins, amelogenins and nonamelogenins Amelogenins account for 90% of the enamel proteins, are hydrophobic and are of low molecular weight. Nonamelogenins (enamelin, ameloblastin and tuftelin) account for 10% of enamel matrix proteins and are high molecular weight proteins. Enamel proteins do not contribute to structuring of enamel.
- ***Inorganic content:*** The inorganic material of enamel is hydroxyapatite $[Ca_{10} (PO_4)_6 (OH_4)_2]$ and various ions such as strontium, magnesium, lead, and fluoride. The crystals of hydroxyapatite are hexagonal in cross-section and are arranged to form enamel rods or prisms. The hydroxyapatite crystal has a central core or C axis of hydroxyl ion around which calcium and phosphorus ions are arranged in the form of triangles.
- Water is present as a part of hydroxyapatite crystal, between crystals and between rods and surrounding the rods.

Q 2. Describe hypocalcified structures of enamel. *(June 2006, Nov. 2009)*

Ans. HYPOCALCIFIED STRUCTURES OF ENAMEL

- Enamel is the hardest calcified tissue of body, forming the outermost covering of tooth crown.
- Hypocalcified structures in enamel are those which have higher organic content than enamel tissue as a whole. These occur due to less removal of organic matrix and water during development. They contribute to the microporosity of enamel.
- These structures are:
  1. Enamel lamellae
  2. Enamel tufts
  3. Enamel spindles
  4. Neonatal line
  5. Lines of Retzius
  6. Cross striations

1. Enamel Lamellae (*SAQ, May 2009, 2010, 2013*)

- They are hypocalcified thin, leaf-like structures that extend from the enamel surface towards the dentinoenamel junction (DEJ) (Fig. 14.2).

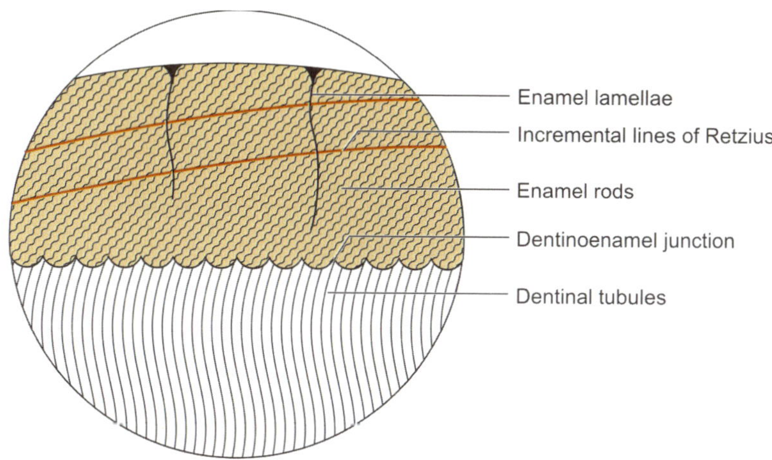

Fig. 14.2: Enamel lamellae

- They consist of organic material but with little mineral content.
- They may extend to and sometimes penetrate into the dentin.
- In ground section, these structures maybe confused with cracks caused by the grinding of the specimen. Crack can be distinguished from lamella by careful decalcification of ground section of the tooth which will cause disappearance of the cracks but lamella will persist.
- Lamellae may develop in planes of tension. When rods cross such a plane, a short segment of rod may not fully calcify. If the disturbance is more severe and occurs in unerupted tooth, a crack may develop that is filled by surrounding cells. If the crack develops after eruption it gets filled by organic substances from the oral cavity.

Types of Lamellae

Three types of lamellae are present:

In type A, lamella is composed of poorly calcified rod segments.

In type B, it consists of degenerated cells.

In type C, the lamellae in erupted teeth are the cracks filled with organic matter from saliva, this type is more common.

Type A and B are produced during enamel formation and type C is produced after eruption. Lamellae of type A are restricted to the enamel, while those of types B and C may reach into the dentin.

Significance

It may be a site of weakness in a tooth and may act as pathways for caries producing bacteria.

2. Enamel Tufts

- Are hypocalcified structures that originate at the DEJ and extend into enamel for about one-third of its thickness.
- Tufts form between groups of enamel rods, which are oriented in slightly different directions at the DEJ which is scalloped. Tufts arise from these scalloped peaks.
- They resemble tufts of grass. They do not spring out from a single small area but are narrow, ribbon-like structures. The impression of a tuft of grass is created by examining such structures in thick sections (Fig. 14.3).

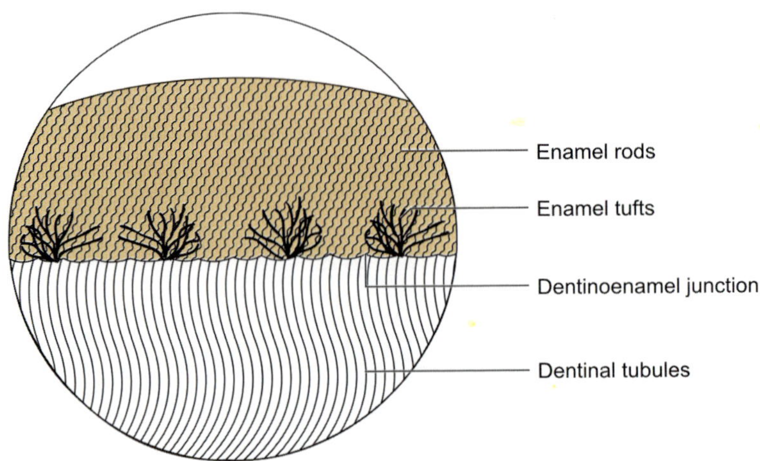

Fig. 14.3: Enamel tufts

- Tufts consist of hypocalcified enamel rods and interprismatic substance. These are areas where young enamel proteins are not completely transformed during maturation.
- Enamel tufts are tubular structures with cross striations as shown by scanning electron microscope.
- They are well-appreciated in cross-sections.
- Developmentally, they are formed due to abrupt changes in the rod direction which leads to different ratio of inter-rod enamel. Their development is a consequence of an adaptation to the spatial conditions in the enamel.

Significance

- At tufts the caries spreads laterally.

3. Enamel Spindles

- They arise at DEJ and extend into enamel. Enamel spindles are the odontoblastic processes that extend into the enamel across DEJ before hard tissue formation (Fig. 14.4).
- They are the only hypocalcified structures of enamel that are not derived ectodermally but are derived from dentin.
- Enamel spindles are channels of about 2 microns in diameter and contain small needle-like crystals or granular and/or amorphosus material, as shown by transmission electron microscope.
- As they are thickened at their ends they are named as enamel spindle. They are found mainly in the cusp tip regions.
- The direction of the spindles corresponds to the original direction of the ameloblast, that is right angles to the surface of dentin. Since the enamel rods are formed at an angle to the axis of the ameloblast, the direction of rod and spindle is divergent.
- Enamel spindles are shorter than the tufts. Enamel spindles, tufts and lamellae contain less calcium and phosphorus than enamel prisms.
- In ground sections of teeth, the organic content of spindle disintegrates and is replaced by air and the spaces appear dark in transmitted light.

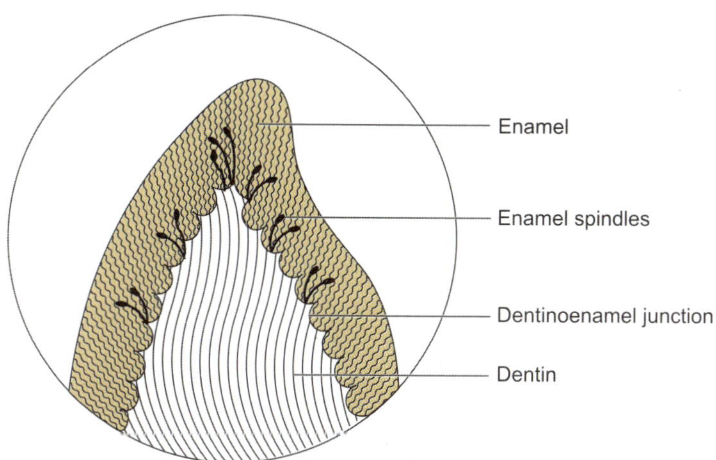

Fig. 14.4: Enamel spindles

4. Lines of Retzius/Incremental Lines (*SAQ, Dec. 2005*)

- They represent the incremental pattern of the enamel.
- They appear as brownish bands in ground section of the enamel.
- They mark the successive apposition of layers of enamel during formation of crown. The mean daily rate of enamel formation is about 3.5 microns. In longitudinal section, incremental lines surround the tip of dentin. In transverse sections of tooth, they appear as concentric circles.
- They have been attributed to periodic bending of the enamel rods, to variations in the basic organic structure or to a physiological calcification rhythm.
- The occurrence of few striae is considered normal but when they are present in great numbers or as a broad band, it indicates periods of metabolic disturbances.
- **Perikymata** are transverse wave-like grooves which are believed to be the external manifestations of lines of Retzius (Fig. 14.5).

5. Neonatal Line

- An accentuated striae which represents the disturbances at birth is the neonatal line or neonatal ring.
- The enamel of deciduous teeth develops partly before and partly after birth. The boundary between the prenatal and postnatal enamel is marked by the neonatal line or neonatal ring.
- It appears to be the result of the abrupt change in the environment and nutrition of the newborn infant.
- Prenatal enamel is better developed than the postnatal. This is explained by the fact that the fetus is developed in a well-protected environment with an adequate supply of all the essential materials, even at the expense of the mother.
- Postnatal enamel has more defects and it is darker.
- Neonatal lines are found more frequently in primary teeth and permanent first molars (Fig. 14.5).

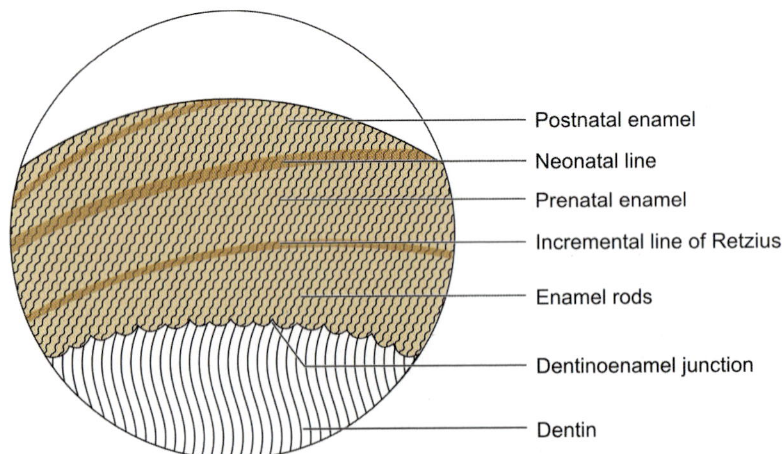

Fig. 14.5: Incremental lines of Retzius and neonatal line

6. Perikymata

- Perikymata are transverse wavelike grooves present on outer surface of newly erupted teeth.
- They are external manifestations of the striae of Retzius.
- Because of the undisturbed and even development of the enamel prior to birth, perikymata are absent in the occlusal parts of deciduous teeth. They are present in the postnatal cervical parts.

7. Cross Striations

- Each enamel rod is build-up of segments separated by dark lines that gives it a striated appearance.
- The rods are segmented because the enamel matrix is laid in a rhythmic manner.
- Cross striations are the structures that mark the daily growth increment in human enamel and are 4 µm apart.
- They run at right angles to the enamel rods.
- They are more pronounced in enamel that is insufficiently calcified.
- In these areas rods show varicosities and variation in composition.

Q 3. What is Nasmyth's membrane? *(May 2008)*

Ans. DEVELOPMENTAL ENAMEL CUTICLE/NASMYTH'S MEMBRANE/DENTAL CUTICLE/PRIMARY ENAMEL CUTICLE

- It is a delicate membrane that covers the entire crown of the newly erupted tooth but is probably soon removed by mastication.
- It is about 0.5 to 1.5 mm thick. It is acellular. It is formed as the final secretory product of ameloblasts. It is basal lamina secreted by ameloblasts.
- This cuticle is apparently secreted by ameloblasts when enamel formation is completed. It is formed after the epithelial enamel organ retracts from the cervical region during tooth development.
- ***Function*** is to protect the enamel from the resorptive activity of the adjacent vascular tissue prior to the eruption of the teeth.

Q 4. What is Tomes' process?

Ans. TOMES' PROCESS

- The surface of ameloblasts facing the developing enamel is not smooth but has a projection penetrating into the enamel matrix, named as **Tomes' process.**
- At first ameloblasts form a structureless enamel layer. Once this structureless enamel layer is formed, ameloblasts migrate away from the dentin surface and each ameloblast develops a short conical projection known as **Tomes' process.** All enamel matrix secretions from then occurs through the Tomes' process.
- Although the cytoplasm of the ameloblasts continues into the Tomes' process, distinction between the process and the cell body is clearly marked by distal terminal bar, which is a distal junctional complex.
- Tomes' process contain secretory granules, rough endoplasmic reticulum and mitochondria.
- Junctional complexes encircle the ameloblast at their distal and proximal ends which serve to control the substances that pass between ameloblast and enamel.

- Secretions from areas close to junctional complexes and from adjacent ameloblasts form the inter-rod enamel. They serve to outline the pit into which secretions from Tomes' process occur later to form the enamel rod.
- This mechanism of enamel formation creates the rod-like structure of enamel.
- Tomes' process persists until the formation of the final few increments of enamel, when it is lost. As a result, the final few increments of enamel are also structureless.

Q 5. Write about Hunter-Schreger bands. *(July 2005)*

Ans. HUNTER-SCHREGER BANDS

Introduction

- These are alternating dark and light strips of varying width that can be seen in longitudinal ground section under oblique reflected light.
- They originate at dentinoenamel junction and pass outward, ending at some distance from the outer enamel surface (Fig. 14.6).

Reason for Appearance

- The change in the direction of rods is responsible for the appearance of the Hunter-Schreger bands.
- The prisms which are cut longitudinally to produce dark bands are called *diazones,* while the prisms which are cut transversely to produce light bands, are called *parazones.* The angle between the parazones and diazones is 40 degrees.
- In the outer third of enamel, the prisms do not bend, hence these bands are absent.
- These structures may not be the sole result of an optical phenomenon but they are actually composed of alternate zones having different permeability and different content of organic material.

Clinical Significance

- The more or less regular change in the direction of the rod may be regarded as functional adaptation, minimizing the risk of cleavage in the axial direction under the influence of occlusal masticatory forces.

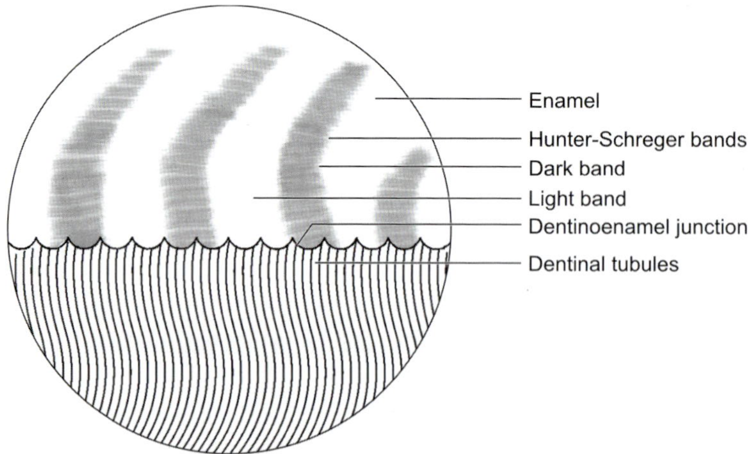

Fig. 14.6: Hunter-Schreger bands

Q 6. Describe surface structures of enamel. *(Oct. 2004)*

Ans. Introduction

Surface Structures of Enamel

Structures seen on the outer surface of enamel are:

1. Aprismatic enamel/structureless layer of enamel
2. Perikymata
3. Enamel rod ends
4. Cracks
5. Cuticle

1. Aprismatic Enamel/Structureless Layer of Enamel/Prismless Enamel

- It is hypermineralized and rodless layer of enamel near the dentinoenamel junction (DEJ), approximately 30 µm thick.
- It is present in almost 70% of permanent teeth and all deciduous teeth.
- It is found commonly towards cervical areas of enamel.
- It is deposited by ameloblasts before formation of Tomes' process.
- All the apatite crystals in it are parallel to one another and perpendicular to the striae of Retzius.

2. Perikymata/Imbrication Lines (June 2004)

- They are transverse wavelike grooves believed to be the external manifestation of the striae of Retzius in enamel.
- They are continuous around a tooth and usually lie parallel to each other and the cementoenamel junction (CEJ).
- There are about 30 perikymata per milliimeter in the region of the CEJ, gradually decrease to 10 per millimeter near the incisal or occlusal surface.
- They are not found in the occlusal third of the deciduous teeth as they are formed prenatally during which time the enamel formation occurs in an undisturbed and even manner.

3. Enamel Rod Ends

- They are concave and vary in depth and shape. They are shallow in cervical region and deepest in occlusal region.

4. Cracks

- Are narrow, fissure like structures. They are the outer edges of the lamellae.
- They extend for varying lengths along the surface at right angles to the DEJ.
- Ultrastructurally, the surface of the enamel appears very uneven. *Pits* of about 1–1.5 µm in diameter and small elevations of about 10–15 µm called *enamel caps* are seen. The surface pits are said to represent the ends of ameloblast and the caps are due to enamel deposition on nonmineralizable debris. Larger enamel elevations are *enamel brochs.*

5. Enamel Cuticle

A. Developmental
B. Acquired

A. ***Developmental enamel cuticle/Nasmyth's membrane/Dental cuticle/Primary enamel cuticle*:**
- It is a delicate membrane that covers the entire crown of the newly erupted tooth but is probably soon removed by mastication.
- It is about 0.5 to 1.5 mm thick. It is acellular. It is formed as the final secretory product of ameloblasts. It is basal lamina secreted by ameloblasts.
- This cuticle is secreted after the epithelial organ retracts from the cervical region during tooth development.

B. ***Acquired*:**
- It is the pellicle that covers erupted enamel which is apparently a precipitate of salivary proteins.
- This pellicle reforms within hours after an enamel surface is mechanically cleaned.
- It becomes colonized by microorganisms to form a bacterial plaque.

Q 7. Write about gnarled enamel. *(June 2001)*

Ans. Gnarled Enamel
- Generally, the enamel rods are oriented at right angles to the dentin surface. The rods are rarely straight, they have a wavy course from dentin to the enamel surface.
- The enamel rods below the cusps and incisal region appear irregularly twisted and interwined. This optical appearance of enamel is called **gnarled enamel** (Fig. 14.7).
- Unlike the Hunter-Schreger bands, gnarled enamel extends throughout the thickness of enamel at the cusp tips and incisal edges.
- It resists the high masticatory loads that the cusps or incisal edges have to bear.

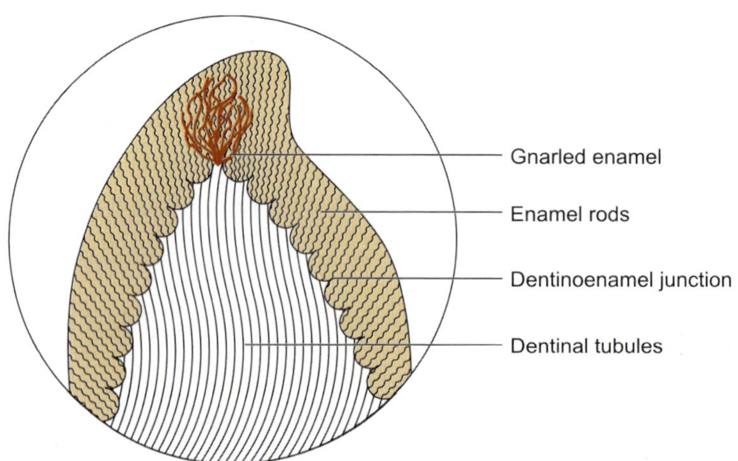

Fig. 14.7: Gnarled enamel

Q 8. What is reduced enamel epithelium (REE)? *(May 2014)*

Ans. Reduced Enamel Epithelium
- During the protective stage in the life cycle of ameloblast, when the enamel is completely developed and has fully calcified, ameloblasts cease to be arranged in a well-defined layer.
- They are no longer differentiated from the cells of the stratum intermedium and outer enamel epithelium.
- These cell layers then form a stratified epithelial covering of the enamel which is known as reduced enamel epithelium (REE).

Functions

- The function of REE is to protect the mature enamel by separating it from the connective tissue until the tooth erupts.
- The epithelial cells elaborate enzymes that are able to destroy connective tissue fibers by desmolysis. This causes fusion of REE with oral epithelium. This helps in eruption of teeth.

Significance

- If reduced enamel epithelium is delayed in its separation from dentin, cementum and dentin do not meet and this result in formation of gap type of cementoenamel junction.
- If REE degenerates prematurely, the connective tissue comes in contact with the enamel and anomalies may develop. Under such conditions, enamel may be either resorbed or covered by a layer of cementum.
- Premature degeneration of the REE may also prevent the eruption of tooth.

Q 9. Describe age changes in enamel.

Ans. **AGE CHANGES IN ENAMEL**

- Enamel is a non-vital tissue and is incapable of replacement.
- Attrition is the most apparent age change in enamel. It is wearing off of the occlusal surface and proximal contact points as a result of mastication. This is evident by a loss of vertical dimension of the crown and by flattening of the proximal contour. The earliest clinical change is the loss of mamelons. Loss of enamel could also be due to mechanical wear (abrasion) and chemical wear (erosion).
- The surfaces of unerupted and recently erupted teeth are covered with pronounced rod ends and perikymata. With age there is generalised loss of rod ends and flattening of perikymata.
- Teeth darken with age which could be due to addition of organic material from environment or due to deepening of dentin color seen through the progressive thinning of translucent enamel.
- Enamel becomes less permeable to fluids with age which could be due to the increase in the size of the crystals which decrease the pores between the crystals. Intake of ions such as nitrogen, fluorine, from oral fluids, accumulates at the surface layers which causes the crystals to become bigger, reducing the pores between them.
- Resistance to decay increases with age.
- Enamel becomes harder with age. However, it tends to become more brittle. Increased hardness is attributable to the uptake of fluoride by the surface layers of enamel.

Q 10. Explain amelogenesis.

Ans. **AMELOGENESIS**

Amelogenesis is the formation of enamel which occurs during advanced stage of tooth development after the first layer of dentin has been laid down.

Enamel formation comprises two stages:

1. Secretion/formation of enamel matrix
2. Mineralisation

Enamel formation differs from other hard tissues like dentin, cementum and bone which are all derived from connective tissue. Enamel is derived from ectoderm and has a unique organic matrix. Noncollagenous proteins are involved in mineralization of enamel whereas collagen plays an important role in mineralization of dentin and bone. Matrix of enamel does not contain collagen while it is present in bone, dentin and cementum. The matrix of enamel is partially mineralized while in other hard tissues matrix is nonmineralized. Enamel lacks a distinct organic phase.

1. Secretion or Formation of Enamel Matrix

- Ameloblasts begin their secretory activity after a layer of dentin has been laid down.
- During tooth development, the low columnar cells of the inner enamel epithelium (IEE) supported by a basement membrane are separated from the acellular zone of the dental papilla.
- When dental papilla cells differentiate into odontoblasts, the IEE cells become tall and columnar and their nuclei become aligned at the proximal end of the cells adjacent to the stratum intermedium. This is *reversal of polarity.*
- Message is sent by preameloblasts to newly differentiated odontoblasts, which lay down predentin. This, in turn, causes the differentiation of secretory ameloblasts which secrete enamel matrix over the newly formed dentin. This is reciprocal epithelial-mesenchymal interaction.
- This matrix immediately becomes partially mineralized. Secretion and partial mineralization continues until almost all of the entire thickness of enamel has been formed.
- As the first increment of enamel is formed, the ameloblasts begin to move away from the dentin surface and soon each cell forms a short conical projection called **Tomes' process** which penetrates into the newly formed enamel.
- There is an interdigitation of the cells and the enamel rod that they produce. This is because the long axes of the ameloblasts are not parallel to the long axes of the rods.
- Four ameloblasts are required for synthesis of one enamel rod.
- Head of each enamel rod is formed by one ameloblast whereas three other ameloblasts contribute to the tail of each rod. Thus, each enamel rod is formed by four ameloblasts and each ameloblast contributes to four different rods.
- When secretion of full thickness of enamel is completed, the ameloblasts shorten, lose their Tomes' processes and become involved in the maturation of the enamel.

2. Enamel Mineralization and Maturation

Mineralization of enamel matrix takes place in two stages:

- In the *first stage* immediate partial mineralization occurs in the matrix segments and the interprismatic substance. Nucleation for mineralization in enamel is initiated by the apatite crystallites of dentin on which enamel is laid. Matrix vesicles are not involved in enamel formation. There is no unmineralized matrix like that of predentin or osteoid during enamel formation. This first formed enamel consists of approximately 65% water, 20% organic material and 15% inorganic material.
- The *second stage* or maturation is characterized by the gradual completion of mineralization, i.e. growth of mineral crystals and withdrawal of substantial amount of protein and water. The original ribbon-shaped crystals increase in thickness than in width. Crystals increase in size from 15 to 25 μm during maturation.
- Maturation begins before the matrix has reached its full thickness.

- Pattern of mineralization/maturation progresses from DEJ towards enamel surface.
- Each rod matures from the depth to the surface of enamel and the sequence of the maturing rods is from cusps or incisal edge toward the cervical line.
- This means incisal and occlusal region reach maturity ahead of the cervical region.
- Maturation is characterized by growth of the crystals. It involves selective removal of proteinaceous material so as to make space for growing mineral crystals.
- Ameloblasts alternate cyclically in developing smooth and ruffled borders in the apical cytoplasm during maturation stage in a cervioocclusal direction. This is modulation. The ruffled ended ameloblasts have their villous surface, packed with mitochondria. They show numerous lysosomes and possess endocyte activity. They also promote calcium entry into the forming enamel. The smooth ended ameloblasts leak small proteins and water into forming enamel.
- In enamel 90% of secreted matrix is absorbed while in other hard tissues there is no absorption of secreted matrix.
- The rate of formation of enamel is 4 µm/day. The rate of formation is more in permanent teeth than in deciduous teeth.
- As the enamel formation continues cells of the outer enamel epithelium, stellate reticulum, and stratum intermedium gradually lose their discrete identities and form a stratified epithelial layer adjacent to the ameloblasts.
- Once the maturation is completed, the ameloblast layer, together with the adjacent stratified layer constitutes the reduced enamel epithelium (REE).
- Though it is no longer involved in the secretion and maturation of enamel, REE continues to cover enamel till tooth eruption and has a protective function.

Clinical Considerations

1. During amelogenesis if matrix formation is affected, *enamel hypoplasia* results. If maturation is lacking or incomplete, *hypocalcification of the enamel* results.
2. Systemic hypocalcification of enamel due to high fluoride content in water is called as mottled enamel.
3. After formation of enamel, ameloblasts undergo apoptosis, hence there is no formation of enamel later in life unlike in other hard tissues.

Q 11. Write about dentinoenamel junction.

Ans. DENTINOENAMEL JUNCTION

- The junction between enamel and dentin is not straight but appears as a scolloped line. (Refer Fig. 14.6)
- The surface of the dentin at the dentinoenamel junction (DEJ) is pitted. Into the shallow depressions of the dentin, fit rounded projections of the enamel. This relation assures the firm hold of the enamel on the dentin.
- The convexities of the scallops of DEJ are directed towards the dentin.
- The pitted dentinoenamel junction is preformed even before the development of hard tissues.
- In the DEJ, the crystals of dentin and enamel mix with each other.
- DEJ is more pronounced in the occlusal area, where masticatory stresses are greater.

Q 12. Describe structure of enamel or ultrastructure of enamel.

Ans. ULTRASTRUCTURE OF ENAMEL

- Enamel is the hardest calcified tissue of body, which forms the outermost covering of the tooth crown.
- It is composed of enamel rods or prisms, rod sheaths, and a cementing interprismatic substance.
- Enamel rods are cylindrical in shape. Their number ranges from 5 million in lower lateral incisors to 12 million in the upper first molars.
- Enamel rods run in oblique direction from dentinoenamel junction (DEJ) to the outer surface of enamel. They have wavy course. Rods located in the cusps are longer than those at the cervical areas of teeth.
- Average diameter of enamel rod is 4 microns but it varies. At the outer surface of the enamel, it is greater than the dentinal surface. The ratio of diameter of rods from the DEJ towards the surface of the enamel is 1:2.
- Rods have a clear crystalline appearance, permitting light to pass through them.
- In cross-section of human enamel, many rods resemble fish scales. Rods have arcade outlines near DEJ and keyhole-shaped outlines at the enamel surface.

Ultrastructure

- Human enamel contains rods or prisms surrounded by rod sheaths and separated by inter-rod substance.
- The enamel prisms appear as segmental rods in longitudinal section and in cross-section they appear as oval, fish scale or keyhole shaped.
- When cut longitudinally, sections pass through the 'heads' or 'bodies' of one row of rods and the tails of an adjacent row.
- Rods are 5 microns in breadth and 9 microns in length.
- Enamel rods have apatite crystals arranged parallel to their long axes in their bodies or heads and deviate about 65 degrees as they fan out into tails of the prims.
- The apatite crystals of human enamel rods are irregular in shape and are about 30 nm in thickness and 90 nm in width.
- Direction of enamel rods: rods are oriented at right angle to the dentin surface. In the cervical and central parts of the crown of a deciduous tooth, they are horizontal while near the incisal edge or cup tips they are almost vertical. In permanent teeth, in cervical region, the rods deviate from horizontal to apical direction.
- Each enamel rod is built-up of segments and are more pronounced in enamel that is insufficiently calcified. The rods are segmented because the enamel matrix is formed in rhythmic manner. In humans these segments are of 4 microns in length.
- The cross striations are due to diurnal rhythm in enamel formation and in these areas rods show variations in composition.
- Ultrastucturally enamel shows certain hypocalcified structures as incremental lines of Retzius, neonatal lines, enamel lamellae, enamel tufts, and spindles.

Clinical Considerations

Course of enamel rods is important in cavity preparation. Close to the cementoenamel junction the rods run in a more horizontal direction. In preparing cavities it is important to remove unsupported enamel rods as they can break and produce leakage.

MULTIPLE CHOICE QUESTIONS (MCQs)

1. The only hard calcified dental tissue derived from ectoderm is
a. Bone b. Dentin
c. Enamel d. Cementum

2. The only dental tissue that is totally acellular
a. Cementum b. Enamel
c. Dentin d. Bone

3. The maximum thickness of enamel is
a. 1.3 mm b. 2.4 mm
c. 2.5 mm d. 3.8 mm

4. The density of enamel is
a. 2.8–3.0 gm/ml
b. 2.5–3.5 gm/ml
c. 1.5–2.0 gm/ml
d. 1.0–0.7 gm/ml

5. The knoop hardness number of enamel is
a. 643 b. 343
c. 243 d. 143

6. The average length of enamel rod at midcrown region is
a. 0.2 mm b. 0.05 mm
c. 0.04 mm d. 0.02 mm

7. The proteins of enamel are unique among mineralized tissues as they are
a. Type I collagen
b. Fibrous collagen
c. Amelogenins and enamelins
d. Type II collagen

8. Enamel lamellae may be confused with cracks caused by grinding of the specimen, decalcification of ground section will cause
a. Disappearance of cracks
b. Disappearance of lamellae
c. No change
d. Both a and b

9. The only high organic containing microscopic structure of enamel that is not derived from enamel is
a. Enamel tuft
b. Enamel spindle
c. Enamel lamellae
d. Cross striations

10. The microscopic structures of enamel that are not lined up as rows are (They do not follow the direction of rods)
a. Lamellae b. Tufts
c. Spindles d. All of the above

11. The hardest tissue in human body is
a. Bone b. Dentin
c. Enamel d. Cementum

12. The color of enamel is
a. Light yellow
b. Dark yellow
c. Light yellow to greyish white
d. Chalky white

13. Mature human enamel is made-up of
a. 96% inorganic and 4% organic material
b. 65% inorganic and 35% organic material
c. 45% inorganic and 55% organic material
d. 30% inorganic and 70% organic

14. The basic structural unit of enamel is
a. Cell b. Fiber
c. Rod/prism d. Tubule

15. The average thickness of enamel rod is
a. 20 mm b. 30 mm
c. 45 mm d. 60 mm

16. From the dentinoenamel junction (DEJ) towards the surface of the enamel, the diameter of the rod
a. Decreases
b. Increases
c. Remains same
d. Alternate increase and decrease

1-c, 2-b, 3-c, 4-a, 5-b, 6-a, 7-c, 8-a, 9-b, 10-c, 11-c, 12-c, 13-a, 14-c, 15-c, 16-b

17. The number of enamel rods in upper first molar are
a. 15 million b. 12 million
c. 2–3 million d. 5000–90,000

18. Incremental lines of enamel are
a. Incremental lines of von Ebner
b. Incremental lines of Salter
c. Incremental lines of Retzius
d. Line of Owen

19. Surface manifestations of lines of Retzius are known as
a. Perikymata and imbrication lines
b. Enamel lamellae
c. Cracks
d. Mamelons

20. Microscopic structures that do not appear to originate at DEJ are
a. Hunter-Schreger bands
b. Enamel tufts
c. Enamel lamellae
d. Spindles

21. The enamel forming cells are
a. Odontoblasts b. Ameloblasts
c. Cementoblasts d. Osteoblasts

22. Ameloblasts are derived from a part of dental organ called
a. Outer enamel epithelium
b. Inner enamel epithelium
c. Stratum intermedium
d. Stellate reticulum

23. The differentiation of ameloblasts require the presence of
a. Enamel b. Pulp
c. Dentin d. Cementum

24. During dentinogenesis, odontoblasts retreat centrally leaving behind formed dentin whereas ameloblasts retreat in
a. Central direction
b. Peripheral direction
c. Mesial direction
d. Distal direction

25. The shape to the crown is given by
a. Outer enamel epithelium
b. Inner enamel epithelium
c. Stellate reticulum
d. Stratum intermedium

26. The diameter and height of ameloblasts is
a. 6–7 mm in diameter and 60 mm high
b. 4–5 mm in diameter and 40 mm high
c. 3–4 mm in diameter and 20 mm high
d. 2–3 mm in diameter and 20 mm high

27. All are hypocalcified structures *except*
a. Enamel tufts
b. Enamel lamellae
c. Enamel rods
d. Inter-rod substances

28. The part of the tooth germ that outlines the root portion does not have the presence of
a. Outer enamel epithelium
b. Inner enamel epithelium
c. Stratum intermedium
d. Stellate reticulum
e. Both c and d

29. The functional unit responsible for the production of enamel
a. Ameloblasts and stratum intermedium
b. Ameloblasts and OEE
c. Ameloblasts and stellate reticulum
d. OEE and IEE

30. On completion of enamel formation, the shortened ameloblasts secrete an organic structureless membrane on the surface of the enamel called
a. Primary cuticle
b. Pellicle
c. Perikymata
d. Membrane preformativa

31. Each enamel rod is formed by
a. One ameloblast
b. Two ameloblasts
c. Three ameloblasts
d. Four ameloblasts

17-b, 18-c, 19-a, 20-c, 21-b, 22-b, 23-c, 24-b, 25-b, 26-b, 27-c, 28-e, 29-a, 30-a, 31-d

32. All of the following are the surface structures of enamel *except*
a. Hunter-Schreger bands
b. Rod ends
c. Enamel crack
d. Perikymata

33. Mesenchymal cells in dental papilla differentiate into odontoblasts under the organizing influence of cells of
a. Outer enamel epithelium
b. Stratum intermedium
c. Inner enamel epithelium
d. All the above

34. The protective covering of the enamel of teeth before its eruption is
a. Enamel cuticle
b. Reduced enamel epithelium
c. Outer enamel epithelium
d. Inner enamel epithelium

35. The largest hydroxyapatite crystals are found in
a. Enamel b. Dentin
c. Cementum d. Bone

36. The cells of dental organ/enamel organ differentiate to form
a. Dentin
b. Enamel
c. Cementum
d. Periodontal ligament (PDL)

37. Cells of dental follicle differentiate to form
a. Cementum and PDL
b. Enamel and pulp
c. Dentin and cementum
d. Pulp and cementum

38. Remnants of dental lamina persist as
a. Enamel pearls
b. Epithelial pearls/cell rests of Serres
c. Cell rests of malassez
d. None of the above

39. Enamel is almost as hard as
a. Granite b. Gold
c. Diamond d. Iron

40. Amount of collagen present in enamel is
a. 2% b. 1%
c. 0.5% d. Nil

41. The successional lamina develops from
a. 6th month *in utero* to 12th month of age
b. 5th month *in utero* to 10th month of age
c. 4th month *in utero* to one year
d. 3rd month *in utero* to one year

42. The development of root begins after the enamel and dentin formation has reached the future
a. Dentinoenamel junction
b. Cementoenamel junction
c. Dentinocemental junction
d. Dentinopredentin junction

43. The direction of the enamel rods in the permanent teeth is
a. Same as in deciduous
b. Inclined in an apical direction in the cervical third of the crown
c. Inclined in an occlusal direction in the cervical third of the crown
d. Horizontal direction

44. The cell rests of Serre represent
a. Remnants of dental lamina
b. Remnants of successional lamina
c. Remnants of Hertwig's epithelial root sheath
d. Remnants of dental follicle

45. The hypocalcified structure of enamel that extends from enamel surface towards dentinoenamel junction (DEJ) is
a. Enamel spindle
b. Enamel tufts
c. Enamel lamellae
d. All of the above

32-a, 33-c, 34-b, 35-a, 36-b, 37-a, 38-b, 39-c, 40-d, 41-b, 42-b, 43-b, 44-a, 45-c

46. The convexities of the scallops of the dentinoenamel junction are directed towards
a. Enamel
b. Dentin
c. Both enamel and dentin
d. Incisal surface

47. Aprismatic enamel is found at
a. Surface layer only
b. DEJ only
c. Surface layer and DEJ
d. None of the above

48. External manifestation of enamel lamellae running longitudinally and in a direction perpendicular to DEJ represents
a. Perikymata
b. Crack
c. Imbrication lines of pickerill
d. Enamel hypoplasia

49. Diameter of enamel rod increase from DEJ towards the surface of the enamel at a ratio of
a. 2:4 b. 2:3
c. 1:4 d. 1:2

50. Permeability of enamel
a. Increases with age
b. Decreases with age
c. Remains same
d. Does not depend on age

51. Enamel can be studied by using
a. Decalcified section
b. Ground section
c. Frozen section
d. All of the above

52. Primary enamel cuticle is also called
a. Nasmyth's membrane
b. Reduced enamel epithelium
c. Preameloblastic layer
d. Pellicle

53. Enamel tufts are
a. Hypercalcified enamel rods
b. Hypocalcified enamel rods
c. Hypocalcified enamel rods and interprismatic substance
d. Accentuated incremental line

54. Under the electron microscope the cut section of enamel rods are seen as
a. Key holes
b. Staggered arches
c. Stacked arches
d. All of the above

55. The dentinal end of ameloblast is also called
a. Mesial end b. Distal end
c. Proximal end d. None of the above

56. The neonatal line is seen in enamel of
a. Deciduous teeth
b. Deciduous and permanent first molar
c. Permanent central incisor
d. Permanent maxillary first molar

57. The neonatal line is seen in dentin of
a. Permanent maxillary first molar
b. Deciduous teeth and permanent first molar
c. Permanent maxillary central incisor
d. Deciduous teeth

58. The enamel spindles are
a. The terminal branches of odontoblasts
b. The terminal branches of odontoblastic processes
c. The terminal branches of odontoblastic process in enamel
d. None of the above

59. The maximum thickness of enamel is
a. At the cusp of molars and premolars
b. At the incisal edge of the newly erupted anterior teeth
c. Cingulum portion of maxillary central incisor
d. At the tip of the crown of maxillary canine

46-b, 47-c, 48-b, 49-d, 50-b, 51-b, 52-a, 53-c, 54-d, 55-b, 56-a, 57-b, 58-c, 59-a

60. Which of the following features does not come under the surface structure of enamel?

a. Perikymata
b. Enamel crack
c. Rod ends
d. Hunter-Schreger bands

61. Process of rhythmic laying down of enamel is called

a. Apposition b. Secretion
c. Deposition d. Calcification

62. The structures of the enamel which are most resistant to the actions of acids are

a. Enamel cuticles
b. Enamel lamellae
c. Enamel spindles
d. Enamel tufts

63. "Seeding" process of mineralization of enamel and dentin is known as

a. Calcification b. Epitaxy
c. Epistaxis d. Phosphorylation

64. All the submicroscopic structures of the enamel are hypocalcified *except*

a. Enamel spindles
b. Enamel lamellae
c. Enamel prisms
d. Enamel tufts

65. All the submicroscopic parts of enamel are of ectodermal in origin *except*

a. Enamel lamellae
b. Enamel tufts
c. Enamel spindles
d. Enamel rod sheath

66. Specific gravity of enamel is

a. 2.8 b. 4.3
c. 6.4 d. 8.2

67. Appositional growth is

a. Additive growth
b. Linear growth
c. Circumferential growth
d. None of the above

68. The formula of the unit cell of hydroxyapatite crystal is

a. $3Ca_3 (PO_4)_2$, : $Ca(OH)_2$
b. $2Ca_3 (PO_4)_2$, : $Ca(OH)_2$
c. $Ca_3 (PO_4)_2$, : $Ca(OH)_2$
d. $Ca_3 (PO_4)_2$, : $3Ca(OH)_2$

69. The other name for inner enamel epithelium in bell stage is

a. Ameloblastic layer
b. Odontoblastic layer
c. Cementoblastic layer
d. Osteoblastic layer

70. On the cusp of human molars and premolars maximum thickness of enamel is about

a. 0 to 1 mm
b. 2 to 3 mm
c. 4 to 5 mm
d. 4 to 6 mm

71. Enamel tufts which arise at the dentino-enamel junction and reach in enamel to about 1/5th to 1/3rd of its thickness are

a. Hypocalcified enamel rods and interprismatic substance
b. Hypocalcified enamel rods only
c. Hypomineralised enamel rods only
d. Similar to surface structures

72. In the life cycle of an ameloblast, the Tomes' process develops during the following stage

a. Morphogenic stage
b. Organizing stage
c. Secretary (formative) stage
d. Maturative stage

73. Each of the following terms is used to describe an enamel structure *except*

a. Prisms
b. Perikymata
c. Striae of Retzius
d. Contour lines of Owen

60-d, 61-a, 62-a, 63-b, 64-c, 65-c, 66-a, 67-a, 68-a, 69-a, 70-b, 71-a, 72-c, 73-d

74. Maturation of enamel is characterized by addition of inorganic content and
a. Addition of water
b. Addition of organic content
c. Removal of water and organic content
d. Removal of water and addition of organic content.

75. Gnarled enamel is most frequently found in
a. Cusps
b. Near the cervical line
c. Around pits and fissures
d. Adjacent to contact areas

76. Perikymata are the result of
a. Enamel hyperplasia
b. Enamel hypoplasia
c. Interstitial growth
d. Normal enamel apposition

77. Direction of enamel rods in deciduous teeth in the cervical third region is inclined
a. Horizontally b. Occlusally
c. Apically d. Vertically

78. One of the following is the optical phenomenon of enamel
a. Enamel crack
b. Perikymata
c. Hunter-Schregar band
d. Enamel spindle

79. Mineralization of enamel takes place in
a. One stage b. Two stages
c. Three stages d. Four stages

80. The percentage of protein found in the enamel of mature teeth is
a. 0.1% b. 0.2%
c. 0.3% d. 0.4%

81. In histological staining reaction, enamel matrix behaves like
a. Keratinized epidermis
b. Non-keratinized mucosa
c. Keratinized mucosa
d. Parakeratinized mucosa

82. The cells leading to differentiation of dentin forming cells are
a. Ameloblasts b. Odontoblasts
c. Cementoblasts d. Osteoblasts

83. Hardness of enamel from surface to inside
a. Increases
b. Decreases
c. Does root changes
d. First increases than decreases

84. All of the following are true regarding incremental lines of Retzius *except*
a. Brownish band in ground section
b. Concentric in transverse section
c. Represents successive apposition of enamel
d. Are present in dentin

85. In protective stage of life cycle of ameloblast, it protects the
a. Osteoblast b. Odontoblast
c. Cementoblast d. Enamel

86. Striations in human enamel appear at a distance of
a. 4 microns b. 5 microns
c. 6 microns d. 7 microns

87. All are age changes in enamel *except*
a. Permeability decreases
b. Resistance to caries decreases
c. Fluoride content at surface increases
d. Enamel becomes harder and darker

88. One of the following is not true regarding Nasmyth's membrane
a. Is also known as primary enamel cuticle
b. It covers the newly formed enamel
c. It disappears with the eruption of tooth due to removal by mastication
d. It forms after tooth eruption

89. The tissue which is lost maximum during decalcification is
a. Bone b. Cementum
c. Dentin d. Enamel

74-c, 75-a, 76-d, 77-a, 78-c, 79-b, 80-a, 81-a, 82-a, 83-b, 84-d, 85-d, 86-a, 87-b, 88-d, 89-d

90. The cell which cannot regenerate is
a. Ameloblast b. Odontoblast
c. Cementoblast d. Fibroblast

91. Which of the following is not true regarding the dentinoenamel junction?
a. Scalloped with convexities towards the dentin
b. Preformed even before the development of hard tissues
c. Hypermineralized zone present at DEJ
d. Hypomineralized zone present at DEJ

92. In organizing stage of amelogenesis, ameloblast resemble
a. Squamous cell
b. Cuboidal cell
c. Flat cell
d. Tall columnar cell

93. The dentinal end of ameloblast can be regarded as
a. Proximal end b. Distal end
c. Mesial end d. Lateral end

90-a, 91-d, 92-d, 93-b

Chapter 15

Dentin

LAQ (10 Marks)

Q 1. Enumerate and describe the hypocalcified structures of dentin. (*May 2002*)

Ans. Dentin provides the bulk and general form of the tooth and is characterized as a hard tissue with tubules throughout its thickness.

***Hypocalcified structures present in dentin are*:**

1. Incremental lines of von Ebner and contour lines of Owen.
2. Neonatal line
3. Interglobular dentin
4. Tomes' granular layer

1. Incremental Lines of von Ebner and Contour Lines of Owen

- Dentin formation proceeds rhythmically with alternate phases of activity and quiescence. These phases are represented in formed dentin as *incremental lines of von Ebner* or imbrication lines. They appear as fine lines or striations in dentin (Fig. 15.1).

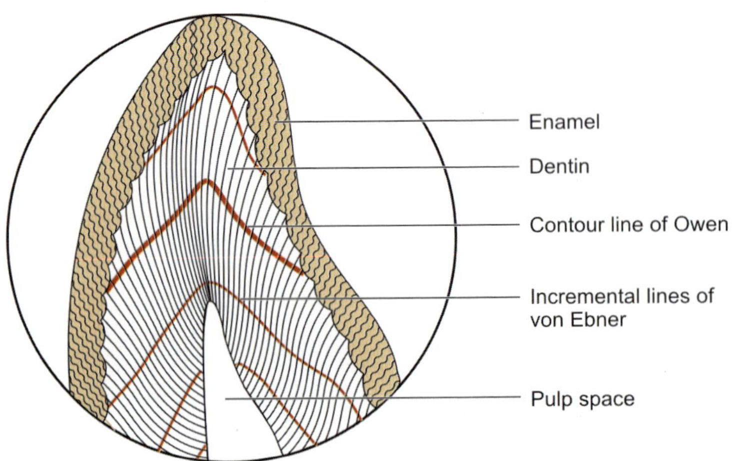

Fig. 15.1: Incremental lines in dentin

- These lines reflect the daily rhythmic recurrent deposition of dentin matrix as well as a hesitation in the daily formative process.
- These are best seen in longitudinal ground section of tooth.
- These incremental lines run at right angles to the dentinal tubules and generally mark the normal rhythmic linear pattern of dentin deposition in an inward and rootward direction. The course of the lines indicates the growth pattern of the dentin.
- The distance between lines varies from 4 to 8 µm in the crown and much less in root.
- Occasionally some of the lines are accentuated because of the disturbance in the matrix and mineralization process. Such lines are readily demonstrated in longitudinal ground section and are known as *contour lines of Owen.* These lines represent hypocalcified bands.

2. Neonatal Line

- This is a hypocalcified structure present in dentin in deciduous teeth and in the first permanent molars, where dentin is formed partly before and partly after birth.
- The prenatal and postnatal dentin in these teeth are separated by an accentuated contour line, a zone of hypocalcification. This is termed as *neonatal line* and is seen in enamel as well as in dentin.
- This line reflects the abrupt change in environment that occurs at birth.
- The dentin matrix formed prior to birth is usually better in quality than that formed after birth.

3. Interglobular Dentin

- This is unmineralized or hypomineralized dentin where in small globular areas of dentin fail to coalesce into a homogenous mass.
- During the mineralization of dentin matrix, the minerals are deposited as globules or calcospherites. In most of the areas, these globules fuse to form a uniformly calcified tissue.
- When some of these globules fail to fuse into a homogenous mass, zones of hypomineralization form between the globules. These zones are known as *globular dentin* or *interglobular spaces* (Fig. 15.2).
- Most often it forms in the crown in the circumpulpal dentin just below the mantle dentin, where the pattern of mineralization is mainly globular.

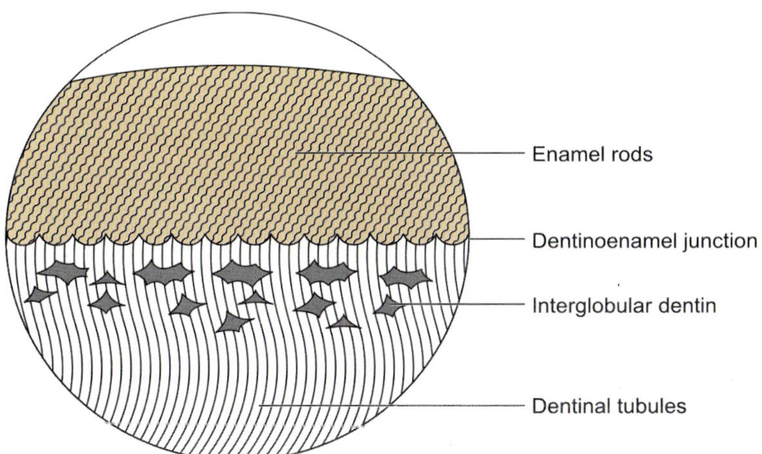

Fig. 15.2: Interglobular dentin

- In areas of interglobular dentin, the architectural pattern of the tubules does not change and the tubules pass through interglobular areas without deviation. This confirms that the formation of interglobular dentin is because of a defect in mineralization and not in matrix formation.
- When ground sections are viewed in transmitted light, interglobular areas appear as dark rounded masses with concave edges.
- Vitamin D deficiency or exposure to high levels of fluoride during dentin formation is thought to be responsible for the failure of fusion of the globules and formation of interglobular dentin.

4. Tomes' Granular Layer

- When dry ground sections of the root dentin are visualized in transmitted light, a zone adjacent to cementum appears granular. This is known as *Tomes' granular layer* (Fig. 15.3).
- This appearance is seen in the root but not in the crown as there is difference in the rate of formation of coronal and radicular dentin.
- It is a hypomineralized region and is found only in root dentin.
- This zone increases in amount from cementoenamel junction to the apex of the root.
- The dentinal tubules in this area branch more profusely leading to coalescing and looping of the terminal branches. This occurs because odontoblasts turn on themselves during early dentin formation. These areas remain unmineralized.
- The air spaces thus created appear dark and granular in ground sections because of internal reflection of transmitted light.
- An alternative explanation for the granular appearance is that it is due to incomplete fusion of calcospherites.
- Recent studies have shown that Tomes' granular layer has a special arrangement of collagen and non-collagenous matrix proteins at the interface between dentin and cementum.
- Among hypomineralized areas, Tomes' granular layer shows highest concentrations of calcium and phosphorus.

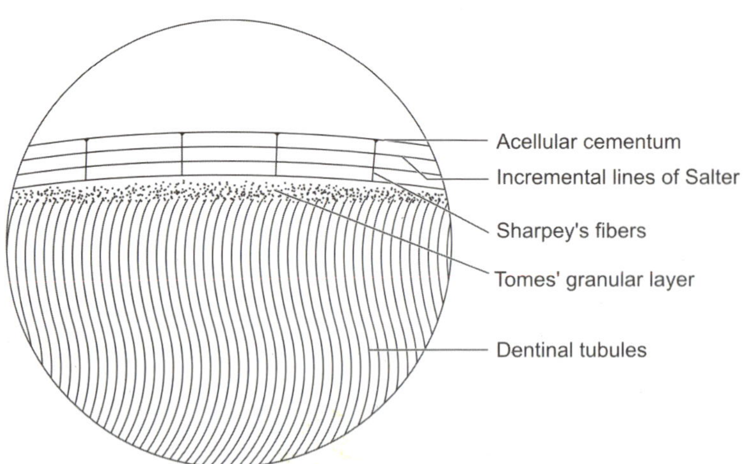

Fig. 15.3: Tomes' granular layer

SAQs (3 Marks)

Q 1. Describe about physical and chemical properties of dentin. *(Oct. 2002, 2004)*

Ans. PHYSICAL PROPERTIES OF DENTIN

- Dentin is a hard tissue of tooth with tubules throughout its thickness. It provides the bulk and general form of the tooth.
- It is sensitive and forms throughout life at the expense of the pulp.
- Even though it resembles bone physically and chemically, morphologically they differ. Bone forming cells (osteoblasts) become entrapped in the matrix to form osteocytes whereas the dentin forming cells remain external to the dentin matrix and only their processes are enclosed in the dentinal tubules.

Colour

Dentin is light yellowish in colour in young individuals. It becomes darker with age.

Permeability

It is a hard tissue with tubules throughout its thickness which makes it more permeable. The permeability decreases with age. Dentinal tubules are filled with tissue fluid.

Hardness

- Dentin hardness varies slightly between tooth types and between crown and root dentin. Dentin is harder in its central part than near the pulp or on its periphery. Dentin of primary teeth is slightly less hard than that of permenant teeth.
- Dentin is viscoelastic and is harder than bone and cementum but softer than enamel. Compared to enamel it has higher compressive strength but lower tensile strength.
- In radiographs, dentin appears more radiolucent (darker) than enamel and more radio-opaque than pulp (lighter).

CHEMICAL PROPERTIES OF DENTIN

Dentin is composed of 65% inorganic material and 35% organic matter and water.

***Organic matter*:** Consists of collagenous fibrils (Type I collagen) embedded in ground substance. Important constituents of ground substane are:

- *Proteoglycans:* Chondroitin sulphates, decorin and biglycan.
- *Glycoproteins:* Dentin sialoprotein, osteonectin, osteopontin.
- *Phosphoproteins:* Dentin phosphoprotein.

  In addition, matrix contains growth factors.

  The matrix components play an important role in mineralisation of dentin.

***Inorganic material*:** Consists of hydroxyapatite.

- Each hydroxyapatite crystal is composed of several thousand unit cells. The unit cell have a formula of $3Ca_3(PO_4)_2$, $Ca(OH)_2$.
- The crystals are plate shaped and much smaller than the hydroxyapatite crystals in enamel.
- Dentin also contains small amount of phosphates, carbonates and sulphates.
- Organic and inorganic substances can be separated by either decalcification or incineration. In the process of decalcification the organic constituents of dentin can be retained and they maintain the shape of dentin.

- Whereas enamel has 95% minerals and therefore, after decalcification enamel is lost. Hence, its histologic visualization is not possible after decalcification. Therefore, enamel can be studied only by ground sections.

Q 2. Describe contents of dentinal tubules. *(Dec. 2005)*

Ans. **CONTENTS OF DENTINAL TUBULES**

- Dentinal tubules are the structural units of dentin. They make the dentin permeable. They are small canal like spaces within the dentin.
- Dentinal tabule contains the odontostastic process surrounded by dentinal fluid.
- The inner wall of dentinal tabule is formed by the highly mineralized intratubular dentin. The space between the odontoblastic process and the intratubular dentin contains the dentinal fluid (tissue fluid), the movement of which forms the basis of dentin sensitivity.
- Dentin producing cell, odontoblast, resides in the peripheral pulp while its process extend into the dentinal tubules. The processes are largest in diameter near the pulp (3–4 µm) and taper to 1 µm into the dentin. The odontoblastic process is composed of microtubules and small filaments and occasionally mitochondria, lysosomes and microvesicles.
- The odontoblastic processes divide near the dentinoenamel junction and may extend into enamel as enamel spindles.
- A thin organic membrane (lining) rich in glycosaminoglycans called the *lamina limitans* is seen on the inner aspect of the intratubular (peritubular) dentin.
- Nerve fibers also accompany the odontoblastic process within dentinal tubules. The fluid movement stimulates the pain mechanism in the tubules by mechanical disturbance of the nerves, thus playing role in pain transmission.

Q 3. What is peritubular dentin/Intratubular dentin? *(May 2015)*

Ans. **INTRATUBULAR/PERITUBULAR DENTIN** (Fig. 15.4)

- The dentin that immediately surrounds the dentinal tubules is termed *peritubular* dentin. Since the deposition of the minerals here occurs in the inner wall of the tubule rather than on the outer walls, the term *intratubular* is more appropriate.
- It is more highly mineralized (about 9%) than intertubular dentin (Fig. 15.4).

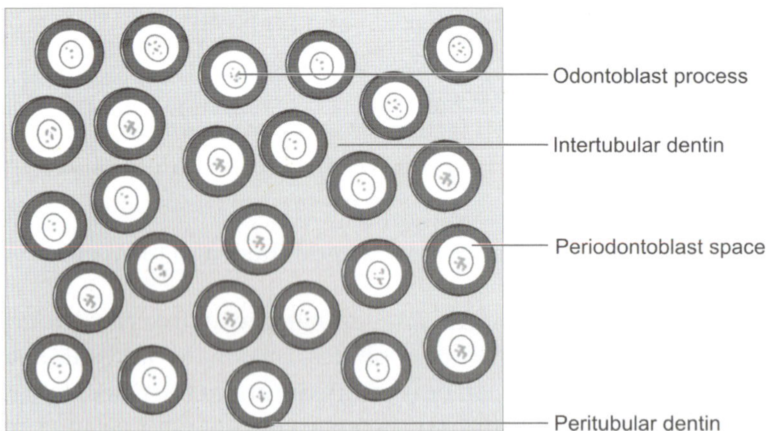

Fig. 15.4: Peritubular and Intertubular dentin

- It is twice as thick in outer dentin than in inner dentin.
- It is absent where the tubules run through the interglobular areas and that portion of dentin which is close to the pulp.
- A very delicate organic matrix has been demonstrated in this dentin that along with the mineral is lost after decalcification. Therefore, after decalcification the odontoblast process appears to be surrounded by an empty space.
- A thin organic membrane (lining) rich in glycosaminoglycans called the **lamina limitans,** is seen on the inner aspect of the peritubular dentin.
- The space between the odontoblastic process and the peritubular dentin contains the dentinal fluid, the movement of which forms the basis of dentin sensitivity.

Q 4. Write about primary and secondary dentin. *(May 2007, 2009, June 2010, 2012)*

Ans. DENTIN

- Dentin is a hard mineralized tissue which provides the bulk and general form to the tooth.
- Based on time of formation physiological types of dentin are: Primary and Secondary dentin.

Primary Dentin

- Primary dentin is the dentin which is formed before root completion (Fig. 15.5).
- It forms most of the tooth and outlines the pulp chamber of the fully formed tooth.
- Primary dentin is of two types: *Mantle dentin* and *Circumpulpal dentin.*

Mantle Dentin

- The outer layer of primary dentin in the crown is called mantle dentin.
- It is about 20 mm thick.
- It is the first formed dentin in the crown underlying the dentinoenamel junction and underlying it is the circumpulpal dentin. It is deposited by the odontoblasts that have just begun to differentiate and have not yet reached their full size.
- This dentin is soft and thus provides cushioning effect to the tooth.
- The organic matrix of mantle dentin is composed of larger collagen fibrils than are present in the rest of the primary dentin. These fibres are oriented perpendicular to the dentinoenamel junction.
- These fibers are argyrophilic (silver stained) and are known as *von Korff's fibers.* They contain mainly type III collagen.
- Compared to circumpulpal dentin it is less mineralized. Mantle dentin has fewer defects than circumpulpal dentin.
- Matrix vesicles are involved in the mineralization of mantle dentin. Mantle dentin undergoes globular mineralization whereas circumpulpal dentin mineralizes either by globular or linear pattern.
- Dentinal tubules branch profusely in the mantle dentin.
- It extends into the root as 5–10 mm thick hyaline layer of Hopewell-Smith. It is the first formed dentin in the root underlying the cementum.
- In the root mantle dentin, the collagen fibres are arranged parallel to the basal lamina.

Circumpulpal Dentin

- The primary dentin that surrounds the pulp is called *circumpulpal dentin.*
- It represents all of the dentin formed before root completion.

- It forms the remaining primary dentin or bulk of the tooth, apart from mantle dentin.
- The circumpulpal dentin before mineralization is termed predentin.
- Collagen fibrils in circumpulpal dentin are smaller in diameter and are closely packed together as compared to the mantle dentin and parallel to the dentinoenamel junction.
- It is slightly more mineralized compared to mantle dentin.
- It is further divided into intertubular and peritubular dentin.
- Intertubular dentin forms the main body of dentin. It is located between the zones of peritubular dentin. Peritubular dentin forms the walls of the dentinal tubules.

Secondary Dentin

- It forms internal to the primary dentin of crown and root. It is a narrow band of dentin bordering the pulp.
- It represents the dentin which is formed after root completion. It develops after the crown has come into clinical occlusal function and the roots are nearly completed.
- It is the most important age-associated change in dentin.
- It represents the continuing, but much slower deposition of dentin by odontoblasts after root formation has been completed.
- It contains fewer tubules than the primary dentin. There is usually a bend in the tubules where primary and secondary dentin interface.
- It is deposited regularly but not uniformly. There is regular arrangement of dentinal tubules. Hence, this dentin is also known as *regular secondary dentin* (Fig. 15.5).
- There is greater deposition of secondary dentin on the roof and floor of pulp chamber, where it protects the pulp from exposure in older teeth.
- The secondary dentin formed is not in response to any external stimuli and it appears very much like primary dentin, but contains fewer tubules.
- The apical dentin shows irregularity in the dentinal tubules of both primary and secondary dentin.
- Secondary dentin scleroses more readily than primary dentin. This tends to reduce the permeability, thereby protecting the pulp.
- It is a physiologic type of dentin whereas tertiary or reparative dentin is formed in reaction to trauma.

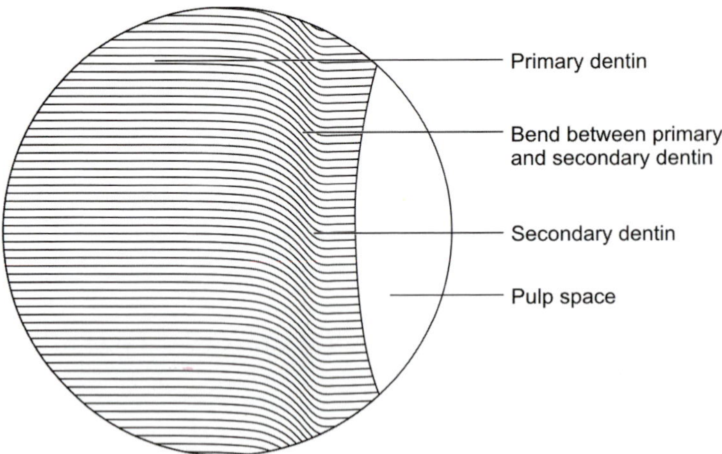

Fig. 15.5: Primary and secondary dentin

Q 5. What is Reparative or Tertiary dentin? *(Oct. 2003, June 2006, Nov. 2010)*

Ans. REPARATIVE OR TERTIARY DENTIN

- Tertiary dentin is reactive, response or reparative dentin.
- It is localized formation of dentin on the pulp-dentin border, formed in reaction to trauma such as caries or restorative procedures, abrasion or erosion.
- Due to trauma depending on the intensity of injury the odontoblasts die or survive.
- If after injury the odontoblasts survive, the dentin that is produced is known as *reactionary* or *regenerated dentin.*
- If after injury the odontoblasts are killed, they get replaced by the migration of undifferentiated mesenchymal cells which differentiate into odontoblasts and form dentin. This dentin is known as *reparative dentin* or *tertiary dentin* (Fig. 15.6).
- It is believed that the origin of the new odontoblasts from cells in the cell-rich zone or from undifferentiated perivascular cells deeper in the pulp.
- Bacteria, living or dead, or their toxic products as well as chemical substances from restorative materials, migrate down the tubules to the pulp and stimulate pulpal response, leading to reparative dentin formation.
- This action to seal off the zone of injury occurs as a healing process initiated by the pulp, resulting in resolution of the inflammatory process and removal of dead cells. The hard tissue then formed is termed *reparative dentin.*
- This reparative dentin has fewer and more twisted dentinal tubules than normal dentin. It is due to irregular nature of the dentinal tubules, this type of dentin is also referred to as *irregular secondary dentin.*
- The quality and quantity of tertiary dentin produced is related to the intensity and duration of the stimulus.
- In rapidly progressing caries, where there is extensive destruction of dentin and considerable pulp damage, tertiary dentin is deposited rapidly and displays a sparse, irregular tubule pattern with frequent cellular inclusions. Tertiary dentin with such cellular inclusions is sometimes called *osteodentin*. In other instances a combination of osteodentin and tubular dentin is seen.

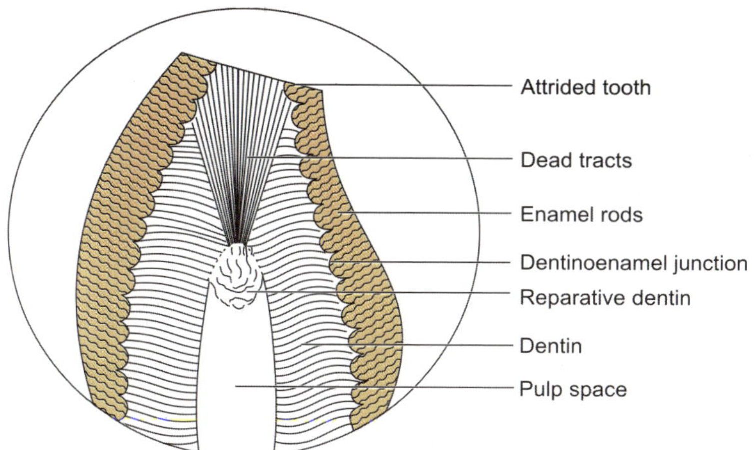

Fig. 15.6: Dead tracts and Tertiary/Reparative dentin

Q 6. Write about dead tracts? *(Nov. 2010)*

Ans. DEAD TRACTS

- In dried ground sections of normal dentin, the odontoblast processes disintegrate and get filled with air. These empty, air-filled tubules appear dark in transmitted light and white in reflected light because of internal reflection.
- Loss of odontoblast processes may also occur in teeth containing vital pulp. Stimuli such as caries, attrition or erosion result in dentin areas characterized by degenerated odontoblastic processes. The dentinal tubules become empty following the retraction of the odontoblastic process or death of odontoblast. These empty dentinal tubules are then sealed by reparative dentin at their pulpal ends.
- These empty dentinal tubules get filled with fluid or gaseous substances. In ground sections, such groups of tubules may entrap air and appear black in transmitted and white in reflected light. Thus, dentin areas characterised by degenerated odontoblast processes give rise to dead tracts (Refer Fig. 15.6).
- Dead tracts are seen more commonly in older teeth and demonstrate reduced sensitivity.
- Dead tracts are considered to be the initial step in the formation of sclerotic dentin.

Q 7. Write about sclerotic/transparent dentin. *(2001)*

Ans. SCLEROTIC/TRANSPARENT DENTIN (Fig. 15.7)

- It refers to the filling up of the dentinal tubules calcified material in response to external stimuli such as slowly progressing caries, attrition or erosion.
- This condition is prevalent in older individuals. It is seen especially in the roots. This may be regarded as an age change.
- Sclerotic dentin formation is a protective change in the existing dentin. It is considered as a defensive reaction because it reduces the permeability of dentin and keeps the pulp vital for a prolonged period.
- In cases of caries, attrition, abrasion, erosion or cavity preparation, sufficient stimuli are generated to cause collagen fibers and apatite crystals to begin appearing in the dentinal tubules. This results in blocking of the tubules which is considered a defensive reaction of dentin.

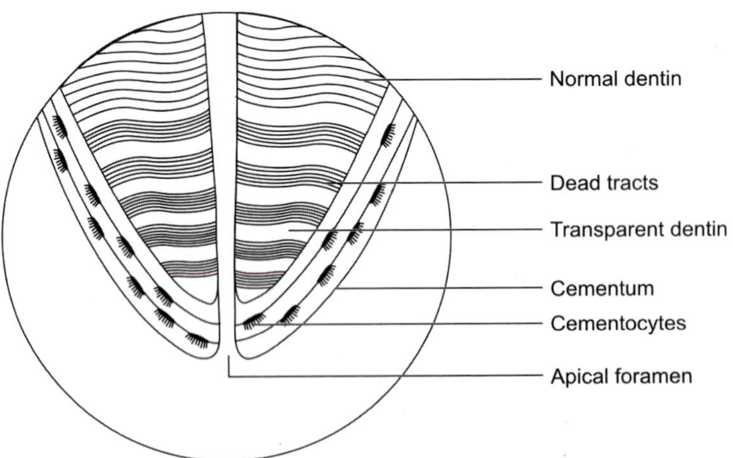

Fig. 15.7: Transparent dentin

- Gradually, the tubule lumen is obliterated with minerals, which appears very much like the peritubular dentin. The refractive indices of dentin in which the tubules are occluded are equalized and such areas become *transparent.*
- It is observed in the teeth of elderly people, especially in roots.
- The deposited mineral is different from that in peritubular dentin. Though the mineral concentration is higher, the size of the crystals in sclerotic dentin is smaller than that in normal dentin.
- Sclerotic dentin is harder, has reduced fracture toughness but same elastic properties as normal dentin.

Significance

- Permeability of dentin becomes reduced while hardness increases in the region of sclerotic dentin.
- It may also be found under slowly progressing caries. Sclerosis reduces permeability of the dentin and may help to prolong pulp vitality.
- It may block the tubules against entry of bacteria.
- Breakage of apical thirds of roots during extraction of teeth of elderly is due to the brittle nature of sclerotic dentin.

Q 8. Describe dentin sensitivity or theories of pain transmission through dentin.

(*June 2005*)

Ans. DENTIN SENSITIVITY OR THEORIES OF PAIN TRANSMISSION THROUGH DENTIN

Innervation of Dentin

- Dentin is highly sensitive tissue. Pulp has numerous myelinated and unmyelinated nerve fibers.
- The unmyelinated nerve fibers end on blood vessels and the myelinated nerve fibers can be followed up to subodontoblastic layer.
- They loose their myelin sheath and go up to odontoblastic layer and form a plexus. Most of the fibers end in contact with odontoblasts in dentinal tubules. These nerve fibers are referred to as intratubular nerves. The nerve endings are packed with small vesicles. Synapse like relation exist between the odontoblast process and nerve fibers.
- The stimulation of dentin by any agent causes a pain like sensation called hypersensitivity.
- There are three basic theories of pain conduction or sensitivity through dentin.
  1. ***Direct neural stimulation:*** According to this theory nerves in the dentin get stimulated. Stimulation in some manner reach the nerve endings in the inner dentin.

     But this theory is not accepted as it is demonstrated that there are no fibres which reach dentinoenamel junction (DEJ). Topical application of local anaesthetics do not abolish sensitivity. Hence this theory is not accepted.
  2. ***Fluid or hydrodynamic theory:*** Dentinal tubules contain odontoblastic processes surrounded by dentinal fluid. Various stimuli such as heat, cold, air blast desiccation or mechanical or osmotic pressure affect fluid movement in the dentinal tubules. This fluid movement either inward or outward, stimulates the pain mechanism in the tubules by mechanical disturbance of the nerve closely associated with the odontoblasts and its process. Thus, nerve endings may act as mechanoreceptors as they are affected by mechanical displacement of the tubular fluid. This is the most accepted theory.

Sensitivity of the dentin is explained by the hydrodynamic theory. This theory explains pain throughout dentin since fluid moment will occur at the DEJ as well as near the pulp.

3. ***Transduction theory:*** This theory presumes that the odontoblast process is the primary structure excited by the stimulus and that the impulse is transmitted to the nerve endings in the inner dentin. This is not a popular theory since there are no neurotransmitter vesicles in the odontoblast process to facilitate the synapse.

Clinical Significance

Treatment of hypersensitivity is done either by blocking the patent tubules or modifying or blocking pulpal nerve response.

Q 9. Describe age and functional changes in dentin. *(Nov. 2009)*

Ans. AGE AND FUNCTIONAL CHANGES IN DENTIN

- Age changes take place in dentin to ensure the function of protection.
- Dentin is able to react to physiological and pathological stimuli because it is a vital tissue due to presence of odontoblastic processes.
- The two most important changes seen in dentin with advancing age are:
  a. Increase in thickness of dentin due to continuous gradual deposition of secondary dentin.
  b. Increased sclerosis or obliteration of dentinal tubules resulting in reduced sensitivity and permeability.
- Dentin is laid down throughout life, although after the teeth have erupted and have been functioning for a short-time, further dentin formation is slow and is called *secondary dentin.* The laying down of dentin is either related to age (secondary dentin formation) or as a response to a stimulus applied to the tooth as in case of tertiary dentin formation.
- Pathological effects of caries, abrasion, attrition or cutting of dentin during operative procedures causes changes in dentin which leads to development of *dead tracts, sclerosis, and reparative dentin* (Refer to Figs 15.6 and 15.7). Secondary dentin and translucent dentin occur due to physiologic age changes.
- Describe dead tracts, sclerotic dentin and reparative dentin as described earlier.

Q 10. Write about dentinogenesis.

Ans. DENTINOGENESIS

- Formation of dentin during development of tooth is dentinogenesis.
- Dentin formation begins when the tooth germ has reached the bell stage of development.
- Dentinogenesis begins at cusp tips after the odontoblasts have differentiated and begin collagen production.
- Initially, the outermost ectomesenchymal cells of the dental papilla are small, undifferentiated and have few organelles and are separated from the inner enamel epithelium by an acellular zone.
- Later, under the organizing influence of the inner enamel epithelium these cells differentiate into odontoblasts. As they differentiate they change from ovoid to columnar shape, nucleus becomes oriented towards the base and there is increased amount of protein-synthesizing organelles.
- Dentinogenesis occurs in a two-phase sequence. Collagen matrix is formed first and then gets calcified. Odontoblasts secrete both collagen and other components of the extracellular matrix.

1. Matrix Formation

- Proteins (proline) appear in the rough surface endoplasmic reticulum and golgi apparatus of odontoblasts. Proline then migrates into the cell process in dense granules and is emptied into the extracellular collagen matrix of the predentin.
- As the matrix formation continues, the odontoblast process lengthens as does the dentinal tubule.
- Initially daily increments of approximately 4 μm of dentin are formed. This continues till the crown is formed and the tooth erupts and moves into occlusion. After which dentin production slows down to 1 μm/day.
- As each increment of predentin is formed along the pulp border, it remains, a day before it is calcified and the next increment of predentin forms.

2. Mineralization

- The mineralization of dentin occurs in relation to collagen fibers as linear deposits (linear mineralization) or by fusion of globules (globular mineralization).
- Matrix vesicles are involved in the mineralization of the mantle dentin.
- These vesicles contain the enzyme alkaline phosphatase, which increases the concentration of phosphates. The phosphate combines with calcium (taken up from the tissue fluid) to form apatite.
- These apatite crystals grow and rupture from the confines of the vesicles to form a cluster of crystallites, which fuse with adjacent clusters to form a continuous layer of mineralized matrix.
- Initially, the apatite crystals are deposited on the surface of collagen fibrils and in the ground substance. Later, the crystals are laid down within the fibrils with their long axis parallel to the long axis of the fibrils.
- In circumpulpal dentin the mineralization is either of globular pattern, if the rate of deposition is fast or the linear pattern, if the rate of deposition is slow.
- The radicular dentin formation compared to coronal dentin, is slower, less mineralised with collagen fibers laid parallel to cementodentinal junction.

Clinical Significance

- Incomplete fusion of globules leads to the formation of interglobular dentin.
- Dentin formation, unlike bone, is not affected by vitamin D deficiency state.

Q 12. Describe predentin.

Ans. PREDENTIN

- Predentin is a band of newly formed unmineralized dentin matrix at the pulpal border of dentin.
- It is the innermost layer of dentin, located adjacent to the pulp tissue and is 2 to 6 μm wide depending on the extent of activity of the odontoblast.
- As the collagen fibres undergo mineralization at the predentin-dentin front, the predentin then becomes dentin and a new layer of predentin forms circumpulpally (Fig. 15.8).
- Predentin is similar to osteoid in bone and is easy to identify in hematoxyline and eosin stained section because it stains less intensely than mineralized dentin.

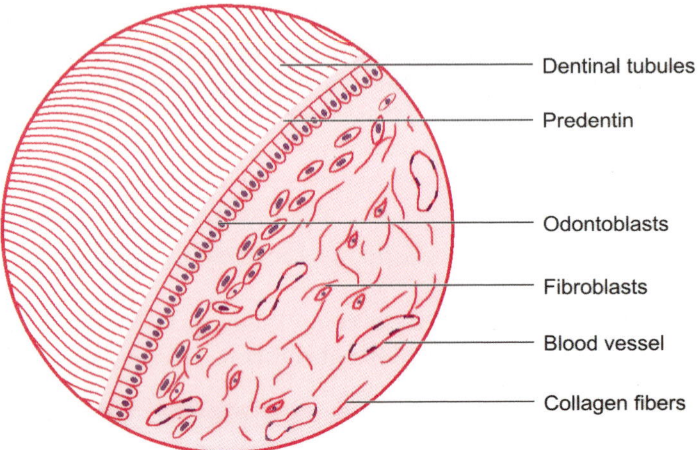

Fig. 15.8: Predentin

- It is thickest cementum layer where active dentinogenesis is occurring.
- Its presence is important in maintaining the integrity of dentin since its absence appears to leave the mineralized dentin vulnerable to resorption by odontoclasts.

Q 13. What is layer of Hopewell and Smith/Intermediate cementum layer?

Ans. HOPEWELL AND SMITH/INTERMEDIATE CEMENTUM LAYER

- Between the Tomes' granular layer and cementum, is found a structureless hyaline layer of 10 µm width; it is called *layer of Hopewell and Smith* or *intermediate cementum layer*. It does not exhibit features of dentin or cementum. It has been suggested that it plays a role in sealing the sensitive root dentin. It is seen in apical two-thirds of roots of molars and premolars. It is considered to be of dentinal origin. It contains no tubules but wide spaces which are thought to be enlarged terminals of dentinal tubules.
- This hyaline layer represents areas where cells of HERS become entrapped in a rapidly deposited dentin or cementum matrix.

MULTIPLE CHOICE QUESTIONS (MCQs)

1. The inorganic component of dentin is studied by
a. Decalcification
b. Electron microscope
c. Roentgen X-ray defraction
d. Scanning electron microscope

2. The most popular theory that explains dentin sensitivity is
a. Direct neural stimulation
b. Hydrodynamic theory
c. Transduction theory
d. None of the above

3. The main histological difference between bone and dentin is
a. Only odontoblasts are entrapped in the matrix
b. Odontoblasts with processes are entrapped in the matrix
c. Only the processes of odontoblasts are entrapped in the matrix
d. None of the above

4. The mineral content is highest in
a. Peritubular/intratubular dentin
b. Intertubular dentin
c. Interglobular dentin
d. Predentin

5. The calcified dentin includes
a. Both odontoblasts and processes
b. Only processes of the odontoblasts
c. Only odontoblasts
d. None of the above

6. The color of the dentin is
a. Yellowish white
b. Grayish white
c. Pale light yellow
d. White

7. The rate of coronal dentin deposition is approximately
a. 1 mm/day b. 2 mm/day
c. 3 mm/day d. 4 mm/day

8. Dentin consists of
a. 35% organic and 65% inorganic
b. 25% organic and 75% inorganic
c. 10% organic and 90% inorganic
d. 4% organic and 96% inorganic

9. The ratio between the outer and inner surface of dentin is about
a. 2:1 b. 4:1
c. 5:1 d. 6:1

10. Intertubular dentin is
a. Dentin in tubules
b. Dentin present between the odontoblastic processes
c. Dentinal tubules which crossover to enamel
d. Dentin between the zones of peritubular dentin

11. Root dentin is distinguished from crown dentin by presence of
a. Mantle dentin
b. Tomes' granular layer
c. Reparative dentin
d. Contour lines of Owen

12. Crown dentin formation begins at
a. Cap stage
b. Early bell stage
c. Late bell stage
d. Bud stage

13. Mineralization of dentin matrix takes place by
a. Immediate mineralization and later maturation
b. Calcospherite calcification
c. Alternate deposition and mineralization
d. None of the above

1-c, 2-b, 3-c, 4-a, 5-b, 6-c, 7-d, 8-a, 9-c, 10-d, 11-b, 12-c, 13-b

14. Completion of root dentin in deciduous teeth takes place
a. 12 months after the tooth erupts
b. 15 months after the tooth erupts
c. 18 months after the tooth erupts
d. 3 years after the tooth erupts

15. The hypocalcified structures of dentin are
a. Mantle dentin and predentin
b. Incremental lines and neonatal line
c. Interglobular dentin and Tomes' granular layer
d. All of above

16. Among two submicroscopic structures seen in dentinal tubules one is odontoblastic process and the other is
a. Nerve ending
b. Collagen fiber
c. Enamel lamellae
d. Fat droplets

17. The first formed hard tissue of the tooth and the vital tissue of the tooth is
a. Pulp b. Enamel
c. Dentin d. Cementum

18. Junction between primary and secondary dentin is characterized by
a. Sharp reduction in number of dentinal tubules
b. Sharp change in direction of dentinal tubules
c. Reversal line
d. Resting line

19. The fibrillar component of mature dentin is
a. Keratin b. Collagen
c. Reticulin d. Elastin

20. Knoop hardness number of dentin is
a. 109 b. 100
c. 68 d. 54

21. The hypercalcified structures of dentin are
a. Intratubular b. Sclerotic dentin
c. Intertubular d. All of the above

22. Transparent dentin is same as
a. Secondary dentin
b. Sclerotic dentin
c. Mantle dentin
d. Predentin

23. The apatite crystal size of dentin is
a. 4 mm thickness and 120 mm length
b. 3 mm thickness and 100 mm length
c. 2 mm thickness and 80 mm length
d. 1 mm thickness and 60 mm length

24. The hard tissue that forms the bulk of the tooth
a. Enamel
b. Dentin
c. Cementum
d. Both enamel and dentin

25. The ratio of number of tubules per unit area on the pulpal and outer surface is about
a. 4:1 b. 3:1
c. 2:4 d. 2:1

26. The dentin retained after decalcification is
a. Intratubular
b. Intertubular
c. Transparent
d. None of the above

27. The dentin which is similar to osteoid in bone and stains light with H and E compared to other dentin is
a. Primary dentin
b. Secondary dentin
c. Predentin
d. Reparative dentin

28. The mineralized dentin is vulnerable to resorption by odontoclasts in the absence of
a. Inner enamel epithelium
b. Odontoblasts
c. Predentin
d. Ectomesenchymal cells

14-c, 15-d, 16-a, 17-c, 18-b, 19-b, 20-c, 21-d, 22-b, 23-b, 24-b, 25-a, 26-b, 27-c, 28-c

29. The outer layer of primary dentin and the first formed dentin, bounded above by DEJ and below by interglobular dentin is
a. Mantle dentin
b. Circumpulpal dentin
c. Layer of Hopewell Smith
d. Secondary dentin

30. The first few layers of dentin in the root which are structure less is called as
a. Tomes' granular layer
b. Hyaline layer
c. Intertubular dentin
d. Interglobular dentin

31. The rhythmic dentin formation with alternate phases of activity and quiescence is represented as
a. Incremental lines
b. Von Ebner lines
c. Imbrication line
d. All the above

32. The accentuated incremental lines in dentin, because of the disturbance in the matrix and mineralization process, are called
a. Neonatal lines
b. Von Ebner lines
c. Contour lines of Owen
d. Lines of salter

33. Dentin areas characterized by degenerated odontoblastic processes give rise to
a. Sclerotic dentin
b. Reparative dentin
c. Dead tracts
d. Secondary dentin

34. Tomes' granular layer is present in
a. Dentin
b. Cementum
c. Enamel
d. Pulp

35. The vitality of dentin is dependent upon the
a. Dentinal tubules
b. Nerve supply of the pulp
c. Odontoblasts
d. Cementoblasts

36. The cells that form secondary dentin are the
a. Mast cells b. Odontoblasts
c. Osteoblasts d. Cementoblats

37. Among the different areas of dentin the area which contains more mineral component is
a. Dentinal tubule
b. Peritubular dentin
c. Intertubular dentin
d. Mantle dentin

38. Osteodentin is a part of dentin in which one of the following are entrapped
a. Osteoid tissue
b. Osteoblasts
c. Odontoblasts
d. Cementoblasts

39. Among two submicroscopic structures seen in the dentinal tubules, one is odontoblastic process and other is
a. Nerve endings
b. Collagen fibers
c. Sharpey's fibers
d. Enamel lamellae

40. Odontoblastic processes are absent in
a. Mantle dentin b. Sclerotic
c. Circumpulpal d. Secondary dentin

41. Dentinoenamel junction at occlusal or incisal third of a tooth is
a. Straight line
b. Scalloped with its convexities towards enamel
c. Scalloped with its convexities towards dentin
d. Irregular

29-a, 30-b, 31-d, 32-c, 33-c, 34-a, 35-c, 36-b, 37-b, 38-c, 39-a, 40-b, 41-c

42. The statement not true about dentin is
a. Dead tracts appear black in transmitted light
b. Sclerotic dentin appears white in transmitted light
c. Sclerotic dentin appears black in reflected light
d. Dead tracts appear black in reflected light

43. The organic and inorganic substance in dentin is separated by
a. Decalcification
b. Incineration
c. Both of the above
d. Frozen section

44. The first convexity of the dentinal tubules is directed towards
a. The apex of the tooth from enamel surface
b. The apex of the tooth from the pulpal surface
c. The coronal part from pulpal surface
d. The coronal part from enamel surface

45. Mantle dentin is the
a. Most peripheral part of primary dentin
b. First formed dentin
c. Contains numerous coarse fibers
d. All of the above are correct

46. Tomes' granular layer is formed
a. By the deposition of the granules by the odontoblasts
b. By looping of the terminal portion of dentinal tubules
c. Due to hypomineralization of the globular dentin
d. None of the above

47. The predominant inorganic element of dentin is
a. Fluorine b. Calcium
c. Phosphorous d. Sodium

48. Transparent dentin is best demonstrated by
a. Scanning electron microscope
b. Electron microscope
c. Dark field microscope
d. Polarized microscope

49. There is decreased permeability in the following types of dentin
a. Reparative
b. Secondary
c. Sclerotic dentin
d. All of the above

50. The calcified tubule wall of dentin has an inner organic lining termed as
a. Lamina dura
b. Lamina limitans
c. Lamina lucida
d. Lamina densa

51. Circumpulpal dentin matrix consists of
a. Dentinal matrix
b. Dentinal fibers
c. Beta fibers
d. Beta and alfa fibers

52. The type of collagen absent in normal adult dentin is
a. Type I
b. Type II
c. Type III
d. All of the above

53. The main body of dentin is
a. Peritubular dentine
b. Intertubular dentin
c. Predentin
d. Tomes' fibers

54. The cytoplasmic extension of the odontoblasts into dentinal tubules is called as
a. Odontoblastic process
b. Tomes' fiber
c. Both a and b
d. None of the above

42-d, 43-c, 44-b, 45-d, 46-b, 47-b, 48-a, 49-d, 50-b, 51-d, 52-b, 53-b, 54-c

55. The first event of dentinogenesis is formation of
a. Enamel
b. Membrana preformativa
c. Mantle dentin
d. Circumpulpal dentin

56. Interglobular dentin is
a. Dentin surrounding the tubules
b. The dentin present between the odontoblastic processes
c. Dentinal tubules which crossover the enamel
d. None of the above

57. Incremental lines of dentin are called
a. Lines of Retzius
b. Lines of Salter
c. Lines of von Ebner
d. None of the above

58. The type of mineralization seen in dentin is
a. Globular
b. Linear
c. Both a and b
d. None of the above

59. The cells that form secondary dentin are
a. Cementoblasts
b. Fibroblasts
c. Odontoblasts
d. Osteoblast

60. The type of dentin that is formed prior to root completion is
a. Intertubular
b. Peritubular
c. Circumpulpal
d. Secondary

61. The pair of calcified tissues that can be considered vital is
a. Dentin and cementum
b. Cementum and bone
c. Enamel and cementum
d. Dentin and bone

62. Structures present in dentinal tubules are
a. Odontoblastic processes
b. Nerve fiber terminals
c. Collagen fibers and fat droplets
d. All of the above

63. Tomes' granular layer is found in
a. Root dentin
b. On pulpal surface
c. In coronal dentin
d. Near cusp tips

64. One of the following is not correct about the dentinal tubule
a. There are more tubules per unit area in the crown than root
b. They richly branched in root dentin
c. Tubules are more in number near the pulpal surface than at periphery
d. They don't arise from odontoblast

65. Circumpulpal and mantle dentin have following facts except one
a. Both are formed before root completion
b. Circumpulpal is more mineralized than mantle dentin
c. Mantle dentin contains Korff's fibers
d. Tertiary dentin is part of mantle dentin

66. The following fact is true about secondary dentin
a. It is found only in permanent dentition
b. It is the first formed dentin below the DEJ
c. It is formed before root completion
d. It represents dentin formed after root completion

67. The following structural changes are found from primary to secondary dentin except
a. Changes in direction of dentinal tubules
b. Reduction in number of dentinal tubules
c. Progressive crowding of odontoblasts in the pulp
d. Increased diameter of odontoblasts

55-c, 56-b, 57-c, 58-c, 59-c, 60-c, 61-d, 62-d, 63-a, 64-d, 65-d, 66-d, 67-d

Chapter 16

Pulp

LAQ (10 Marks)

Q 1. Write structural elements of pulp. Write the functions and clinical considerations. (*May 2008*)

Ans. Pulp is delicate, soft, richly vascularised and innervated connective tissue which is present at the center of the tooth and is bounded by dentin. It reflects the tooth vitality.

Various structural elements of pulp are (Flowchart 16.1):

1. Cells such as odontoblasts, undifferentiated mesenchymal cells, fibroblasts, various defense cells, and pulpal stem cells
2. Intercellular/extracellular substance
3. Fibers
4. Blood vessels, lymph vessels, and nerves

Flowchart 16.1: Structural elements of dental pulp

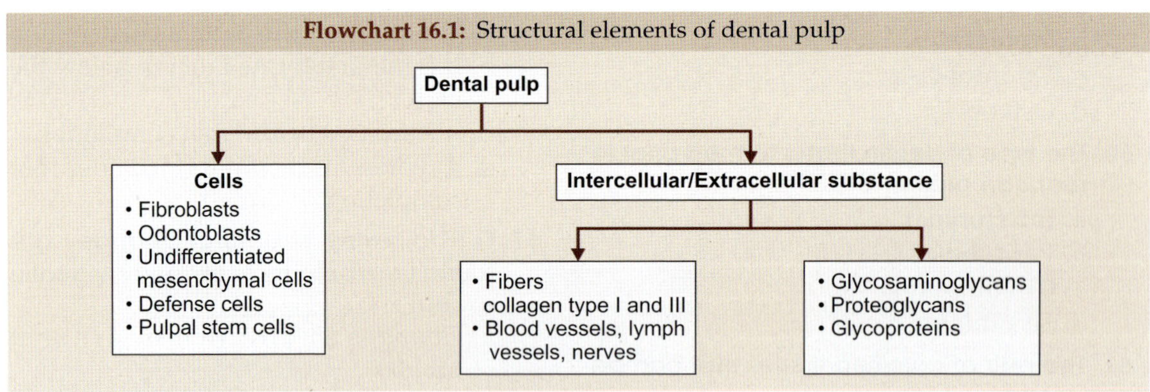

When viewed under microscope pulp shows two regions.

1. The *pulp at periphery* which is composed of three zones.
   a. **Odontoblastic zone:** The outermost zone, adjacent to the pulp-dentin border.
   b. **Cell-free zone:** The middle cell-free zone, Weil's zone, is the space that is seen between the odontoblastic zone and the cell rich zone.
   c. **Cell-rich zone:** It is restricted to the coronal regions.

2. The *pulp at center* : The central region of both the coronal and the radicular pulp contains large nerve trunks and blood vessels (Flowchart 16.2).

Flowchart 16.2: Pulp at center and periphery

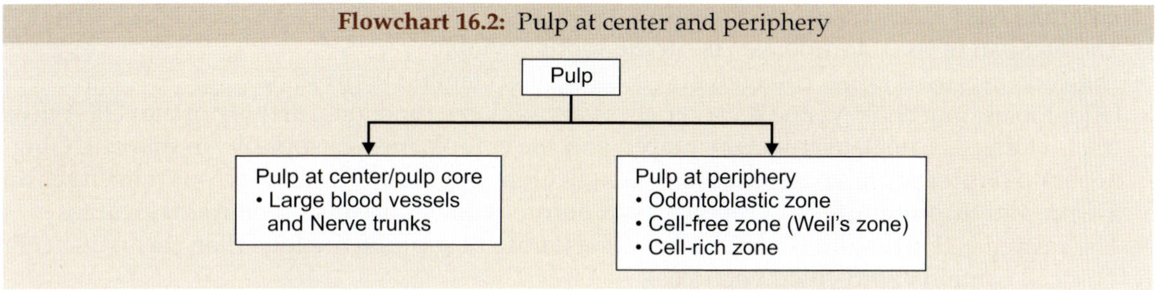

1. Pulp at Periphery (Fig. 16.1)

a. Odontoblastic Zone

- As the name suggests, this zone shows the presence of odontoblasts, the dentin forming cells arranged in a palisading manner. These cells are seen at the periphery of the pulp, adjacent to unmineralized dentin called predentin.
- Odontoblasts are the second most prominent cells in the pulp with cell bodies in the pulp and cell processes in the dentinal tubules.
- They are 5–7 µm in diameter and 25–40 µm in length.
- Though these cells are arranged in a single row, sometimes they crowd and appear pseudo-stratified, as if arranged in two to three rows. The crowding of the odontoblasts is seen because of the reduction in surface area when the odontoblasts move inward and produce secondary dentin.
- The number of the odontoblasts may range from 59,000–76,000/mm^2.
- There is some variation in the morphology, size, and number of odontoblasts in different parts of the tooth. The number and size of the odontoblasts is greater in the coronal pulp as compared with the root.

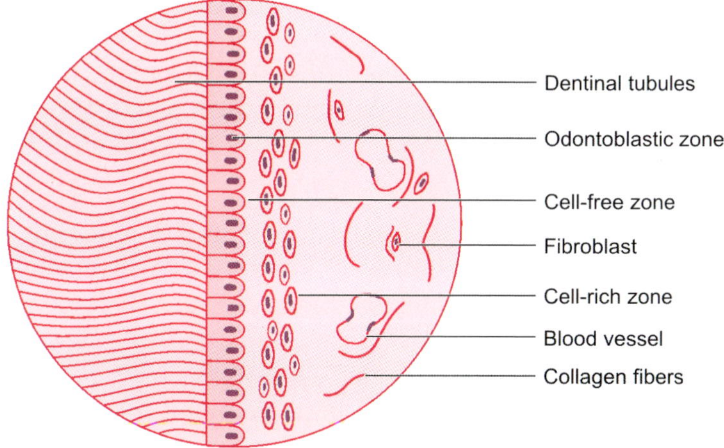

Fig. 16.1: Zones of pulp at periphery

- The cells are columnar in the crown, cuboidal in the mid portion and spindle-shaped in the apical part of the tooth.
- Cell junctions such as gap junction, tight junction, and junctional complexes are seen between odontoblasts.
- The lifespan of the odontoblasts is till the tooth is viable.
- Odontoblasts synthesize collagen and some non-collagenous proteins.
- Odontoblast morphology and its organelles vary with the functional activity of the cell. Active cell is elongated, nucleus is basally placed and the cytoplasm is basophilic. In this cell, Golgi apparatus is prominent, rough endoplasmic reticulum is abundant and numerous mitochondria are present throughout the cytoplasm. Numerous vesicles are also seen in the process.
- The resting cell is devoid of organelles. It has more basophilic nucleus than the active cell. This cell contains lipid-filled vacuoles.
- In the transitional or intermediate stage, the cells are narrower, have fewer organelles and contain autophagic vacuoles.
- Since the odontoblasts are highly differentiated cells, they do not divide. Thus, formation of the reparative dentin happens by the differentiation of undifferentiated mesenchymal cells into the odontoblasts.

***Odontoblastic process*:**

- It is an extension of the odontoblast cell.
- The process measures about 3–4 μm in diameter at their pulpal end and is present inside the dentinal tubule. Junctional complexes are present at this zone.
- Majority of the odontoblastic processes extend to about two-thirds of the lengths of the dentinal tubules.
- The odontoblastic process is devoid of major cell organelles. There are numerous micro-tubules and filaments arranged along the length of the process.
- The space between the odontoblastic process and the dentinal tubule contains fluid called as dentinal fluid. This fluid movement stimulates the pain mechanism in the tubules by mechanical disturbance of the nerves closely associated with the odontoblast and its process.

b. Cell-free Zone of Weil

- This zone appears as a space between the odontoblastic zone and the cell-rich zone. In this space, odontoblasts move more pulpward during tooth development and to a limited extent in functioning teeth.
- There are no cells in this zone. However, there are a few fibres which run through this zone.
- Peripheral axons of myelinated and somatic nerves form a network of nerves within cell-free zone, termed as parietal layer of nerves, also known as ***plexus of Raschkow.***

c. Cell-rich Zone

- This zone is composed principally of fibroblasts and undifferentiated mesenchymal cells and is restricted to the coronal pulp.
- During early dentinogenesis there are many young collagen fibers in this zone.

  1. *Fibroblast*:

  - Fibroblasts are the most numerous cell type in pulp.
  - They function in collagen fiber formation throughout the pulp during the life of the tooth.
  - They are stellate-shaped and have extensive cytoplasmic processes which contact and are joined by intercellular junctions to the processes of other fibroblasts.

  - In young pulp, they divide and are active in protein synthesis, but in older pulp they appear rounded or spindle-shaped with short processes and exhibit fewer organelles and are termed fibrocytes.
  - They synthesise and degrade collagen.
  - They also play role in inflammation and healing.
  - The size of these cells decreases as age advances, while fibrous components predominate.

2. ***Undifferentiated mesenchymal cells*:**
  - Undifferentiated mesenchymal cells are the primary cells in very young pulp.
  - These are totipotent cells which can differentiate into odontoblasts, fibroblasts or macrophages when the need arises.
  - They are larger than fibroblasts and are polyhedral in shape with peripheral processes and large oval nuclei.
  - Apart from cell rich-zone, they are also found along pulp vessels and throughout the central pulp.
  - Number of these cells decreases with age.

- ***Other cells of pulp are*:**
  - Pulp shows a variety of defence cells such as histiocytes, macrophages, dendritic cells, mast cells, and plasma cells.
  - In addition, there are blood vascular elements such as neutrophils (PMNs), eosinophils, basophils, lymphocytes, and monocytes. These migrate from pulpal blood vessels and develop in response to inflammation.

***Defence cells*:**

- *Histiocyte or macrophage* is an irregularly shaped cell with short blunt process and has function of phagocytosis in inflammation. It has small, round, dark staining nucleus and granular cytoplasm. It can be stained by toluidine blue stain.
- *Plasma cells* have eccentrically placed nucleus and abundant cytoplasm and they have function of antibody production. Chromatin of their nucleus is adherent to the nuclear membrane and gives the cell a cartwheel appearance. The cytoplasm is basophilic with light stained Golgi zone adjacent to the nucleus.

Dendritic cells:

- They are found in close relation to the endothelial cell.
- They present the antigen to the T-cells.
- They play an important role in immunosurveillance and their number is increased in areas affected by caries, attrition or restorative procedures.

Lymphocytes, eosinophils and mast cells:

- Lymphocytes and eosinophils are found extravascularly in the normal pulp.
- Their number increases during inflammation.
- Most of the lymphocytes present in pulp are T-lymphocytes.
- Mast cells are seen along the vessels in inflamed pulp. They have a round nucleus and contain many dark staining granules in the cytoplasm.

***Pulpal stem cells*:**

- These are pluripotent cells present in pulp.
- They undergo proliferation and migrate to the site of injured odontoblasts and produce dentin.

- *Clinical significance:* The pulp tissue of the third molars may serve as a suitable source of stem cells for future stem cell based therapies as they are viable after cryopreservation.

2. The Pulp at Centre

Central region of pulp contains large nerve trunks and blood vessels.

Blood Vessels

- Pulp organ is extensively vascularised and vitality of the tooth is due its blood supply.
- The circulation in pulp facilitates rapid transport of metabolites.
- Blood vessels of the pulp and the periodontium arise from the inferior or superior alveolar artery and also drain by the same veins.
- There is communication of the vessels of the pulp with the periodontium through apical foramen and accessory canals due to which the infection has a potential to spread.
- When the vessels enter the pulp, they become thinner walled. Small arteries and arterioles enter the apical canal and along their course to the coronal pulp they give off numerous branches in the radicular pulp. These pass peripherally to form a plexus in the odontogenic region.
- Pulpal blood flow is more rapid than in most areas of the body. Pulpal pressure is among the highest of body tissues.
- *Arteries* possess three layers, the ***tunica intima*** consisting of squamous or cuboidal endothelial cells, ***tunica media*** consisting of one to three layers of smooth muscle cells and the third and the outer layer, the ***tunica adventitia*** made-up of collagen fibers.
- Arterioles are present throughout the coronal pulp and the terminal arterioles are present peripherally in the pulp.
- *Veins* and *venules* are larger than the arteries and appear in the central region of the root pulp. They exhibit much thinner walls in relation to the size of the lumen with much flatter endothelial cells.
- Blood *capillaries,* endothelium-lined tubes, form a network in the coronal pulp. They are involved in rapid transport of metabolites during dentinogenesis.

Lymph Vessels

- The lymphatic vessels are endothelium-lined tubes that join thin-walled lymph venules or veins and are more numerous in the central part of the pulp.
- Lymph vessels draining the pulp and periodontal ligament of the anterior teeth pass to the submental lymph nodes while those of the posterior teeth pass to the submandibular and deep cervical lymph nodes.

Nerves

- Abundant nerve supply in the pulp follows the distribution of the blood vessels. Blood vessels and nerves enter and leave through apical foramen.
- Majority of them are unmyelinated and many are sympathetic. They have role in vasoconstriction.
- The large myelinated fibers mediate the sensation of pain.
- The peripheral axons of the myelinated and somatic nerves form a network of nerves adjacent to the cell-rich zone. This is termed the ***parietal layer of nerves,*** also known as ***plexus of Raschkow.***
- Nerve axons from the parietal zone pass through the cell-rich and cell-free zones and terminate adjacent to the odontoblast processes in the dentinal tubules. These are sensory receptors. They play important role in pain transmission.
- Since, pulp contains only free nerve endings all forms of sensory stimuli result in pain sensation.

Intercellular Substance

- It is composed of acid mucopolysaccharides, protein polysaccharides, and glycoproteins.
- The ground substance lends support to the cells of the pulp. It also transports nutrients from the blood vessels to the cells as well as transport metabolites from cells to blood vessels.

Fibers

- Main type of collagen in pulp is type I. Type III is also present.
- They exhibit typical cross striations at 64 nm and range in length from 10–100 nm.
- They are diffuse or in bundles.
- Bundles of collagen fibers increase as the pulp matures.
- They are prevalent in root-canals, especially at apex.

Functions

Functions of the pulp are inductive, formative, nutritive, protective and reparative.

1. ***Inductive***:

- Primary role of pulp anlage is to interact with the oral epithelial cells, which leads to differentiation of the dental lamina and enamel organ formation, leading to formation of enamel.
- The pulp anlage also interacts with the developing enamel organ as it determines a particular type of tooth.

2. ***Formative***: Pulp contains dentin forming cells, the odontoblasts. They secrete organic matrix of dentin and also take part in its calcification.

3. ***Nutritive***: Pulp is richly vascular. It nourishes dentin through the odontoblasts and their processes and by means of the blood vascular system of the pulp.

4. ***Protective***: The pulp is supplied by sensory nerves. These respond to various thermal, chemical, and physical stimuli in the form of pain and protect the tooth from injury.

5. ***Defensive or reparative***:

- Pulp has capacity to repair injury.
- It responds to irritation, whether mechanical, thermal, chemical or bacterial by producing reparative dentin and mineralizing any affected dentinal tubule *(sclerotic dentin formation)*.
- After injury to the mature tooth, the fate of odontoblast varies according to the intensity of the injury. Milder injury can result in functional activity leading to focal secretion of reactionary dentin called *Regeneration.* If the injury is greater, death of odontoblasts can result. Differentiation of the totipotent cells from subodontoblastic zone then takes place resulting in formation of new odontoblasts which then form *Reparative dentin.*
- Both, the reparative dentin formed in the pulp and the sclerosis in the dentinal tubules are attempt to wall off the pulp from its source of irritation.
- Pulp has macrophages, lymphocytes, neutrophils, monocytes and plasma and mast cells, which aid in the process of repair of the pulp.

SAQs (3 Marks)

Q 1. Write about age changes in pulp or regressive changes in pulp.

Pulp stones/denticles or diffuse/linear calcifications.

Ans. Introduction

Pulp is the soft connective tissue present at the center of the tooth and is surrounded by dentin. With age, size of pulp reduces due to continuous deposition of dentin.

In aging pulp the changes are seen in both cellular and extracellular components as:
1. Cellular changes
2. Fibrosis
3. Vascular changes
4. Pulp stones (denticles)
5. Diffuse calcification

1. Cellular Changes

Ageing pulp shows decrease in the number of cells with decrease in their size and number of cytoplasmic organelles.

2. Fibrosis

- In the ageing pulp accumulation of diffuse fibrillar components and bundles of collagen fibers appear (Fig. 16.3).
- In radicular pulp, fiber bundles are arranged longitudinally while in coronal pulp they are more diffuse.
- Any external trauma such as dental caries or deep restorations usually cause a localized fibrosis.
- Collagen gets deposited in medial and adventitial layers of blood vessels.

3. Vascular Changes

- Atherosclerotic plaques may appear in pulpal vessels.
- Calcifications are found in the walls of blood vessels and surrounding the vessels.
- Blood flow decreases with age.

4. Pulp Stones (Denticles)

- Pulp stones or denticles are nodular, calcified masses appearing in either or both the coronal and root portions of the aging pulp (Figs 16.2A and B).
- Tooth with pulp stones appears normal and is asymptomatic unless they impinge on nerves or blood vessels.
- They are seen in functional or embedded unerupted teeth as well.
- Types according to their structure are: (a) True denticles, (b) False denticles.
- Depending on the relation with dentin, pulp stones can be grouped as: (i) Free, (ii) Attached, (iii) Embedded.

True denticles (Fig. 16.2A)	*False denticles* (Fig. 16.2B)
1. **Structure:** These are similar in structure to dentin as they have dentinal tubules and contain processes of odontoblasts.	1. Do not exhibit dentinal tubules but appear as concentric layers of calcified tissue in the centre of which there appear remnants of necrotic and calcified cells.
2. **Location:** These are rare and located close to the apical foramen.	2. Appear within bundle of collagen fibers or arise around vessels or necrotic tissue.
3. **Formation:** True pulp stones are formed because of the inclusion of remnants of Hertwig's epithelial root sheath into the pulp. These cells induce differentiation of pulpal cells into odontoblasts and further lead to deposition of dentin.	3. Remnants of necrotic and calcified cells or calcification of thrombi in blood vessels, phleboliths, serve as nidi for false denticles.

***Free, attached or embedded pulp stones*:**

- Depending on the relationship of denticles to the dentin, they can be free, attached on embedded. The free denticles are entirely surrounded by pulp tissue, attached denticles are partly fused with the dentin and embedded denticles are entirely surrounded by dentin.
- All are formed free in the pulp and later they become attached or embedded as dentin formation progresses.

Clinical Significance

1. Pulp stones lying at the opening of the root canal can cause difficulty in locating the canals during root canal treatment.
2. A statistically significant relationship has been found between patients with cardiovascular disease (CVS) and presence of pulp stones. This suggests the usefulness of dental radiograph to identify patients with CVS disease for further evaluation.

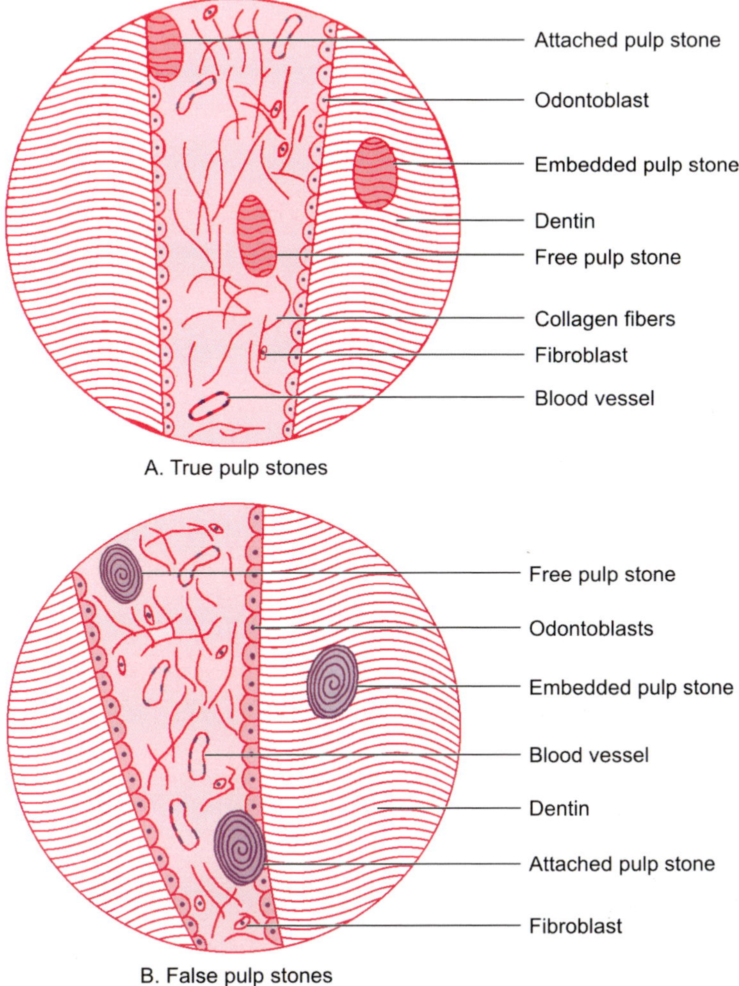

Figs 16.2A and B: Types of pulp stones/Denticles—true and false

5. Diffuse or Linear Calcifications

- These appear as irregular calcific deposits in the pulp tissue.
- Usually seen around collagenous fiber bundles or blood vessels.
- Are found in the root canals while denticles are commonly found in the coronal pulp.
- These are dystrophic type of calcifications (Fig. 16.3).
- With increasing age the volume of pulp and reparative capabilities of pulp decreases. The blood flow is reduced. There is increase in the number of calcified tissues in pulp.
- All these changes contribute to a decrease in pulp resilience and its ability to sense and react to insult.

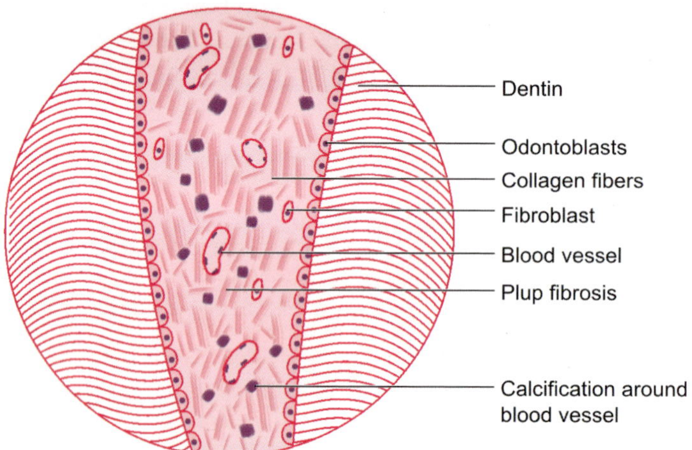

Fig. 16.3: Pulp fibrosis and calcification

Q 2. Write about vitality of pulp.

Ans. VITALITY OF PULP

- Pulp organ is extensively vascularized and the vitality of the pulp depends on its blood supply.
- In clinical practice, instruments called *vitalometers*, which test the reaction of the pulp to electrical stimuli or thermal stimuli (heat or cold) are often used to test the vitality of the pulp.
- However, these methods provide information about the status of the nerves supplying the pulp tissue and therefore check the *"sensitivity"* and not the *"vitality"* of pulp.
- The vitality of the pulp depends on its blood supply.
- In traumatized teeth, there can be damage to the nerves but the blood supply can be normal. Such pulps do not respond to electrical or thermal stimuli but are completely viable.

Q 3. Write clinical considerations of pulp.

Ans. CLINICAL CONSIDERATIONS

- Pulpitis, inflammation of pulp, is a response of the traumatized pulp, due to dental caries or physical trauma to the tooth structure. Mild pulpal inflammation, focal reversal pulpitis, if left untreated may progress to acute or chronic pulpitis. Pulp polyp or chronic hyperplastic pulpitis, a type of chronic pulpitis is seen with well-vascularized pulpal apex. This requires endodontic theraphy or open extraction of tooth.

- Internal resorption or pink tooth, is the outward resorption of dentinal walls which results in the pulpal tissue appearing pink through thin, transulent enamel.
- For all operative procedures the shape of the pulp chamber and its extension into the pulpal horns is important. Wide pulp chamber and higher pulp horns in the tooth of a young person will make a deep cavity preparation hazardous, and it should be avoided. X-ray will help to determine the size of the pulp cavity.
- Since dehydration causes pulpal damage, operative procedures producing this condition should be avoided. An appropriate cavity liner should be used below deep restorations. Pulp has to be protected from damage due to heat transmission by metallic restorations by the use of bases.
- In older person, due to excessive deposition of dentin at the roof and floor of the pulp chamber, it is difficult to locate the root canals. In such cases it is advisable to advance toward the distal root in the lower molar and toward the palatal root in the upper molar to avoid perforation of the floor of the pulp chamber.
- In the anterior teeth, the coronal part of the pulp chamber may be filled with secondary dentin and pulp stones lying at the opening of the root canal make location of the root canal difficult.
- The shape and location of apical foramen may play an important role in the treatment of root canal.
- When accessory canals are located near the coronal part of root or in the bifurcation are, a deep periodental pocket may cause inflammation of dental pulp. Conversely, a necrotic pulp can cause spread of disease to periodontium.
- Pulpal and periodontal disease may spread by their common blood supply. Pulpal infection can spread into periodontal ligament causing abssesses and cysts.
- Most of the compounds containing Ca(OH) readily induce reparative dentin underlying a cavity. Enamel matrix derivative is also shown to be promoting reparative process in the wounded pulp. Mineral trioxide aggregate (MTA) is shown to be with effective as pulp capping agent.
- In clinical practice, instrument called vitalometer is used to test the vitality of the pulp. It tests the reaction of pulp to electrical or thermal stimuli. These methods provide information about the status of the nerves supplying the pulpal tissue and therefore check the sensitivity of the pulp and not its vitality.
- The vitality of pulp depends on its blood supply. The thickness of remaining dentin is shown to be an import factor in maintaining the vitality of pulp. A minimum thickness of 5 mm or greater has a powerful influence on pulp vitality.
- Since the pulp contains only free nerve endings all forms of sensory stimuli like touch, pressure or temperature to the pulp result in pain sensation only. Pain is the only symptom of pulpitis.

MULTIPLE CHOICE QUESTIONS (MCQs)

1. The total number of pulp organs in every person is
a. 20 b. 28
c. 32 d. 52

2. The total volume of all the permanent teeth pulp organs is
a. 0.50 cc b. 0.42 cc
c. 0.38 cc d. 0.28 cc

3. As the age advances the pulp becomes
a. Smaller
b. Larger
c. Remains of same size
d. None of the above

4. The average size of the apical foramen of the maxillary teeth in the adult is
a. 0.2 mm b. 0.3 mm
c. 0.4 mm d. 0.5 mm

5. In the mandibular teeth the average size of the apical foramen is
a. 0.4 mm b. 0.3 mm
c. 0.2 mm d. 0.1 mm

6. The cells occurring in the greatest number in the pulp are
a. Plasma cells
b. Odontoblasts
c. Fibroblasts
d. Macrophages

7. The pulp is the only specialized connective tissue which lacks
a. Precollagenous fibers
b. Collagenous fibers
c. Elastic fibers
d. All of the above

8. As the pulp matures, the number of bundles of collagen fibers
a. Increases
b. Decreases
c. Remains same
d. Disappear

9. Close to the apex of the adult tooth, the odontoblasts appear like osteoblasts, they can be recognized as odontoblasts
a. Due to their ovoid shape
b. Due to their spindle shape
c. Due to their processes extending into the dentin
d. Due to their large nucleus

10. Compared to the pressure in other body tissue the pressure in the pulp is
a. Higher
b. Lower
c. Moderate
d. Same as in other tissues

11. The capillary associated fibroblasts are
a. Fibrocytes b. Pericytes
c. Mast cells d. Lymphocytes

12. The change that occurs in pulp due to aging is
a. Increase in vascularity
b. Increase in number of collagen
c. Increase in size of pulp chamber
d. Calcification and vascularity decreases

13. The sensation felt by pulpal nerves is that of
a. Temperature b. Pressure
c. Pain d. Proprioception

14. Rich nerve plexus in the subodontogenic cell-free zone is known as
a. Parietal plexus
b. Plexus of Rashkow
c. Circum odontoblastic plexus
d. All of the above

15. The pulp responds to irritation because of its remarkable reparative ability by
a. Producing reparative dentin in the pulp
b. Calcification of dentinal tubules
c. Both a and b
d. None of the above

1-d, 2-c, 3-a, 4-c, 5-b, 6-c, 7-c, 8-a, 9-c, 10-a, 11-b, 12-b, 13-c, 14-d, 15-c

16. The cells of the pulp which aid in the process of repair of the pulp are
a. Macrophages and mast cells
b. Lymphocytes and monocytes
c. Neutrophils and plasma cells
d. All of the above

17. As each tooth matures, the number of odontoblasts
a. Decreases
b. Increases
c. Remains the same
d. Degenerates

18. The collagen fibers in the pulp are secreted (produced) by
a. Fibroblasts b. Odontoblasts
c. Both a and b d. Osteoblasts

19. Degradation of fibers in pulp takes place by
a. Odontoblasts b. Fibroblasts
c. Both a and b d. Osteoblasts

20. Plexus of Rashkow is the name given to plexus of
a. Nerve fibers around blood vessels in periodontal ligament (PDL)
b. Periodontal fibers in PDL
c. Nerve fibers in peripheral pulp
d. Gingival fibers around the cervix of a tooth

21. True pulp stones exhibit structure of
a. Concentric layers of calcification
b. Tubular arrangement like in dentin
c. Homogeneous mass of calcification
d. Cells of remnants of Hertwig's epithelial root sheath

22. Diffuse, minute foci of calcification in the pulp are termed
a. Pulp stones
b. Diffuse calcification
c. Pulp polyps
d. False denticles

23. In pulp, the cells which are believed to be totipotent are
a. Pericytes
b. Odontoblasts
c. Undifferentiated mesenchymal
d. Fibroblasts

24. As age advances pulp becomes smaller because of
a. Continuous deposition of collagen fibers
b. Continuous deposition of dentin
c. Increase in the cells of the pulp
d. Calcification

25. The location and shape of apical foramen may undergo changes as a result of
a. Functional influence on the teeth
b. Continuous deposition of dentin
c. Continuous deposition of cementum
d. Continuous deposition of bone

26. Fibers which are found in pulp are
a. Collagen and oxytalan
b. Collagen and elastic
c. Collagen
d. Collagen and reticulin

27. The cart wheel appearance of nuclear chromatin is seen in
a. Mast cells b. Macrophages
c. Basophils d. Plasma cells

28. All of the following cells are present in pulp *except*
a. Fibroblast
b. Fat cells
c. Odontoblasts
d. Undifferentiated mesenchymal cells

29. Histologically the dental pulp at centre most closely resembles
a. Nerve tissue
b. Vascular tissue
c. Granulation tissue
d. Loose connective tissue

16-d, 17-a, 18-c, 19-b, 20-c, 21-b, 22-b, 23-c, 24-b, 25-a, 26-c, 27-d, 28-b, 29-d

30. Which one of the following structures is not found in a living pulp?
a. Collagen fibers
b. Haversian canals
c. Nonmyelinated nerves
d. Odontoblasts

31. All the following fibers are seen in the dental pulp *except*
a. Elastic fibers
b. Collagen fibers
c. Argyrophilic fibers
d. Nerve fibers

32. Total volume of pulp tissue combined in all permanent teeth is
a. 0.38 cc b. 0.68 cc
c. 0.95 cc d. 2.23 cc

33. Histiocytes in the pulp are also called
a. Fibroblasts
b. Resting wandering cells
c. Undifferentiated mesenchymal cells
d. Mast cells

34. Perivascular granulocyte found in inflamed pulp is
a. Histiocyte
b. Lymphocyte
c. Plasma cell
d. None of the above

35. True denticles are present
a. Near apical foramen
b. In pulp chamber
c. In coronal third of the root
d. In apical third of the root

36. Accessory canals result from
a. Defects in cementogenesis
b. Dividing epithelial bridges
c. Break in Hertwig's root sheath
d. Adherent epithelial rests

37. The principal cell of pulp tissue is
a. Fibroblast b. Odontoblast
c. Defence cell d. Histiocyte

38. Nerve supply of pulp is
a. Sympathetic afferent
b. Sympathetic efferent
c. Parasympathetic afferent
d. Parasympathetic efferent

39. Pulp formation starts at
a. 6th week b. 8th week
c. 10th week d. 14th week

40. Space occupied by dental pulp is called
a. Pulp chamber b. Pulp cavity
c. Pulp canal d. Any of above

41. The total volume of pulp organ of maxillary first molars is
a. 0.006 cc b. 0.007 cc
c. 0.068 cc d. 0.38 cc

42. The total volume of pulp organ of mandibular central incisor is
a. 0.006 cc b. 0.007 cc
c. 0.012 cc d. 0.014 cc

43. Weil's zone of pulp is a
a. Cell-rich zone
b. Cell-free zone
c. Fibroblast zone
d. Mesenchymal cell zone

44. In young pulp the cells which divide and are active in protein synthesis are known as
a. Fibroblasts b. Fibrocytes
c. Odontoblasts d. Histiocytes

45. The anastomosis which occurs in pulp is
a. Venous-venous
b. Arteriole-venous
c. Both a and b
d. None of the above

46. The second most prominent cell in pulp is
a. Fibroblast
b. Cementoblast
c. Odontoblast
d. Neutrophil

30-b, 31-a, 32-a, 33-b, 34-a, 35-a, 36-c, 37-a, 38-a, 39-b, 40-b, 41-c, 42-a, 43-b, 44-a, 45-c, 46-c

47. Sensation of pain in pulp is mediated by
a. Large myelinated fibers
b. Large unmyelinated fibers
c. Small unmyelinated fibers
d. None of the above

48. The peripheral axons form a network of nerves located adjacent to the cell-rich zone in pulp is known as
a. Parietal layer of nerves
b. Plexus of Rashkow
c. Zone of Weil
d. Both a and b

49. In which week of intrauterine life nerve fibers in dental follicles are first seen
a. Sixth week
b. Eleventh week
c. Eighteenth week
d. Twenty fourth week

50. In which week of intrauterine life nerve fibers in dental papillae are first seen
a. Sixth week
b. Twelfth week
c. Eighteenth week
d. Twenty fourth week

51. Wandering cells of pulp are
a. Lymphoid wandering cells
b. Histiocytes
c. Fibroblasts
d. Undifferentiated mesenchymal cells

52. Calcification in the walls of blood vessels in aging pulp is found most often in the region near the
a. Coronal portion of root
b. Cementoenamel junction of root
c. Apical foramen
d. Pulp chamber

53. The tooth pulp is initially called the
a. Predentine
b. Dental papilla
c. Subpulpal dentin
d. Pulp polyp

54. Protein secreted by odontoblast is
a. Chitin b. Keratin
c. Collagen d. Elastin

55. Dystrophic calcification is seen most commonly in
a. Enamel b. Pulp
c. Dentin d. PDL

56. In a developing tooth, the junction of the dental papilla and the inner enamel epithelium becomes the
a. Zone of Weil
b. Dentinoenamel junction
c. Cementoenamel junction
d. Primitive epithelial layer

57. Pulp chamber is that part of pulp cavity where the external surface of dentin is covered by
a. Cementum
b. Enamel
c. Both cementum and enamel
d. None of the above

58. Pulp canal or root canal space is that part where the external surface of dentin is covered by
a. Cementum
b. Enamel
c. Both a and b
d. None of the above

59. The cellularity of pulp within the pulp chamber is
a. More than the pulp in the canal
b. Less than the pulp in the canal
c. Same as in the canal
d. None

60. The odontoblasts are cuboidal in pulp chamber but as the apex is approached they are
a. Still cuboidal
b. Columnar
c. Flatter
d. Hexagonal

47-a, 48-d, 49-b, 50-c, 51-b, 52-c, 53-b, 54-c, 55-b, 56-b, 57-b, 58-a, 59-a, 60-c

61. Lateral root canals in anterior teeth are most commonly found in
a. Apical third of the root
b. Middle third of the root
c. At cervical line
d. Cervical third of the root

62. In a tooth the entire space occupied by pulp organ is
a. Pulp cavity
b. Pulp chamber
c. Pulp canal
d. None of the above

63. Pulp stones are usually seen in
a. Young pulp organ
b. Aged pulp organ
c. Traumatized pulp
d. Infected pulp

64. Pulp communicates with peripheral tissues through
a. Apical foramen
b. Pulp canals
c. Mental foramen
d. Dentinoenamel junction

65. The pulp cavities of deciduous teeth are
a. Proportionately smaller than in permanent teeth
b. Proportionately larger than in permanent teeth
c. Have long pulp horns
d. Are same as that of permanent teeth

66. The term fibrocytes is applied to
a. Fibroblasts active in protein synthesis
b. Fibroblasts with fewer intracellular organelles
c. The undifferentiated mesenchymal cells
d. Fibroblasts undergoing calcification

67. The average length of time a primary pulp functions in the oral cavity is
a. 8.3 years b. 9.3 years
c. 7.3 years d. 6.3 years

68. All the following are true regarding blood supply to the pulp *except*
a. Blood flow is more rapid and highest amongst body tissues
b. Blood capillaries form dead ends in the pulp
c. Blood vessels form rich anastomosing network in the odontogenic region
d. Blood supply increases as the age increases

69. All the facts are true regarding nerve supply *except*
a. Supplied by branches of trigeminal nerve
b. A nerve plexus of Rashkow near cell-rich zone
c. Nerve fibers are sympathetic and nonmyelinated
d. Nerve fibers are parasympathetic and myelinated

61-a, 62-a, 63-b, 64-a, 65-c, 66-b, 67-a, 68-d, 69-d

Chapter 17

Cementum

LAQs (10 Marks)

Q. 1. Define cementum. Give functions and its properties. Add a note on cementogenesis.
(Nov. 2010)

Ans. Introduction

- Cementum is a mineralized, avascular connective tissue covering the anatomic roots of the human teeth.
- It furnishes the medium for the attachment of collagen fibers that bind the tooth to the surrounding structures.

Physical Properties

- ***Colour***: Cementum is light-yellow in colour and can be distinguished from enamel by its lack of luster and its darker hue.
- ***Hardness***: Its hardness is less than that of dentin.
- ***Permeability***: It is permeable to a variety of materials. It is more permeable than dentin.
- ***Thickness***: It varies in thickness. It is thinnest at cementoenamel junction (20 to 50 μm) and thickest at apex (150 to 200 μm).

Chemical Properties

- ***Chemical composition***: It contains 45 to 50% inorganic substance and 50 to 55% organic substance and water.
- Inorganic portion consists mainly of calcium and phosphate in the form of hydroxyapatite.
- Organic portion consists of type I collagen and protein polysaccharides. The noncollagenous proteins in cementum have role in matrix deposition, initiation, and control of mineralization and matrix remodeling. These proteins are bone sialoprotein and osteopontin.
- Proteoglycans present in cementum are chondroitin sulfate, heparan sulfate, etc.
- Cementum has the highest fluoride content of all the mineralized tissues.

Cementogenesis

(SAQ, Oct. 2002, Nov. 2010)

- The process of formation of cementum is known as cementogenesis and the cells which form cementum are cementoblasts (Fig. 13.4B).

- Cementum formation in developing tooth is preceded by the deposition of dentin along the inner aspect of *Hertwig's epithelial root sheath (HERS).* HERS induces cells of dental papilla to differentiate into odontoblasts, which form root dentin.

Cementoblasts

- Once dentin formation is underway, HERS breaks, allowing the newly formed dentin to come in direct contact with the connective tissue of dental follicle.
- Cells derived from dental follicle then differentiate into cementoblasts which form *cellular intrinsic fiber cementum (CIFC).* Cementoblasts derived from dental follicle have a similar phenotype to osteoblasts.
- One more source of cementoblasts is HERS. Cementoblasts derived from HERS are involved in the formation of *acellular extrinsic fiber cementum.*
- Cementoblasts have numerous mitochondria, a well-formed golgi apparatus and large amount of granular rough endoplasmic reticulum.
- Cementoblast synthesize collagen and protein polysaccharides, which make-up the organic matrix of cementum.

Formation of Acellular Cementum

- Acellular cementum formation is preceded by mineralization of first formed dentin after which the root sheath breaks.
- Cementoblasts derived from HERS come in contact with dentin and lay down ground substance and collagen fibrils forming acellular cementum.
- Acellular cementum extends from cervical margin to apical one-third.

Formation of Cellular Cementum

- Celluar cementum is deposited over acellular cementum. It is less mineralized than acellular cementum.
- The cementoblasts derived from dental follicle secrete the collagen fibers and ground substance which form the intrinsic fibers of cellular cementum.
- Matrix secretion occurs from different regions of these cementoblasts (multipolar) and the rate of deposition of matrix is fast. Uncalcified matrix of cementum is **cementoid.**
- This results in entrapment of cementoblasts in its own matrix resulting in formation of cellular cementum.
- Incremental lines called *lines of Salter* are seen in cementum during cementogenesis as there are periods of rest and activity. These lines are closer in acellular cementum.

FUNCTIONS OF CEMENTUM *(SAQ, MAY 13)*

- Cementum is a mineralized, avascular connective tissue covering the anatomic roots of the human teeth.
- Though different functions have been attributed to the different types of cementum, cementum functions as a single unit.

1. Anchorage

- Primary function of cementum is to furnish a medium for the attachment of the collagen fibers that bind the tooth to the alveolar bone.

- Connective tissue fibers from periodontal ligament (PDL) pass between the cementoblasts into the cementum. These fibers, known as *Sharpey's fibers* are embedded in the cementum and they serve to attach the tooth to surrounding bone providing anchorage to teeth.
- In hypophosphatasia, which is characterized by absence of cementum, there is loosening and premature loss of teeth.
- Continuous formation of cementum helps to maintian the width of periodontal ligament.

2. Adaptation

- Cementum is a tissue that makes functional adaptation of teeth possible.
- Deposition of cementum in an apical area compensates for loss of tooth substance from occlusal wear.
- Continuous deposition of cementum is of considerable importance. As the most superficial layer of cementum ages a new layer of cementum is deposited to keep the attachment apparatus intact.

3. Repair

- Cementum serves as a major reparative tissue for root surfaces.
- Damage to roots such as fractures and resorption can be repaired by deposition of new cementum.
- Cementum formed during repair is cellular cementum.

SAQs (3 Marks)

Q. 1. Describe formation of acellular cementum. *(2000, June 2006)*

Ans. Acellular cementum extends from cervical margin to apical one-third.

- Hertwig's epithelial root sheath (HERS) shows close relationship with cementoblasts during acellular cementum formation.
- Acellular cementum formation is preceded by mineralization of first layer of dentin and is associated with secretion of cementum related proteins such as bone sialoprotein, osteopontin and fibrillar collagen.
- Cementoblasts derived from HERS form a fibrous fringe over the layer of first formed dentin. The periodontal ligament (PDL) fibers get attached to this fibrous fringe to form *acellular extrinsic fiber cementum* (Fig. 17.1).
- Connective tissue fibers from PDL pass into cementum and they serve to attach the tooth to the surrounding bone. These are called as *Sharpey's fibers*. These are the extrinsic fibers seen in acellular cementum. The main function of this type of cementum is anchorage especially in single rooted teeth.
- In permanent teeth, this acellular extrinsic fiber cementum is formed after the tooth is erupted, when two-thirds of the root would have been formed. Before this the acellular cementum lining the root, is *acellular intrinsic fiber cementum.*
- *Acellular aftrillar cementum* is the one which is formed when there is premature loss of the reduced enamel epithelium protecting the newly formed enamel at the cervical margin of the tooth.
- Uncalcified cementum matrix is called **cementoid tissue.**
- Growth of cementum is rhythmic process and as new layer of cementoid is formed the old one calcifies.

- A thin layer of cementoid is usually observed on the cemental surface. It is lined by cementoblasts.
- After cementoid is laid down, its mineralization begins. Calcium and phosphate ions present in tissue fluids are deposited into the matrix and are arranged as unit cells of hydroxyapatite.
- Osteocalcin and osteonectin act as nucleators for mineralization and alkaline phosphatase promotes mineralization while osteopontin regulates growth of apatite crystals.
- Incremental lines called as *lines of Salter*, are seen during cementogenesis as there are periods of rest and activity. The periods of rests are associated with these lines. The lines are closer in acellular cementum as it is formed slowly.

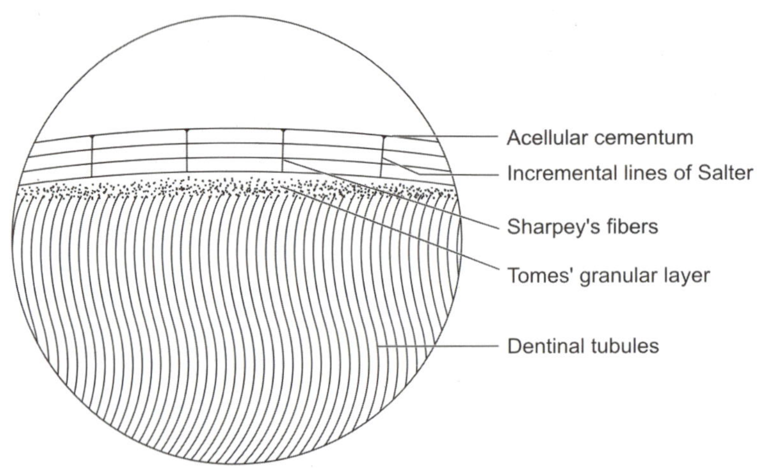

Fig. 17.1: Acellular cementum/Sharpey's fibers

Q. 2. Describe types of cementum, acellular and cellular cementum.

(2000, June 2006, May 2007)

Ans. Introduction

- Cementum is a mineralized, avascular connective tissue covering the anatomic roots of human teeth. It furnishes a medium for the attachment of collagen fibers that bind the tooth to the alveolar bone.
- Cementum of different types differ from one another in their location, structure, function, rate of formation, biochemical composition and degree of mineralization.

On the basis of presence of cementocytes cementum can be classified as:

1. Cellular
2. Acellular cementum.

On the basis of types of fibers, cementum can be classified as:

1. Intrinsic fiber cementum
2. Extrinsic fiber cementum
3. Afibrillar cementum.

- **Intrinsic fibers** are produced by cementoblasts, smaller, and are usually oriented parallel to the surface.

- The **extrinsic fibers** are produced by periodontal ligament (PDL) fibroblasts and are larger bundles and are oriented perpendicular to the surface.
- Thus, by combining the types of fibers, extrinsic and intrinsic, presence or absence of cementocytes, different types of cementum are described as:
  1. Acellular extrinsic fiber cementum (AEFC)
  2. Cellular intrinsic fiber cementum (CIFC)
  3. Acellular afibrillar cementum (AAC).

In addition, acellular intrinsic fiber, cellular and acellular mixed fiber and cellular mixed stratified cementum have also been described.

1. ***Acellular extrinsic fiber cementum (AEFC):***
   - It is regarded as **primary cementum** (Fig. 17.2) as it forms first.
   - It extends from cervical margin to apical third.
   - It is the only type of cementum seen in single rooted tooth.
   - It is formed by cementoblasts which is derived from Hertwig's epithelial root sheath.
   - Cementocytes are not seen. The extrinsic collagen fibers are formed by fibroblasts of PDL and they run perpendicular to the surface of cementum and are known as *Sharpey's fibers.* They are mineralized except for their inner cores.
   - The noncollagenous proteins fill up the space between the extrinsic fibers.
   - This type of cementum is formed slowly and regularly. Therefore, the incremental lines *(lines of Salter)* run parallel to the surface and are closer together.
   - Cementoid is not observed in AEFC.
   - Main function of this type of cementum is anchorage especially in single rooted teeth.
2. ***Cellular cementum (Fig. 17.2):***
   - It is also known as **secondary cementum** as it is formed later than AEFC.
   - It is found in apical third and furcation of roots of teeth.
   - It is of two types:
     a. *Cellular mixed fiber cementum*: It forms the bulk of the secondary cementum and occupies the apical interradicular regions. It contains both types of fibers, that is derived from PDL fibroblasts and the cementoblasts.
     b. *Cellular intrinsic fiber cementum (CIFC)*: It is present in the middle and apical third.
   - These types are mainly involved in adaptation and repair.
   - Cementocytes are present, which lie in lacunae.
   - They have cell processes or canaliculi which anastomose with those of neighbouring cells.
   - Most of the canaliculi are directed toward the PDL surface of the cementum.
   - Cementoblasts forming this type of cementum are derived from dental follicle.
   - Noncollagenous proteins and proteoglycans are present in matrix.
   - Both cellular and acellular cementum are separated by incremental lines into layers which indicate periodic formation.
   - These incremental lines are highly mineralized with less collagen and more ground substance.
   - Incremental lines counted in ground sections are of value in age estimation.
   - As cellular cementum is rapidly formed the incremental lines in it are placed further apart than in AEFC.

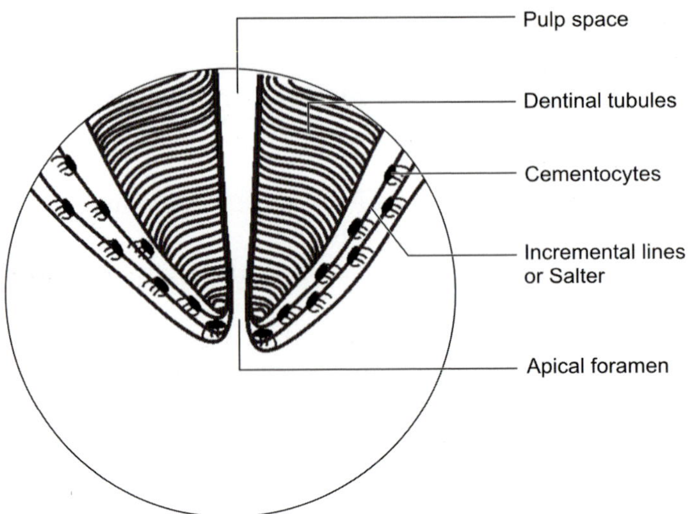

Fig. 17.2: Cellular cementum

3. *Acellular afibrillar cementum:*
   - It is formed when there is premature loss of the reduced enamel epithelium protecting the newly formed enamel at the cervical region. It is deposited as a thin layer on the enamel at the cervical margin of the tooth.
   - It is mineralized ground substance containing no cells and is devoid of extrinsic and intrinsic collagen fibers.

Differences between AEFC and CIFC

	Acellular extrinsic fiber cementum	Cellular intrinsic fiber cementum
1. **Location**	Cervical to apical third of root.	Apical third and furcation.
2. **Formation**	Formed earlier, hence *primary cementum.*	Formed later and during repair, hence named as *secondary cementum.*
3. **Composition**	Noncollagenous proteins are absent. Growth factors are not seen. Proteoglycons are not identified in matrix.	Noncollagenous proteins are present. Growth factors are seen. Proteoglycans are present in the matrix.
4. **Cementoid**	It is usually absent	It is seen on the surface.
5. **Fibers present**	Contain extrinsic fibers of the PDL formed by fibroblast.	Contain intrinsic fibers produced by cementoblasts.
6. **Rate of formation**	Slow	Rapid
7. **Incremental lines of Salter**	These are regular and close together.	These are irregular and far apart.
8. **Presence of Cementocytes**	Cementocytes are not seen.	Cementocytes are present.
9. **Origin of cementoblasts**	Derived from HERS.	Derived from inner cells of dental follicle, cementoblasts are phenotypically similar to osteoblasts.
10. **Expression of parathormone receptor**	Cementoblasts do not express.	Cementoblasts express.
11. **Present in which teeth**	Single rooted teeth.	Absent in single rooted teeth.
12. **Function**	Anchorage	Adaptation and repair

Q. 3. Write about cementocytes. *(2001)*

Ans. CEMENTOCYTES

- Cementum is a mineralized dental tissue covering the anatomic roots of teeth.
- It furnishes a medium for attachment of collagen fibers of periodontal ligament (PDL) that bind the tooth to alveolar bone.
- Cellular or secondary cementum, a type of cementum found in the apical third of the root, is characterized by presence of cementocytes.
- Cementocytes are the cementoblasts which get incorporated into this type of cementum during its formation.
- In cellular cementum, since the matrix secretion occurs from different regions of the cementoblast and it forms fast, cementoblasts get entrapped in their own matrix. These entrapped cells are cementocytes. They are phenotypically similar to osteocytes.
- They lie in spaces called *lacunae.*
- They have numerous cell processes called *canaliculi.* These processes branch and anastomose with those of neighbouring cells.
- These processes are directed towards the PDL surface of cementum for nutrition as cementum is avascular.
- Cytoplasm of cementocytes in deeper layer of cementum contains few organelles, dilated endoplasmic reticulum and sparse mitochondria, suggesting that they are marginally active cells.
- In deeper layers, lacunae appear empty suggesting their degeneration.

Function

They play role in cementum formation and repair.

Q. 4. Write about cementoenamel junction (CEJ). *(July 2005, 2016)*

Ans. CEMENTOENAMEL JUNCTION

- The relation between cementum and enamel at the cervical region of the tooth is cementoenamel junction (CEJ) and is variable (Fig. 17.3).
- Three types of cementoenamel junctions are described :

1. Gap junction:
   - In 10% of the teeth, enamel and cementum do not meet.
   - This occurs when enamel epithelium in the cervical portion of the root is delayed in its separation from dentin.
   - There is no CEJ in such cases and therefore, a zone of root is devoid of cementum and is, for a time, covered by reduced enamel epithelium.

2. Edge-to-edge junction:
   - In 30% of the teeth, cementum meets the cervical end of the enamel in a sharp line.

3. Overlap type of junction:
   - In 60% of the teeth, cementum overlaps the cervical end of enamel for a short distance.
   - This occurs when the enamel epithelium degenerates at its cervical termination, permitting connective tissue to come in direct contact with the enamel surface, which results in formation of afibrillar cementum.

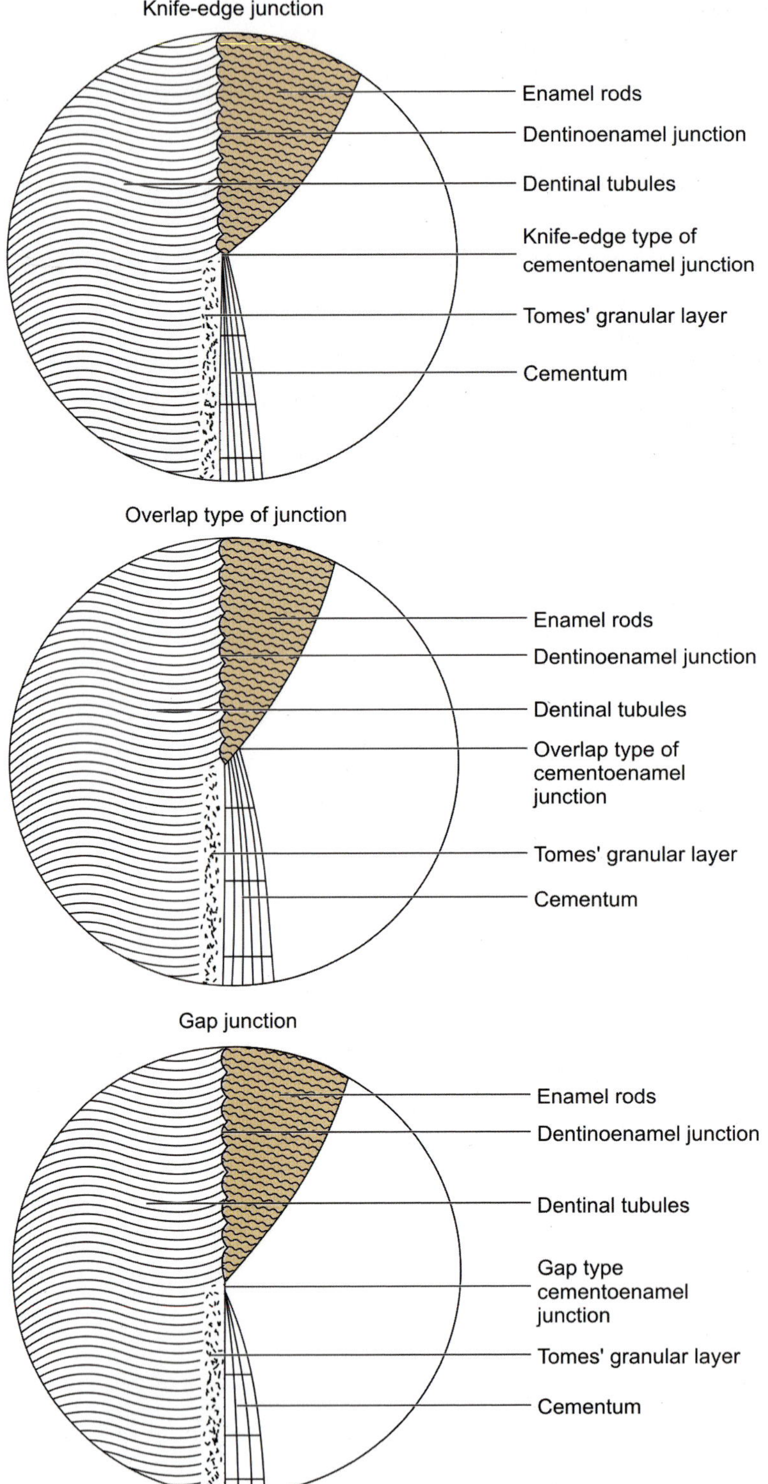

Fig. 17.3: Types of cementoenamel junction

- Afibrillar cementum is so named because it does not possess collagen fibrils with 64 nm periodicity. If such afibrillar cementum remains in contact with connective tissue for long-time, fibrillar cementum is deposited on its surface.
- Recently a fourth type of CEJ has been described in which enamel overlaps the cementum.
- CEJ may exhibit all of these patterns in teeth of an individual.
- In deciduous teeth, edge-to-edge junction is more common, followed by overlap junction.

Q. 5. Write about Sharpey's fibers.

Ans. **SHARPEY'S FIBERS**

- Periodontium is a connective tissue organ, that attaches the tooth to the bone of the jaws.
- This function is furnished by collagen fibers of periodontal ligament (PDL) that are embedded into cementum on one side of the periodontal space and into alveolar bone on the other side. These embedded fibers are termed as *Sharpey's fibers* (Fig. 17.1).
- Sharpey's fibers are the terminal portions of the principal fibers of PDL embedded in cementum and bone.
- They are more numerous but smaller at their attachment into cementum than alveolar bone.
- They are oriented perpendicular to the surface of cementum.
- Each Sharpey's fiber is composed of numerous collagen fibrils that pass well into the cementum.
- Sharpey's fibers in primary acellular cementum are fully mineralized, while those in cellular cementum and bone are generally mineralized only partially at their periphery.
- They are associated with abundance of noncollagenous proteins.
- The mineralization is at right angles to long axis of fibers, indicating that in function the fibers are subjected to tensional forces.
- Few Sharpey's fibers pass uninterruptedly through the bone of the alveolar process, termed *transalveolar fibers,* which may serve as a mechanism to connect adjacent teeth.

Q. 6. Write about intermediate cementum layer (Hyaline layer of Hopewell Smith).

Ans. **INTERMEDIATE CEMENTUM LAYER**

- At cementodentinal junction, sometimes dentin is separated from cementum by a zone known as **intermediate cementum layer**.
- This does not exhibit characteristic features of either dentin or cementum.
- This is predominantly seen in the two-thirds of roots of permanent molars and premolars and is rarely seen in permanent incisors or deciduous teeth.
- This layer represents areas where cells of Hertwig's epithelial root sheath become trapped in a rapidly deposited dentin or cementum matrix.
- It is considered to be of dentinal origin. It contains no tubules but wide spaces which are thought to be enlarged terminals of dentinal tubules.
- **Functions:** It may act as permeability barrier and may be precursor for cementogenesis in wound healing.
- **Clinical significance:** Relates to regeneration of the periodontium following periodontal surgery.

Q. 7. Write about hypercementosis. *(May 2002, 2009)*

Ans. **HYPERCEMENTOSIS**

- It is an abnormal thickening of cementum. It is excessive formation of cementum (Fig. 17.4).

Types

1. ***Generalised*:** When it affects all teeth of the dentition

   or

2. ***Localised*:** When it is confined to a single tooth or even only parts of one tooth.
   - Hypercementosis can be **diffuse** or **circumscribed.**
   - There can be **hypertrophy** or **hyperplasia.** When excessive deposition of cementum improves the function of a tooth, it is known as cementum hypertrophy. Excessive deposition of cementum in non-functional teeth is known as cementum hyperplasia.

Reasons for Hypercementosis

- Excessive cementum formation can occur due to physiological causes like in accelerated eruption of teeth or pathological causes like secondary to chronic periapical infection, Paget's disease.
- ***In localized hypertrophy*** tooth exposed to more stress may form a spur or prong-like extension of cementum to provide firmer anchorage to the subjected tooth.
- ***Localized hypercementosis*** is sometimes seen in areas where enamel drops have been developed on the dentin.
- ***Excementosis*** is knob-like projection of hyperplastic cementum which has developed around degenerated epithelial rests.
- Extensive deposition of cementum associated with chronic periapical inflammation is circumscribed and it surrounds the root like a cuff.
- Thickening of cementum is observed in non-functioning teeth which may extend around the entire root or may be localized. Hypercementosis in non-functioning tooth has reduction in the number of Sharpey's fibers embedded in the root.
- Thickening of cementum around the apex of all teeth and in the furcation of multirooted tooth may be found in embedded and in newly erupted teeth.
- Sometimes irregular overgrowth of cementum with spike like extensions and calcification of Sharpey's fibers accompanied by numerous cementicles may be observed as a sequela of injuries to the cementum.

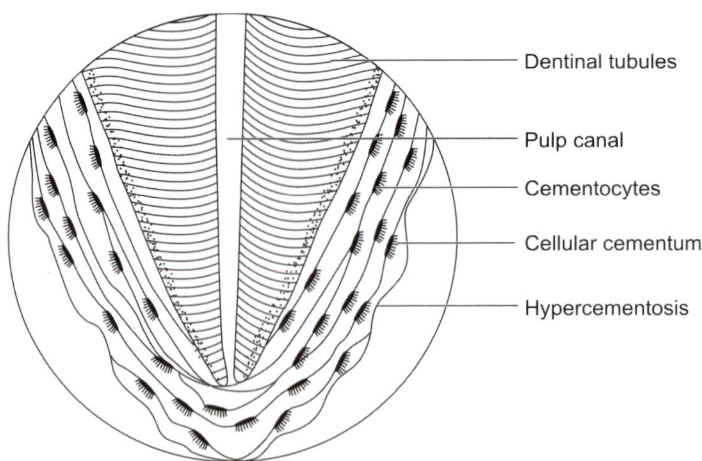

Fig. 17.4: Hypercementosis

- With progressive age, cemental hyperplasia can reach almost three-fold of the normal thickness of cementum.
- Hypercementosis can be seen in some of the neoplastic and non-neoplastic diseases.
- **Generalized thickening** of cementum is seen in **Paget's** disease.
- **Localized thickening** is seen in benign cementoblastoma, florid cemento-osseous dysplasia, acromegaly, calcinosis and some form of arthritis.

Clinical Significance

Hypercementosis results in anchoring the teeth tightly to the socket of jaw and therefore a part of jaw may be fractured in an attempt to extract the tooth. Therefore, it is necessary to take the radiographs of the tooth before extraction.

Q. 8. Write clinical considerations of cementum. *(June 2004, Nov. 2014)*

Ans. Introduction

- Cementum is a mineralized dental tissue covering the anatomic root of human teeth.
- It furnishes a medium for the attachment of collagen fibers that attaches the tooth to the surrounding structure.

Clinical Considerations

- Cementum is avascular and is therefore more resistant to resorption than bone. Because of this property of cementum, the orthodontic tooth movement is possible. When the tooth is moved by orthodontic appliance, bone is resorbed on the side of the pressure and the new bone is formed on the side of tension while minimum cementum resorption is seen.
- Cementum resorption can occur after trauma or excessive occlusal forces and resorption can continue into dentin. The damage is usually repaired either by formation of cellular or acellular cementum or both. When the former outline of root surface is restored, repair is called **anatomic repair.** When a thin layer of cementum is deposited, a bay-like recess remains. In such cases the periodontal space is restored to normal width by formation of a bony projection for proper functional relationship. This type of repair is known as **Functional repair.**
- Transverse fractures of root may heal by formation of new cementum.
- Hypercementosis occurs secondary to periapical inflammation or extensive occlusal stress. Extraction of such teeth may necessitate removal of bone.
- Extensive excementosis anchors the tooth tightly to socket because of which a part of jaw can fracture during extraction of such teeth. Therefore, radiograph should be taken before extraction.
- In periodontal pockets, plaque can cause alterations in pathologically exposed cementum. In periodontal therapy, this altered cementum is intentionally removed so that periodontal regeneration can occur. Commercially available enamel matrix proteins are coated on cleaned and planed root surface for new cementum deposition.
- Cementum is found to be thick in type-2 diabetes.
- Abnormal deposition of cementum can lead to fusion of bone and cementum called as **ankylosis.**
- Counting of the incremental lines in cementum can be useful in age determination in forensic dentistry.

MULTIPLE CHOICE QUESTIONS (MCQs)

1. **The highest content of fluoride of all the mineralized tissues is found in**
   a. Bone
   b. Enamel
   c. Dentin
   d. Cementum
2. **The cellular cementum can be best differentiated from acellular cementum due to presence of**
   a. Embedded Sharpey's fibers
   b. Incremental growth pattern
   c. Separate and distinct functions
   d. Lacunae
3. **The percentage of inorganic and organic contents of cementum is**
   a. 50–55% inorganic and 45–50% organic
   b. 45–50% inorganic and 50–55% organic and water
   c. 40% inorganic and 60% organic
   d. 30–40% inorganic and 60–70% organic
4. **The hardness of fully mineralized cementum compared to dentin is**
   a. Less
   b. More
   c. Equal
   d. Almost equal
5. **Color of cementum is**
   a. Dark yellow
   b. Light yellow
   c. White
   d. Gray
6. **The organic portion of cementum consists of**
   a. Type I collagen and proteoglycans
   b. Type II collagen
   c. Type III collagen
   d. All of the above
7. **When compared to dentin, cementum color is**
   a. Lighter
   b. Darker
   c. Same as dentin
   d. None of these
8. **The characteristic of cementum that is important clinically in the orthodontic treatment is**
   a. Its similarity with bone
   b. Its lusterless light yellow color
   c. Its function of attachment of periodontal ligament fibers
   d. Its resistance to resorption
9. **The thickness of cementum is least at**
   a. Cementoenamel junction
   b. Cementodentinal junction
   c. Middle of the root
   d. At the apex
10. **The cementodentinal junction (CDJ) in permanent teeth is**
    a. Smooth
    b. Scalloped
    c. Zigzag
    d. None of the above
11. **The cementodentinal junction in deciduous teeth is**
    a. Smooth
    b. Scalloped
    c. Zigzag
    d. None of the above
12. **In decalcified and stained sections compared to dentin, cementum stains**
    a. Darker
    b. Lighter
    c. Same as dentin
    d. Does not take stain

1-d, 2-d, 3-b, 4-a, 5-b, 6-a, 7-a, 8-d, 9-a, 10-a, 11-b, 12-a

13. The cementum and enamel meet edge to edge in
a. 40% of teeth
b. 30% of teeth
c. 25% of teeth
d. 20% of teeth

14. Presence of gap between cementum and enamel at cementoenamel junction is found in
a. 10% of teeth
b. 15% of teeth
c. 20% of teeth
d. 25% of teeth

15. Cementum overlaps enamel in
a. 70% of teeth
b. 60% of teeth
c. 40% of teeth
d. 20% of teeth

16. Human cementum is
a. Highly vascular
b. Less vascular
c. Avascular
d. None of the above

17. Under normal conditions cementum undergoes
a. Alternate resorption and formation
b. Resorption and no new formation
c. No resorption
d. No change

18. On the teeth that are not in function, it is observed that cementum gets
a. Thinner
b. Thicker
c. Remains same
d. None of the above

19. Cementum can replace resorbed
a. Enamel only
b. Dentin only
c. Bone only
d. Dentin and cementum

20. Cellular cementum is present along the
a. Coronal third of the root
b. Middle third of the root
c. Apical third of the root
d. All the above

21. Accessory canals result from
a. Defect in cementogenesis
b. Dividing epithelial bridges
c. Breaks in Hertwig's epithelial root sheath (HERS)
d. Adherent epithelial rests

22. Cementicles are the submicroscopic structures present mostly in
a. Acellular cementum
b. Periodontal ligament
c. Cellular cementum
d. Tomes' granular layer

23. Epithelial cell rests of Hertwig's epithelial root sheath may be present in
a. Periodontal ligament
b. Pulp
c. Cementum
d. None

24. The remnants of HERS are known as
a. Epithelial pearls
b. Epithelial islands
c. Epithelial cell rests of Malassez
d. Epithelial knots

25. Incremental lines which indicate periodic formation of cementum are
a. Less mineralized
b. Highly mineralized
c. Both a and b
d. Not mineralized

26. Sharpey's fibers are seen in
a. Ground section
b. Decalcified section
c. Both
d. None of the above

13-b, 14-a, 15-b, 16-c, 17-c, 18-b, 19-d, 20-c, 21-c, 22-b, 23-a, 24-c, 25-b, 26-a

27. If overgrowth of cementum inspires the functional abilities of cementum it is termed as:
a. Hyperplasia
b. Hypoplasia
c. Hypertrophy
d. Hypotrophy

28. Absence of cementum is found in
a. Hypophosphatasia
b. Hyperparathyroidism
c. Hyperthyroidism
d. Mongolism

29. Cementum formation is
a. Not a continuous process
b. Always results in cellular cementum
c. A continuous process
d. Present only during development of tooth

30. Cellular cementum is thickest
a. Around the root apex
b. At cementoenamel junction
c. At middle one-third of the root
d. At coronal one-third of the root

31. Cementum is thinnest at
a. Apical third of root
b. Middle third of root
c. Cementoenamel junction
d. Apical foramen

32. Acellular cementum is thickest at
a. Apical foramen
b. Coronal one-third of the root
c. Middle one-third of the root
d. Apical one-third of the root

33. Cementum deposited on enamel of tooth is
a. Acellular b. Cellular
c. Fibrillar d. Afibrillar

34. Transeptal fibers are present in
a. Between cementum of two teeth
b. Septal area
c. Inter-radicular area
d. Apical area

35. Extrinsic fibers in cementum are secreted by
a. Periodontal ligament fibroblasts
b. Cementoblasts
c. Osteoblasts
d. Cementocytes

36. The commonest type of CEJ is the
a. Knife edge junction
b. Gap junction
c. Enamel overlapping cementum
d. Cementum overlapping enamel

37. Intermediate cementum is also known as
a. Hyaline layer
b. Mixed fiber cementum
c. Hyaline layer of Hopewell Smith
d. None of the above

38. The type of cementum predominantly involved in the process of attachment with the periodontal ligament
a. Cellular
b. Acellular
c. Both a and b
d. None of the above

39. Functional repair of cementum is
a. Repair without a defect restoring the normal anatomy
b. Repair with a bay-like defect
c. Formation of a bony projection by the alveolar bone to establish the normal physiologic width of the periodontal attachment
d. Both b and c

27-c, 28-a, 29-c, 30-a, 31-c, 32-b, 33-d, 34-a, 35-a, 36-d, 37-c, 38-b, 39-c

Chapter 18

Periodontal Ligament

LAQs (10 Marks)

Q. 1. Describe different fibers of periodontal ligament. Enumerate functions of periodontal ligament. *(May 2012)*

Ans. Periodontal ligament (PDL) is a fibrous connective tissue which provides continuity between cementum and alveolar bone and primarily serves to support the teeth in the bony socket.

It is a soft, fibrous, vascular and cellular connective tissue that surrounds the roots of the teeth and joins the root cementum with the socket wall. The extracellular substance of the PDL comprises of fibers and ground substance (Table 18.1).

The connective tissue fibers are mainly collagenous but there are small amounts of oxytalan and reticulin fibers, and in some species, elastin fibers.

Table 18.1: Extracellular substance of PDL

Fibers	*Ground substance*
1. Collagen	1. Glycosaminoglycans
2. Elastic-oxytalan	2. Proteoglycans
3. Reticular	3. Glycoproteins
4. Secondary	
5. Indifferent fiber plexus	

I. COLLAGEN PRINCIPAL FIBERS OF PDL *(SAQ, JUNE 2006)*

The connective tissue fibers of PDL are mainly collagenous.

The collagen fibrils in PDL are of mean diameter 45–55 nm. They are gathered to form bundles of 5 μm in diameter. The main types of collagen in PDL are type I and type III.

Bundles of collagen in PDL are termed *principal fibers.* The principal fiber group is the *alveolodental ligament* which consists of five fiber groups:

1. Alveolar crest group
2. Horizontal group

3. Oblique group
4. Apical group
5. Interradicular group in multirooted teeth.

Principal group of fibers help the periodontal ligament to support the tooth in the bony socket (Figs 18.1A and 18.1B).

1. Alveolar Crest Group

- Extend obliquely from the cementum just beneath the junctional epithelium to the alveolar crest.
- These fibers resist tilting, intrusive, extrusive, and rotational forces.

2. Horizontal Group

- They are immediately apical to the alveolar crest fiber group and run at right angles to the long axis of the tooth from cementum to bone.

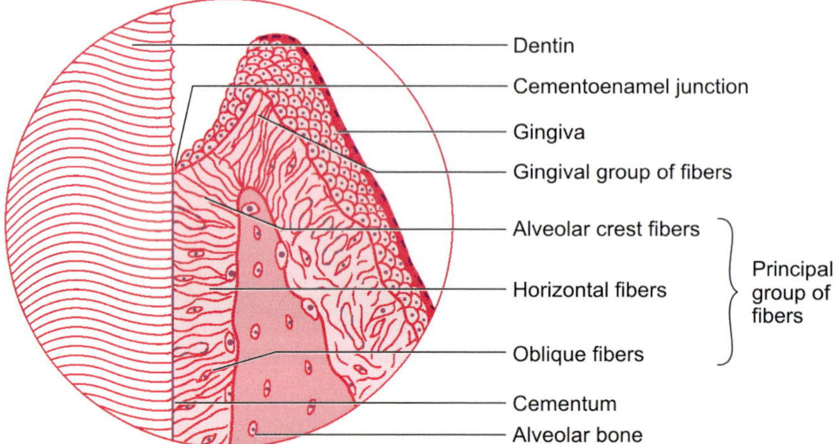

Fig. 18.1A: Principal fibers of periodontal ligament

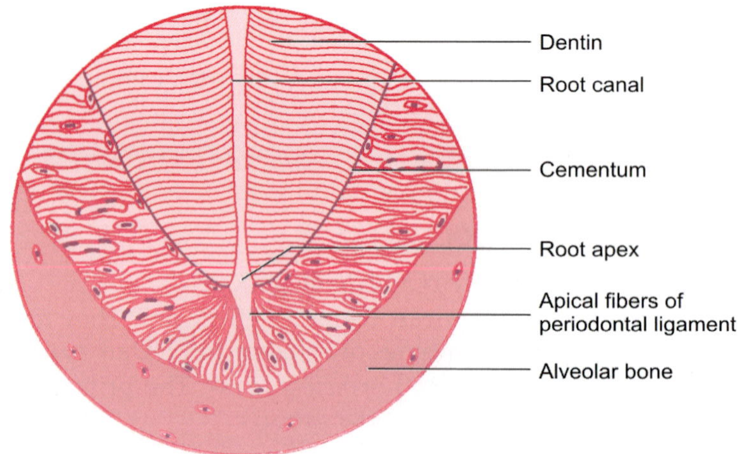

Fig. 18.1B: Principal fibers of periodontal ligament: Apical group of fibers

- They pass from their cemental attachment across the periodontal ligament space to become inserted in the alveolar process as Sharpey's fibers.
- These fibers resist horizontal and tipping forces.

3. Oblique Group

- These are the most numerous and occupy nearly two-thirds of the ligament.
- They run obliquely and coronally from cementum to alveolar bone.
- They resist vertical and intrusive forces.

4. Apical Group

- They traverse from the cementum at the root tip through the periodontal space to the fundus of the bony socket.
- They resist forces of luxation, may prevent tooth tipping and protect delicate blood and lymph vessels and nerves.

5. Interradicular Group

- They are inserted into the cementum from the crest of interradicular septum in multirooted teeth.
- They resist tooth tipping, torquing and luxation.
- They are lost in age related gingival recession when the furcation area is exposed.
- In chronic inflammatory periodontal disease, there occurs total loss of these fibers.

Gingival Group of Fibers (Fig. 18.2) *(SAQ, July 2005)*

- These are found within lamina propria of the marginal gingiva, attaching the gingiva firmly to the teeth.
- They support the marginal gingival tissues and maintain their relationship to the tooth.
- They are referred as gingival ligament and they serve to support the free gingiva, bind attached gingiva to the alveolar bone, tooth, and link one tooth to another (Fig. 18.2). They are divided into:

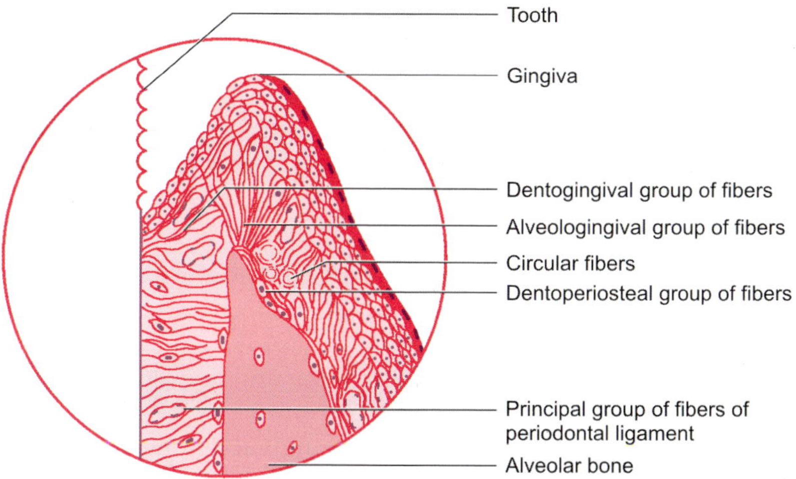

Fig. 18.2: Gingival fibers of periodontal ligament

Gingival group of fibers

1. **Dentogingival:** Extend from the cervical cementum into the lamina propria of the gingiva. They constitute the most numerous group of gingival fibers.
2. **Alveologingival:** They arise from the alveolar crest and extend into the lamina propria.
3. **Circular:** These are small group of fibers that encircle the tooth and interlace with other fibers.
4. **Dentoperiosteal:** They traverse from the cementum into the periosteum of the alveolar crest and of the vestibular and oral surfaces of the alveolar bone.

Transseptal fibers

- These are accessory fibers that extend interproximally between adjacent teeth and they make-up the interdental ligament (Fig. 18.3).
- Apart from all these fibers, semicircular, vertical and transgingival fiber groups also exist.

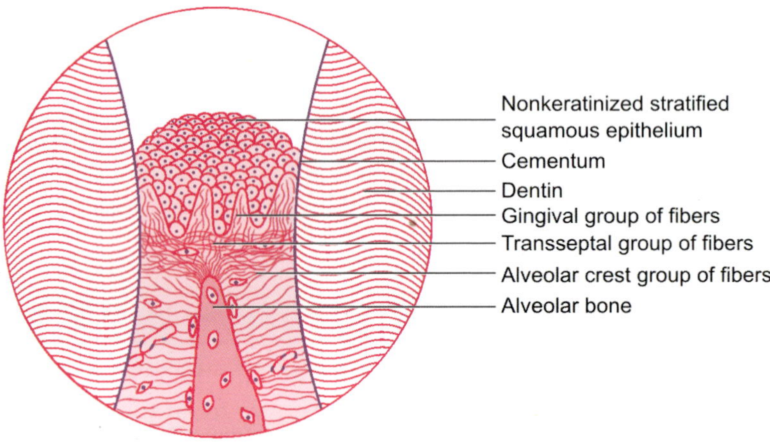

Fig. 18.3: Transseptal fibers

Sharpey's fibers

- These are the terminal portions of the principal fibers embedded into cementum on one side of the periodontal space and into alveolar bone on the other.
- Few Sharpey's fibers pass through the bone of the alveolar process to continue as principal fibers of PDL and are termed as *transalveolar* fibers. They connect adjacent teeth.

II. ELASTIC FIBERS

- There are three types of elastic fibers elastin, elaunin, and oxytalan fibers.
- Elastin are the mature elastic fibers while elaunin and oxytalan are immature. These fibers are present in the walls of afferent blood vessels.
- Elastin meshwork in PDL is composed of many elastin lamellae with peripheral oxytalan fibers and elaunin fibers.
- Elaunin fibers are found within the fibers of the gingival ligament.
- **Oxytalan fibers** *(SAQ, Oct. 2002, July 2005)*: These are a type of immature elastic fibers associated with PDL. They are 0.5 mm to 2.5 mm in diameter. They consist of microfibrillar

component only. Light microscopic demonstration of oxytalan fibers is possible if the tissue is oxidized prior to staining. In electron microscope, they resemble elastic fibers.

Orientation of these fibers is different from that of collagen fibers. They run in axial direction, one end being embedded in cementum or bone and the other in the wall of a blood vessel. At the apex of the tooth they form a complex network.

Functions: They play a part in supporting the blood vessels of the periodontal ligament. They are thicker and more numerous in teeth subjected to high loads. Thus, they have a role in tooth support.

III. RETICULAR FIBERS

They are fine immature collagen fibers with argyrophilic properties. They are related to basement membrane of blood vessels and epithelial cells which lie within PDL.

Functions of PDL *(SAQ, May 2008, Nov. 2010)*

Periodontal ligament is a fibrous connective tissue which provides continuity between cementum and alveolar bone, and primarily serves to support the teeth in the bony socket.

It has following functions:

1. Supportive
2. Sensory
3. Nutritive
4. Homeostatic
5. Eruptive

1. Supportive

PDL collagen fibers, vasculature and its ground substance, all contribute to the tooth support.

When a tooth is moved in its socket as a result of forces acting on it as during mastication, part of the periodontal space will be narrowed and the periodontal ligament contained in these areas will be compressed. Other parts of periodontal space will be widened. The collagen fibers in the compressed ligament, act as a cushion for the displaced tooth. The pressure of blood in the vessels (vascular pressure) also provides a hydraulic cushion for the support of the teeth. Biochemical analysis of the proteoglycans in the PDL has shown that the degree of aggregation/disaggregation of the ground substance may have a role of tooth support. Thus, PDL behaves as a suspensory ligament.

2. Sensory

PDL through its nerve supply provides a most efficient proprioceptive mechanism. PDL can detect the application of the most delicate forces to the teeth and very slight displacement of the teeth.

Mechanoprotection protects both supporting structures of the tooth and the crown from excessive masticatory forces.

3. Nutritive

PDL contains blood vessels, which provide nutrition to its cells, cementocytes and superficial osteocytes of alveolar bone.

4. Homeostatic

PDL has the capacity to resorb and synthesize the extracellular substance of the connective tissue of ligament, alveolar bone, and cementum. This results in maintaining the width of PDL throughout life which functions under physical forces of mastication. This is done by formation or resorption of bone, formation of cementum, formation and degradation of collagen fibers, the ground substance, and detachment and reattachment of collagen fibers to their new locations. Failure of homeostatic mechanism, that is if the balance between synthesis and resorption is disturbed, it may lead to tooth ankylosis and/or tooth resorption and can result in loss of function by the tooth.

5. Eruptive

The cells, vascular elements, and extracellular matrix proteins of the PDL function collectively to enable eruption.

6. Physical

Physical function of PDL entails protection of vessels and nerves of PDL from mechanical forces and also offers resistance to impact from occlusal forces. PDL transmits occlusal forces to the bone by acting as shock absorber.

Q. 2. Describe cells of periodontal ligament.

Ans. CELLS OF PERIODONTAL LIGAMENT

- The periodontium is a connective tissue organ, covered by epithelium that attaches the teeth to the bones of the jaws and provides a continually adapting apparatus for support of the teeth during function. It comprises of cementum, periodontal ligament, bone lining the tooth socket (alveolar bone) and that part of the gingiva facing the tooth (dentogingival junction).
- Periodontal ligament is a fibrous connective tissue which provides continuity between cementum and alveolar bone, and primarily serves to support the tooth in the bony socket.

CELLS OF PDL

- PDL is a fibrous connective tissue that is noticeably cellular.
- The principal cells of the healthy, functioning PDL are concerned with the synthesis and resorption of alveolar bone and the fibrous connective tissue of the ligament and cementum.

Cells of PDL are

I. Synthetic cells

1. Fibroblasts
2. Osteoblasts
3. Cementoblasts

II. Resorptive cells

1. Fibroblasts
2. Osteoclasts
3. Cementoclasts

III. Progenitor cells

IV. Epithelial cell rests of Malassez

V. Defense cells
1. Mast cells
2. Macrophages
3. Eosinophils

I. Synthetic Cells

- These cells synthesize proteins for extracellular substance of connective tissue.
- In light microscope, these cells show a large, open faced or vesicular nucleus with prominent nucleoli (due to increased transcription of RNA and production of ribosomes).
- These cells show cytoplasmic basophilia due to large quantities of rough endoplasmic reticulum (RER) covered by ribosomes. Increased RER and golgi membrane is for translation and transport of proteins.
- Such cells are:
  1. **Osteoblasts:** Synthesizing cells present at the periodontal surface of the alveolar bone.
  2. **Fibroblasts:** Synthesizing cells lying in the body of the soft connective tissue.
  3. **Cementoblasts:** Synthesizing cells found in cementum.

1. Osteoblasts

- Osteoblasts, the bone forming cells, cover the periodontal surface of the alveolar bone or line the tooth socket.
- These cells are cuboidal in shape with prominent round nucleus present at their basal end.
- These are active cells with abundant rough endoplasmic reticulum, mitochondria, and vesicles.
- Cells contact one another and also with the underlying osteocytes through their cytoplasmic processes.

2. Fibroblasts:

- Fibroblasts, the predominant cell in the PDL, are ectomesenchymal in origin. These are different from the fibroblasts which are present in other connective tissues.
- The role of fibroblasts is to produce the structural connective tissue proteins, collagen and elastin, as well as glycoproteins, and glycosaminoglycans that comprise the PDL ground substance.

  Fibroblasts of PDL are characterised by rapid turnover of extracellular matrix, particularly collagen.
- These cells are responsible for the formation and remodelling of the PDL fibers, and a signalling system to maintain the width of PDL by preventing encroachment of bone and cementum into PDL space.
- They are fusiform with extensive cytoplasm and abundant organelles. They are arranged parallel to collagen fibers.
- Presence of actin network endows PDL fibroblasts with a degree of contractility with which it can exert tractional forces on extracellular matrix.

3. Cementoblasts:

- These cells line the surface of cementum.
- They lay down cementum which helps in attachment of tooth.

- They are cuboidal with large vesicular nucleus and abundant cytoplasm. Cementoblasts actively depositing cellular cementum exhibit abundant basophilic cytoplasm and cytoplasmic processes and folded nuclei while those depositing acellular cementum do not have prominent cytoplasmic processes.

II. Resorptive Cells

1. **Osteoclasts:**
   - These are multinucleated giant cells, derived from blood monocytes.
   - They resorb bone and have abundant eosinophilic cytoplasm and numerous cytoplasmic organelles.
   - They appear in *Howship's lacunae* on the surface of the bone to be resorbed.
   - They have ruffled plasma membrane which is separated from the rest of the plasma membrane by *clear zone.*
   - The area of bone to be resorbed is sealed by the ruffled border and is exposed to acidic pH due to pumping of protons by osteoclasts which brings about resorption.
2. **Fibroblasts:**
   - These cells show rapid degeneration of collagen by phagocytosis and that is the basis for fast turnover of collagen in periodontal ligament.
   - Degradation of collagen includes both intracellular and extracellular events.
   - Collagen is degraded extracellularly by matrix metalloproteinases after which there occurs intracellular digestion of collagen with the help of lysosomal cysteine proteinases.
3. **Cementoclasts:**
   - Resemble osteoclasts and are occasionally found in normal functioning PDL.
   - Though cementum does not undergo resorption normally but under certain circumstances its resorption can occur and in these instances cementoclasts located in Howship's lacunae are found on the surface of the cementum.

III. Progenitor Cells (SAQ)

- PDL being a connective tissue, contain progenitors for synthetic cells that have capacity to undergo mitotic division.
- These progenitor cells replace differentiated cells dying at the end of their lifespan or as a result of trauma.
- They are small in size, nucleus is close faced and have very little cytoplasm.
- These cells divide in response to normal biologic requirement or to wounding of PDL.
- They are located predominantly in the vicinity of blood vessels.
- Within this group, mesenchymal stem cells are present and are responsible for tissue homeostasis. They can generate cementoblasts, osteoblasts, and fibroblasts.

IV. Epithelial Rests of Malassez *(SAQ, 2000, Oct. 2003, May 2007)*

Introduction

- These are the epithelial cells that are found close to the cementum in periodontal ligament.
- These were described by Malassez in 1884 and are the remnants of Hertwig's epithelial root sheath.

- At the time of cementum formation, the continuous layer of epithelium that covers the surface of the newly formed dentin breaks into lace like strands which are *epithelial rests of Malassez*.

Location

- They are present near and parallel to the root surface lying about 25 µm from the cementum surface in PDL.
- Their distribution varies as per the site and age. They are numerous in children. They are commonly found in apical region up to the second decade and later are mainly located cervically in the gingiva above alveolar rest.

Histological features

- The epithelial rests persist as a network, strands, islands or tubule like structures near and parallel to the surface of the root.
- In cross-section they appear cluster like and are separated from the surrounding connective tissue by a basal lamina.
- These are cuboidal cells with deeply stained nucleus and with scanty cytoplasm having less number of cytoplasmic organelles, indicating lack of protein synthesis.

Function

- It is not clear but they could be involved in periodontal repair and regeneration.

Significance

- These cells may proliferate to form cysts and tumor.
- These cells may undergo calcification to become cementicles.

V. Defence Cells

1. **Mast cells:**
    - Mast cells are seen occasionally in healthy PDL.
    - They are small round cells often associated with blood vessels.
    - Cells are characterised by numerous cytoplasmic granules which are dense, membrane bound vesicles.
    - These granules stain with basic dyes and are readily demonstrated by metachromatic dye, Azure A. They are also stained by PAS stain.
    - *Function:* These granules contain heparin and histamine. Histamine plays role in inflammatory reaction and its release into extracellular environment causes proliferation of endothelial cells and mesenchymal cells resulting in regulation of their population in PDL.
2. **Macrophages:**
    - Are predominantly located adjacent to blood vessels in PDL.
    - They phagocytose dead cells and secrete growth factors that regulate the proliferation of adjacent fibroblasts and endothelial cells.
3. **Eosinophils:**
    - They are occasionally seen in PDL and are capable of phagocytosis.
    - Balance between the synthesis and resorption of tissues by synthetic and resorptive cells in PDL helps to maintain tissue homeostasis in PDL and maintains its width throughout life.

SAQs (3 Marks)

Q. 1. Write about homeostatic function of PDL. *(June 2004)*

Ans. HOMEOSTATIC FUNCTION

- Homeostatic function is one of the important functions of PDL.
- PDL has the capacity to resorb and synthesize the extracellular substance of the connective tissue of the ligament, alveolar bone, and cementum. This results in maintaining the width of PDL throughout life which functions under physical forces of mastication.
- This is done by formation or resorption of bone, formation of cementum, formation, and degradation of collagen fibers, the ground substance and detachment and reattachment of collagen fibers to their new locations.
- The preservation of the PDL width throughout mammalian life-time is an important measure of PDL homeostasis.
- The ability of the PDL cells to synthesize and secrete a wide range of regulatory molecules is an essential component of tissue remodeling and PDL homeostasis. PDL cells can induce mitogenic effect and can also downregulate osteoblastic activity and differentiation of PDL cells. They can also regulate bone formation.
- Loss of balance between synthesis and resorption results in failure of homeostatic mechanism.
- Failure of homeostatic mechanism may lead to tooth ankylosis and/or tooth resorption and can result in loss of function by the tooth.
- Homeostatic function of PDL is also related to tooth function.
- In non-functional tooth much of the extracellular substance of the ligament is lost due to diminished synthesis of substances required to replace structures resorbed during normal turnover. This results in decreased width of the PDL. With this there occurs increased deposition of cementum and decrease in alveolar bone. The process is irreversible if the tooth is returned to function.

Q. 2. Enumerate the principal fibers of PDL and functions of PDL. *(Dec. 2005)*

Ans. Same as answer of LAQ 1.

Q. 3. Write about evolution of periodontal ligament. *(May 2009)*

Ans. EVOLUTION OF PERIODONTAL LIGAMENT

- There is a fundamental difference between the attachment of reptilian and mammalian teeth.
- In the ancestral reptiles the teeth were ankylosed to the bone. In mammals they are suspended in their socket by ligaments.
- The evolutionary step from reptile to mammal included a series of coordinated changes in the jaws.
- In reptiles, the mandible consists of a series of bones united by sutures. The dentary, the uppermost bone, carries the ankylosed teeth.
- During transition from advanced types of reptiles to the first mammals, dentary occupied the large part and the other mandibular bones were reduced in size. Finally, only the dentary formed the mammalian mandible.
- Other components are lost or changed into two ossicles of the middle ear.

- The evolutionary change replaces the ankylosis of teeth and bone to a ligamentous suspension with tooth.

Q. 4. Write about development of periodontal ligament.

Ans. **DEVELOPMENT OF PERIODONTAL LIGAMENT**

- Development of periodontal ligament (PDL) begins with root formation, prior to tooth eruption.
- It develops from dental follicle.
- Dental follicle cells located between the developing alveolar bone and the Hertwig's epithelial root sheath are composed of two subpopulation of cells, mesenchymal cells of *dental follicle proper* and the *perifollicular mesenchyme*.
- As the tooth formation continues, mesenchymal cells in the perifollicular area actively synthesize and deposit collagen fibrils and glycoproteins in the developing PDL.
- Developing PDL contain undifferentiated stem cells that retain the potential to differentiate into osteoblasts, cementoblasts and fibroblasts.
- **Development of principal fibers:** Immediately before tooth eruption, active fibroblasts adjacent to cementum of the coronal third of the root, align in an oblique direction and the first collagen fiber bundles of the ligament appear, *alveolar crest fiber* bundle. By the time of first occlusal contact of the tooth with its antagonist, the *horizontal* group are developed. As eruption continues and definite occlusion is established, *oblique* fiber bundles mature.

  With the formation of the apical fiber group, the definitive PDL architecture is established.
- **Development of cells:** With the onset of root formation, the cells of the follicle show increasing number of cell organelles. Collagen and ground substance formation begins and fills the extracellular spaces. Stem cells, which give rise to cementoblasts, osteoblasts, and fibroblasts are seen in a perivascular location.

Q. 5. Write about cementicles.

Ans. **CEMENTICLES:**

- These are calcified bodies found in periodontal ligament.
- They are seen in older individuals, and they may remain free in the connective tissue, they may fuse into large calcified masses, or they may be joined with the cementum.
- As the cementum thickens with advancing age, it may develop these bodies.
- When they are adherent to the cementum they form excementoses.
- Degenerated epithelial cells form the nidus for calcification and these bodies may form.

Q. 6. Write about Sharpey's fibers?

Ans. **SHARPEY'S FIBERS** *(Refer fig. 17.1)*:

- Collagen fibers of PDL are embedded into cementum on one side and into alveolar bone on the other. These terminal portions of the principal fibers embedded in cementum and bone are termed Sharpey's fibers.
- Sharpey's fibers are more numerous but smaller at their attachment into cementum than alveolar bone.
- Once embedded in either the wall of the alveolus or the tooth, Sharpey's fibers calcify to a certain degree.
- Each Sharpey's fiber is composed of numerous collagen fibrils.

- Sharpey's fibers in primary cellular cementum are mineralized fully while those in cellular cementum and bone are mineralised partially at their periphery.
- Bundles of Sharpey's fibers are anchored in the bundle bone of alveolar bone proper.
- Few Sharpey's fibers pass uninterruptedly through the bone of the alveolar process and are termed as *transalveolar fibers.* They can continue as principal fibers of the adjacent PDL or they may mingle buccally and lingually with fibers of the periosteum that cover the outer cortical plates of the alveolar process.
- Transalveolar fibers may serve as a mechanism to connect adjacent teeth.
- **Function of Sharpey's fibers:** They serve to attach the tooth to surrounding bone.

MULTIPLE CHOICE QUESTIONS (MCQs)

1. Periodontal ligament (PDL) is found in
a. Reptiles b. Mammals
c. Amphibians d. Both a and b

2. PDL consists of the following synthetic cells except
a. Osteoblast b. Osteoclast
c. Cementoblast d. Fibroblast

3. PDL is
a. Thickest at cervical third of root
b. Thinnest at middle third of root
c. Thickest at apical third of root
d. Uniform throughout the root

4. The cells usually not found in PDL are
a. Osteoblasts and fibroblasts
b. Cementoblasts and osteoclasts
c. Cementoclasts
d. Odontoblasts

5. The cells that resemble osteoclasts are
a. Cementoblasts
b. Cementoclasts
c. Odontoblasts
d. Fibroblasts

6. The most numerous fibers found in PDL are
a. Apical group
b. Gingival group
c. Horizontal group
d. Oblique group

7. Cells of the dental follicle give rise to
a. Cementoblasts
b. Fibroblasts
c. Osteoblasts
d. All of the above

8. Human PDL is made-up of
a. Collagen fibers
b. Elastic fibers
c. Nerve fibers
d. Argyrophylic fibers

9. Intermediate plexus of PDL is a distinct zone of
a. Fibers from bone to cementum
b. Site of rapid remodeling
c. Site allowing small movement of teeth
d. An artifact due to tissue sectioning

10. Oxytalan is a type of fiber largely restricted to the walls of blood vessels in humans. It is a type of
a. Elastic fibers
b. Collagen fibers
c. Nerve fibers
d. Argyrophylic fibers

11. Cementicles, calcified bodies found in PDL, are possibly formed by
a. Degenerated epithelial cells
b. Blood vessels
c. Fibers
d. Osteoblasts

12. The width of PDL ranges from
a. 0.12 mm to 0.25 mm
b. 0.15 mm to 0.38 mm
c. 0.18 mm to 0.39 mm
d. 0.20 mm to 0.41 mm

13. The cell that is responsible for remodeling of collagen in PDL is
a. Fibroblast b. Epithelial cell
c. Osteoblast d. Cementoblast

14. The majority of collagen fibers in PDL are arranged in definite and distinctive fiber bundles. They are called
a. Principal fibers
b. Bundle fibers
c. Group fibers
d. Gingival fibers

15. The richest supply of proprioceptive nerve endings found in PDL is in
a. Incisors b. Molars
c. Canines d. Premolars

1-b, 2-b, 3-b, 4-d, 5-b, 6-d, 7-d, 8-a, 9-d, 10-a, 11-a, 12-b, 13-a, 14-a, 15-c

16. The cells of PDL which have synthesizing and resorbing function are
a. Osteoblasts
b. Fibroblasts
c. Cementoblasts
d. Fibrocytes

17. Cementicles are found in
a. Pulp b. Dentin
c. PDL d. Cementum

18. Which is a part of periodontium
a. Gingiva
b. Alveolar bone
c. PDL
d. All of the above

19. Which of the following cells of PDL are epithelial in origin
a. Fibroblasts
b. Rests of Malassez
c. Osteoblasts
d. Osteoclasts

20. PDL fibers that help to maintain arch integrity are
a. Transseptal fibers
b. Oblique fibers
c. Horizontal fibers
d. Apical fibers

21. Which of the following has proprioceptive mechanism
a. Pulp b. Dentin
c. Cementum d. PDL

22. Fibers of PDL are arranged at
a. 64° striated pattern
b. 90° striated pattern
c. 30° striated pattern
d. Straight with no striations

23. Nerve supply of PDL is by
a. Unmyelinated nerves
b. Myelinated nerves
c. Both
d. None

24. PDL is thickest at
a. Apical region
b. Alveolar crest region
c. Furcation region
d. Mid-root region

25. Desmodont is another name for
a. The tooth with one wall pocket
b. Tooth with three walled pocket
c. Periodontal ligament
d. Dehiscence

26. The blood supply of PDL is derived from
a. Branches from apical vessel that supply dental pulp
b. Branches from intraalveolar vessel
c. Branches from gingival vessels
d. All of the above

27. A particular glycoprotein which occurs in filamentous form in PDL is called
a. Fibronectin
b. Proline
c. Hydroxyproline
d. Chitin

28. What is most appropriate about intermediate plexus in PDL
a. It may appear as fibers arising from cementum and bone joined in the mid region of periodontal space
b. It provides a site where rapid remodelling of fibers occur
c. It is an artifact
d. All of the above

29. PDL appears to be made-up of
a. Type I and Type II collagen
b. Type I and Type III collagen
c. Type II and Type III collagen
d. Only Type III collagen

30. The function of PDL is/are
a. Support and nutrition
b. Synthesis and resorption
c. Proprioception
d. All of the above

16-b, 17-c, 18-d, 19-b, 20-a, 21-d, 22-a, 23-c, 24-b, 25-c, 26-d, 27-a, 28-c, 29-b, 30-d

31. The periodontium comprise of how many connective tissues
a. 2 b. 3
c. 4 d. 5

32. The interradicular group of fibers is present
a. Between two roots of multirooted teeth
b. In the apex
c. In between two teeth
d. All of the above

33. The following group of fibers of the PDL is most likely to be found in the middle third of the root
a. Apical b. Oblique
c. Horizontal d. Transseptal

34. The following fibers of the PDL provide the major support to the tooth during function
a. Apical
b. Oblique
c. Horizontal
d. Alveolar crest
e. Interradicular

35. PDL develops from
a. Enamel organs
b. Dental papilla
c. Dental follicle
d. Perifollicular mesenchyme

36. Transseptal fibers are present between
a. Cementum of two teeth
b. Septal areas
c. Interradicular area
d. Apical area

37. The principal fibers of PDL are
a. Reticular b. Elastic
c. Collagenous d. Oxytalan

38. The periodontal fibers not attached to bone are
a. Horizontal
b. Circular
c. Oblique
d. Apical

39. Gingival fibers seen in free gingiva are
a. Alveologingival group
b. Dentogingival group
c. Circular group
d. Transseptal group

40. The ageing of PDL leads to
a. Widening of the ligament
b. Narrowing of the ligament
c. Loss of ligament
d. All of the above

41. The cells of PDL include all except
a. Fibroblasts
b. Cell rests of Malassez
c. Defense cells
d. Langerhans cells

42. Fibers of PDL which prevent intrusion are
a. Apical
b. Interradicular
c. Oblique
d. None of the above

43. The type of collagen present in PDL is
a. II and III
b. III and IV
c. I and III
d. Both a and b

44. Procollagen formation is dependent on
a. Vitamin A
b. Vitamin C
c. Vitamin E
d. All of the above

31-c, 32-a, 33-b, 34-b, 35-d, 36-a, 37-c, 38-b, 39-c, 40-b, 41-d, 42-c, 43-c, 44-b

Chapter 19

Bone

LAQ (10 Marks)

Q. 1. Describe the histological structure of alveolar process. (Oct. 2004)

Ans. Introduction

Alveolar process is that part of the maxilla and the mandible that forms and supports the sockets of the teeth.

Anatomically there is no distinct boundry between the body of the maxilla or mandible and their respective alveolar processes. As a result of its adaptation to function, two parts of the alveolar process can be distinguished:

A. **Alveolar bone proper**, which consists of thin lamella of bone that surrounds the root of the tooth and gives attachment to principal fibers of the periodontal ligament. The second part is
B. **Supporting alveolar bone**, the bone that surrounds the alveolar bone proper and gives support to the socket.

A. Alveolar Bone Proper

It consists partly of *lamellated* and partly of *bundle* bone and is about 0.1–0.4 mm thick.

a. Lamellated bone

Some lamellae are arranged parallel to the surface of the adjacent marrow spaces, whereas others form Haversian systems.

b. Bundle bone

It is that bone in which the principal fibers of the periodontal ligament are anchored.

It is termed as 'bundle' because the bundles of the principal fibers continue into the bone as Sharpey's fibers (Fig. 19.1).

As bundle bone contains fewer fibrils than lamellated bone, it appears dark in hematoxylin and eosin stained sections and lighter in preparation with silver.

Bundle bone is formed in areas of apposition and lines of rest are seen in it.

Radiographically, bundle bone is referred to as **lamina dura** because of increased radiopacity.

This is due to the presence of thick bone without trabeculations that X-rays have to penetrate.

Alveolar bone proper forming the inner wall of the socket is perforated by many openings. These carry branches of the interalveolar nerves and blood vessels into the periodontal ligament and is therefore called *cribriform plate.*

Bone between the teeth is composed of cribriform plate entirely and is called *interdental septum.*

The interdental and interradicular septa contain the perforating *canals of Zuckerkandl and Hirschfeld* (nutrient canals) which house the interdental and interradicular arteries, veins, lymph vessels and nerves.

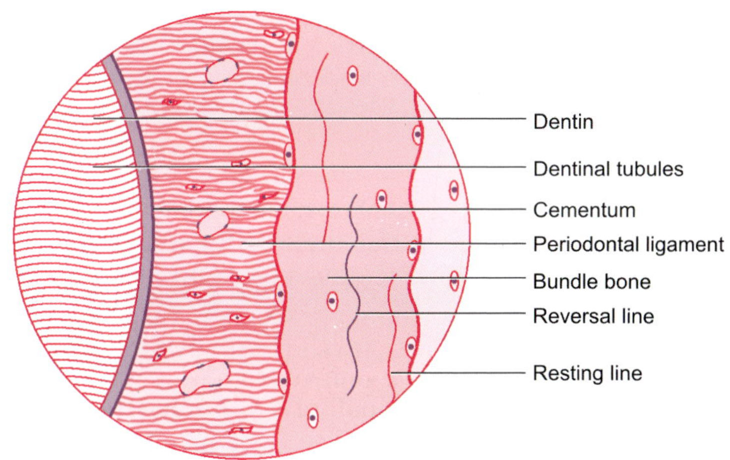

Fig. 19.1: Bundle bone, Resting and Reversal lines

B. Supporting Alveolar Bone

Consists of two parts:

a. Cortical plates
b. Spongy bone

a. Cortical plates

Consists of compact bone and forms the outer and inner plates of the alveolar processes and are covered by gingiva. They are continuous with the compact layers of the maxillary and mandibular body.

They are thinner in the maxilla than in mandible and are thickest in the premolar and molar region of the lower jaw, especially on the buccal side.

Histologically:

The cortical plates consists of longitudinal lamellae and Haversian systems.

Both cribriform plate and cortical plate are compact bone separated by spongy bone.

b. Spongy bone

This fills the area between the cortical plates and the alveolar bone proper.

Histologically:

The bony substance in spongy bone consists of large trabeculae of lamellar bone. These are surrounded by marrow that is rich in adipocytes and pluripotent mesenchymal cells. Trabeculae are arranged along the lines of stress to withstand the forces applied to bone. The marrow spaces in spongy bone are large and trabeculae surround them to derive the nutrition. Trabeculae buttress the functional forces to which alveolar bone proper is exposed. The cancellous component in maxilla is more than in the mandible.

Spongiosa of the alveolar process is classified radiographically into two types.

i. Type I: In this type the interdental and interradicular trabeculae are regular and horizontal in a ladder-like arrangement.
   This is most often in the mandible and fits into the trajectory pattern.
ii. Type II: Show irregularly arranged, numerous, delicate interdental, and interradicular trabeculae. This lacks trajectory pattern and has greater number of trabeculae. This arrangement is common in maxilla.

Marrow Tissue

Marrow space in the alveolar process many contain hematopoietic marrow but usually contain fatty marrow. In the condylar process, in the angle of the mandible and in the maxillary tuberosity, hematopoietic cellular marrow is found.

Crest of Alveolar Septa

In a healthy mouth, the distance between the cementoenamel junction and the free border of the alveolar bone proper is constant and is usually 1.5 to 2 mm.

Clinical Significance

1. Bone is sensitive to pressure, whereas tension acts as a stimulus to new bone formation. This quality of bone is utilised in orthodontic tooth movement.
2. Periodontal disease is associated with horizontal and vertical resorption of bone which is related to bacteria present in plaque.
3. Resorption of alveolar bone occurs after tooth loss. In maxilla, resorption is upwards and inwards whereas in mandible it is downwards and outwards.
4. Lamina dura is important diagnostic landmark in determining health of the periapical tissue. Loss of density usually means infections, inflammation and resorption of bony socket.
5. In the anterior teeth region, the supporting bone is very thin and the cortical plate is fused with alveolar bone proper. In this area and in the premolar and molar regions of the maxilla, defects of outer alveolar wall are common.

SAQs (3 Marks)

Q. 1. Describe histology of mature bone.

Ans. Introduction

- Bone is a living tissue and is one of the hardest structures of human body.
- Bone can be histologically classified as mature and immature bone.
- Mature bone is further classified as *compact* and *cancellous* bone.

Mature Bone

- All mature bones have a dense outer sheet of *compact bone* and a central medullary cavity which is filled with red or yellow marrow.
- This cavity shows a network of bony trabeculae, termed as *trabecular*, *spongy* or *cancellous* bone.

a. Compact bone

- Outer aspect of compact bone is surrounded by *periosteum* which has an outer fibrous layer and an inner osteogenic layer, next to the bone surface consisting of bone cells, their precursors, and a rich vascular supply.
- The inner surfaces of compact and cancellous bone are covered by a thin cellular layer, *endosteum.*
- At the periosteal and endosteal surfaces, *circumferential lamellae* are present, while deep to these, the lamellae are arranged as small concentric layers around a central vascular canal, *Haversian canal.*
- *Haversian (vascular) canal* and the *concentric lamellae* together is known as ***osteon* or *Haversian system***, which is the basic metabolic unit of bone.
- ***Interstical lamella***: These are remnants of osteons, left behind during remodeling.
- ***Reversal line*** *(Refer Fig 19.1)*: The cement line of mineralized matrix, *reversal line,* delineates the Haversian system. It marks the limit of bone erosion prior to formation of osteon. It appears irregular and is basophilic due to more glycoproteins and proteoglycans.
- ***Resting line*** *(Refer Fig. 19.1)*: A more regular and eosinophilic line which denotes the period of rest during formation of bone is *resting line.*
- ***Volkman's canals***: Adjacent Haversian canals are interconnected by Volkman's canals, which contain blood vessels. This creates a rich vascular network, throughout the compact bone.
- ***Cells***: Osteocytes are present in lacunae at the junctions of lamellae. Small canaliculi radiate from lacunae to Haversian canal, which connect all the osteocytes in an osteon together. Osteoblasts, cells responsible for synthesis of organic matrix of bone, are found on the surface of growing or remodeling bone (Fig. 19.2).

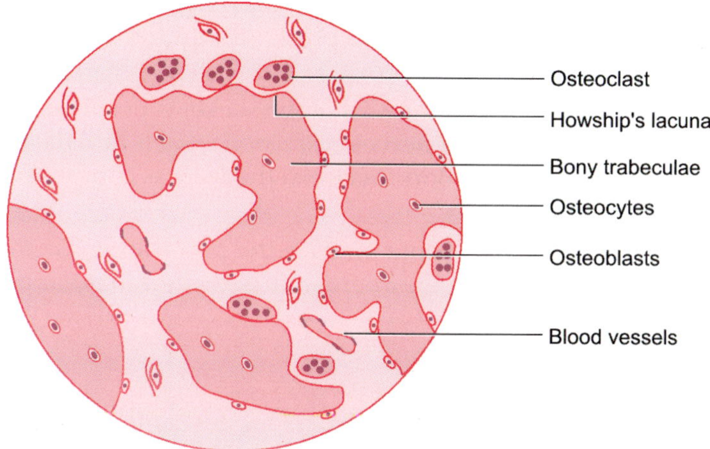

Fig. 19.2: Osteoblasts, Osteocytes and Osteoclasts

b. Spongy bone

- Spongy bone and compact bone have the same cells and intercellular matrix, but differ in the arrangement of components. In spongy bone, bony substance is arranged in the form of large slender spicules called *trabeculae* with large marrow spaces in between.
- In jaw bone, the alveolar process has *alveolar bone proper,* which is partly lamellated and partly bundle bone and *supporting bone* which has cortical plates. Spongy bone is present between the buccal and lingual cortical plates.

Q. 2. Describe alveolar bone proper. *(Oct. 2002, May 2009)*

Ans. ALVEOLAR BONE PROPER

Alveolar process is that part of maxilla or mandible that forms and supports the sockets of teeth. Anatomically there is no distinct boundary between the body of maxilla or mandible and their respective alveolar processes. As a result of its adaptation to function, two parts of alveolar process can be distinguished:

A. Alveolar bone proper

B. Supporting alveolar bone

Alveolar bone proper consists partly of *lamellated* and partly of *bundle* bone *(Refer Fig. 19.1).*

a. Lamellated bone

Some lamellae are arranged parallel to the surface of the adjacent marrow spaces, whereas others form Haversian systems.

b. Bundle bone

It is that bone in which the principal fibers of the periodontal ligament are anchored.

The term 'bundle' because, the bundles of the principal fibers continue into the bone as Sharpey's fibers.

As bundle bone contains fewer fibrils than lamellated bone, it appears dark in hematoxylin and eosin stained sections and lighter in preparation with silver. Bundle bone is formed in areas of apposition and lines of rest are seen in it.

Radiographically bundle bone is referred to as ***lamina dura*** because of increased radiopacity. This is due to the presence of thick bone without trabeculations, that X-rays have to penetrate.

Alveolar bone proper forming the inner wall of the socket is perforated by many openings. These carry branches of the interalveolar nerves and blood vessels into the periodontal ligament and is therefore called *cribriform plate.* Bone between the teeth is composed of cribriform plate entirely and is called *interdental septum.*

The interdental and interradicular septa contain the perforating *canals of Zuckerkandl and Hirschfeld* (nutrient canals) which house the interdental and interradicular arteries, veins, lymph vessels and nerves.

Clinical Significance

Lamina dura is an important diagnostic landmark in determining health of the periapical tissue. Loss of density usually means infections, inflammation and resorption of bony socket.

Q. 3. Write about woven bone/immature bone. *(June 2004)*

Ans. Introduction

- Bone is a living tissue and is one of the hardest structures of human body.
- Histologically, bones are classified as mature and immature bone or woven bone.
- Woven bone is the first formed bone with irregularly oriented collagen fibers of varying diameters.

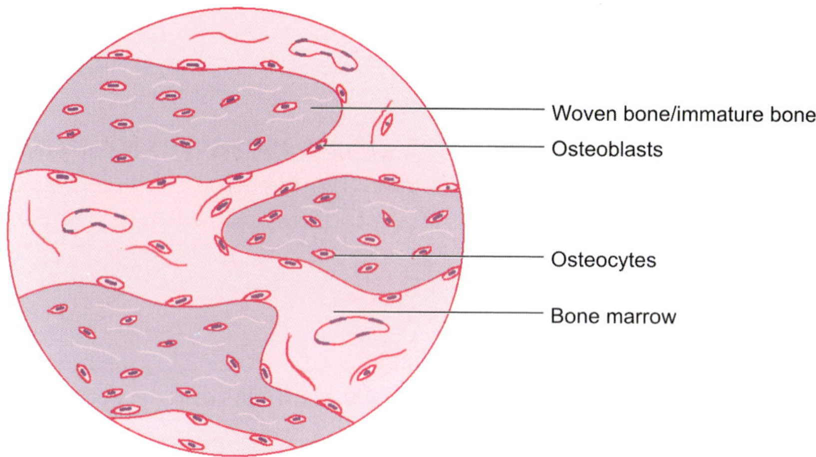

Fig. 19.3: Immature/Woven bone

Location

This type of bone is usually not seen after birth. It is seen only in the alveolar bone and during healing of fractures.

Composition: Mineral density is lower and water content is higher in woven bone.

Histology (Fig. 19.3)

- Woven bone is an immature bone characterized by interwined collagen fibers oriented in many directions, hence the name *woven*.
- It has greater number, size, and irregular arrangement of osteocytes as its rate of formation is fast.
- In woven bone, there is more interfibrillar space that is occupied by mineral crystals and acidic proteins.
- Mineral density is lower and water content is high in woven bone matrix.
- Woven bone is enriched in BAG-75 (bone acidic glycoprotein-75) and BSP (bone sialoprotein).

Bone Deposition and Resorption

- Rate of deposition and mineralization is higher and matrix vesicles participate in initiation of mineralization of woven bone.
- Woven bone can be entirely removed by osteoclasts, whereas only a portion of lamellar bone is resorbed at one time.

Staining

The matrix of woven bone in hematoxylin and eosin stained section is tinged with blue as it has higher proteoglycan content.

X-ray Features

On roentgenogram, immature bone appears more radiolucent as it has greater number of osteocytes and reduced volume of calcified intercellular substance.

Clinical Significance

During healing of fractures or extraction wounds, this embryonic bone is formed which later gets replaced by mature bone.

Q. 4. Write about osteoblasts and osteocytes. *(June 2006)*

Ans. OSTEOBLASTS AND OSTEOCYTES

- Bone is a connective tissue composed of cells, fibers, and ground substance.
- Cells present in bone are:
  - **Osteoblasts**
  - **Osteocytes**
  - **Osteoclasts.**

OSTEOBLASTS

- They are mononucleated cells responsible for the synthesis and secretion of organic matrix of bone.

Origin

- They are derived from osteoprogenitor cells of mesenchymal origin which are present in the bone marrow and other connective tissue. Periosteum also serves as an important reservoir of osteoblasts.

Morphology

- They are mononucleated, basophilic, plump, cuboidal cells.
- They are found on the forming surface of growing or remodeling bone.
- They produce organic matrix of bone which consists of collagenous and non-collagenous proteins.
- They exhibit abundant and well-developed protein synthesis organelles.
- The intense cytoplasmic basophilia is due to abundance of rough endoplasmic reticulum (RER).
- The procollagen and other organic constituents of bone matrix are synthesized by RER and are transferred to golgi complex and are assembled in golgi complex in secretory granules.
- These granules release their contents on the surface of forming bone where it assembles extracellularly as fibrils to form osteoid. Noncollagenous proteins are also released along the surface of osteoblasts which participate in regulating mineral deposition.
- Nucleus of these cells is situated eccentrically in the cell, away from the adjacent bone surface.
- The organic matrix is deposited around the cell bodies and their cytoplasmic processes resulting in the formation of canaliculi.
- Osteoblasts contact one another by adherence and gap junctions. Osteoblastic layer completely covers the osteoid surface and functions in a coordinated manner.
- They contain bundles of actin, myosin and cytoskeletal proteins which are associated with maintenance of cell shape, attachment and motility.

Functions

1. Formation of new bone by synthesis of various proteins and polysaccharides.
2. Regulation of bone remodeling and mineral metabolism.
3. Mineralization of osteoid.

Regulation of osteoblast activity

- Parathormone and vitamin D enhance bone resorption at high concentration but support bone formation at low concentration by their action on osteoblasts.
- Various other hormones and proteins like growth harmone, insulin, bone morphogenetic proteins, fibroblast growth factor, etc. help to maintain the overall integrity of bone.

Bone lining cells

- Once osteoblasts have completed their function they are either entrapped in bone matrix and become osteocytes or remain on the surface as lining cells. Osteoblasts flatten, when bone is not forming and extend along the bone surface. They contain very few organelles but retain their vitality.

OSTEOCYTES (Refer Fig. 19.2)

- As the osteoblasts form the bone matrix, they get entrapped within the matrix they secrete and are called *osteocytes.*
- The number of osteoblasts that become osteocytes depend on the rapidity of bone formation. Embryonic (woven) bone and repair bone, show more osteocytes, than lamellar bone, as they are formed rapidly.
- Within the bone matrix, the osteocytes reduce in size, creating a space around it, called the *osteocytic lacuna.*
- Lacunae could be ovoid or flattened. Narrow extension of these lacunae form channels called *canaliculi.* Osteocytic processes are present within these canaliculi. These processes contact the processes of the adjacent cell, i.e. other osteocytes in the same system. They also maintain contact with osteoblasts and bone lining cells at the surface. This interconnecting system maintains the bone integrity and bone vitality.
- Canaliculi penetrate the bone matrix and permit diffusion of nutrients, gases, and waste products between osteocytes and blood vessels.
- Osteocytes possess an ellipsoid cell body with long axis parallel to the lamellae. Nucleus is oval with a narrow rim of faintly basophilic cytoplasm. Cell has few organelles, but contain sufficient RER and large golgi region which suggests that these cells are capable of keeping the bone matrix in a state of good repair.
- Osteocytes secrete few matrix proteins.
- Old osteocytes when die, their lacunae and canaliculi get plugged with debris. The death of osteocytes leads to resorption of the matrix by osteoclasts.

Functions

- Osteocytes sense the changes in environment and send signals that affect the response of cells to bone remodeling.
- The interconnecting system of osteocytes through canaliculi maintains bone integrity and bone vitality. Failure of this leads to sclerosis and death of bone.

Q. 5. Describe about osteoclasts. *(May 2009, Nov. 2010, May 2013)*

Ans. Introduction

The word **osteoclast** is derived from the Greek word for "bone and broken". Osteoclast is a type of bone cell that removes bone tissue by removing the mineralized matrix of bone.

Origin

- Osteoclasts are derived from hemopoietic cells of monocyte macrophage lineage.

Morphology *(Refer Fig. 19.2)*

- Osteoclast is a physiological multinucleated giant cell responsible for bone resorption.
- They are found in bay-like depressions called *"Howship's lacunae"*.
- They are large, about 40–100 µm in diameter with 15–20 closely packed nuclei. Number of nuclei is related to the activity of the cell.
- Osteoclasts with many nuclei resorb more bone than osteoclasts with few nuclei.
- They are variable in shape due to their motility.
- Cytoplasm shows acid-phosphatase containing vesicles and vacuoles. Mitochondria and golgi complex are extensive and arranged in stacks. Rough endoplasmic reticulum is sparse. Cathepsin containing vesicles are present close to the ruffled border.
- They are rich in acid phosphatase, which distinguishes them from other multinucleated giant cells.

Function

- It resorbs bone by removal of minerals and organic components of extracellular matrix of bone. They develop a ruffled border and area devoid of organelles and containing smooth plasma membrane called *sealing zone* close to the resorbing surface of bone. There is dissolution of the minerals by the action of hydrochloric acid. Protons are released by osteoclast across the ruffled border into the resorption zone which leads to fall in pH and therefore dissolution of mineralized component of bone. Degradation of organic matrix occurs by action of enzymes released by osteoclasts.

Regulation of Osteoclastic Activity

- Interaction between (receptor activator of nuclear factor kB RANK) ligand and RANK on the surface of osteoclast precursors is necessary for the differentiation of the osteoclast. Factors regulating osteoclast activity are estrogen, paratharmone, vitamin D3 and calcitonin.

Q. 6. Describe resorption of alveolar bone. *(Nov. 2010)*

Ans. Introduction

- Bone is a highly dynamic connective tissue with a capacity for continuous remodeling and the two principal cell types, osteoclast and osteoblast are the major effectors in this process.
- Bone remodeling is the 'coupling' of bone synthesis and bone resorption.
- Bone resorption is the removal of mineral and organic components of extracellular matrix of bone.
- Cells responsible for bone resorption are *osteoclasts*.

Sequence of Events in Bone Resorption

- First phase is formation of osteoclast progenitor in the hematopoietic tissues, followed by their vascular dissemination and generation of resting preosteoclasts and osteoclasts in the bone itself.

- Second phase is activation of osteoclasts.
- Third phase involves resorption of bone by activated osteoclasts.
- They create cavities for themselves known as *'Howship's lacunae'* on the surface of the bone to be resorbed *(Refer fig. 19.2)*.
- Resorption involves alterations in the osteoclast, dissolution of hydroxyapitite, degradation of organic matrix and removal of degradation products.

1. *Alterations in the osteoclast*

- Immediately before resorption, osteoclasts undergo changes which facilitate bone resorption.
- There is development of ruffled border and a *'sealing zone'* of the plasma membrane of the cell that is next to the bone surface.
- The ruffled border (Fig. 19.4) consists of many infoldings of the cell membrane, resulting in finger-like projections of the cytoplasm. This increases the surface for an intensive exchange between the cell and bone.
- Adjacent to the ruffled border, cell cytoplasm is devoid of cell organelles but contain contractile actin microfilaments. This region is called the *clear (sealing) zone* (Fig. 19.4). This zone serves to attach the cell very closely to the surface of the bone to be resorbed.
- This creates an isolated microenvironment in which resorption takes place without diffusion of the hydrolytic enzymes into adjacent tissues.

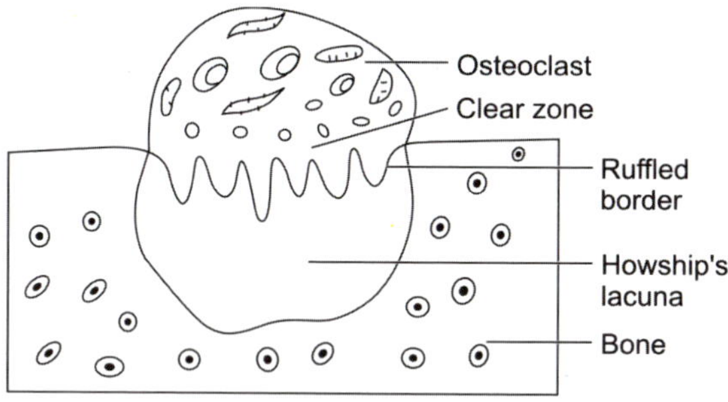

Fig. 19.4: Osteoclast

2. *Dissolution of mineralized component of bone*

- At the resorption site, osteoclast cell membrane attaches to the bone matrix at the sealing zone.
- There is dissolution of the minerals by the action of hydrochloric acid.
- Protons for the acid arise from the activity of cytoplasmic carbonic anhydrase II, synthesized in the osteoclast.
- Protons are then released across the ruffled border into the resorption zone, which leads to a fall in pH in the osteoclast resorption space and dissolution of the mineralized component of bone.

3. *Degradation of organic matrix*

- Next step involves digestion of organic components of bone matrix.
- Protolytic enzymes cathepsin–K and matrix metalloproteinase-9 are synthesized by osteoclast. These enzymes are released into the sealed compartment where they degrade collagenous and non-collagenous proteins of bone matrix.

4. Removal of degradation products

- Once liberated from bone, the free organic and non-organic particles of bone matrix are taken in or endocytosed from the resorption lacunae, across the ruffled border into the osteoclast.
- These are then packed into membrane-bound vesicles which are passed across the cell and released by exocytosis into extracellular space.
- Following resorption, osteoclast undergoes apoptosis, limiting the resorption activity.
- Resorbing surface of bone appears scalloped and exhibits scattered osteoclasts.

Q. 7. Write about bundle bone? *(May 2012)*

Ans. Introduction

Bundle bone is a part of alveolar bone proper. Alveolar bone proper is that part of alveolar process which surrounds the roots of the teeth. It consists partly of lamellated and partly of bundle bone.

Bundle bone is that bone in which principal fibers of the periodontal ligament are anchored.

Histology *(Refer Fig. 19.1)*

- The term bundle was chosen because the bundles of the principal fibers continue into the bone as *Sharpey's fibers.*
- Bundle bone is characterised by scarcity of fibrils in the intercellular substance. These fibrils are arranged at right angle to Sharpey's fibers.
- In some areas, the alveolar bone proper consists mainly of bundle bone.
- Bundle bone is formed in areas of recent bone apposition and lines of rest are seen in it.
- Alveolar bone proper forming the inner wall of the socket is perforated by many openings that carry branches of interalveolar nerves and blood vessels into the periodontal ligament and is therefore called *cribriform* plate. The perforating canals are called as *canals of Zuckerkandl and Hirschfeld* (nutrient canals).

Staining

- Bundle bone has fewer fibrils than lamellated bone and therefore it appears dark is routine hemotoxylin and eosin stained sections and lighter in preparations stained with silver than lamellated bone.

X-ray Features

- Radiographically, bundle bone is referred as the **lamina dura**, because of increased radiopacity.
- This is due to the presence of thick bone without trabeculations, that X-rays have to penetrate and not due to any increased mineral content.

Clinical Significance

- Lamina dura is an important diagnostic landmark in determining the health of the supporting tissues of teeth.
- Loss of density of lamina dura means infection, inflammation and resorption of bone socket.

Q. 8. Write about resting and reversal lines.

Ans. **Introduction**

- Bone, a living tissue, is one of the hardest structures of human body.
- All bones have a dense outer sheet of compact bone and central medullary cavity, which shows a network of bony trabeculae called as **trabecular spongy** or **cancellous bone.**
- In order to maintain its integrity and stability, bone undergoes constant remodeling, that is, 'coupling' of bone resorption and formation.
- Bone shows irregularly appearing *reversal lines* and regularly appearing *resting lines.*

Reversal Line

- Lamellated bone has a Haversial system or osteon. Osteon is the basic metabolic unit of bone.
- A cement line of mineralised matrix delineates the Haversian system. This is a *reversal line.*
- Reversal line denotes the junction between bone resorption and bone formation.
- It contains little or no collagen, and is strongly basophilic, due to high content of glycoproteins and proteoglycans.
- Reversal line marks the limit of bone erosion prior to the formation of osteon.
- This line is irregular as it is formed by the scalloped outline of the Howship's lacunae.

Resting Line

- The production and mineralization of the organic matrix of bone is phasic, i.e. it stops and starts again. During these alternating periods of activity and quiscence, the character of the organic matrix varies and also there is variation in the degree of mineralisation.
- This phasic formation of bone is reflected in its structure as *resting lines.* Resting line denotes the period of rest during the formation bone.
- It is more regular and is eosinophilic.
- These are seen in ground section because of variation in mineralization and also in a mineralized section due to variation in matrix composition (Refer Fig. 19.1).

Q. 9. Describe histology of alveolar socket of permanent maxillary first molar. *(June 2008)*

Ans. Bone that forms and supports the sockets of teeth is alveolar process bone. As a result of its adaptation to function, two parts of alveolar bone are:

1. **Alveolar bone proper:** Which consist of a thin lamellae of bone that surrounds the roots of the teeth and gives attachment to principal fibers of the periodontal ligament.
2. **Supporting alveolar bone:** It is the bone that surrounds the alveolar bone proper and gives support to socket.

Describe alveolar bone proper as described in answer of LAQ.1 (Refer Fig. 19.1).

Supporting alveolar bone has cortical plates and spongy bone. In maxillary premolar and molar region, no spongy bone is found and the cortical plate is fused with the alveolar bone proper.

In maxilla, cortical plates are much thinner.

In maxilla, interdental and interradicular trabeculae show irregular arrangement known as type II.

(Describe compact and spongy bone as described in LAQ.1)

Q. 10. Explain buccolingual section through dentulous mandible.

Ans. BUCCOLINGUAL SECTION THROUGH DENTULOUS MANDIBLE

- Buccolingual section through dentulous mandible will show buccal and lingual cortical plates enclosing spongy bone. Bone which forms and supports the sockets of teeth is alveolar process.
- Describe entirely the histology of alveolar bone as described in LAQ.1.

Q. 11. Write functions of alveolar bone. *(Oct. 2002, May 2009)*

Ans. FUNCTIONS OF ALVEOLAR BONE

- Alveolar bone is that part of maxilla or mandible that forms and supports the sockets of the teeth.
- As a result of its adaptation to function, two parts of alveolar process can be distinguished, the alveolar bone proper and the supporting alveolar bone.

Functions of alveolar bone are:

1. It houses the roots of the teeth.
2. Anchors the roots to the alveoli through Sharpey's fibres.
3. Helps the tooth to move for better occlusion.
4. Helps to absorb and distribute occlusal forces generated during tooth contact.
5. Supplies vessels to the periodontal ligament.
6. Houses and protects developing permanent teeth while supporting primary teeth..
7. Organizes eruption of primary and permanent teeth.

Q. 12. What are differences between mature and immature bone? *(June 2007)*

Ans. Introduction

- Bone, a living tissue, is one of the hardest structures of human body.
- Histologically, bone is classified as mature bone and immature or woven bone.
- Woven bone is the first formed bone which is usually not seen after birth except in the alveolar bone and during healing of fractures.
- Mature bone is of two types, compact and cancellous.

Differences between mature and immature bones

MATURE BONE (*Lamellar/trabecular bone*)	*IMMATURE BONE* (*Woven bone*)
1. **Distinctive, orderly arrangement:** Mature bone which is due to repeated addition of uniform lamellae to bony surfaces during appositional growth.	1. Immature bone is characterized by **interwined collagen fibers** oriented in many directions, hence the name woven.
2. **Direction of collagen fibrils:** In a lamella mature bone lies at right angles to that of the fibrils in the adjacent lamella.	2. Collagen fibers are oriented in many directions.
3. **Interfibrillar space is less.**	3. It is **more** and is occupied by mineral crystals and acidic proteins.
4. **Chemical composition:** • Mineral density is high and water content is low. • Mature bone is enriched in osteocalcin.	4. **Chemical composition:** • Mineral density is low and water content is high. • Immature lone is enriched in bone acidic glycoprotein-75 and bone sialoprotein.

(Contd.)

Differences between mature and immature bones (*Contd.*)

MATURE BONE (*Lamellar/trabecular bone*)	*IMMATURE BONE* (*Woven bone*)
5. Staining: In H and E stained section lamellar bone shows uniform acidophilic staining of the matrix.	**5. Staining:** The matrix of woven bone is tinged with blue indicating that it has higher proteoglycan content.
6. Bone formation: • Rate of deposition and mineralization is slow. • Collagen mediated mechanism is operative in calcification of lamellar bone.	**6. Bone formation:** • Rate of deposition and mineralization is faster. • Matrix vesicles participate in initiation of mineralization of woven bone.
7. X-ray features: • More radiopaque.	**7. X-ray features:** • More radiolucent due to less mineral density
8. Clinical significance: Bone is a vascularised connective tissue which is one of the hardest tissue of human body but highly plastic as well.	**8. Clinical significance:** It is not seen after birth except for alveolar bone proper and at the sites of fractures.

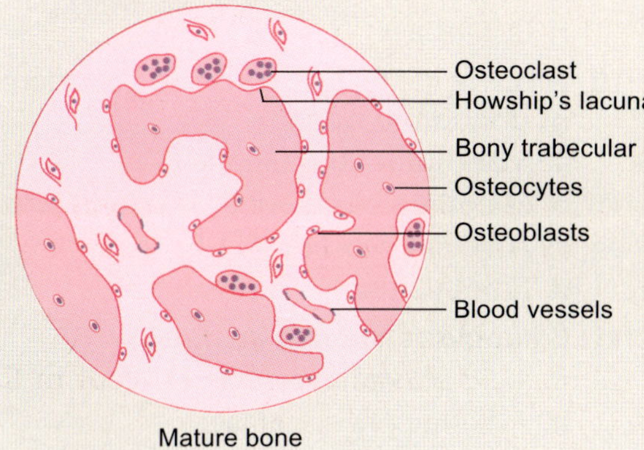

Mature bone

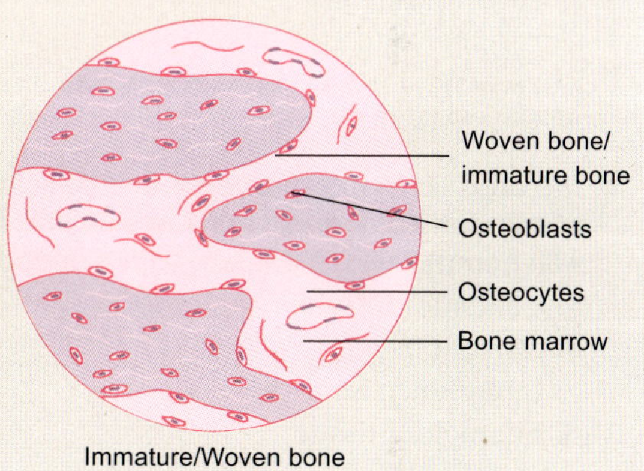

Immature/Woven bone

MULTIPLE CHOICE QUESTIONS (MCQs)

1. The supporting bone (cortical plate and spongy bone) is very thin in the
a. Anterior region of mandible
b. Posterior region of mandible
c. Anterior region of maxilla
d. Anterior teeth of both the jaws

2. The inorganic and organic constituents of bone are
a. 65% inorganic and 35% organic
b. 55% inorganic and 45% organic
c. 65% organic and 35% inorganic
d. 40% inorganic and 60% organic

3. Organic material of bone is
a. Type I collagen
b. Type II collagen
c. Type III collagen
d. Type I and type III collagen

4. The organic matrix of bone that is devoid of mineral salts and stains eosinophilic with hematoxylin and eosin stain is called
a. Cementoid tissue
b. Osteoid tissue
c. Lymphoid tissue
d. Enameloid tissue

5. The interdental and interradicular septa contain the perforating canals which have the interdental and interradicular arteries, veins, nerves, and lymph vessels. These are
a. Zuckerkandl canals
b. Hirschfeld canals
c. Nutrient canals
d. All of the above

6. The successive processes that occur during bone resorption are
a. Decalcification
b. Degradation of matrix
c. Transport of soluble products
d. All of the above are correct

7. During healing of fractures or extraction wounds, the type of bone that is formed is
a. Embryonic bone
b. Immature bone
c. Coarse fibrillar bone
d. All of the above

8. Lamina dura is same as
a. Bundle bone
b. Cribriform plate
c. Alveolar bone socket
d. All of the above

9. High level of enzyme acid phosphatase is a characteristic feature of
a. Osteocyte b. Chondrocyte
c. Osteoclast d. Mast cell

10. Which of the following can be considered as chondroid bone
a. Mandibular basal bone
b. Maxillary basal bone
c. Alveolar process
d. Frontal bone

11. Osteoclasts are rich in
a. Acid phosphatase
b. Alkaline phosphatase
c. Citrases
d. Peroxidase

12. The bone immediately surrounding the roots and giving support for insertion of periodontal fibers is
a. Supporting bone b. Alveolar bone
c. Spongy bone d. Woven bone

13. Odontoclasts help in resorption of
a. Dentin b. Bone
c. Cementum d. All of the above

14. Supporting bone is
a. Spongy bone
b. Woven bone
c. Immature bone
d. None of the above

1-d, 2-a, 3-a, 4-b, 5-d, 6-d, 7-d, 8-d, 9-c, 10-c, 11-a, 12-b, 13-a, 14-a

15. Growth of alveolar bone depends on presence of

a. Ramus b. Condyle
c. Teeth d. None of the above

16. In a healthy mouth, the alveolar process is thinnest at

a. Lingual to maxillary central incisor
b. Labial to mandibular central incisor
c. Lingual to maxillary canine
d. Lingual to mandibular first molar

17. Fusion of alveolar bone to tooth is called as

a. Ankylosis
b. Hypercementosis
c. Gomphosis
d. None of the above

18. The shape of the outline of the crest of the alveolar septa in radiogrpah is dependent on

a. Anatomy of alveolar process
b. Position of gingival margin
c. Position of adjacent teeth
d. Amount of underlying trabecular bone

19. The external most layer of the alveolar process is colectively called

a. Spongy layer
b. Cortical plate
c. Cribriform plate
d. Cancellous bone

20. Thinnest cortical bone occurs at

a. Facial surface of mandibular incisors
b. Facial surface of maxillary incisors
c. Buccal plate of maxillary canine
d. Buccal plate of mandibular first molar

21. The bone that is not found in anterior part of both jaws is

a. Spongy bone
b. Supporting bone
c. Compact bone
d. Cortical bone

22. All the following enzymes are essential for bone formation except

a. Alkaline phosphatase
b. Acid phosphatase
c. ATPase
d. Pyrophosphates

23. The cortical plates are thickest in the region of

a. Anterior maxillary
b. Anteror mandibular
c. Posterior maxillary
d. Posterior mandibular

24. The space in which developing tooth is present in the jaw bone is called

a. Alveolar bone
b. Alveolar process
c. Bony crypt
d. Supporting bone

25. The canal which houses, interdental and interradicular nerves and vessels is

a. Retzius
b. Von Ebner
c. Salter
d. Zuckerkandl and Hirschfeld

26. The alveolar bone seen between the first molar teeth is called the

a. Interdental septum
b. Interalveolar septum
c. Interradicular septum
d. Both a and b

27. The density of the alveolar bone is more in the

a. Anterior region of the maxilla
b. Anterior region of the mandible
c. In the posterior region of maxilla and mandible
d. Both a and b

28. The distance between the cemento-enamel junction and the crestal margin of the alveolar bone is

a. 2–5 mm b. 5–7 mm
c. 1.5–2 mm d. 2.5–3 mm

15-c, 16-b, 17-a, 18-c, 19-b, 20-b, 21-a, 22-b, 23-d, 24-c, 25-d, 26-c, 27-d, 28-c

Chapter

20

Oral Mucous Membrane

LAQs (10 Marks)

Q. 1. Classify and give functions of oral mucous membrane, describe macro and microscopic features of gingiva. or *(Nov. 2010)*

Classify and give functions of oral mucous membrane. *(SAQ, Oct. 2007)*

Ans. Surface of oral cavity is lined by mucous membrane.

- Based on the *functional criteria,* the oral mucosa is divided into three major types:
  1. Masticatory mucosa (gingiva and hard palate)
  2. Lining or reflecting mucosa (lip, cheek, vestibular fornix, alveolar mucosa, floor of mouth and soft palate)
  3. Specialized mucosa (dorsum of the tongue and taste buds)
- Based on the *type of epithelium,* oral mucosa can be divided into :
  1. **Keratinized areas:**
     a. Masticatory mucosa
     b. Specialized mucosa
     c. Vermilion zone of lip
  2. **Nonkeratinized areas:**
     a. Lining mucosa
- Masticatory mucosa is bound to bone and does not stretch. It bears forces generated when food is chewed.
- Lining mucosa covers the musculature and is distensible, adapting itself to the contraction and relaxation of the muscles.
- Specialized (sensory) mucosa is so called because it bears the taste buds, which have a sensory function.

Oral Mucosa has many Important Functions

1. **Defence:** Integrity of the oral epithelium is an effective barrier for the entry of the microorganisms. Oral mucosa is impermeable to bacterial toxins. It also secretes antibodies and has an efficient humoral and cell mediated immunity.

2. **Lubrication:** Saliva keeps the oral cavity moist thereby ensuring an intact oral epithelium which helps in speech, mastication, swallowing and in the perception of taste.
3. **Sensory:** Oral mucosa is sensitive to touch, pressure, pain and temperature. The sensation of taste is a unique sensation, felt only in anterior two-thirds of the dorsum of the tongue. Swallowing, gagging, retching, and salivating reflexes are intiated by receptors in the oral mucosa.
4. **Protection:** Oral mucosa protects the deeper tissues from mechanical forces resulting from mastication and from abrasive nature of foodstuffs.

GINGIVA

- Gingiva is keratinized and constitutes masticatory mucosa along with hard palate.
- Gingiva is that part of oral mucosa which covers the alveolar processes. It extends from the dentogingival junction to the alveolar mucosa.
- It is limited on the outer surface of both jaws by the mucogingival junction, which separates it from the alveolar mucosa.
- It can be divided into *free gingiva, attached gingiva* and the *interdental papilla.* The dividing line between the free gingiva and the gingiva is the *free gingival groove,* which runs parallel to the margin of the gingiva at a distance 0.5 to 1.5 mm.

Macroscopic Features of Gingiva

- Gingiva is pink but sometimes has a grayish tint.
- The surface may be translucent or transparent permitting the colour of the underlying tissues to be seen.
- Gingiva can be divided into the free gingiva, the attached gingiva and the interdental papilla. The dividing line between the free gingiva and the gingiva is the *free gingival groove* which runs at a distance of 0.5 to 1.5 mm from the margin of gingiva.
- **Free or marginal gingiva** is the unattached portion of gingiva that forms and surrounds the teeth in a collar like fashion. It is coronal most portion of gingiva and it follows a scalloped line on the facial and lingual surface of the teeth. It forms the soft tissue wall of the gingival sulcus.
- **Gingival sulcus** is a shallow crevice between inner aspect of gingiva and the tooth. Normal gingival sulcus depth is 2 mm. The bottom of the gingival sulcus corresponds to the free gingival groove.
- The **attached gingiva** is 4–6 mm. It is firm, resilient immobile portion of gingiva which is tightly bound to the alveolar bone. It extends from free gingival groove to mucogingival junction.
- Attached gingiva is stippled. This is because portions of epithelium are elevated, between these elevations, there are shallow depressions. Disappearance of stippling is an indication of edema, an expression of an involvement of the gingiva in gingivitis. Males have more heavily stippled gingiva than females.
- Intedental grooves are the vertical folds present on the gingiva between adjacent teeth.
- The **interdental papilla** is that part of the gingiva that fills the space between two adjacent teeth.
- The interdental papilla between anterior teeth is pyramidal and that between posterior teeth appears tent shaped. In this tent shaped interdental papilla, the central concave area

below the oral and the vestibular corners is depressed, valley like and is called *col.* Col is covered by thin nonkeratinized epithelium and is more vulnerable to periodontal disease.

- The **mucogingival junction** seperates the gingiva from the alveolar mucosa. Mucogingival junction is 3–5 mm below the level of the crest of the alveolar bone.

Microscopic Features of Gingiva

Gingiva is subjected to the friction and pressure of mastication. Morphology of both epithelium and connective tissue indicates the adaptation to these forces.

Epithelium

- Stratified squamous epithelium of gingiva is parakeratinized in 75%, orthokeratinized in 15% and nonkeratinized in 10% of the population.
- In **parakeratinized** epithelium, superficial cells retain pyknotic nuclei and show some signs of being keratinized. The stratum granulosum is absent. In **keratinized** (orthokeratinized) epithelium, the superficial cells form scales of keratin and lose their nuclei. Stratum granulosum is present in it.
- Keratinized gingival epithelium has stratum basale, stratum spinosum, stratum granulosum and stratum corneum.
- Inflammation which is frequently seen in gingiva, interferes with keratinization.
- In **nonkeratinized** epithelium, surface cells are nucleated and show no signs of keratinization.
- The epithelium of the gingiva is keratinized but epithelium of the col and that lining the sulcus is nonkeratinized.
- Presence of melanin pigment in the epithelium gives it brown to black coloration. Pigmentation is most abundant at the base of the interdental papilla. It may increase in various pathologic states.
- The epithelium of gingiva interdigitates with underlying connective tissue by long, narrow rete ridges.

Lamina propria

- Papillae of the connective tissue are long, slender, and numerous.
- Underlying lamina propria of gingiva is dense connective tissue that does not contain large vessels.
- Collagen fibers of the lamina propria may either insert into the alveolar bone and the cementum or blend with the periosteum.
- Lamina propria contains few elastic fibers, most of which are confined to the walls of the blood vessels. Oxytalan fibers are also present. Elastic fibers are more numerous in submucosa and are thick also.
- Gingival fibers of the periodontal ligament enter into the lamina propria attaching the gingiva firmly to the teeth.
- The collagen fibers in the lamina propria of the gingiva are arranged in various groups, referred as the **gingival ligament.** They serve to support the free gingiva, bind attached gingiva to the alveolar bone and link one tooth with the other.
- These gingival fibers are *dentogingival, alveologingival, circular, dentoperiosteal* and *transseptal.* Apart from these, semicircular, vertical and transgingival fiber groups are also described.

- Gingiva is firmly attached to the periosteum of the alveolar bone and this arrangement is referred as *mucoperiosteum.* Here a dense connective tissue, consisting coarse collagen bundles extends from the bone to the lamina propria.
- The lamina propria of gingiva differs from other regions in arrangement of collagen fibers, in its composition and response of its matrix to the stimuli and also, in the nature of the fibroblast.
- Fibroblasts of gingiva have less contractile protein and also lack alkaline phosphatase. Matrix contains less of type III collagen, more of hyaluron and has a lower turnover rate. They release more prostaglandins in response to histamine.
- Small number of lymphocytes, plasma cells, and macrophages are present in the connective tissue of gingiva which are involved in defense and repair.

Sulcular Epithelium

- It lines the gingival sulcus.
- Sulcular epithelium is nonkeratinized with flat interface with the underlying connective tissue.

Junctional or Attachment Epithelium

- The epithelium of the gingiva which gets attached to the tooth is junctional or attachment epithelium. The union between this epithelium and tooth is referred to as *epithelial attachment.*
- Junctional epithelium is nonkeratinized. It has the highest turnover rate of 5–6 days (Fig. 20.1).

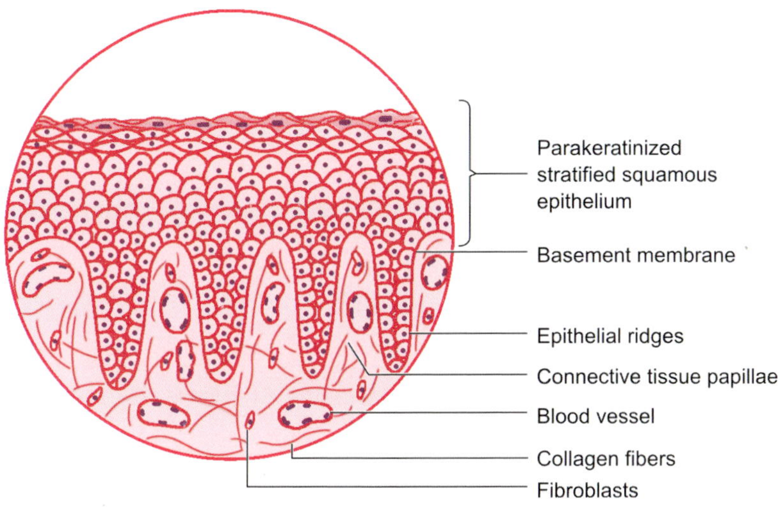

Fig. 20.1: Gingiva

Clinical Considerations of Gingiva

1. Metal poisoning (lead, bismuth) causes characteristic discoloration of the gingival margin.
2. Periodontal disturbances produce a deepened gingival sulcus, called periodontal pocket, as a response to plaque toxins.

Q. 2. Describe anatomy of dorsum of the tongue, histology of anterior two-thirds of the tongue and nerve supply of tongue. or *(Oct. 2003)*

Classify oral mucous membrane, give its functions and describe in detail about specialized mucosa. or *(May 2013)*

Describe in detail specialized mucosa. *(May 2009)*

Ans. Introduction

- The surface of oral cavity is lined by mucous membrane. Structure of oral mucous membrane varies in different regions as per the adaptation to function.
- Superior surface of tongue is rough and irregular and is lined by the specialized (sensory) mucosa as it bears the taste buds, which have a sensory function. However, the mucous membrane of the inferior surface of tongue is smooth, thin and nonkeratinized.
- A 'V' shaped line divides the superior surface into an anterior two-thirds part, or body and posterior one-third part, or base.

Anterior two-thirds of dorsum of tongue: Papillae of tongue/lingual papillae.

(SAQ, June 2004, Oct. 2004)

- Anterior part of tongue is termed 'papillary' as it has numerous, fine pointed, cone shaped papillae, while the posterior third of tongue is called **lymphatic portion.**
- The dorsolingual mucosa has numerous papillae many of which contains taste buds which helps in the perception of taste and therefore regarded as specialized mucosa.
- Papillae are epithelial projections with a core of connective tissue.
- Papillae present on tongue are filiform, fungiform and vallate. On the lateral border of the posterior part of the tongue, large foliate papillae are present.

Filiform (thread-shaped) papillae (Fig. 20.2A)

- These are the most numerous papillae, but they do not contain taste buds. They are fine pointed, cone shaped papillae that give a velvet like appearance.
- They are epithelial structures containing a core of connective tissue from which secondary papillae protrude towards the epithelium.
- Their epithelium is keratinized and forms tufts at the apex of the dermal papilla.

Fungiform (mushroom shaped) papillae (Fig. 20.2A)

- These are interspersed between filiform papillae.
- These are round, reddish prominences on tongue. Their red colour is due to rich capillary network visible through the relatively thin epithelium.
- They contain 1–3 taste buds, present on their dorsal surface.

Circumvallate (walled) papillae (Fig. 20.2B) *(SAQ, 2000, 2001)*

- These are present in front of the dividing 'V' shaped terminal sulcus.
- They are 8–10 in number.
- They do not protrude above the surface of the tongue and are bounded by a deep circular furrow.
- Their free surface shows numerous secondary long papillae that are covered by a thin, smooth epithelium.

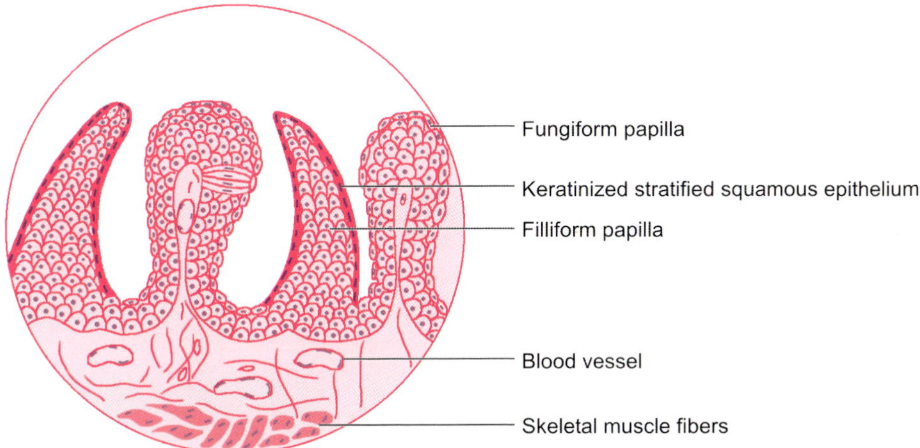

Fig. 20.2A: Filliform and fungiform papillae

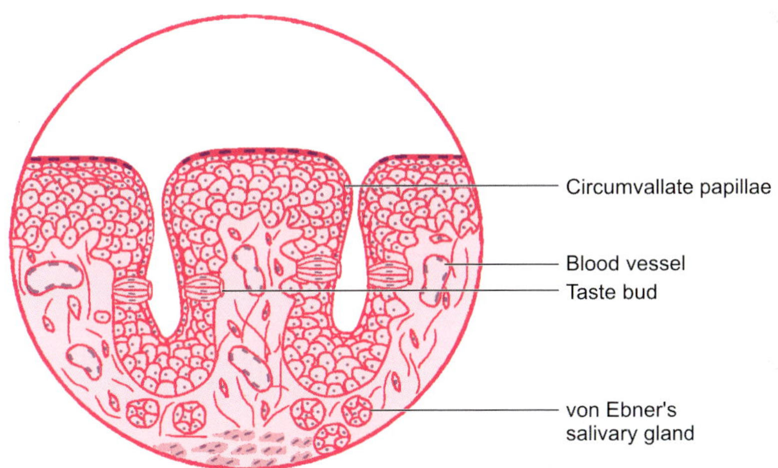

Fig. 20.2B: Circumvallate papillae

- On the lateral surface, they have numerous taste buds, which are responsible for taste perception.
- The ducts of small serous glands called von Ebner's glands open into the trough.

Foliate papillae

- They are present on the lateral border of the posterior part of the tongue.
- They contain taste buds.

Taste buds (Fig. 20.3) *(SAQ, Oct. 2004, May 2012)*

- These are small ovoid or barrel shaped intraepithelial organs present within the papillae of tongue.
- They are responsible for the perception of taste.

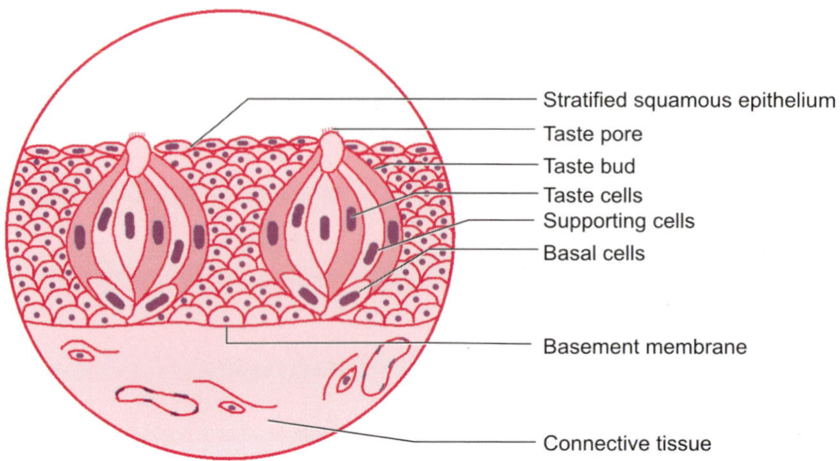

Fig. 20.3: Taste buds

- They are numerous on the inner wall of the trough surrounding the vallate papillae, in the folds of the foliate papillae, on the posterior surface of epiglottis and on some of the fungiform papillae at the tip and the lateral borders of the tongue. They are not present on fungiform papillae.
- They are 80 μm high and 40 μm thick. They extend from the basal lamina to the surface of the epithelium.
- Their outer surface is covered by a few flat epithelial cells, which surround a small opening, the *taste pore.* The pore leads into a narrow space lined by the supporting cells of the taste bud.
- The outer supporting cells are arranged like the staves of a barrel. The inner and shorter ones are spindle shaped. Between these, 10 to 12 neuroepithelial cells are arranged. These are the receptors of taste stimulus. These are slender, dark-staining cells that carry finger like processes at their superficial end.
- A rich plexus of nerves is found below the taste buds. Some fibers enter the epithelium and contact with the sensory cells of the taste bud.
- Taste sensation is perceived in different regions of the tongue. Sweet taste is perceived at the tip, salty at the lateral border of the tongue, bitter and sour on the palate and also in the posterior part of the tongue bitter in the middle and sour in the lateral areas of the tongue.
- Bitter and sour taste sensations are mediated by the glossopharyngeal nerve, and sweet and salty taste are mediated by chorda tympani.
- *Foramen cecum* is located at the angle of the 'V' shaped terminal groove on the tongue. It is the remnant of the thyroglossal duct.
- Posterior to this, surface of tongue shows *lingual follicles* each of which shows one or more lymph nodules. Lingual follicles together form the *lingual tonsil*.

BLOOD AND NERVE SUPPLY OF TONGUE

(SAQ, MAY 2007)

Blood Supply

- The tongue and floor of the mouth are supplied by lingual artery.
- The lingual artery is a branch of external carotid artery.

- Its dorsal lingual branch supplies the base of the tongue.
- The deep lingual branch supplies the body and apex of the tongue.
- One of its terminal branches communicates with the deep lingual artery of the opposite side and is called the arcus raninus.
- Venous drainage of tongue is quite peculiar and is from two different routes for two different parts of tongue. The dorsal surface and side of the tongue drains into lingual vein, ventral surface drains into deep lingual veins.
- Venous blood from lingual vein drains into facial vein and later into internal jugular veins.

Nerve Supply

- The tongue is developed from the contribution of different arches which is reflected in its nerve supply.
- Mucous membrane of anterior two-thirds of the tongue is supplied by mandibular branch of trigeminal nerve.
- Lingual branch of the mandibular branch of trigeminal nerve supplies the anterior two-thirds of the tongue for general sensation of pain, temperature, touch, etc.
- Chorda tympani branch of the 7th cranial nerve, supplies the anterior two-thirds for special sensation of taste.
- Posterior one-third of the tongue is supplied by glossopharyngeal nerve, the ninth cranial nerve which carries the taste and general sensation from the posterior part.
- Posterior most part of the tongue is innervated by vagus nerve via internal laryngeal branch.
- The hypoglossal nerve, the 12th cranial nerve supplies the voluntary muscles of tongue, except for palatoglossus which is supplied by cranial part of accessory nerve through the pharyngeal plexus.

Clinical Considerations of Tongue

Changes of the tongue are sometimes diagnostically significant.

1. In scarlet fever, atrophy of the lingual mucosa causes redness of tongue, known as *stawberry tongue.*
2. Systemic diseases such as pernicious anemia, and vitamin deficiencies, especially vitamin B-complex lead to characteristic changes such as *magenta tongue* and *beefy red tongue.*

SAQs (3 Marks)

Q. 1. Describe histology of keratinized oral mucous membrane. *(Dec. 2005)*

Ans. Introduction

- Based on the type of epithelium, oral mucous membrane is either keratinized or nonkeratinized.
- Keratinized areas in oral mucosa are masticatory mucosa, that is gingiva and hard palate, and vermilion border of lip.
- In keratinized oral epithelium, four cell layers are seen (Fig. 20.1):

Stratum Basale

It is made-up of a single layer of cuboidal cells. These cells synthesize DNA and undergo mitosis. The basal and parabasal spinous cells are referred to as the *stratum germinativum.*

Basal cells are made-up of two populations of cells. One population is serrated and heavily packed with tonofilaments, which are adopted for attachment and the other is non-serrated and consists of slowly cycling *stem cells.* Basal cells are attached to the connective tissue through hemidesmosomes while they are connected to adjacent cells by desmosomes.

Stratum Spinosum

These cells are polyhedral and larger than basal cells. Cells are joined by intercellular bridges. Tonofibrils course from cell to cell across these bridges. The tonofilament network and desmosomes make-up a tensile supporting system for the epithelium. The intercellular spaces of the spinous cells in keratinizing epithelia are large or distended thus making desmosomes more prominent which gives prickly appearance. The spiny appearance of the spinous layer is due to shrinkage of cells during tissue processing causing them to separate at points where desmosomes do not anchor them together. Spinous cells are most active in protein synthesis which is required for keratinization.

Stratum Granulosum

This layer has flatter and wider cells. They are known as granulosum due to presence of the basophilic **keratohyalin** granules in them. Nuclei show signs of degeneration and pyknosis. Protein synthesis rate is low in these cells. Tonofilaments are more dense and are associated with keratohyaline granules. A lamellar granule, known as **keratinosome, Odland body** or **membrane coating granule** is formed in the upper spinous and granular cell layer. These lamellar granules discharge their contents into the intercellular space forming an intercellular lamellar material which contributes to the permeability barrier. At the same time a highly resistant electron dense cornified envelop is formed by proteins *involucrin* and *loricrin,* just beneath the plasma membrane.

Stratum Corneum

It is made-up of keratinized squamae. Cellular organelles disappear. Layer is acidophilic and histologically amorphous. Keratohyaline granules disappear. Ultrastructurally, the cells are composed of densely packed filaments developed from the tonofilaments, altered, and coated by basic protein of keratohyalin granule, *filagrin.* Filagrin causes aggregation of filaments in these cells. Cross linking of tonofilaments by disulfide bonds facilitates close packing of the filaments and gives mechanical and chemical resistance to this layer. The keratinized cell becomes compact and dehydrated and is closely applied to adjacent squamae. In parakeratinization, the cells retain pyknotic and condensed nuclei and contain partially lysed cell organelles until they desquamate.

Q. 2. Describe histology of hard palate.

Ans. Introduction

- Hard palate is lined by masticatory mucosa.
- Masticatory mucosa is bound to bone and does not stretch.
- It bears forces generated when food is chewed.

Histology of Hard Palate

The mucous membrane of the hard palate is tightly attached to the underlying periosteum and is pink in colour. It has following zones.

1. Gingival region—which is adjacent to teeth.
2. Palatine raphe or median area—extends from the incisive or palatine papillae posteriorly.
3. Anterolateral area or fatty zone—between the raphe and gingiva.
4. Posterolateral area or glandular zone—present between the raphe and gingiva.

1. **Lingual/gingival region:** Here the palatine tissue is identical with the gingiva and shows the same structure as gingiva. Epithelium is well-keratinized. Only lamina propria and periosteum are present below the epithelium and submucosa is absent.
2. **Palatine raphe:** Structure is same.
3. **Anterolateral** and **posterolateral parts of hard palate:** (Figs 20.4A and B)
   - Epithelium of hard palate is keratinized.
   - The mucous membrane is immovably attached to the periosteum of the maxillary and palatine bones by dense bands and trabeculae of fibrous connective tissue.

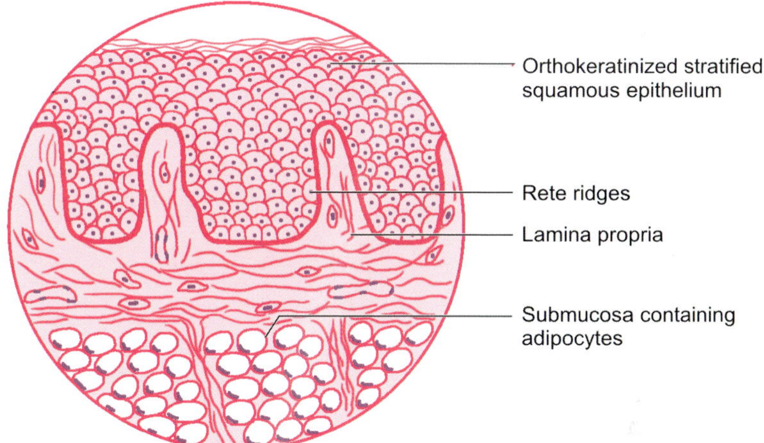

Fig. 20.4A: Hard palate (anterolateral area/fatty zone)

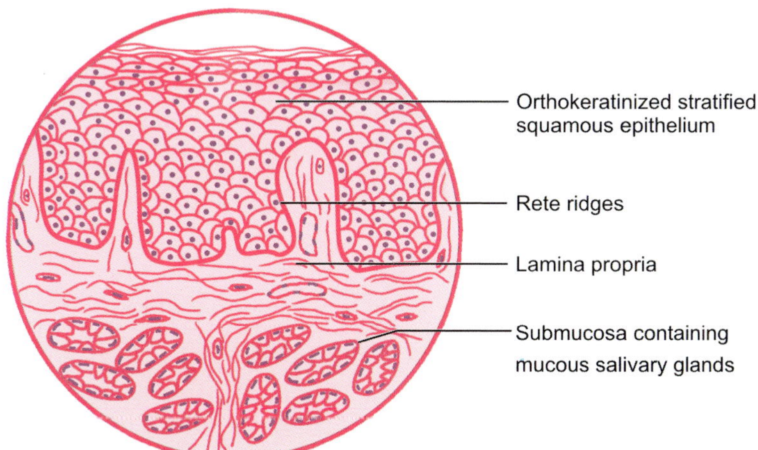

Fig. 20.4B: Hard palate (posterolateral area/glandular zone)

- The lamina propria is thicker in the anterior than in the posterior parts of the palate and has numerus long papillae.
- The submucous space is divided into irregular intercommunicating compartments. In anterolateral part, they are filled with adipose tissue and in posterior part with mucous glands.
- Laterally, at the junction of the alveolar process and the horizontal plate of the hard palate, the anterior palatine vessels and nerves course in loose connective tissue. This wedge-shaped area is smaller in anterior part and larger in posterior part.

Significance: Presence of fat or glands act as a cushion.

Incisive papilla: Oral incisive (palatine) papilla contains the oral parts of the vestigeal nasopalatine ducts, which are lined by simple or pseudostratified columnar epithelium rich in goblet cells.

Functions: In mammals, together with Jacobson's organ, nasopalatine ducts are considered as auxiliary olfactory sense organs.

Palatine rugae: They are ridges of mucous membrane extending laterally from the incisive papilla and the anterior parts of the raphe.

Epithelial pearls: They are present in the midline, in the region of incisive papilla. They are found in lamina propria. They consist of concentrically arranged keratinized epithelial cells.

They are remnants of the epithelium found in the line of fusion between the palatine processes.

Clinical Considerations

1. Due to firmness of attachment of masticatory mucosa to the underline bone, infiltration of local anesthesia into it is difficult and causes pain.
2. Palatine torus when present has thinner mucous membrane. While constructing denture, this area has to be relieved.
3. In the region of incisive papilla, small mucous glands open into the lumen of the nasopalatine ducts which may become cystic, resulting into formation of nasopalatine duct cysts.

Q. 3. Write about nonkeratinocytes. *(July 2005, May 2013, 2016)*

Ans. Introduction

Epithelial cells that keratinize are called **keratinocytes.** However, epithelium contains a smaller population of cells that do not possess cytokeratin filaments, hence do not keratinize. These group of cells are termed **nonkeratinocytes.**

Characteristics of Nonkeratinocytes

1. They do not have cytokeratine filaments, hence cannot keratinize.
2. They do not show mitotic activity.
3. They do not undergo maturative changes or desquamate.
4. They are not arranged in layers.
5. They do not form desmosomal attachments with adjacent keratinocytes.
6. They are usually dendritic and appear unstained or clear in hematoxylin and eosin stain and therefore are referred as clear cells.

7. They are identified by special stains or by immunocytochemical methods.
8. They migrate to oral epithelium from neural crest or from bone marrow.

Nonkeratinocytes are (Flowchart 20.1)

1. Melanocytes
2. Langerhans' cells
3. Merkel cells are the nonkeratinocytes found in oral epithelium.
4. Inflammatory cells such as lymphocytes and neutrophils found in certain regions of epithelium, are also considered as nonkeratinocytes.

Flowchart 20.1

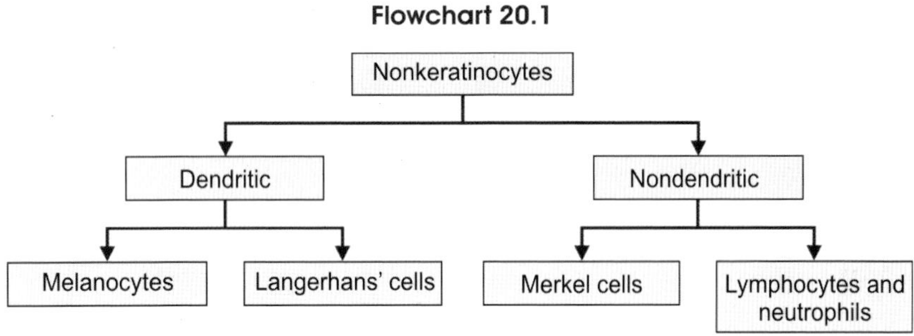

1. Melanocytes

Location

They reside in basal layer of epithelium.

Origin

- They are derived from the embryologic neural crest and migrate into the epithelium.
- Each melanocyte establishes contact with 30–40 keratinocytes through their dendritic processes.
- Keratinocytes release mediators essential for normal melanocyte function.

Functions

- Melanin produced by the melanocytes is transferred through their dendritic processes to the adjacent basal cell keratinocytes which store pigment in the form of melanosomes.
- Variation in the degree of pigmentation in different regions is related to the activity of melanosomes and not to their numbers.

Appearance

- Melanocytes appear as clear cells in hematoxylin sections and their dendritic appearance is revealed by silver stains. Hence are called as clear or dendritic cells.

Special stains

a. Silver stain reveals their spider like (dendritic) appearance and dye the melanin pigment.
b. They are also stained by Mason-Fontana stain.
c. Oral pigmentation can be studied by use of dopa reaction.
    - Melanin pigment dispersed in connective tissue is phagocytosed by macrophages, melanophages, which also stain positively with dopa.

2. Langerhans' cell

Location: It is another clear or dendritic cell found in the upper layers of the skin and mucosal epithelium, restricted to zones of orthokeratinization.

Structure: Cell has a convoluted nucleus and characteristic rod-like granules in the cytoplasm, termed *Birbeck granules.*

It has vimentin type intermediate filaments.

Origin: It is of hematopoietic origin. It penetrates epithelium from lamina propria.

Special stains: It stains with gold chloride, ATPase, and immunofluorescent markers.

Functions: It is involved in immune response. In presence of antigenic challenge by bacterial plaque, Langerhans' cells migrate into the gingiva. They present the antigen to helper T-cells.

Epithelium of skin and oral mucosa have immunologic functions and for this, it interacts with the lymphoid system in concert with the Langerhans' cells.

3. Merkel Cells

Location: They are found among the basal cells. They are commonly seen in masticatory mucosa but are absent in lining mucosa.

Structure: They are not dendritic. Ultrastructurally, the nucleus shows a deep invagination and characteristic electron-dense granules that are located at the side of cytoplasm in contact with axon terminals.

Origin: These cells migrate from the neural crest.

Special stain: They are stained by PAS stain.

Function: They are specialized neural pressure sensitive receptor cells. They respond to touch sensation.

4. Lymphocytes and Polymorphonuclear Leukocytes

They are found at various levels of the epithelium. These cells are transient and can pass through the epithelium to the surface.

Function: Immune function.

A comparative study of nonkeratinocytes

	Melanocytes	*Langerhans cell*	*Merkel cell*	*Inflammatory cells such as lymphocytes and neutrophils*
Location	Basal layer of epithelium	Upper layer of skin and mucosa	Among basal cells of epithelium	Various levels of epithelium
Origin	Neural crest	Hematopoietic	Neural crest	Hematopoietic
Structure	Dendritic or clear cells	Dendritic cells have convoluted nucleus and Birbeck granules	Non-dendritic cells with electron-dense granules	Non-dendritic

(*Contd.*)

A comparative study of nonkeratinocytes (*Contd.*)				
	Melanocytes	*Langerhans cell*	*Merkel cell*	*Inflammatory cells such as lymphocytes and neutrophils*
Special stain	Silver stains, Mason-Fontana, Dopa reaction	Gold chloride, ATPase, Immunofluorescent markers	PAS	Seen in hematoxyline and eosin stained sections
Functions	Transfer melanin to adjacent basal keratinocytes.	Immune response, presents antigen to helper T-cells.	Neural pressure sensitive receptor cell. They respond to touch sensation.	Immunity

Q. 4. Write about vermilion border of lip. *(May 2008)*
Write about transitional zone of lip. *(Nov. 2010, IIrd B.D.S. old course)*

Ans. Introduction

- The transitional zone between the skin of the lip and the mucous membrane of the lip is the *red zone* or the *vermilion zone* (Fig. 20.5).
- **Vermilion border** is the line that separates the skin from the vermilion zone.
- It is found only in humans.
- The zone is present between the skin on the outer surface of the lip and the inner aspect of the lip.
- **Skin on the outer surface of the lip:** It is covered by a moderately thick, keratinized epithelium with a thick stratum corneum. The papillae of the connective tissue here are few and short. Many sebaceous glands are found with hair follicles. Sweat glands are present in between them.
- **Transitional zone:** Has thick, mildly keratinized epithelium and numerous densely arranged, long papillae of the lamina propria reaching deep into the epithelium and carrying large capillary loops close to the surface.
  Thus, blood is visible through the thin parts of the translucent epithelium which gives the red colour to the lips.

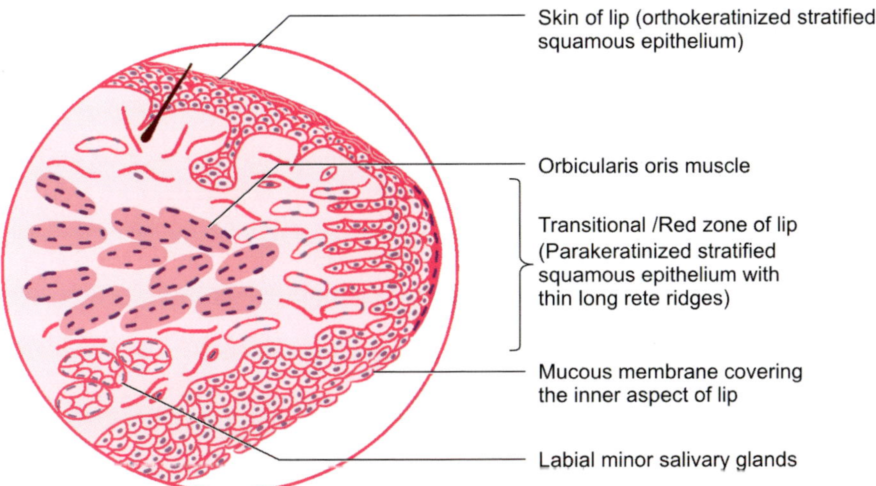

Fig. 20.5: Vermilion/Transitional/Red zone

- **Inner aspect of the lip:** Keratinization decreases towards the lips, but the thickness of epithelium increases. Here the epithelium is thicker and nonkeratinized.

Significance of Transitional Zone

- Like skin, the transitional zone is exposed to the atmosphere but it has no glands to keep it moist or prevent it from drying. It is for this reason, lips become dry easily and we lick our lips to moisten it.

Q. 5. What is gingival stippling? *(May 2008)*

Ans. GINGIVAL STIPPLING

- Gingiva is characterized by a surface that appears stippled. Portions of the epithelium appear to be elevated and between these elevations there are shallow depressions, the net result of which is stippling. Attached gingiva, a part of gingiva attached to bone or teeth, appears specifically stippled.
- They are probably functional adaptations to mechanical impacts.
- Degree of stippling varies with the age and sex. Males have more heavily stippled gingiva than do females.
- Histologically in stippled gingiva, depressions in between the elevations correspond to the center of heavy epithelial ridges.

Significance

Disappearance of stippling is an indication of edema, an indication of an involvement of the gingiva in progressing gingivitis.

Q. 6. Explain shift of dentogingival junction. *(Nov. 2014)*

Ans. Introduction

- Dentogingival junction is the junction between the gingiva and the tooth. It is a unique junction as it is an attachment of epithelium with the hard tissue.
- The epithelium of the gingiva which gets attached to the tooth is called **junctional** or **attachment epithelium.**
- The union between the attachment/junctional epithelium and the tooth is referred to as **epithelial attachment.**

Structure of Epithelial/Junctional Epithelium

- The firmness and mechanical strength of the dentogingival junction is though mainly attributable to the connective tissue attachment, the attachment of the epithelium to the enamel is also strong.
- The junctional epithelium extends up to 2 mm on the surface of the tooth.
- It has highest turnover rate of 5–6 days, hence regenerates readily.
- It structurally resembles reduced enamel epithelium. It has a basal layer and few layers of flattened cells. It is nonkeratinized.
- It is highly permeable and has large intercellular spaces.

Epithelial attachment *(SAQ, 2004)*

- The union between the junctional/attachment epithelium of the tooth is referred as epithelial attachment.

- It is submicroscopic, 40 nm wide and formed by attachment epithelium.
- The reduced ameloblasts and gingival epithelial cells form an electron microscopic basal lamina on enamel and cementum. Hemidesmosomes of the epithelial cells attach to this basal lamina.
- The adhesive forces in this zone are molecular in nature and act across a distance smaller than 40 nm.

Clinical Significance of Dentogingival Junction

- Dentogingival junction is of great physiologic and clinical importance.
- The dense, and resilient lamina propria take up impacts produced during mastication. When the connective tissue is injured, fibroblasts form collagen and ground substance contributing to repair.
- Lymphocytes and plasma cells found in the connective tissue below the junctional epithelium, contribute to defense against the bacterial injury.
- The lysosomes of the junctional epithelium have a phagocytic function. These defense reactions constitute barrier against invasion of bacteria and the penetration of toxins.

Development of Dentogingival Junction

- After completion of enamel formation, the crown of unerupted tooth is covered by reduced enamel epithelium (REE). During eruption, the tip of the tooth approaches the oral mucosa and the REE and the oral epithelium meet and fuse.
- The epithelium that covers the tip of the crown degenerates in its center, and the crown emerges through this perforation into the oral cavity.
- The REE remains organically attached to the part of the enamel that has not erupted yet. Once the tip of the crown has emerged, the REE is termed as *primary attachment epithelium.*
- A shallow groove, the gingival sulcus develops between the gingiva and the surface of the tooth and extends around its circumference.
- Gingival sulcus is bounded by the attachment epithelium at its base and by the gingival margin laterally. It deepens as a result of separation of the reduced dental epithelium from the actively erupting tooth.
- Later, the reduced enamel epithelium gets gradually replaced by the growth of gingival epithelium and this is known as *secondary attachment epithelium.*

Shift of Dentogingival Junction

- The position of the gingiva on the surface of the tooth changes with time.
- The tooth erupts until it reaches the plane of occlusion. The attachment epithelium separates from the enamel surface while the crown emerges into the oral cavity.
- **Active eruption:** The actual movement of the tooth toward the occlusal plane is *active eruption.*
- **Passive eruption** *(SAQ, 2000)*: The separation of the primary attachment epithelium from the enamel is *passive eruption.* Further, recession exposing the cementum may occur.
- Passive eruption describes various levels of attachment that may occur as the gingiva recedes onto the cementum.
- Crown exposure involving passive eruption and further recession is described in *four stages.* First two stages are considered normal while the last two are pathologic.
  1. *First stage:* In this stage, the bottom of the gingival sulcus remains in the region of the enamel-covered crown and the apical end of the attachment epithelium stays at the

cementoenamel junction. This relation persists in primary teeth almost up to 1 year of age before shedding and in permanent teeth, usually to the age of 20 or 30 years.

2. *Second stage*: In this stage, the bottom of the gingival sulcus is on the enamel and the apical end of the attachment epithelium has shifted to the surface of the cementum. This shift of dentogingival junction occurs by destruction of fiber bundles that were anchored in the cervical parts of the cementum and an apical shift of the gingival and transseptal fibers. This stage of tooth exposure lasts to the age of 40 years or later.
3. *Third stage:* In this stage, the enamel-covered crown is fully exposed, the gingival sulcus is at the cementoenamel junction and the epithelial attachment is entirely on the cementum. This exposure of tooth is regarded as the body's attempt to maintain an intact dentogingival junction in the face of factors that cause its deterioration.
4. *Fourth stage*: This stage represents recession of the gingiva caused pathologically. The entire attachment is on cementum and the clinical crown appears larger than anatomic crown.

- The shift of dentogingival junction occurs because the junctional epithelium moves apically due to detachment of basal lamina. It then replicates a new basal lamina. The epithelial cells then migrate along this basal lamina.
- The hemidesmosomes hold the cells to this structure so that the strength of the attachment is not diminished despite of migration. Thus, the epithelial attachment re-establishes and the shift occurs.

Clinical Significance

- If there occurs difference in the position of the top of the epithelial attachment relative to the marginal gingiva resulting in deepened gingival sulcus, a periodontal pocket develops. This occurs as a response to plaque toxins.
- The level of the gingival attachment to the tooth plays an important role in restorative dentistry.
- With gingival recession and exposure of the cervical part of anatomic crown, cemental caries or abrasion may occur.

MULTIPLE CHOICE QUESTIONS (MCQs)

1. The arrangement of tonofibrils in keratinized epithelium is
a. In bundles
b. Dispersed
c. End to end
d. Whorl pattern

2. The connective tissue component of the oral mucosa that supports the overlying epithelium is called
a. Submucosa
b. Dermis
c. Lamina propria
d. Reteplase

3. Which of the following cells are non-keratinocytes
a. Melanocytes
b. Langerhans' cells
c. Merkel cells
d. All of the above

4. Basket cell is a synonym used for
a. Myoepithelial cell
b. Mucous cells
c. Serous cells
d. None of the above

5. Ectopic location of sebaceous glands in the buccal mucosa represents
a. Koplik's spots
b. Fordyce spot
c. Linea alba
d. None of the above

6. The only minor serous salivary gland found in oral mucosa
a. Labial salivary gland
b. Von Ebner's salivary gland
c. Glands in the posterolateral zone of hard palate
d. None of the above

7. One of the distinguishing features of an epithelial cell, regardless of its function is that one of the components of its cytoskeleton is
a. Keratin intermediate filaments
b. Desmin
c. Vimentin
d. None of the above

8. Epithelial cell is also known as
a. Keratinocyte
b. Keratosome
c. Odland body
d. Hyaline body

9. Nonkeratinized epithelium does not have
a. Basal layer
b. Prickle cell layer
c. Granular layer
d. Intermediate layer

10. The distinguishing feature of squamous epithelial cell is that it contains
a. Tonofilaments
b. Desmosomes
c. Keratin filament
d. All of the above

11. Adhesion between epithelium and lamina propria is provided by
a. Desmosomes
b. Hemidesmosomes
c. Plasma membrane
d. Pellicle

12. The functions of the oral epithelium are
a. Permeability
b. Protection
c. Sensation
d. All of the above

13. The oral epithelium does not have the following function
a. Permeability b. Absorptive
c. Secretive d. Formative

1-a, 2-c, 3-d, 4-a, 5-b, 6-b, 7-a, 8-a, 9-c, 10-d, 11-b, 12-d, 13-b

14. All nonkeratinocytes, except one type of cell has desmosomal attachment to adjacent cells
a. Melanocytes
b. Langerhans' cells
c. Merkel cells
d. Inflammatory cells

15. Gingiva is attached to the tooth by the
a. Epithelial attachment
b. Pellicle
c. Periodontal ligament
d. Reduced enamel epithelium

16. Macrophages are also termed as
a. Mast cells
b. Monocytes
c. Histiocytes
d. Lymphocytes

17. Principal functions of macrophages are
a. Ingestion of damaged tissue
b. Stimulation of fibroblast proliferation for repair
c. Formative
d. Both a and b

18. Von Ebners salivary glands at the base of circumvallate papillae are
a. Mucous glands
b. Serous glands
c. Mixed glands
d. None of the above

19. Basal lamina is an
a. Electron microscopic structure
b. Light microscopic structure
c. Macroscopic structure
d. Both a and b

20. Lamina propria consists of
a. Collagen fibers
b. Elastic fibers
c. Oxytalan fibers
d. Both a and b

21. Unlike collagen fibers elastic fibers
a. Run in bundles
b. Branch and anastomose
c. Run singly
d. Both b and c

22. The feature that contributes to the more rapid healing of the oral mucosa when compared with skin is due to
a. Rich blood supply
b. Rich anastomoses of arterioles and capillaries
c. Arteriovenous shunts
d. Both a and b

23. The specialized mucosa which is non-keratinized and contains taste buds is
a. Fungiform papillae
b. Filiform papillae
c. Lateral walls of circumvallate papillae
d. Both a and c

24. The primitive oral cavity comes to be lined by epithelium at about
a. 24 days *in utero*
b. 25 days *in utero*
c. 26 days *in utero*
d. 30 days *in utero*

25. Membrane-coating granules are also known as
a. Fordyce granules
b. Desmosomes
c. Keratinosomes
d. Tonofibrils

26. Masticatory mucosa is made-up of
a. Gingiva b. Hard palate
c. Soft palate d. Both a and b

27. Anterior two-thirds of the tongue is supplied by
a. Trigeminal nerve (lingual branch)
b. Glossopharyngeal nerve
c. Temporal nerve
d. Occulomotor nerve

14-c, 15-a, 16-c, 17-d, 18-b, 19-a, 20-d, 21-d, 22-d, 23-d, 24-c, 25-c, 26-d, 27-a

28. Posterior third of the tongue is supplied by
a. Glossopharyngeal nerve
b. Trigeminal nerve
c. Temporal nerve
d. Occulomotor nerve

29. The area of masticatory mucosa which does not have submucosa is
a. Gingiva
b. Lateral areas of hard palate
c. Median raphe
d. Both a and c

30. The sulcular epithelium gets renewed in
a. 5 days b. 8 days
c. 10 days d. 12 days

31. General oral mucosa gets renewed in
a. 8–10 days
b. 10–12 days
c. 12–13 days
d. 15–20 days

32. Gingiva is parakeratinized in
a. 75% of normal population
b. 72% of normal population
c. 60% of normal population
d. 50% of normal population

33. Epithelium of *col* of interdental papilla is
a. Parakeratinized
b. Nonkeratinized
c. Hyperkeratinized
d. Keratinized

34. The width of the basement membrane is
a. 1–4 mm b. 2–3 mm
c. 2–5 mm d. 3–6 mm

35. Racial pigmentation present in gingiva is the result of
a. Size of the melanin granule
b. Difference in number of melanocytes
c. Difference in ratio of melanin production
d. All of the above

36. The outermost layer of oral epithelium of buccal mucosa is called
a. Stratum granulosum
b. Stratum basale
c. Stratum corneum
d. Stratum superficiale

37. Gingiva is attached to the tooth by
a. Periodontal ligament
b. Pellicle
c. Reduced enamel epithelium
d. Epithelial attachment

38. Epithelium covering the mucosa on the dorsal surface of the tongue is
a. Specialized mucosa
b. Keratinized mucosa
c. Parakeratinized mucosa
d. Nonkeratinized mucosa

39. Mucous membrane of the posterior part of tongue gets its nerve supply by
a. Lingual nerve
b. Glossopharyngeal nerve
c. Superior laryngeal nerve
d. Inferior laryngeal nerve

40. The connective tissue component of the anterior two-thirds of the tongue is derived from
a. First arch mesenchyme
b. Second arch mesenchyme
c. Third arch mesenchyme
d. Fourth arch mesenchyme

41. Stippling is a feature present in
a. Attached gingiva
b. Alveolar mucosa
c. Free gingiva
d. All of the above

42. The lining mucosa is the one that lies the
a. Hard palate
b. Dorsum of the tongue
c. Gingiva
d. Soft palate

28-a, 29-d, 30-c, 31-c, 32-a, 33-b, 34-a, 35-d, 36-d, 37-d, 38-a, 39-b, 40-a, 41-a, 42-d

43. The type of collagen fibers of the basement membrane are
a. Type IV b. Type I
c. Type III d. All of the above

44. Minor salivary gland in the oral cavity are present in all tissues except
a. Alveolar mucosa
b. Lip
c. Palate
d. Gingiva

45. Mucous membrane of soft palate is
a. Keratinized
b. Nonkeratinized
c. Parakeratinized
d. Orthokeratinized

46. Programmed cell death is also known as
a. Shedding b. Exfoliation
c. Apoptosis d. None of the above

47. Connective tissue of lamina propria of the oral mucosa is derived from
a. Neural crest cells
b. Mesoderm
c. Endoderm
d. Ectoderm

48. Stratum spinosum is also known as
a. Basal cell layer
b. Superficial layer
c. Granular layer
d. Prickle cell layer

49. The function of Odland body is
a. Nutrition
b. Sensory
c. Exchange of fluids
d. Permeability barrier

50. The part of gingiva that is susceptible to infection and nonkeratinized is
a. Palatal gingiva
b. Sulcular gingiva
c. Attached gingiva
d. Marginal gingiva

51. Epithelial cells which ultimately get keratinized are
a. Keratinosomes
b. Keratinocytes
c. Nonkeratinocytes
d. All of the above

52. Which component of oral mucous membrane contains glands and adipose tissue
a. Epithelium
b. Lamina propria
c. Submucosa
d. All

53. Of all the four layers of epithelium the layer which is more active in protein synthesis is
a. Spinous layer
b. Granulosum
c. Stratum Corneum
d. Basal cell layer

54. Clear cells of epithelium of oral mucous membrane are
a. Keratinocytes
b. Keratinosomes
c. Nonkeratinocytes
d. None

55. Nonkeratinocyte that does not have desmosomal attachment is
a. Melanocyte
b. Langerhans cell
c. Merkel cell
d. Both a and b

56. The nonkeratinocytes referred as dentritic cells are
a. Melanocytes b. Langerhans cell
c. Merkel cell d. Both a and b

57. The only nonkeratinocyte having desmosomal attachment is
a. Langerhans cell
b. Merkel cell
c. Melanocyte
d. Lymphocyte

43-a, 44-d, 45-b, 46-c, 47-a, 48-d, 49-d, 50-b, 51-b, 52-c, 53-a, 54-c, 55-d, 56-d, 57-b

58. Racket-shaped Birbeck granules are found in
a. Langerhans cells
b. Merkel cells
c. Melanocytes
d. Both b and c

59. Taste buds are not present in
a. Filiform papillae
b. Fungiform papillae
c. Circumpallate papillae
d. None of the above

60. Langerhans cells can be studied by using
a. Silver stain
b. Dopa reaction
c. Gold chloride
d. Hemotoxylin and eosin stain

61. Melanocytes can be studied using
a. Silver stain
b. Mason-Fontana
c. Dopa reaction
d. All of the above

62. The component of oral mucous membrane which contains glands and adipose tissue is
a. Epithelium b. Lamina propia
c. Submucosa d. All of the above

63. Neurosecretory cells are
a. Melanocytes b. Merkel cells
c. Keratinocytes d. Lymphocytes

64. Richest nerve sensation is in
a. Anterior two-thirds of tongue
b. Posterior one-third of tongue
c. Lateral border of tongue
d. Tip of the tongue

65. Dentogingival junction is
a. Primary attachment epithelium
b. Secondary attachment epithelium
c. Attachment epithelium
d. All of the above

66. Free gingiva is made-up of
a. Circular group of fibers
b. Transseptal fibers
c. Dentogingival fibers
d. All of the above

67. The boundaries that define the attached gingiva are
a. From the gingival crest to the interdental groove
b. From the mucogingival junction to the free gingival groove
c. From the epithelial attachment to cementoenamel junction
d. From the free gingival groove to the gingival crest.

68. The embrassure surrounding the contact area of anterior teeth is
a. Gingival, cervical, facial, lingual
b. Incisal, cervical, facial, lingual
c. Incisal, cervical, facial only
d. Cervical and lingual only

69. Gingival sulcus is deepest on
a. Incisal surface of incisors
b. Lingual suface of incisors
c. Mesial surface of incisors
d. Distal surface of incisors

70. Oral mucous membrane is thinnest in
a. Soft palate
b. Labial mucosa
c. Buccal mucosa
d. Floor of the mouth

71. Bitter and sour taste are mediated by
a. Chorda tympani
b. Glossopharyngeal nerve
c. Hypoglossal nerve
d. None of the above

72. The papillae responsible to recognize sour taste is
a. Vallate papillae
b. Foliate papillae
c. Fungiform papillae
d. Filiform papillae

58-a, 59-a, 60-c, 61-d, 62-c, 63-b, 64-a, 65-c, 66-d, 67-b, 68-b, 69-b, 70-d, 71-b, 72-b

73. The number of circumvallate papillae ranges from
a. 20–25
b. 15–20
c. 8–10
d. 4–5

74. The most numerous group of gingival fibers is
a. Dentoperiosteal
b. Dentogingival
c. Alveogingival
d. Circular

75. The disappearance of stippling occurs due to
a. Trauma
b. Old age
c. Progressive gingivitis
d. None of the above

76. Jacobson's organ is also known as
a. Vomeronasal organ
b. Considered as auxillary olfactory
c. Ellipsoidal structure lined with olfactory epithelium
d. All of the above

77. Of the four layers, the cells most active in protein synthesis are of
a. Stratum corneum
b. Stratum granulosum
c. Stratum spinosum
d. Stratum basale

78. The epithelium of the cheek and sublingual tissue is
a. Nonkeratinized
b. Parakeratinized
c. Keratinized
d. None of the above

79. The epithelium in gingiva is
a. Parakeratinized
b. Nonkeratized
c. Keratinized
d. Any of the above

80. The epithelium of the oral mucous membrane is
a. Stratified columnar
b. Simple squamous epithelium
c. Stratified squamous
d. Non-stratified squamous

81. The specialized mucosa is present on
a. Lips and cheeks
b. Gingiva and hard palate
c. Dorsum of the tongue and taste buds
d. Floor of the mouth and soft palate

82. Majority of the taste buds are found on the
a. Filiform papillae
b. Fungiform papillae
c. Circumvallate papillae and the adjacent trench wall
d. All of the above

83. The oral epithelium is
a. Nervous tissue
b. Muscle tissue
c. Connective tissue
d. Avascular tissue

84. Lamina propria of the oral mucous membrane contains
a. Ectoderm b. Bone
c. Keratin d. Blood vessels

85. The last organic material secreted by the ameloblast is
a. Primary enamel cuticle
b. Secondary cuticle
c. Enamel tufts
d. Tomes' process

86. The papillae of the tongue which are keratinized and do not have taste buds are
a. Fungiform
b. Filiform
c. Vallate papillae
d. Both b and c

73-c, 74-b, 75-c, 76-d, 77-c, 78-a, 79-d, 80-c, 81-c, 82-c, 83-d, 84-d, 85-a, 86-b

87. The sebaceous glands lateral to the corner of the mouth and often seen opposite the molars are called
a. Fordyce spot
b. Hutchinson spot
c. Koplik's spot
d. Miller's spot

88. Vermilion border, which is transitional zone between the skin of the lip and the mucous membrane of the lip, is also know as
a. White zone
b. Red zone
c. Violet zone
d. Pink zone

89. The gingiva is
a. 75% parakeratinized
b. 15% keratinized
c. 10% nonkeratinized
d. All of the above

90. The pigmentation is more abundant at the
a. Buccal gingiva
b. Labial gingiva
c. Lingual gingiva
d. Base of the interdental papilla

91. Filaggrin protein is present in
a. Periodontal ligament
b. Pulp
c. Oral epithelium
d. All of the above

92. The only purely serous minor salivary gland is located in the lamina propria of the
a. Tongue b. Hard palate
c. Soft palate d. Buccal mucosa

93. Keratohyaline granules are found in
a. Granulosum
b. Spinosum
c. Basal cell layer
d. Prickle cell layer

94. The labial masticatory mucosa is narrowest on the following mandibular tooth
a. First molar
b. Second molar
c. First premolar
d. Central incisor

95. The following type of mucosa characterizes attached gingiva
a. Free b. Alveolar
c. Specialized d. Masticatory

96. Oral mucosa exhibits
a. Humoral immunity
b. Cell mediated immunity
c. Both of the above
d. None of the above

97. Lining mucosa includes all except
a. Lip
b. Cheeks
c. Floor of mouth
d. Dorsum of tongue

98. Oral mucosa is lined by the
a. Stratified squamous epithelium
b. Cuboidal
c. Columnar
d. None of the above

99. Mucoperiosteal attachment is seen in the
a. Gingiva b. Lips
c. Cheeks d. All of the above

100. The epithelium of oral cavity is derived from
a. Ectoderm
b. Endoderm
c. Mesoderm
d. None of the above

101. Hemidesmosomes help in
a. Adhesion between epithelium and connective tissue
b. Adhesion between cells of epithelium
c. Both a and b
d. None of the above

87-a, 88-b, 89-d, 90-d, 91-c, 92-a, 93-a, 94-a, 95-d, 96-c, 97-d, 98-a, 99-a, 100-a, 101-a

102. Desmosomes are
- a. Two-attachment plaque
- b. One attachment plaque
- c. Three-attachment plaque
- d. Four-attachment plaque

103. Odland body is seen in the
- a. Stratum spinosum
- b. Stratum granulosum
- c. Stratum intermedium
- d. Stratum superficiale

104. Most prominent finding in stratum granulosum is
- a. Presence of keratinosome
- b. Keratohyaline granules
- c. Langerhans cells
- d. All of the above

105. Characteristic features of melanocytes are
- a. Clear cells
- b. Spider-like appearance in silver stains
- c. Production of melanin pigment
- d. All of the above

106. Characteristic of Langerhans cells are
- a. Presence of Birbeck granules
- b. Antigen presenting cells
- c. They are derived from bone marrow
- d. All of the above

107. Basal lamina has
- a. Type I collagen
- b. Type II collagen
- c. Type IV collagen
- d. All of the above

108. The epithelium present in the intermediate zone is
- a. Nonkeratinized
- b. Orthokeratinized
- c. Parakeratinized
- d. None of the above

102-a, 103-a, 104-b, 105-d, 106-d, 107-c, 108-c

Chapter 21

Salivary Glands

LAQ (10 Marks)

Q. 1. Describe histology of parotid/submandibular/sublingual gland. Major salivary glands.

Ans. Salivary glands are a group of compound exocrine glands secreting saliva.

They are classified as:

1. *Based on size*:
   - **Major:** Major salivary glands are three bilaterally paired major salivary glands namely, *parotid, submandibular* and *sublingual.*
   - **Minor:** Minor salavary glands are located beneath the epithelium in oral cavity except gingiva, anterior raphe region of hard palate, and anterior two-thirds of the dorsum of the tongue.

     (*e.g.* labial glands, buccal glands, lingual glands, palatine, and glassopalatine glands, etc.)

     Major salivary glands are located, extraorally and their secretions reach the mouth by long ducts. While minor salivary glands consist of several small groups of secretory units which open via short ducts directly into the mouth.

2. *Based on histochemical nature of secreting product*:
   - **Serous**
   - **Mucous**

Parotid gland is a pure serous gland, the submandibular and the sublingual glands are mixed glands. While, submandibular gland is predominantly serous and the sublingual gland is predominantly mucous gland.

PAROTID GLAND

- **Introduction:**
  - It is the largest major salivary gland.
  - It has: (a) *superficial portion*—located subcutaneously in front of the external ear.
    (b) *deeper portion*—lies behind the ramus of the mandible.
  - It measures 5.8 cm craniocaudally and 3.4 cm ventrodorsally. It weighs between 14–28 grams.

- **Excretory duct:** It is *Stenson's duct*, which opens at a papilla at the buccal mucosa opposite the maxillary second molar.
- **Blood and nerve supply:**
  - *Blood supply*—branches of the external carotid artery.
  - *Parasympathetic nerve supply*—ninth cranial nerve reaching the gland via otic ganglion and the auriculotemporal nerve.
  - *Sympathetic innervation*—for all salivary glands is by postganglionic fibers from superior cervical ganglion.
  - *Lymphatic drainage*—is to the superficial and deep cervical lymph nodes.
- **Histology :**
  - Parotid gland is enclosed in a well-defined connective tissue capsule which sends septa into the gland, separating it into lobes and lobules.
  - It is a **pure serous gland** (Fig. 21.1).
  - Describe serous cells histology as described in answer of SAQ 2.
  - The intercalated ducts of the parotid are long and branching.
  - Striated ducts are numerous.
  - Connective tissue septa in the parotid contain numerous fat cells which increase with age.

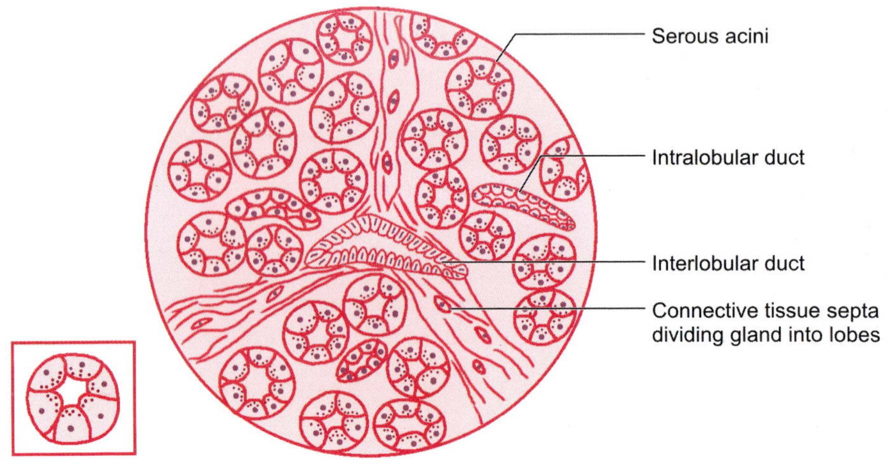

Fig. 21.1: Serous salivary gland

SUBMANDIBULAR GLAND

(SAQ, NOV. 2011)

- **Introduction:**
  - It is the second largest major salivary gland.
  - It is also called as **submaxillary salivary gland.**
  - It is located on the medial aspect of the body of the mandible in the submandibular triangle, posterior and superficial to the mylohyoid muscle.
- **Excretory duct**—It is *Wharton's duct* which runs forward above the myolohyoid muscle lying just below the mucosa of the floor of the mouth. It opens at the sublingual papillae, caruncula sublingualis, lateral to the lingual frenum.

- **Blood and Nerve supply:**
  - *Blood supply*—from the lingual and facial arteries.
  - *Parasympathetic innervation*—from 7th cranial nerve reaching the gland through lingual nerve.
  - *Lymphatic drainage*—to the deep cervical and jugular chain of nodes.
- **Histology:**
  - It is a branched tubuloacinar gland of **mixed** type (Fig. 21.2).
  - It has a well defined capsule.
  - It has both serous and mucous secretory units. ***Serous*** units ***predominate***.
  - Describe both serous and mucous acini as described in answer of SAQ 3.
  - Mucous terminal portions are capped by demilunes of serous cells.
  - Intercalated ducts are shorter than those of the parotid and striated ducts are usually longer.

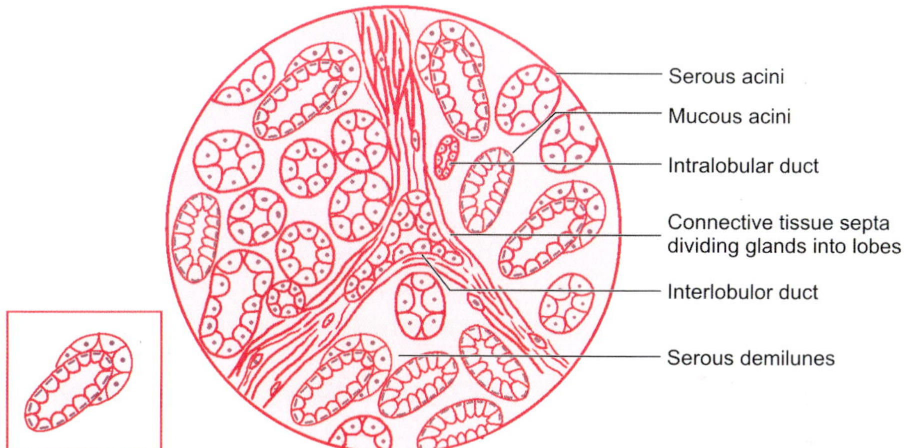

Fig. 21.2: Mixed salivary gland

SUBLINGUAL GLAND

- **Introduction:**
  - It is the smallest of the major salivary glands.
  - It is almond shaped and lies between the floor of the mouth, below the mucosa and above the mylohyoid muscle.
- **Excretory duct:**
  - *Bartholin's duct* is the main duct which opens with or near the submandibular duct.
  - Several small ducts; duct of Rivinus, open independently along the sublingual fold.
- **Blood and nerve supply:**
  - *Blood supply* – from the sublingual and the submental arteries.
  - *Parasympathetic nerve supply* – from the 7th cranial nerve.
  - *Lymphatic drainage* – is to thc submandibular lymph nodes.
- **Histology:**
  - It is composed of one main gland with several small glands.

- It is a **mixed** gland (Fig. 21.2), with ***mucous*** secretory units seen ***predominantly.***
- Mucous cells are arranged in a tubular pattern.
- Serous demilunes may be present.
- Describe the histology of mucous cells as described later in SAQ.
- The intercalated and striated ducts are poorly developed.

Clinical Significance

1. Salivary glands are subject to a number of pathologic conditions. These include inflammatory diseases such as viral, bacterial or allergic sialadenitis, a variety of benign and malignant tumors, autoimmune diseases such as Sjögren's syndrome and genetic diseases. One of the most common surface lesions of the oral mucosa is mucocele, which is produced from the severance of the duct of a minor salivary gland and pooling of saliva in the tissues.
2. A loss of salivary function or reduction in volume of saliva secreted is called **xerostomia.** This leads to dryness of the mouth resulting in caries, mucosal ulceration and oral infection.

SAQs (3 Marks)

Q. 1. Write differences between serous and mucous acini. *(Oct. 2004)*

Ans. DIFFERENCES BETWEEN SEROUS AND MUCOUS CELLS

Differences between serous and mucous cells

Serous cells	*Mucous cells*
1. Serous acini are spherical.	1. Mucous acini are tubular.
2. Serous acini have smaller lumen.	2. Mucous acini have larger lumen.
3. Serous cells are pyramidal with a broad base on the basement membrane.	3. Mucous cells are also pyramidal but are larger and have a broader luminal surface.
4. Has spherical nucleus placed at the basal region.	4. Has oval or flat nucleus pressed against the base of the cell.
5. Apex of the cell has zymogen granules. Apical portion stains strongly with H and E.	5. Cells show large amount of mucous secretory product at the apical cytoplasm. Apical portion stains weakly with H and E.
6. Serous secretion has enzymatic activity. It is watery and thin.	6. Has little or no enzymatic activity. It is thick and viscid.
7. Contributes less to the lubrication.	7. Has main function as lubrication and protection of the oral tissues.
8. Carbohydrate content is less in secretion. Zymogen granules are glycolated proteins.	8. Carbohydrate to protein ratio is greater.
9. Secretion is by exocytosis.	9. Secretion is by fusion of the membrane of mucous droplets to the apical plasma membrane.
10. Special stain: Apical portion shows numerous eosinophilic secretory granules which stain with toluidine blue.	10. Apical portion stains strongly with carbohydrate stains like PAS and Alcian blue.

(Contd.)

Differences between serous and mucous cells *(Contd.)*

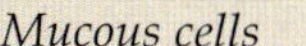

Serous cells	*Mucous cells*
11. Electron microscopy: Extensive RER in parallel aggregates, lateral and basal to nucleus. Golgi regions are located apical to nucleus. Secretory granules are smaller, seen at apical area and are covered by unit membrane (Fig. 21.3).	11. Prominent golgi regions are located between nucleus and secretory droplets. Secretory droplets are irregular and larger than serous (Fig. 21.4).

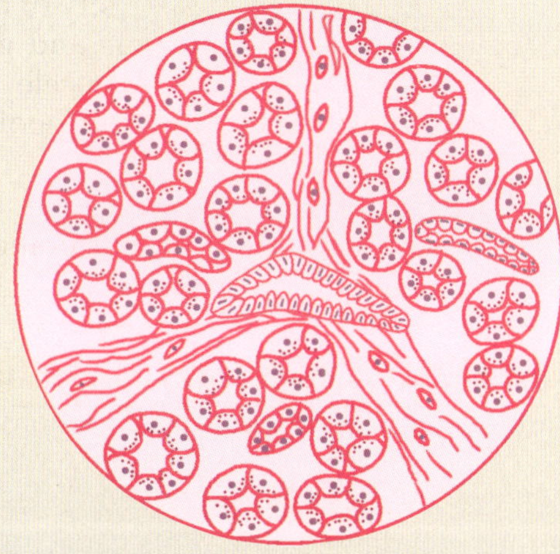

Fig. 21.3: Serous salivary gland

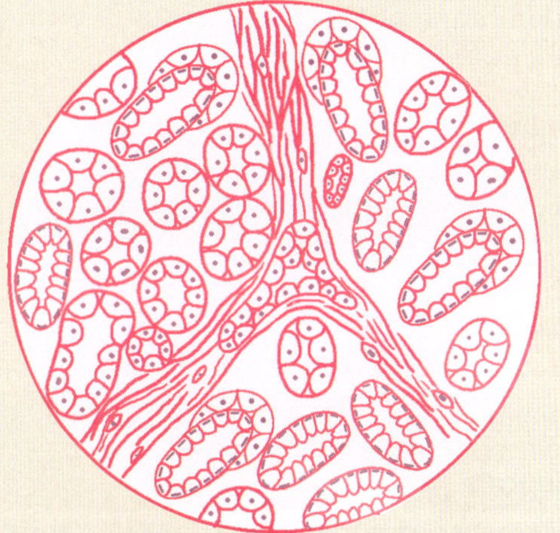

Fig. 21.4: Mucous salivary gland

Q. 2. Write about serous acini. *(July 2006, 2012, May 2012)*

Ans. SEROUS ACINI

- Salivary glands are a group of compound exocrine glands secreting saliva. Saliva regulates a healthy environment in oral cavity.
- The basic functional unit of a salivary gland is the terminal secretory unit called acini, which is made-up of epithelial secretary cells, namely serous and mucous cells.
- Serous or mucous cells along with myoepithelial cells are arranged in an acinus with a roughly spherical or tubular shape and a central lumen.

Serous Cell Histology *(Refer Fig. 21.1)*

- Serous acini are roughly round in shape.
- Serous cells are main secretory cells in parotid and submandibular major salivary gland and in von Ebner's minor salivary gland.
- Serous secretory cells are pyramidal with a broad base on the basement membrane and the apex faces the lumen.
- They have a spherical nucleus placed at the basal region.
- Apical cytoplasm of these cells shows accumulation of secretory granules, which are 1 μm in diameter with a distinct limiting membrane. These are **zymogen granules** and are formed by glycolated proteins. They can be stained by toluidine blue.

- Serous cell is a typical protein secreting cell. Basal cytoplasm of serous cells is packed with protein synthesizing organelles like ribosomes and rough endoplasmic reticulum. It also shows good number of mitochondria.
- Newly synthesized proteins are sent to the Golgi apparatus, which are located apically and laterally to the cell nucleus. In the Golgi saccules, they are packed into vacuoles. These are the forming secretory granules. These presecretory immature granules increase in size and density to mature.
- Many secretory proteins undergo structural modification prior to their secretion.
- The mature granules stored at the apex of the cell are emptied into the lumen by exocytosis. Membrane of the granules fuses with the plasma membrane of the cell and contents are released into lumen.

Staining

- With hematoxylin and eosin, apical portion stains strongly.
- Apical portion shows numerous eosinophilic secretory granules, zymogen granules, which stains with *toluidine blue.*

Secretion

- Serous secretion is thin and watery. Zymogen granules are glycolated proteins. Secretion is rich in enzymatic and non-enzymatic proteins and contain small amount of carbohydrate.

Functions

- Serous secretion has enzymatic activity. The serous cell devote 80% of its capacity in the production of secretory granules, zymogen granules.
- Lysosomes are seen with hydrolytic enzymes in these cells, which help to destroy foreign material and worn out cell organelles.
- Serous cells are considered to be powerhouses for numerous synthetic and transportation proceses.

Q. 3. Write histology of mucous salivary gland. *(Nov. 2014)*

Ans. MUCOUS CELL HISTOLOGY (Fig. 21.5)

- Mucous cells are the predominant secretory cells in the sublingual glands and majority of minor salivary glands in oral cavity.
- Mucous acini are tubular and have larger lumen than serous acini.
- Mucous cells are specialized for the synthesis, storage, and secretion of a secretory product.
- They are pyramidal in shape, larger than serous cells, and have broader luminal surface.
- Nucleus of the mucous cell is oval or flattened. The nucleus and a thin rim of cytoplasm are compressed against the base of the cell.
- Mucous cell shows accumulation of large amounts of secretory product at the apical cytoplasm.
- Mucous cells have rough endoplasmic reticulum, mitochondria and large Golgi apparatus which adds large amount of carbohydrate to the secretion.
- Secretion of mucous cells occurs by fusion of the membrane of the mucous droplets with the apical plasma membrane of the cell. After this, the separating membrane may fragment and is lost with the discharge of mucous or the droplet may be discharged with the membrane intact.

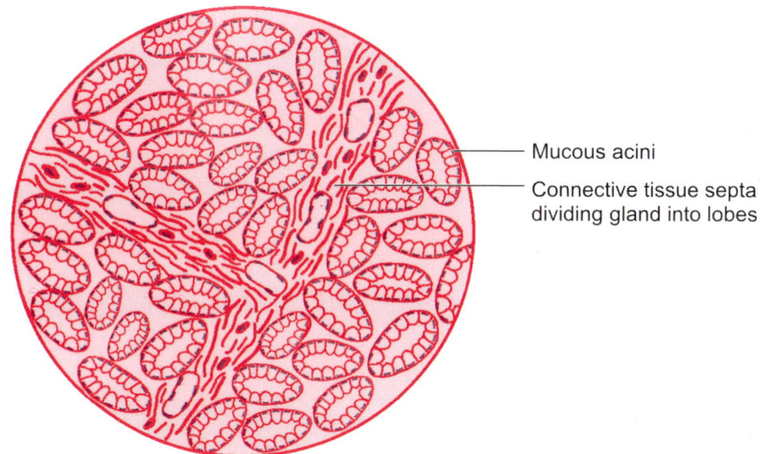

Fig. 21.5: Mucous salivary gland

Staining

In hematoxylin and eosin stained section, apical portion of mucous cells appears empty. Basal cytoplasm appears basophilic. Special stain such as *Mucicarmine* or *Periodic Acid Schiff stain* or *Alcian blue* can be used to reveal the secretory granules.

Secretion

- They have no enzymatic activity and serve mainly for lubrication and protection of the oral tissues.
- The secretion is rich in glycoproteins and is thick.
- Ratio of carbohydrate to protein is greater and larger amounts of sialic acid and sulfated sugars are present.

Function

1. Due to presence of large amount of glycoproteins, main function is lubrication therefore, protection of the oral tissues.
2. Well-lubricated oral tissues facilitates speech and deglutition.

Q. 4. Write about myoepithelial cells. *(June 2007, 2008)*

Ans. **MYOEPITHELIAL CELLS**

Introduction

Salivary glands are a group of compound exocrine glands secreting saliva.

Myoepithelial cells are contractile cells closely related to the secretory and intercalated duct cells of salivary glands.

Location

They are located around the terminal secretory units and the first portion of the duct system. They are situated between the basal plasma membrane of parenchymal cells and basement membrane supporting the secretory unit or duct.

Histology

They are stellate or spider-like, with a flattened nucleus, scanty cytoplasm and long branching processes that embrace the secretory and duct cells.

In intercalated ducts they are more fusiform in shape and have short processes.

They resemble a basket cradling the secretory unit, hence they are also termed as **'basket cells'.**

They contain cytokeratin, intermediate filament and contractile actin filaments. The plasma membrane of the myoepithelial cell closely parallels the basal membrane of the parenchymal cell and are joined by desmosomes. Numerous micropinocytotic vesicles are located on the plasma membrane of these cells.

They are innervated through the parasympathetic motor nerve.

Origin

They are similar to smooth muscle cells but are derived from epithelium. Presence of cytokeratin confirms their epithelial origin.

Identification

- They are difficult to identify in routine histologic preparations. They can be detected by histochemical tests that can demonstrate ATPase reaction.
- Presence of cytokeratin and actin helps in identification of these cells by immunohistochemistry.

Functions

Structural details of myoepithelial cells indicate their contractile property.

1. They accelerate the initial outflow of the saliva from acini.
2. They reduce luminal volume.
3. Contribute to secretory pressure in the acini or duct.
4. Support the underlying parenchyma and reduce the back permeation of fluid.
5. Help salivary flow to overcome increase in peripheral resistance of the ducts.
6. They produce a number of proteins that have tumor suppressor activity, which act as barriers against invasive epithelial neoplasms.

Q. 5. Write about minor salivary glands. *(June 2008, Nov. 2010)*

Ans. MINOR SALIVARY GLANDS:

Minor salivary glands consist of several small groups of secretory units opening via short ducts directly into the mouth. They contribute to 5–10% of the total saliva secreted.

They are located beneath the epithelium in almost all parts of the oral cavity except for gingiva, anterior raphe of hard palate and anterior two-thirds of dorsum of tongue.

Minor salivary glands are:

1. Labial and buccal glands
2. Glossopalatine glands
3. Palatine glands
4. Lingual glands
5. von Ebner's glands.

1. **Labial and buccal glands:**
   - Glands of the lips and cheeks are mixed consisting of mucous tubules with serous demilunes.
2. **Glossopalatine glands:**
   - They are pure mucous glands and are located in the region of glossopalatine fold and may extend to soft palate.
3. **Palatine glands:**
   - These are pure mucous.
   - They are located in the posterolateral region of the hard palate and in the submucosa of the soft palate and uvula.
4. **Lingual glands:**

   The glands of the tongue can be divided as:

   a. *Anterior lingual glands (Glands of Blandin and Nuhn)*:
      - They are located near the apex of the tongue.
      - The anterior regions of the glands are chiefly mucous whereas the posterior portions are mixed.
      - Ducts open on the ventral surface of the tongue near the lingual frenum.

   b. *Posterior lingual mucous glands*:
      - These are located lateral and posterior to vallate papillae.
      - These are purely mucous.
      - Ducts open onto the dorsal surface of tongue.
5. **von Ebner's glands (posterior lingual serous glands):**
   - These are group of posterior lingual serous glands.
   - They are purely serous and are located between the muscle fibers of the tongue below the vallate papillae.
   - Their ducts open into the trough of the vallate papillae.
   - **Functions:**
     - Secretion by minor salivary glands is thick and mucous.
     - The secretion is rich in proteins and they have an important role in innate immunity.

     1. Serves to wash out the trough of the papillae and ready the taste receptors.
     2. Has protective and digestive functions.
     3. Has antibacterial enzymes, peroxidase and lysozyme.
     4. Has secretory enzyme with lipolytic activity. It has lingual lipase, which has an acidic pH and therefore is capable of hydrolyzing triglycerides in the stomach.

Q. 6. Write about ductal system of salivary glands.

Ans. **DUCTAL SYSTEM OF SALIVARY GLANDS** (Fig. 21.6)

- Salivary glands are a group of compound exocrine glands secreting saliva.
- The parenchymal elements of the gland consist of terminal secretory units leading into ducts that open into the oral cavity.
- Ductal system is a pipeline or conduit for the passageway for the saliva and it participates in the production and modification of saliva.

- In a major gland, the smallest ducts are the *intercalated ducts* connecting the terminal secretary units, acini, to the next larger duct, the *striated ducts.* In the interlobar tissue the ducts continue to join one another increasing in size until the main *excretory duct* is formed.
- Intercalated and striated ducts are intralobular ducts while excretory ducts are interlobular.

1. **Intercalated ducts:** They are lined by a single layer of low cuboidal cells. They modify the saliva through secretory and resorptive process. They contribute components like lysozymes and lactoferrin. They also house undifferentiated cells which undergo differentiation to replace damaged or dying cells.

2. **Striated ducts:** They receive saliva from intercalated ducts. They are lined by a layer of tall columnar epithelial cells with large, spherical, centrally placed nuclei. Cytoplasm is abundant and shows striations at the basal ends due to infoldings of the plasma membrane, which are packed with mitochondria.

   These ducts are site of electrolytic reabsorption especially of sodium and chloride and secretion of potassium and bicarbonate, which results into a hypotonic luminal fluid.

3. **Excretory ducts:** Striated ducts join each other to form larger intralobular ducts. Along the path, the duct becomes large to become the excretory interlobular duct. It has two layers, the mucosa and the outer connective tissue adventitia which allow passive stretching of the duct to allow and accommodate varying volumes of saliva. Lining epithelium of the duct is pseudostratified columnar with occasional goblet and ciliated cells.

   Main excretory duct of parotid gland is **Stensen's duct** which opens at the buccal mucosa opposite the maxillary 2nd molar. **Wharton's duct,** is the main excretory duct for submandibular gland which opens at the sublingual papillae at the floor of the mouth. Bartholin's duct, excretory duct of sublingual gland, opens near **submandibular duct.**

   In contrast to major salivary gland, where their secretions reach to, mouth by long ducts, minor salivary glands have short ducts which open directly in mouth.

Function

- Ductal system of salivary gland helps in passage and formation of saliva.
  Formation of saliva occurs in two stages.
  - In the *first stage*, cells of the secretory end pieces and intercalated ducts produce primary saliva, which is an isotonic fluid containing most of the organic components and all of

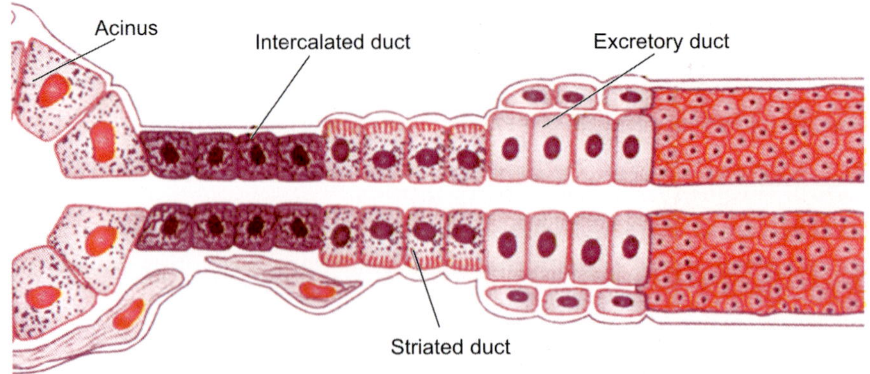

Fig. 21.6: Ductal system of salivary glands

the water secreted by the salivary glands. In the *second stage*, the primary saliva is modified as it passes through the striated and excretory ducts by reabsorption and secretion of electrolytes, so the final saliva is hypotonic. Thus, ductal system of salivary gland acts as conduit for passage of saliva and also participates in production and modification of saliva.

Q. 7. What are demilunes?

Ans. DEMILUNES

- Salivary glands are compound exocrine glands, main function being secretion of saliva.
- The basic functional unit of a salivary gland is the terminal secretory unit called **acini,** which is made-up of epithelial secretory cells, namely serous and mucous cells.
- Sometimes mucous acini have bonnet or crescent shaped covering which is made of serous cells. These are called **demilunes** (demilune-half moon).
- However, the presence of demilunes is questioned. It has been shown that demilunes are a result of an artifact during tissue processing.
- Recent advanced techniques have shown that serous cells align with mucous cells to surround a common lumen.

Q. 8. Elaborate functions of saliva.

(2000, 2001, May 2009, Oct. 2002, Nov. 2010, Old course, IInd B.D.S.)

Ans. FUNCTIONS OF SALIVA

- Saliva is a complex fluid, produced by the salivary glands, the most important function of which is to maintain the well-being of the mouth.
- There are three pairs of major salivary glands, which are located extraorally. While minor salivary glands are located in almost all parts of oral cavity.

Functions

Protection is the main function of salivary gland while, the other functions are being assisting in digestion, speech, mastication, taste, and tissue repair.

1. **Protection of the oral cavity and oral environment:**
   - Constant secretion of saliva prevents dessication of the oral tissues.
   - It washes/flushes away debris and non-adherent bacteria.
   - Mucin and glycoproteins provide lubrication to the oral, oropharyngeal and esophageal tissues. The mucins also form a barrier against toxicologic stimuli, microbial toxins, and minor trauma.
   - Saliva protects mucosa from chemical and thermal insults.
   - It causes dilution of detritus and oral acid neutralization.
   - It maintains high pH, which is nonconducive for cariogenic bacteria to survive, ferment carbohydrate, and produce acid. Thus, preventing tooth decay.
   - It promotes remineralization of the tooth enamel. Remineralization of the initial carious lesions can be enhanced by fluoride ions in saliva.
   - **Antimicrobial property of saliva:**
     It contains many antimicrobial substances like lysozymes, lactoferrins calprotectin, lactoperoxidase, immunoglobulins, etc. High molecular weight glycoproteins of saliva aggregate microorganisms and facilitate their clearance.

Acinar cells and ductal system secrete thiocyanate which establishes bactericidal system. Saliva has antibacterial protein in it, lysozyme, which hydrolyzes the polysaccharide of bacterial cell walls resulting in cell lysis.

Predominant salivary immunoglobulin is IgA which inhibits adherence of microorganisms.

Saliva has antibacterial substance, lactoferrin, which enhances the inhibitory effect of the antibody on microorganisms.

Antifungal action of saliva is exerted by histatins, chromogranin A and immunoglobilins.

2. **Digestion:**
   - Saliva solubilizes food and taste substances through digestive enzyme, amylase.
   - Amylase acts on ingested carbohydrates to produce glucose and maltose.
   - Lingual lipase produced by lingual serous glands initiate digestion of dietary lipids.
3. **Mastication and deglutition:**
   - Saliva moistens food and breaks it down into smaller particles.
   - It helps in bolus formation and facilitates deglutition.
   - It moistens dry food and reduces temperature of hot foods.
4. **Taste perception:**
   - Food is emulsified in saliva and is dissolved which is a prerequisite for perception of taste.
   - This is due to the presence of water and lipocalins in saliva.
5. **Speech:**
   - Saliva keeps oral cavity moist and lubricated which facilitates speech and deglutition.
6. **Tissue repair:**
   - Growth factors and trefoil proteins in saliva promote tissue growth, differentiation, and wound healing.
7. **Excretion:**
   - Many substances from blood reach saliva, thus saliva can be considered as a route of excretion.
   - Due to this property, electrolytes and drug concentrations can be assessed in saliva.

Q. 9. Describe factors influencing the flow of saliva. *(May 2002)*

Ans. FACTORS AFFECTING THE FLOW OF SALIVA

Saliva is a complex fluid, produced by the salivary glands, the most important function of which is to maintain the well-being of the oral cavity.

Secretion of saliva depends on many factors.

1. Physiologic control of salivary gland secretion is mediated by ANS, particularly parasympathetic nervous system. Postganglionic fibers of both, sympathetic and parasympathetic divisions, innervate the secretory cells, myoepithelial cells, intercalated and striated duct cells. Release of neurotransmitter from the vesicle in the nerve terminals adjacent to parenchymal cells stimulates them to discharge their secretory granules, secrete water and electrolytes and cause contraction of myoepithelial cells. Secretion elicited in response to sympathetic stimulation differ in protein and electrolyte from that due to parasympathetic.

2. Blood vessels in the salivary glands are innervated. Vascular response elicited by the autonomic stimulation determines the availability of water, electrolytes and metabolic substances during secretory activity.
3. Control of secretion is also linked to changing taste and smell. Secretion of saliva can alter from 0.1 ml/min at rest to 4.0 ml/mm at actively stimulated times.
4. Secretion of saliva also depends on age, duration and nature of stimulus. Secretion of saliva is minimum at birth and does not contain salivary amylase. In old age the secretory reserve becomes decreased.
5. Proportion of the components of saliva depends on the sources of saliva, the nature and the intensity of the secreting stimulus and the time of the day.
6. Saliva produced by major salivary gland differ from others. Parotid gland secretes a watery saliva rich in enzymes while submandibular gland has higher proportion of glycosylated substances such as mucin.
7. Other factors affecting the composition of saliva are flow rate, differential gland contribution, circardian rhythm, duration of stimulus, nature of stimulus and diet.

Each of these factors is capable of modifying the amount and consistency of the salivary secretion. Gustatory stimulus is more important than masticatory stimulus for salivary secretion.

Q. 11. Write about composition of saliva.

Ans. **COMPOSITION OF SALIVA**

- Most important function of the salivary gland is the production and secretion of saliva. Protection of the oral cavity is the major function of saliva, though it also serves other function such as digestion, speech, mastication, taste, and tissue repair.
- Saliva consists of 99% water. Iorganic ions, secretory glycoproteins of serum constituents and other substances account for 1% or less (Flowchart 21.1).

Flowchart 21.1

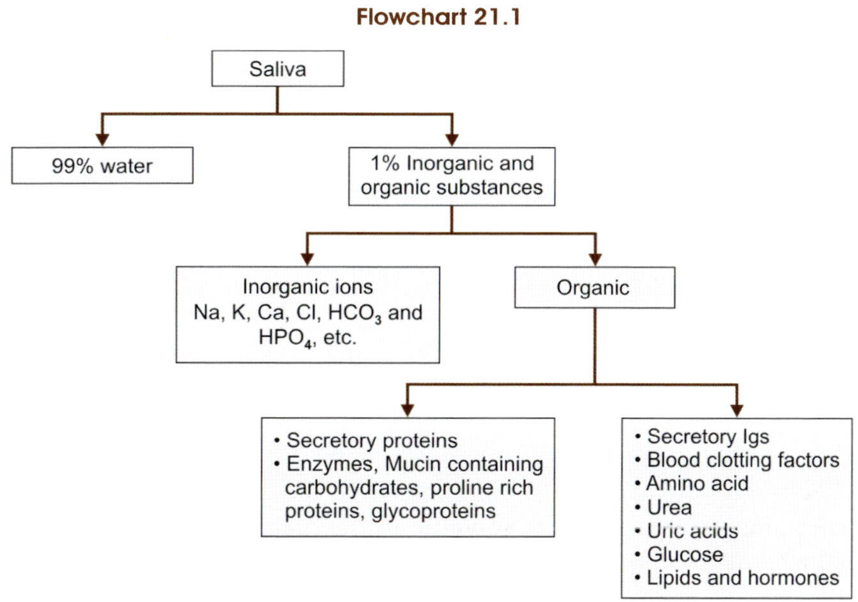

- Main electrolytes of saliva are Na, K, Ca, Cl, HCO_3^- and HPO_4^-. Other electrolytes are Mg, SO_4^-, F, SCN and I.
- Main organic substances found in saliva are secretory proteins. These include enzymes such as amylase, ribonuclease, kallikrein, peroxidase, lysozymes, lactoferrin and acid phosphatase. Mucin containing large amount of bound carbohydrates, proline rich proteins and glycoproteins are also present.
- Other organic constituents of saliva include secretory immunoglobulins like IgG and IgM, blood clotting factors, amino acids, urea, uric acid, glucose, various lipids and hormones.
- Saliva produced by secretory end pieces and intercalated duct is primary saliva. It is isotonic containing most of the organic components and all of water secreted by the salivary glands. The primary saliva is modified as it passes through the striated and excretory ducts, mainly by reabsorption and secretion of electrolytes.
- Proportion of the components of saliva are variable depending upon the source of saliva, the nature and intensity of the secretory stimulus and the time of the day.

Whole Saliva (Mixed Saliva)

- It is the secretion of all the minor and major salivary glands. In addition to the components derived by the gland, the whole saliva also contains desquamated oral epithelial cells.
- Total volume of saliva is 750-1000 ml/day of which submandibular accounts for 60%, parotid for 30% and sublingual about 5% and 1% is desired from minor salivary glands.
- Saliva produced by parotid gland is watery and is rich in enzymes such as amylase, proteins and glycoproteins. Secretion by submandibular gland contains higher proportion of mucin. Sublingual gland produces viscous saliva rich in mucin.
- Resting flow rate of whole saliva is 0.2 to 0.4 ml/min.
- pH of whole saliva is 6.4 to 7.4.

Clinical Significance

1. In elderly individuals, parenchyma of salivary glands is replaced by fatty tissue resulting in its decreased secretory activity.
2. *Xerostomia*: It is loss of salivary function or reduction in volume of saliva. It is due to various reasons like Sjögren's syndrome, chemotherapy, radiation therapy or as a result of variety of medications. Decreased salivary secretion leads to caries, mucosal ulceration and oral infection.
3. *Ptyalism or sialorrhea*: Excessive salivary secretion.
4. Salivary glands are affected by many pathologic conditions like viral, bacterial, or allergic sialdenitis, benign and malignant tumors, autoimmune diseases and genetic diseases.
5. *Mucocele*: It is a lesion produced by severance of the duct of a minor salivary gland and pooling of the saliva in the tissues.
6. Salivary gland and sialochemistry is of value in the diagnosis of glandular and systemic diseases. Sialochemistry is also used to monitor plasma concentration of certain therapeutic drugs.

Q. 12. Write about anticaries property of saliva. *(July 2005)*
or
Write about antimicrobial property of saliva. *(Oct. 2002, Dec. 2005)*

Ans. ANTICARIES PROPERTY OF SALIVA

Protection of the oral cavity is the major function of saliva. It has anticaries property.

- It flushes away debris and nonadherent bacteria.
- Saliva is supersaturated with calcium and phosphate ions. The solubility of these ions is maintained by calcium binding proteins, i.e. acidic proline rich proteins and statherin. At the tooth surface, the high concentraction of calcium and phosphate results in a posteruptive maturation of the enamel, increasing its surface hardness and resistance to demineralization.
- Remineralization of initial carious lesion is enhanced by the presence of fluoride ions in saliva.
- Saliva helps in maintaining a high pH. Primary buffering system of saliva is formed by bicarbonates, phosphate ions and salivary proteins. This high pH prevents survival of cariogenic bacteria, fermentation of carbohydrates and acid production, thus preventing tooth decay.
- Anticaries activity of saliva is also due to its antimicrobial action. In addition to the barrier effect provided by mucins, saliva contains many antibacterial substances like lysozymes, lactoferrins, calprotectin, lactoperoxidose, immunoglobulins, etc. The major salivary immunoglobulin, secretory IgA, causes agglutination of specific microorganisms preventing their adherence to oral tissue.

Q. 13. Enumerate differences among major salivary glands.

Ans. DIFFERENCES AMONG MAJOR SALIVARY GLANDS

Sr. No.	*Characteristic features*	*Parotid*	*Submandibular*	*Sublingual*
1.	Type of gland	Purely serous	Mixed, predominantly serous	Mixed, predominantly mucous
2.	Secretion	Serous (watery)	Seromucous	Mucous (thick and viscous)
3.	Contribution to saliva	25%	70%	Minimum
4.	Excretory duct	Stenson's duct, opens at buccal mucosa opposite to maxillary 2nd molar	Wharton's duct, opens at sublingual papillae lateral to lingual frenum	• Bartholin's duct, opens near submandibular gland duct. • Ducts of Rivinus, open in the floor of the mouth
5.	Nerve supply	Presynaptic-glosso-pharyngeal post-synaptic-auriculote-mporal nerve	Facial nerve-chorda tympani	Facial-chorda tympani
6.	Blood supply	External caroid artery	Lingual/facial artery	Sublingual/submental arteries
7.	Lymphatic drainage	Paraparotid/intraparo-tid nodes which drain to deep cervical nodes	Deep cervical, jugular nodes.	Submandibular lymph-nodes
8.	Function	Enzymatic activity is more. Amylase activity is maximum	• Serves mainly for lubrication and pro-tection of tissues • Lysozymeactivity is also seen.	• Serves for lubrication and protection of oral tissues

Q. 14. Enumerate differences between major and minor salivary glands.

Ans. DIFFERENCES BETWEEN MAJOR AND MINOR SALIVARY GLANDS

Sr. No.	*Characteristic features*	*Major salivary glands*	*Minor salivary glands*
1.	Number	3, parotid, submandibular, and Sublingual	600–1000
2.	Location	Extraoral	**Intraoral:** Labial and buccal glossopalatine, palatine, lingual and von Ebner's glands. Minor salivary glands are not present in gingiva, anterior raphe of hard palate and anterior two-thirds of the dorsum of the tongue.
3.	Contribution to whole saliva	90–95%	5–10%
4.	Excretory duct	Single, long	Multiple, short
5.	Type of secretion	• Thin, watery • Mostly mixed except parotid which is purely serous	• Thick, mucous • Mucous or mixed except von Ebner's gland which is serous
6.	Function	• Rich in enzymes, mucous and proteins • Therefore, helps in digestion, lubrication and protection	• Rich in proteins • Has important role in innate immunity

MULTIPLE CHOICE QUESTIONS (MCQs)

1. The largest salivary gland, situated in front of the ear, weighing 14ñ28 g, is
a. Submandibular
b. Sublingual
c. Parotid
d. None of the above

2. The main excretory duct of the parotid gland is
a. Wharton's duct
b. Stenson's duct
c. Bartholin's duct
d. Thyroglossal duct

3. All the minor salivary glands are mucous glands except
a. Labial b. Palatine
c. Von Ebner d. Buccal

4. The smallest of the three paired major salivary glands is
a. Parotid
b. Submandibular
c. Sublingual
d. None of the above

5. Total volume of saliva secreted daily by humans is
a. 300–500 ml b. 500–750 ml
c. 750–1000 ml d. 1000–2000 ml

6. About 60% of total saliva is secreted by
a. Parotid salivary gland
b. Submandibular
c. Sublingual
d. Minor salivary gland

7. The proportion of water to other constituents in the saliva is
a. 50% H_2O: 50% inorganic + organic substance
b. 85% H_2O: 15% inorganic + organic substance
c. 90% H_2O: 10% inorganic + organic substances
d. 99% H_2O: 1% inorganic + organic substance

8. The pH of whole saliva varies from
a. 6.8–7.8
b. 6.7 to about 7.4
c. 6.5 to 7.5
d. 6.4–7.0

9. Minor salivary glands are seen everywhere in the oral cavity except
a. Anterior part of hard palate and gingiva
b. Tongue
c. Soft palate
d. Buccal mucosa

10. Serous cells primarily secrete
a. Mucus b. Amylase
c. Lipids d. Sialic acid

11. The function of the myoepithelial cells which are found around acini is
a. Secreting mucus
b. Secreting amylase
c. Releasing secretory material from the acinor cells
d. Secreting lipids

12. The substance produced by the connective tissue of salivary gland, having bactericidal property is
a. Peroxidase b. Lysozyme
c. IgA d. Amylase

13. Blandin and Nuhn glands are
a. Anterior lingual minor salivary gland
b. Posterior lingual minor salivary gland
c. Purely mucous glossopalatine
d. Purely mucous palatine glands

14. Reduction of salivary flow is seen in following conditions
a. Sicca syndrome or Sjögren's syndrome
b. After irradiation of head and neck region
c. Because of use of certain therapeutic drugs
d. All of the above

1-c, 2-b, 3-c, 4-c, 5-c, 6-b, 7-d, 8-b, 9-a, 10-b, 11-c, 12-c, 13-a, 14-d

15. Sialochemistry (quantity and composition) of saliva is of value in the diagnosis of
a. Glandular or systemic diseases
b. Monitoring of plasma concentration of drugs
c. To determine ovulation time
d. All of the above

16. Sialography is useful in the diagnosis of
a. Tumors
b. Sjögren's syndrome
c. Salivary calculi
d. All

17. Mucoceles may be found throughout the oral cavity wherever minor salivary glands are present, but most common on the
a. Soft palate
b. Tongue
c. Lower lip
d. Upper lip

18. Salivary duct stones are more common in
a. Stenson's duct
b. Wharton's duct
c. Bartholin's duct
d. All of the above

19. The salivary glands that produce only a serous secretion are the
a. Parotid glands
b. Minor salivary glands on the floor of the mouth
c. Submandibular glands
d. Sublingual gland

20. The average specific gravity of saliva is
a. 1.001 b. 1.003
c. 1.010 d. 1.012

21. The secretion from submandibular salivary gland is
a. Serous only
b. Mucous only
c. Predominantly mucous
d. Predominantly serous

22. The principal immunoglobulin found in the saliva is
a. IgA b. IgM
c. IgG d. All of the above

23. Parotid gland is a
a. Pure serous gland
b. Mucous gland
c. Mixed gland
d. Predominantly serous gland

24. Submandibular and sublingual both are
a. Mucous b. Serous
c. Mixed d. Predominantly mucous

25. Carancula sublingualis is the opening of
a. Wharton's duct
b. Stenson's duct
c. Bartholin's duct
d. None of the above

26. The Stensen's duct opens into the oral cavity
a. On the floor of the mouth
b. Near the lower lip
c. Opposite the maxillary second molar
d. None of the above

27. The Wharton's duct opens
a. Opposite maxillary second molar
b. Near the mandibular second molar
c. At the carancula sublingualis
d. None

28. Basket cell is a
a. Mucous cell
b. Serous cell
c. Myoepithelial cell
d. None

29. Demilunes that are found in mixed salivary gland are
a. Serous cells capped by crescents of mucous cells
b. Mucous cells capped by crescents of serous cells
c. Both
d. None

15-a, 16-d, 17-c, 18-b, 19-a, 20-b, 21-d, 22-a, 23-a, 24-c, 25-a, 26-c, 27-c, 28-c, 29-b

30. The shape of the basket cell is

a. Cuboidal b. Columnar
c. Stellate d. Squamous

31. Pure mucous glands are

a. Labial and buccal gland
b. Glossopalatine gland
c. Sublingual gland
d. Lingual gland

32. Total number of minor salivary glands in oral cavity are

a. 1000 b. 500
c. 100 d. 800

33. Salivation is controlled by

a. Hormonal system
b. Neural system
c. Both
d. None of the above

34. Serous crescent is also known as

a. Crescent of Giannuzzi
b. Demilune of Heidenhain
c. Both of the above
d. None of the above

35. Salivary glands are derived from

a. Mesoderm b. Ectoderm
c. Endoderm d. Both b and c

36. Saliva contains

a. 99% water b. 80% water
c. 70% water d. 60% water

37. The three bilaterally paired major salivary glands are located

a. Extraorally
b. Intraorally
c. In tongue
d. In neck

38. Human parotid gland produces a hormone which is known as

a. Serotonin
b. Parotin
c. Prohormone
d. None of the above

39. The enzyme which plays major role in starch digestion is

a. Amylase
b. Maltase
c. Lactase
d. All of the above

40. Which of the following are purely serous in nature

a. von Ebner and parotid
b. Sublingual and submandibular
c. Submandibular and von Ebner
d. Sublingual and von Ebner

41. Salivary glands arise from

a. Hypobranchial eminence
b. Oral mesenchyme
c. Oral epithelium
d. Dental lamina

42. The structure of salivary gland may be described as

a. Mixed or compound tubuloalveolar
b. Simple tubuloalveolar
c. Compound acinar
d. Simple tubular

43. Most viscous saliva is present in

a. Parotid salivary gland
b. Sublingual salivary gland
c. Submandibular salivary gland
d. Minor salivary gland

44. Circumvallate papillae contain a minor salivary gland in its trough called

a. Blandin and Nuhn
b. Zuckerkandl
c. Stenson's
d. von Ebner

45. Saliva contains one of the following digestive enzymes

a. Peptin
b. Amylase
c. Lysozome
d. Insulin

30-c, 31-b, 32-b, 33-b, 34-c, 35-d, 36-a, 37-a, 38-b, 39-a, 40-a, 41-c, 42-d, 43-c, 44-d, 45-b

46. Primordia of submandibular and parotid salivary glands appear during
a. 6th week of foetal life
b. 7th week of foetal life
c. 8th week of foetal life
d. 9th week of foetal life

47. Parasympathetic ganglion associated with parotid salivary gland is
a. Otic b. Geniculate
c. Submandibular d. Trigeminal

48. Zymogen granules are seen commonly in
a. Serous cell
b. Mucous cell
c. Myoepithelial cell
d. All of the above

49. Neutralization of saliva is due to
a. Mucin
b. Ammonia
c. Aminoacids
d. Bicarbonates

50. Striations seen in striated duct are due to
a. Basal cell membrane infoldings
b. Lysosomes
c. Mitochondria
d. Both a and c

51. Lingual lipase enzyme is secreted by the
a. Parotid gland
b. Submandibular salivary gland
c. Parotid and von Ebner's salivary glands
d. None of the above

52. Antifungal property is present in
a. Peroxidase
b. Mucins
c. Lactoferrin
d. Histatin

46-a, 47-a, 48-a, 49-d, 50-d, 51-c, 52-d

Chapter 22

Tooth Eruption

LAQs (10 Marks)

Q. 1. Define eruption and explain physiologic tooth movement.

or

What are the various patterns of tooth movement?

Ans. Introduction

- **Eruption** is the axial or occlusal movement of the tooth from its developmental position within the jaw to its functional position in the occlusal plane.

  It is a part of total pattern of physiologic tooth movement. Physiologic tooth movement is required to bring the teeth into occlusal plane, to maintain their position in the growing jaws and to compensate for masticatory wear.
- **Physiologic tooth movement** is described as consisting of :
  - I. Preeruptive tooth movement
  - II. Eruptive tooth movement
  - III. Posteruptive tooth movement

I. Preeruptive Tooth Movement

- These are the movements made by both deciduous and permanent tooth germs within the jaws before they begin to erupt.
  These movements position the tooth and its crypts within the growing jaws at the correct position for eruption.
- Preeruptive movements occur due to bodily movement of the tooth germ and its eccentric growth. Tooth germ is present in bony crypt. Bodily movement of tooth germ results from resorption of the bony crypt on one side and deposition on other side.
- In eccentic growth, base of the tooth germ is fixed while rest of it continues to grow causing a shift in the centre of the tooth germ. Eccentric growth of tooth germ exerts pressure which results in resorption of bone on the required side and movement of the tooth germ.

Pattern of preeruptive tooth movement

- When deciduous tooth germs first differentiate they are very small and space is present between them. This space is used because of the rapid growth of the tooth germs and crowding results.

- This crowding is relieved by the growth of jaws. This permits drifting of anterior tooth germs forward and posterior tooth germs backwards which involves bodily movement of these tooth germs.
- *Anterior region*: Initially, permanent teeth are lingually placed to their predecessors in the same bony crypt. As the jaws increase in size and primary teeth erupt, permanent tooth germs move and occupy lingual and apical position to the roots of primary teeth.
- *Posterior region*: Premolar tooth germs move and reside between the roots of primary molars.
  - Permanent molar tooth germs move distally and occupy their position within the jaws.
  - Initially due to lack of space, the occlusal surface of maxillary molar is positioned distally and the mandibular molar is positioned mesially. This gets corrected as jaws further grow in size.

Histology of preeruptive tooth movement

- It involves drifting or growth of the tooth germs.
- It requires remodeling of the bony wall of the crypt.
- Deposition and removal of bone results from osteoblastic and osteoclastic activity.
- Skeletal morphogenesis is also involved in determining the tooth position before eruption.

II. Eruptive Tooth Movement (Prefunctional Eruptive Movement)

Eruption is the axial or occlusal movement of the tooth from its developmental position within the jaws to its functional position in occlusion.

Direction or pattern of movement

Axial or occlusal is the principal direction of movement in eruption. But movement other than axial is superimposed on eruptive movement.

Histology of eruptive movement

- Significant developmental events occur along with eruptive tooth movement which bring the tooth into the oral cavity.
- This includes formation of roots, formation and organization of periodontal ligament and remodeling of bone.

Mechanism of tooth movement

- Mechanism that brings about tooth movement is likely to be a combination of a number of factors.
- Theories which have been put forth to explain this process of eruption are:
  1. Root formation theory
  2. Bone remodeling theory
  3. Vascular pressure theory
  4. Periodontal ligament traction theory

1. Root formation theory:

- This theory proposes that the eruptive tooth movement in axial or occlusal direction is mainly because of the formation of root.
- According to this theory, the growth of root impinges upon a sling of connective tissue, cushion-hammock ligament to produce the necessary thrust for tooth eruption.

- *But, root formation is unlikely to be the cause of tooth eruption because*:
  It is found that some teeth move a greater distance than the length of their fully formed roots.
  Eruptive tooth movement can occur even after the root formation is complete.
  In certain developmental disturbances, rootless teeth erupt into oral cavity.
  Teeth with completely formed roots and impacted teeth do not erupt.
  Onset of root formation is not synchronous with the onset of axial tooth movement.
  If it has to be believed that the root formation results in an eruptive force, then the apical growth of the root needs to be translated into occlusal movement for which a fixed base is required. But, no such fixed base exists. The bone at the base of the socket cannot act as a fixed base because pressure on bone results in its resorption.
  Advocates of the root growth theory, proposed that there exists a ligament, the **cushion-hammock ligament** at the base of the socket which provides a fixed base against which the growing root can react. But, this ligament was found to be a pulp delineating membrane and cannot act as a fixed base.
- These facts indicate that root formation cannot be responsible for eruptive tooth movement. It could be a prerequisite for eruption.

2. **Bone remodeling theory:**
   - According to this theory, resorption of the bone at the site of pressure and deposition of bone at the site of tension may cause eruption.
   - Bone remodeling is important to permit tooth movement during eruption.
   - However, bone remodeling that occurs around the teeth, causes or is the effect of tooth movement is not clear.
   - Through experiments it was found that dental follicle is an absolute requirement to achieve bone remodeling and tooth eruption.
3. **Vascular pressure theory:**
   - According to this theory, local volume changes in arteries can produce tooth movement.
   - It was found that increase of hydrostatic pressure induced by hypotensive drugs, increases the rate of eruption.
   - Though vascular pressure can play an important role by generating an eruptive force, whether these pressures are primarily responsible for eruption is not proved.
4. **Periodontal ligament traction theory:**
   - Evidence through experiments has suggested that the eruptive force resides in the **dental follicle-periodontal ligament complex.**
   - This theory states that the fibroblasts of the dental follicle by their contraction can generate a force which can pull the teeth into occlusion. The fibroblasts have their processes attached to the collagen fibers by a sticky protein called **fibronectin** and as their processes are in contact with each other, it produces a summative force. This force is transmitted to the extracellular compartment via fibronexus and to collagen fiber bundles.
   - These collagen fiber bundles are inclined at an angle to bring about tooth movement resulting in eruption of tooth.
   - The dental follicle plays an important role in tooth eruption. It produces factors for promoting osteoclastic bone resorption in the coronal part and by promoting bone formation in the apical part.

- It was found that when the tooth germ is removed experimentally and the dental follicle is left intact, an eruptive pathway forms in the overlying bone.
- If silicon replica is substituted for the tooth germ, it also erupts.
- Abnormalities of dental follicle as seen in certain diseases are associated with delayed permanent teeth eruption.
- Drugs that interrupt the proper formation of collagen in the ligament also interfere with eruption.
- All these experiments show that as long as dental follicle or developing periodontal ligament exist tooth eruption can occur.
- It is said that eruptive movement is multifactorial like vascular pressure at the apex along with contractile force generated by the dental follicle playing an important part and bone formation and resorption facilitating the process.

III. Posteruptive tooth movement

Functional eruptive movement

- Posteruptive tooth movements are those that maintain the position of the erupted tooth, while the jaw continues to grow. This movement occurs in an axial direction to keep pace with the increase in height of the jaws.
- *This movement compensates for occlusal and proximal wear:*
  - Occlusal and proximal wear of teeth occurs after the teeth have erupted in the oral cavity.
  - To compensate for occlusal wear the same mechanism responsible for moving the tooth axially during eruption, is most likely to be used.
  - The movement which compensates for the proximal wear of teeth and maintain their position, consists of mesial migration of teeth called as **physiologic mesial drift.**
  - Mesial or proximal drift involves a combination of two separate forces resulting from occlusal contact of teeth and contraction of transseptal ligaments between teeth.
  - *Forces causing mesial drift are multifactorial and include*:

    a. Occlusal force.

    b. Contraction of the transseptal ligament between teeth.

    Mesial drift is achieved by contraction of transseptal fibers and enhanced by occlusal forces.

    a. *Occlusal force*:

    When teeth are brought into contact (*e.g.* in clenching of the jaws), force is generated in a mesial direction because of summation of cuspal planes and because many teeth have a mesial inclination. An anterior component of this occlusal force is responsible for mesial drift.

    b. *Contraction of transseptal fibers*:

    Periodontal ligament plays an important role in maintaining tooth position.

    Transseptal ligament fibers running between teeth across the alveolar process, draw neighboring teeth together and maintain them in contact.
- Thus, physiologic mesial drift helps to compensate for proximal wear.

Q. 2. Prepare a table exhibiting normal eruption age and sequence of all deciduous and permanent teeth. *(2005, Nov. 2009)*

Ans. Eruption is the axial or occlusal movement of the tooth from its developmental position within the jaw to its functional position in the occlusal plane.

- Timely initiation and eruption of teeth into oral cavity is important for healthy dentition.
- Human beings have two sets of dentition where deciduous dentition is replaced by permanent dentition due to increase in the size of jaws and increasing masticatory forces.
- Deciduous teeth eruption starts at the age of 6–7 months of life.
- Sequence of eruption of deciduous teeth is

AB	D	C	E
A	B	D	CE

Age of eruption of deciduous teeth

Teeth	*Maxillary*	*Mandibular*
Central incisors	7 months	6 months
Lateral incisors	9 months	7 months
First molars	14 months	12 months
Canines	18 months	16 months
Second molars	24 months	20 months

Sequence of eruption of permanent dentition

6	1	2	4	5	3	7	8
6	1	2	3	4	5	7	8

Age of eruption of permanent dentition

Teeth	*Maxillary*	*Mandibular*
First molars	6–7 years of age	6–7 years of age
Central incisors	7–8 years	6–7 years
Lateral incisors	8–9 years	7–8 years
First premolars	10–12 years	10–11 years
Canine	11–12 years	9–10 years
Second premolar	10–12 years	11–12 years
Second molar	12–13 years	11–13 years
Third molar	17–21 years	17–21 years

Q. 3. Write about gubernacular cord.

Ans. GUBERNACULAR CORD

- Eruption is the axial or occlusal movement of the tooth from its developmental position within the jaw to its functional position in the occlusal plane.
- Significant histologic changes occur in the tissue overlying the erupting tooth.
- Bone removal is necessary for permanent teeth to erupt.

- In case of those teeth with deciduous predecessors, there is an additional anatomic feature, the *gubernacular canal* and its contents, the *gubernacular cord.*
- When the successional tooth germ first develops within the same crypt as its deciduous predecessor, bone surrounds both tooth germs but does not completely close over them.
- As the deciduous tooth erupts, the permanent tooth germ becomes situated apically and is entirely enclosed by bone except for a small canal, *gubernacular canal.*
- This canal is filled with connective tissue and often contains epithelial remnants of the dental lamina. This connective tissue mass is termed as *gubernacular cord.*
- Thus, the dental follicle that surrounds the succedaneous tooth germ is connected to the lamina propria of the oral mucous membrane by the gubernacular cord. This may have an influence on eruptive tooth movement.
- The cord of tissue is believed to be the remnant of the dental lamina.

Functions

- It may have function in guiding the permanent tooth as it erupts.
- As the permanent tooth starts erupting through the gubernacular canal, local osteoclastic activity is seen around the canal to widen it so that the tooth erupts into the oral cavity.

SAQs (3 Marks)

Q. 1. Define eruption. Decribe any two theories. *(Oct. 2004)*

or

Enumerate various theories of eruption of tooth and explain the most accepted theory of tooth eruption. *(May 2009)*

Enumerate theories of eruption, describe periodontal ligament traction theory.

or *(June 2006)*

Define eruptive tooth movement and enumerate various theories. *(Dec. 2000)*

or

Describe eruptive tooth movement or describe prefunctional eruptive movement.

Ans. Eruption is the axial or occlusal movement of the tooth from its developmental position within the jaws to its functional position in occlusion.

Direction or Pattern of Movement

Axial or occlusal is the principal direction of movement in eruption. But, movement other than axial movement is superimposed on eruptive movement.

Histology of Eruptive Movement

- Significant developmental events occur along with eruptive tooth movement which brings the tooth into the oral cavity.
- This includes formation of roots, formation and organization of periodontal ligament and remodeling of bone.

Mechanism of Tooth Movement

- Mechanism that brings about tooth movement is likely to be a combination of a number of factors.

- Theories which have been put forth to explain this process of eruption are :
  1. Root formation theory
  2. Bone remodeling theory
  3. Vascular pressure theory
  4. Periodontal ligament traction theory.
- Explain various theories of tooth eruption as described in answer of LAQ 1.

Q. 2. What is physiologic mesial drift? *(May 2008)*

or

Describe posteuptive movement.

or

Describe functional eruptive movement.

Ans. POSTERUPTIVE TOOTH MOVEMENT

Functional Eruptive Movement

- Posteruptive tooth movements are those that maintain the position of the erupted tooth while the jaw continues to grow. This movement is like eruptive movement which occurs in an axial direction to keep pace with the increase in height of the jaws. Physiologic mesial drift is a part of posteruptive tooth movement.
- Posteruptive tooth movement also compensates for occlusal and proximal wear :
  - Occlusal and proximal wear of teeth occurs after the teeth have erupted in the oral cavity.
  - To compensate for occlusal wear the same mechanism responsible for moving the tooth axially during eruption, is most likely to be used.
  - The movement which compensates for the proximal wear of teeth and maintain their position consists of mesial migration of teeth and is called as **physiologic mesial drift.**
  - Mesial or proximal drift involves a combination of two separate forces resulting from occlusal contact of teeth and contraction of transseptal ligament between teeth.
  - Forces causing mesial drift are multifactorial and include:
    a. Occlusal force.
    b. Contraction of the transseptal ligament between teeth.
- Physiologic mesial drift is achieved by contraction of transseptal fibers and enhanced by occlusal forces.

  a. ***Occlusal force*:**
  When teeth are brought into contact (*e.g.* in clenching of the jaws), force is generated in a mesial direction because of summation of cuspal planes and because many teeth have a mesial inclination. An anterior component of this occlusal force is responsible for mesial drift.

  b. ***The contraction of transseptal fibres*:**
  Periodontal ligament plays an important role in maintaining tooth position.
  Transseptal ligament fibers running between teeth across the alveolar process draw neighboring teeth together and maintain them in contact.
- Physiologic mesial drift helps to compensate for proximal wear.
- Histologically mesial drift is seen as a selective deposition and resorption of bone on the socket walls by osteoblasts and osteoclasts respectively and by collagen remodeling in the periodontal and transseptal ligament.

Chapter

23

Shedding of Deciduous Teeth

SAQs (3 Marks)

Q. 1. Describe mechanism of resorption and shedding. *(Oct. 2004)*

Describe process of shedding. Describe process of shedding of deciduous teeth. *(June 2006)*

Ans. Introduction

The physiologic process resulting in elimination of deciduous dentition is called **exfoliation** or **shedding.**

Shedding is the result of progressive resorption of the roots of teeth and their supporting tissue, periodontal ligament (PDL).

Factors Responsible for Resorption

- Pressure from erupting tooth.
- Forces of mastication applied on deciduous teeth.
  - Increasing masticatory forces in growing individual exert forces on deciduous tooth greater than its PDL can withstand. This results in trauma to PDL and initiation of resorption.
  - As there is resorption of roots, there is progressive loss of surface area for attachment of PDL. This weakening of tooth support results in exfoliation.

Mechanism and Histology of Shedding

- Shedding is a physiological process by which deciduous teeth roots and parts of crown undergo resorption by multinucleated giant cells called **odontoclasts.**

  It involves:

  a. Resorption of dental hard tissues.

  b. Resorption of soft tissues.

  a. Resorption of dental hard tissues:

  - Odontoclasts (dentinoclast) are multinucleated giant cells responsible for removal of dental hard tissues.

- Pressure from erupting successional tooth plays a key role in resorption.
- Odontoclasts appear at sites of pressure.
- These cells occupy resorption bays on the surface of dental hard tissue to be resorbed.
- Its surface near the hard tissue forms a ruffled border.
- Peripheral to the ruffled border, is a clear or a sealing zone in which the cytoplasm is devoid of organelles but rich in contractile proteins, actin and myosin.
- Sealing zone helps in attaching the odontoclast to the hard tissue surface, thereby creating a sealed space in which odontoblasts pump hydrogen ions.
- This results in fall in pH and therefore dissolution of minerals. Thus, dental hard tissue is degraded.
- Primary lysosomes of odontoclasts secrete their enzymatic contents to degrade the organic matrix.

b. Resorption of dental soft tissues:

- Apoptotic cell death (programmed cell death) is involved in resorption of dental soft tissues, the pulp and the PDL.

Clinical Considerations

- *Remnants of deciduous teeth*: Sometimes parts of the roots of deciduous tooth may escape resorption and its remnants remain embedded in the jaw, more frequently with mandibular second molars.
- *Overretained deciduous teeth*: More often deciduous maxillary lateral incisors, less frequently mandibular second molars and rarely mandibular central incisor are retained for a long-time beyond their usual shedding schedule. Frequently, upper permanent canine is embedded and therefore, deciduous canine remains overretained.
- *Submerged teeth*: Trauma to deciduous tooth results in ankylosis. These ankylosed deciduous teeth cannot continue to erupt like adjacent teeth. Hence, they lie below occlusal plane and are referred to as submerged teeth. Submerged deciduous teeth should be removed as they can prevent eruption of their permanent successors or force them from their position.

Q. 2. Write differences in resorption of single rooted and multirooted teeth.

Ans. The physiologic process resulting in elimination of deciduous dentition is called **exfoliation** or **shedding.**

Exfoliation of Single Rooted Tooth

- Because of the developmental position of the permanent incisors and canine tooth germs and their subsequent movement in an occlusal and vestibular direction, resorption of the roots of the deciduous incisors and canine begins on their lingual surfaces. Later these permanent teeth occupy a position directly apical to the deciduous tooth and they erupt in the position of their deciduous predecessors.
- However, the apical positioning of the tooth germs of the permanent mandibular incisors may not occur and they frequently erupt lingual to the still functioning deciduous teeth.
- Single rooted teeth are usually shed before root resorption is complete.

Exfoliation of Multirooted Teeth

- Resorption of the roots of deciduous molars begins on their inner surface because the early developing bicuspids are formed between them. Resorption of the roots of deciduous molars occurs long before they are shed due to the expansion of their growing permanent successors.

- In multirooted teeth, the roots are usually completely resorbed and the crown is also partially resorbed before exfoliation.

Q. 3. What are overretained deciduous teeth?

Ans. Introduction

These are the deciduous teeth which are retained for a long-time beyond their usual shedding schedule.

- These teeth are invariably out of function.
- Upper lateral incisors are the most commonly overretained deciduous teeth. Less frequently mandibular second molar and rarely the lower central incisor are overretained.

Etiology

- Either there is no permanent successor or the permanent successor is impacted.
- Ankylosed or impacted permanent teeth. This is seen most commonly with deciduous and permanent canine.
- Presence of supernumerary tooth or an odontogenic tumor may prevent eruption of permanent teeth. In such cases, ankylosis of the deciduous tooth may occur.

Clinical Significance

Overretained deciduous tooth can affect function and esthetics.

Q. 4. What are submerged deciduous teeth?

Ans. SUBMERGED DECIDUOUS TEETH

- Trauma can result in damage to either the dental follicle or periodontal ligament. This prevents eruption of the tooth and it becomes ankylosed to the bone of the jaw.
- Due to the continuous eruption of the adjacent teeth and increased height of alveolar bone, the ankylosed tooth remains submerged in the alveolar bone.
- Submerged deciduous tooth prevents the eruption of its permanent successor or force it to erupt in an abnormal position.
- Such submerged deciduous teeth should be extracted.

Q. 5. Explain shedding of deciduous 2nd mandibular molar. *(May 2008)*

Ans. Introduction

- The physiologic process resulting in the elimination of the deciduous dentition is called **shedding** or **exfoliation.**
- Decidous teeth exfoliate because a second dentition consisting of larger and more teeth is required for the larger jaws of the adult.
- Shedding involves progressive resorption of the roots of teeth and their supporting tissue, periodontal ligament.
- There is difference in shedding of single rooted and multirooted teeth.
- Resorption of roots of mandibular deciduous second molars begin on the inner surface because the early developing bicuspids are formed between them.
- Its resorption occurs long before the deciduous molar is shed due to expansion of their growing permanent successor, second premolar.

- In molars, the roots are completely resorbed and the crown is also partially resorbed before exfoliation.
- Shedding involves resorption of dental hard tissues by odontoclasts and resorption of soft tissues.
- Remnants of mandibular deciduous second molar are frequently found embedded in the jaw. The reason is that the roots of the lower second deciduous molar are strongly curved or divergent. The mesiodistal diameter of the second premolar is much smaller than the greatest distance between the roots of the deciduous molar.

MULTIPLE CHOICE QUESTIONS (MCQs)

1. **Early in the preeruptive phase, the successional permanent teeth develop**
   a. Labial to and near the apical level of their primary predecessors
   b. Lingual to and near the incisal or occlusal level of their primary predecessors
   c. Both are correct
   d. Both are incorrect

2. **At the end of the preeruptive phase the successional permanent teeth develop lingual to deciduous teeth at**
   a. Incisal or occlusal level
   b. Middle third level
   c. Apical third level
   d. Occlusal level

3. **The change in the position of the permanent tooth germ is due to**
   a. Apical movement of permanent tooth germ
   b. Eruption of primary teeth
   c. Increase in height of supporting tissues
   d. Both b and c

4. **The tooth moves more rapidly in the socket during**
   a. Preeruptive phase
   b. Prefunctional phase
   c. Posteruptive phase
   d. Postfunctional phase

5. **The permanent teeth which have no deciduous predecessors are**
   a. Mandibular and maxillary second premolars
   b. Mandibular and maxillary first premolars
   c. Mandibular and maxillary molars
   d. Maxillary and mandibular canines

6. **The resorption of deciduous molars initially takes place on**
   a. Inner surface of the root below furcation
   b. At the apex of the root
   c. Outer surface of the root at the cervical level
   d. Outer surface of the root below furcation

7. **The permanent incisors develop**
   a. Labial to the roots of deciduous teeth
   b. Lingual to the roots of deciduous teeth
   c. Mesial/distal to the deciduous roots
   d. Below the apices of deciduous roots

8. **An anatomic feature having influence on eruptive tooth movement of successional teeth is**
   a. Enamel cord
   b. Gubernacular cord
   c. Epithelial cord
   d. Enamel knot

9. **The remarkable property of the principal supporting tissues of the tooth (PDL and bone) is**
   a. Elasticity
   b. Plasticity
   c. Stretchability
   d. Resiliency

10. **The mesial drift is achieved by**
   a. Oblique ligament
   b. Alveolar ligament
   c. Transseptal ligament
   d. Horizontal ligament

11. **Resorption of the roots of the deciduous incisors and canines begins on their**
   a. Labial surface
   b. Lingual surface
   c. Apical surface
   d. All the surfaces

1-b, 2-c, 3-d, 4-b, 5-c, 6-a, 7-b, 8-b, 9-b, 10-c, 11-b

12. Most common congenitally missing teeth are
a. Permanent upper lateral incisor
b. Permanent lower lateral incisors
c. Permanent lower first molars
d. Permanent upper canine

13. The cells responsible for removal of dental hard tissue are
a. Odontoclasts
b. Odontoblasts
c. Osteoblast
d. Fibroblasts

14. Most frequently the remnants of deciduous teeth are found in association with
a. Maxillary canines
b. Mandibular incisors
c. Premolars
d. Maxillary laterals

15. The most often retained deciduous teeth are
a. Lower central incisors
b. Upper canines
c. Upper lateral incisors
d. Lower canines

16. The most frequently retained deciduous tooth due to the impaction or ankylosis of its permanent successor is
a. Deciduous central incisor
b. Deciduous lateral incisor
c. Deciduous canine
d. Deciduous molars

17. The most common primary teeth to remain/appear submerged are
a. Primary canines
b. Primary first molars
c. Primary mandibular second molars
d. Primary incisors

18. The deciduous maxillary canine exfoliates at the age of
a. 6–7 years b. 2–3 years
c. 10–11 years d. 11–12 years

19. Maxillary primary root resorption begins at
a. 4 years b. 5 years
c. 6 years d. 7 years

20. Maxillary premolars erupt at
a. 8–9 years b. 9–10 years
c. 10–12 years d. 13–14 years

21. The most likely factor responsible for tooth eruption is
a. Vascular pressure
b. Developing periodontal ligament (PDL)
c. Bone growth
d. Growing root

22. The most accepted theory for tooth eruption is
a. Root growth theory
b. Pulp constriction theory
c. Periodontal ligament traction theory
d. Pulp growth theory

23. When a successional tooth germ is missing, shedding of deciduous teeth is
a. Premature
b. Normal
c. Delayed
d. None of the above

24. The upper first permanent molars develop in the tuberosity of the maxilla and in the beginning their occlusal surfaces faces
a. Labially b. Lingually
c. Mesially d. Distally

25. At first the occlusal surface of the permanent mandibular molar faces
a. Mesially b. Distally
c. Lingually d. Labially

26. The PDL fibers which has a key role in maintaining tooth position is
a. Horizontal group fibers
b. Apical group
c. Oblique group
d. Transseptal ligament fibers

12-a, 13-a, 14-c, 15-c, 16-c, 17-c, 18-c, 19-a, 20-c, 21-b, 22-c, 23-c, 24-d, 25-a, 26-d

27. The transseptal ligament fibers connect
a. Bone to bone
b. Cementum to bone
c. Gingiva to bone
d. Cementum of one tooth to the cementum of the adjacent tooth

28. The actual eruptive movement occurs in
a. Horizontal direction
b. Rotational way
c. In an axial direction
d. All of the above

29. Final position of the tooth in the oral cavity is determined by
a. Pressure exerted by tongue and teeth
b. Pressure exerted by the adjacent teeth
c. Both of the above
d. None of the above

30. In case of delayed resorption of primary incisors, the permanent incisors may be expected to erupt
a. Facial to the normal arch form
b. Lingual to the normal arch form
c. Mesial to the normal arch form
d. Distal to the normal arch form

31. The following movement of a tooth through the surrounding tissue due to which the clinical crown appears longer is
a. Eruption
b. Exfoliation
c. Mastication
d. Longitudinal development

32. The percentage of root calcification completed at the time of eruption is
a. 25%
b. 50%
c. 75%
d. 100%

33. The resorption of the roots of primary molars begins at about the age of
a. 6 years
b. 7 years
c. 8 years
d. 9 years

34. Posteruptive tooth movement is to compensate for
a. Occlusal and proximal wear
b. Occlusal wear only
c. Proximal wear only
d. Cervical abrasion

35. Time taken for root completion of primary teeth after eruption is
a. 3 years
b. 2 years
c. 6 months
d. 1 year

36. Time taken for root completion of permanent teeth after eruption is
a. 0.5–1 year
b. 2–3 years
c. 4–5 years
d. 6–7 years

37. The cell which resorbs dentin is
a. Fibroblast
b. Ameloblast
c. Odontoclast
d. Osteoclast

38. Fibronexus is seen in
a. PDL
b. Alveolar bone
c. Pulp
d. Gingiva

39. Shedding is
a. Pathologic
b. Physiologic
c. Anatomical
d. All of the above

40. Odontoclasts are
a. Resorptive cells
b. Formative cells

27-d, 28-c, 29-c, 30-b, 31-a, 32-d, 33-d, 34-a, 35-d, 36-b, 37-c, 38-a, 39-b, 40-a

c. Blood forming cells
d. Defence cells

41. Howship's lacuna is
a. Resorption bay
b. Elevated area
c. Clear zone
d. Attachment apparatus

42. Origin of odontoclasts is from
a. Lymphocytes
b. Macrophages
c. Dendritic cells
d. Circulating monocytes

43. Resorption is a
a. Continuous process
b. Active process
c. Period of activity and intervening rest period
d. None of the above

44. Submerged teeth
a. Appear at a lower level
b. Force their permanent successors from their position
c. Prevent eruption of permanent successor
d. All of the above

41-a, 42-d, 43-c, 44-d

Chapter 24

Preparation of Specimen for Histologic Study

LAQ (10 Marks)

Q. 1. Different steps in the preparation of a slide for staining of a soft tissue biopsy.

(Nov. 2009)

Describe in detail the method of preparation of histological section of a soft tissue specimen by paraffin embedding technique.

Ans. Introduction

- The morphologic study of tissue involves the preparation of tissue sections for microscopic examination.
- Tissue processing is the treatment of tissue necessary to keep them in as life like manner as possible and to impregnate them with a solid medium so as to give them enough rigidity to facilitate the production of sections for microscopy.
- The most commonly used method of preparing soft tissues for study with an ordinary light microscope is that of embedding the specimen in paraffin and then cutting 4–6 microns thick sections. The sections are mounted on microscope slides, stained and then viewed under microscope.

Steps in preparation of soft tissue specimen for sectioning:

1. **Obtaining the specimen**
2. **Fixation of the specimen:**
    - Immediately after removal of the specimen, it must be placed in a fixing solution to prevent autolysis and putrefaction.
    - Most commonly used fixative is neutral 10% buffered formalin.
    - The purpose of fixation is to coagulate the proteins so as to reduce alteration by subsequent treatment and to make the tissues more readily permeable to the subsequent application of reagents.
    - After fixation, the tissue is washed overnight in running water.
3. **Dehydration of the specimen:**
    - After being washed in formalin, the specimen is gradually dehydrated in alcohol to remove water. This is done because paraffin, in which the tissue is to be embedded and water in which the tissue is washed after fixation are not miscible.

- For dehydration, tissue is passed through a series of increasing percentages of alcohol, 40%, 60%, 80%, 95% and absolute.

4. **Clearing of the specimen:**
   - Since alcohol and paraffin are not miscible, the specimen is passed from alcohol through two changes of xylene, a clearing agent which is miscible with both alcohol and paraffin.
   - This step helps in improving the refractive index of the tissue. Tissue appears clear and it allows light to pass through, hence the procedure is called **clearing.**
5. **Infiltration of the specimen with paraffin:**
   - Now the tissue is removed from the xylene and placed in a dish of melted paraffin at about 60°C.
   - **Embedding the specimen:** When the specimen is completely infiltrated with paraffin, it is embedded in the center of a block of paraffin.
   - For this either a small paper box, or two 'L' shaped metallic pieces, usually made of brass or aluminium are used.
   - The tissue should be properly oriented and placed in the paper box or 'L' shaped pieces containing paraffin.
6. **Cutting the sections of the specimen:**
   - After cooling the hardened paraffin block is removed, is trimmed and sectioned on a microtome.
   - Sections are usually 4–6 mm thick.
7. **Mounting the cut sections on slides:**
   - A microscope slide is coated with a thin film of Meyer's albumin adhesive.
   - A short length cut paraffin ribbon with tissue sections is floated in a pan of warm water.
   - The prepared slide is then slipped under the ribbon and is then lifted from the water with the ribbon.
   - The slide is then placed on a constant temperature drying table at about 42°C, so that the sections adhere to the slide.
8. **Staining the sections:**
   - For routine microscopic study hematoxylin and eosin stain is commonly used.
   - The stained slides are mounted with DPX. Once DPX is hardened, the slide is ready for microscopic examination.

SAQs (3 Marks)

Q. 1. Write about fixatives? *(2001, Oct. 2002)*
Write about tissue fixation? *(May 2009)*

Ans. FIXATION

- It is the technique to maintain the tissue in as much a life-like state as possible, by preventing autolysis and putrefaction.
- The principle is to coagulate the tissue proteins, thus reducing alteration of tissue by subsequent treatment and to make it more readily permeable to the subsequent application of reagents.
- This is accomplished by using optimum osomotic conditions, cold temperatures, controlled pH of the fixing solutions, and minimum possible exposure to the fixative.

Techniques and fixatives used are:

1. Chemical fixatives
   - Formaldehyde
   - Acrolein and glutaraldehyde: Electron microscopy
   - Rossman's fliud: For glycogen, glycoproteins, and proteoglycans
   - Carnoy's fliud: Nucleic acids
2. Fresh frozen sections
3. Freeze drying—Liquid nitrogen
   - The most commonly used fixative is 10% formalin.
   - Formaldehyde is considered to be one of the ideal fixatives, especially for enzymes and other proteins. This is due to its ability to react with major reactive groups of proteins to form polymeric or macromolecular networks.

Q. 2. Write about ground section. *(Oct. 2003, May 2008, Nov. 2009)*

Ans. GROUND SECTION

Decalcification of bone and teeth often obscures the structures. Teeth in particular are damaged because tooth enamel, being about 96% mineral substance, is usually completely destroyed by ordinary methods of decalcification. Undecalcified teeth and undecalcified bone may be studied by making thin ground sections of the specimens.

This can be done by slicing the undecalcified specimen, which is ground down to a section of about 50 mm on a revolving stone or disc.

Equipment required: The equipment used for making ground section includes a laboratory lathe, a coarse and a fine abrasive lathe wheel, a stream of water, a wooden block, adhesive tape, a camel's hair brush, ether, mounting medium, microscope slides and cover slips.

Procedure: Before making of ground section, extracted tooth should be preserved in 10% formalin. Using coarse abrasive lathe, the tooth is ground down to the level of the desired section. The coarse wheel is then exchanged for a fine abrasive lathe wheel so that the rough surfaces are removed. The cut surface of the tooth is ground until the level of the desired section is reached. The tooth is ground down to a thickness of about 0.5 mm. Throughout the procedure, the specimen should be protected from heat and should not be allowed to dry. The finished ground section is dried and mounted on a slide with mounting media. For making sections out of enamel, hard tissue microtomes are used.

Q. 3. Write about decalcification. *(June 2010)*

Ans. DECALCIFICATION

- Specimens that contain teeth and bone cannot be cut with a microtome knife unless these calcified tissues are made soft by decalcification.
- Decalcification is the removal of the calcified substance from hard tissues like bone and teeth to make them soft for sectioning.
- This is usually done by using 5% nitric acid.
- After fixation, the specimen is decalcified. One of the methods is to suspend the specimen in about 400 ml of 5% nitric acid. The acid is changed daily for 8–10 days and then the specimen is tested for complete decalcification. One way to test is by piercing it with a needle, another way is to test it by precipitation method.

- After decalcification the procedure is same as that of soft tissue processing.
- Instead of embedding in puraffin wax, decalcified tissues can be embedded in parlodian which is purified nitrocellulose dissolved in ether-alcohol. Parlodian embedding gives better sectioning, but the procedure is cumbersome.
- Except enamel all hard tissues can be processed by these methods and studied.

Q. 4. Write about hematoxylin and eosin stain. *(Nov. 2009)*

Ans. Hematoxylin and eosin stain is the most commonly used stain for routine microscopic study of tissue specimens.

HEMATOXYLIN AND EOSIN STAIN

Principle

Hematoxylin is basic stain which stains nuclei whereas eosin is acidic stain which stains cytoplasm. Hematoxylin is converted to hematin by oxidation.

Hematoxylin stains section regressively with a stain at sufficient power and for long enough to ensure some overstaining of nuclei. Excess stain is removed by treatment with acid-alcohol.

This is most popular stain and is called **routine stain.**

Solutions

Hematoxylin is a natural product obtained from logwood of Mexican tree.

Eosin is chemically or artificially prepared in laboratory.

i. Harri's alum hematoxylin
ii. 1% eosin
iii. 1% acid-alcohol

Procedure

i. **Deparaffinization:** First dip in xylene to remove paraffin, then dip in alcohol to remove xylene, then wash in running water for 5 minutes.
ii. **Rinsing:** Rinse in water for 15 minutes.
iii. **Staining:** Put sections in hematoxylin jar for 10–15 minutes (stains the neclei).
iv. **Decolorization:** 1–2 drops in 1% acid-alcohol (to decolorize section).
v. **Counter staining:** Counter staining with 1% eosin for 2 minutes (stains cytoplasm).
vi. **Dehydration:** Dehydrate with absolute alcohol (dehydrate sections and remove excess alcohol).
vii. **Clearing:** One dip in xylene (clears alcohol).
viii. Blot dry and mount in DPX.

Results

Nuclei	–	**Blue**
Cytoplasm	–	**Pink**
Connective tissue	–	**Pink**
Blood vessels	–	**Pink**
Collagen fibers	–	**Pink**

Application

Hematoxylin and eosin stain is most commonly used stain for routine microscopic study of tissue specimens as well as for cytological smears.

Q. 5. Write about periodic acid Schiff (PAS) stain. *(May 2007)*

Ans. PERIODIC ACID SCHIFF (PAS) STAIN

This is the most frequently used stain for detection of carbohydrates.

Principle

1% periodic acid oxidizes the glycol groups of carbohydrates to aldehydes. These aldehydes then react with Schiff's solution (reagent) giving magenta red color.

Solution

i. 1% periodic acid
ii. Schiff's reagent
iii. Hematoxylin reagent (Iron Hematoxylin)

Procedure

i. **Deparaffinization:** First dip to deparaffinize the section.
ii. **Oxidation:** Oxidize in PAS solution for 5 minutes
iii. Place in Schiff's reagent for 20–30 minutes.
iv. **Rinsing:** Rinse in water and blot dry.
v. Wash in running water for 5 minutes to develop pink color.
vi. Stain with iron hematoxyline for 4–5 minutes.
vii. Wash in water, then counter stain with saturated solution of picric acid.
viii. **Dehydration:** Dehydrate, clear and mount in DPX.

Results

Nucleus – **Blue black**
Basement membrane – **Magenta red**
Glycogen content – **Magenta red**
Background – **Yellow** (due to picric acid)
Acid mucopolysaccharide – **Magenta red**

Applications

It is a special stain for acid mucopolysaccharides present in basement membrane. They take up magenta red color on staining.

The break in basement membrane can be well-observed and studied by PAS in case of suspicion of oral squamous cell carcinoma.

MULTIPLE CHOICE QUESTIONS (MCQs)

1. **The methods used for the preparation of oral tissues for microscopic examination are**
   a. Paraffin embedding
   b. Parlodion embedding
   c. Ground sections of mineralized tissues
   d. Frozen sections
   e. All of the above
2. **The most commonly used method for preparing specimens of gingiva, cheek and tongue is**
   a. Ground section
   b. Frozen section
   c. Paraffin embedding
   d. All of the above
3. **During tissue processing water from tissue is removed by using solution of**
   a. Xylene
   b. Alcohol
   c. Formalin
   d. Saline
4. **The clearing solution used in tissue processing is**
   a. Xylene
   b. Alcohol
   c. Water
   d. Saline
5. **The most commonly used method for preparing specimens of hard tissues is by embedding in**
   a. Paraffin
   b. Parlodion
   c. Celloidin
   d. All of the above
6. **The decalcifying solution used is**
   a. 10% formalin
   b. 10% nitric acid
   c. 5% nitric acid
   d. 5% formalin
7. **The method to determine the end of decalcification procedure is**
   a. Probing with a needle
   b. Radiography
   c. Precipitation test
   d. All of the above
8. **Special stain used for keratin is**
   a. Van Gieson's stain
   b. Masson trichrome stain
   c. Mallory stain
   d. Periodic acid Schiff stain
9. **Hematoxylin is a**
   a. Counter stain
   b. Basic stain
   c. Acidic stain
   d. None of the above
10. **Eosin is a**
    a. Counter stain
    b. Basic stain
    c. Acidic stain
    d. None of the above
11. **Special stain used for basement membrane is**
    a. Van Gieson's stain
    b. Periodic acid Schiff stain
    c. Prussian blue
    d. Hematoxylin and eosin
12. **Extracted teeth should be preserved in**
    a. 10% formalin
    b. 10% alcohol
    c. Normal saline
    d. Hydrogen peroxide
13. **For decalcification of bone the solution used is**
    a. Xylene
    b. Formalin
    c. Alcohol
    d. Nitric acid

1-e, 2-c, 3-b, 4-a, 5-b, 6-c, 7-d, 8-c, 9-b, 10-c, 11 – b, 12-a, 13-d

14. The most ideal fixative is
a. Sodium hypochlorite
b. Formaldehyde
c. Acetaldehyde
d. H_2SO_4

15. Formaldehyde as a fixative is used as
a. 10% solution
b. 20% solution
c. 30% solution
d. 40% solution

16. The special stain used for glycoprotein is
a. Silver stain
b. Alcian blue
c. Ninhydrin stain
d. Hematoxylin and eosin stain

17. Dehydration of the specimen for embedding in paraffin is carried out by passing through
a. Decreasing percentage of alcohol
b. Increasing percentage of alcohol
c. Increasing percentage of ether
d. Increasing percentage of xylene

18. Special stain used to demonstrate mucin is
a. Mallory
b. Von Gieson
c. Mucicarmine
d. Massons' trichrome

19. The most commonly used fixative for light microscopy is
a. Formalin
b. Glutaraldehyde
c. Acetone
d. Ether

20. The most commonly used fixative for electron microscopy is
a. Formalin
b. Glutaraldehyde
c. Acetone
d. Ether

21. Most commony used mountant is
a. DPX b. Glycerine
c. Araldite d. Balsam

22. The thickness of section obtained in routine tissue processing is
a. 3–5 mm b. 13–15 mm
c. 23–25 mm d. 33–35 mm

23. The thickness of ground section is
a. 10 mm b. 50 mm
c. 100 mm d. 150 mm

24. The instrument used to obtain frozen sections is
a. Cryostat
b. Microscope
c. Microtome
d. Tissue floatation both

25. The thickness of frozen section is
a. 10–15 mm
b. 100–150 mm
c. 10–15 mm
d. 100–150 mm

26. Which of the following is the aim of fixation
a. Preserve tissues in a lifelike manner
b. Prevent autolysis and putrefaction
c. Prevent change in shape or volume of tissue
d. All of the above

27. Fixation for demonstration of lipids should be done by
a. Formaldehyde
b. Carnoy's solution
c. Freeze drying
d. Formol calcium

28. Fixative used for demonstration of nucleic acid is
a. Acrolein
b. Glutaraldehyde
c. Formaldehyde
d. Carnoy's solution

14-b, 15-a, 16-b, 17-b, 18-c, 19-b, 20-b, 21-a, 22-a, 23-b, 24-a, 25-a, 26-d, 27-c, 28-d

29. Demonstration of nucleic acid is done by
a. Sudan Black B
b. Feulgen technique
c. PAS technique
d. Mucicarmine method

30. The best known staining method for studying carbohydrate is
a. Mallory
b. Von Gieson
c. Mucicarmine
d. PAS

31. The maximum thickness of ground section is
a. 1 mm b. 0.5 mm
c. 0.2 mm d. 0.1 mm

32. The correct order of steps in tissue processing is
a. Fixation, embedding, clearing, Dehydration
b. Fixation, dehydration, clearing, embedding
c. Fixation, clearing, embedding, dehydration
d. Fixation, dehydration, embedding, clearing

33. The minimum volume of fixative required is
a. Five times more than the volume of the tissue
b. Fifteen times more than the volume of the tissue
c. Forty-five times more than the volume of the tissue
d. Hundred times more than the volume of the tissue

34. Which of the following is a fixative
a. DPX b. Formalin
c. Paraffin wax d. Xyline

35. The instrument used to obtain thin sections is
a. Cryostat b. Microscope
c. Microtome d. Tissue floatation bath

29-b, 30-d, 31-b, 32-b, 33-b, 34-b, 35-a

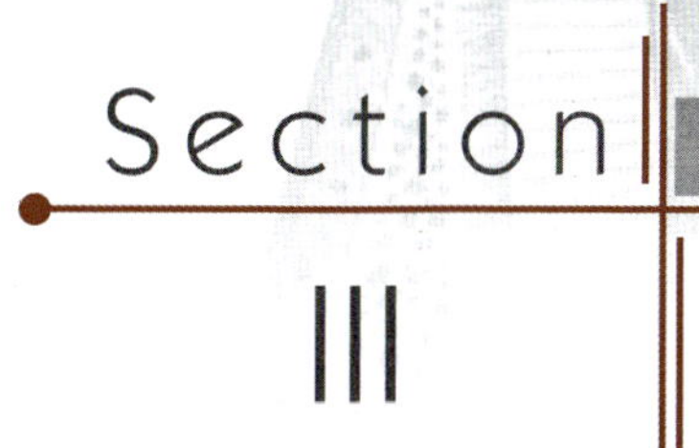

Section III

Practical Guide

Chapter 25

Carving of Teeth

MEASUREMENT OF TEETH (in mm)								
		Length of Crown	*Length of Root*	*Total Length of Tooth*	*MD at contact area*	*MD at cervix*	*Labio-lingual at crest of curvature*	*Labio-linguo at cervix*
MAXILLARY								
CI	P	10.5	13	23.5	8.5	7	7	6
	D	6	10	16	6.5	4.5	5	4
LI	P	9	13	22	6.5	5	6	5
	D	5.6	11.4	17	5.1	3.7	4	3.7
C	P	10	17	27	7.5	5.5	8	7
	D	6.5	13.5	20	7	5.1	7	5.5
PM	P	8.5	14	22.5	7	5	9	8
First								
M	D	5.1	10	15.1	7.3	5.2	8.5	6.9
PM	P	8.5	14	22.5	7	5	9	8
Second								
M	D	5.7	11.7	17.4	8.2	6.4	10	8.3
First								
M	P	7.5	12 13	20.5	10	8	11	10
Second		B L						
M	P	7	11 12	19	9	7	11	10
MANDIBULAR								
CI	P	9	12.5	21.5	5	3.5	6	5.3
	D	5	9	14	4.2	3	4	3.5
LI	P	9.5	14	23.5	5.5	4	6.5	5.8
	D	5.2	10	15.2	4.1	3	4	3.5
C	P	11	16	27	7	5.5	7.5	7
	D	6	11.5	17.5	5	3.7	4.8	4
PM	P	8.5	14	22.5	7	5	7.5	6.5
First								
M	D	6	9.8	15.8	7.7	6.5	7	5.3
PM	P	8	14.5	22.5	7	5	8	7

(Contd.)

MEASUREMENT OF TEETH (in mm) (*Contd.*)								
		Length of Crown	*Length of Root*	*Total Length of Tooth*	*MD at contact area*	*MD at cervix*	*Labio-lingual at crest of curvature*	*Labio-linguo at cervix*
MANDIBULAR								
Second M	D	5.5	11.3	16.8	9.9	7.2	8.7	6.4
First M	P	7.5	14	21.5	11	9	10.5	9
Second M	P	7	13	20	10.5	8	10	9

P = Permanent **M** = Molar **C** = Canine **D** = Deciduous **PM** = Premolar

LEARNING TOOTH MORPHOLOGY

- **Tooth carving:** It is one of the best methods for learning tooth morphology because it gives a three dimensional understanding of the details of tooth form.
- It cannot be mastered in a day. It can be learnt only with practice and patience.
- Good carving skills come handy in clinical practice, especially during restoration of lost tooth structure.

Materials Required for Carving

- Standard size wax block made of paraffin wax 3 × 1.25 × 1.25 cm
- Lecron carver
- Six inches metal scale ruler
- A gauze piece
- Soap, water, cotton wool for final polishing.

Lecron Carver: (Fig. 25.1)

- It is double ended stainless steel tool. It has a handle and two working ends.
- The shaft is generally serrated to facilitate firm grip of the instrument.
- One working end is knife-shaped which has both straight and curved part. This working end is used for major part of carving.
- The other working end is spoon-shaped/scoop like which is generally used for carving depressions/fossa.
- It is used with **modified pen-grip** for almost all the steps in carving except when big chunks of wax have to be removed or major reduction is required then the **palm-grip** is used.

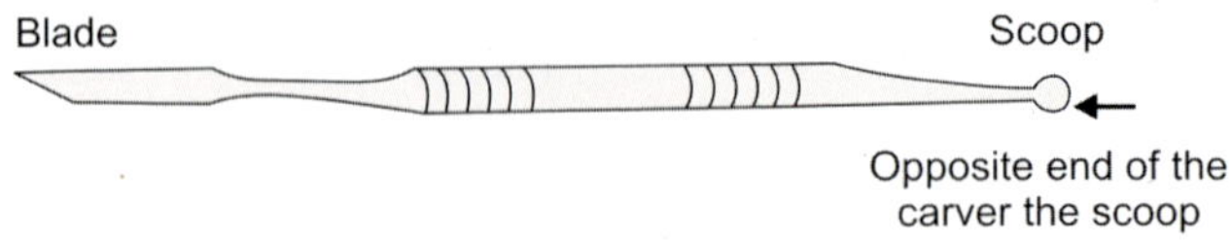

Fig. 25.1

Modified Pen-grip

- In modified pen-grip, the carver is held at its neck with the thumb, index finger and middle finger.
- Middle finger is placed closer to the blade.
- Index-finger bends at its second joint.
- The neck is held with thumb and index finger.
- Blade is supported with the middle finger.
- Middle finger rests on the ring finger and little finger.
- Support is gained by resting the ring finger and little finger on the fingers of the block holding hand.

Before carving a tooth the student can practice some imaginary carvings like carving of single dumbbell, a ball, a pencil, a doll, a dice, a flower, or any other object one can think of.

This will help the student to learn how to hold the carver, how much pressure to apply on wax, how to cut, shape and polish wax. It will help the student to learn the properties of wax. It is a basic process of learning.

We have tried to give some guidelines for a few objects.

EXERCISE–1

BLOCK

Carve a Block of dimension 3 cm × 1 cm × 1 cm.

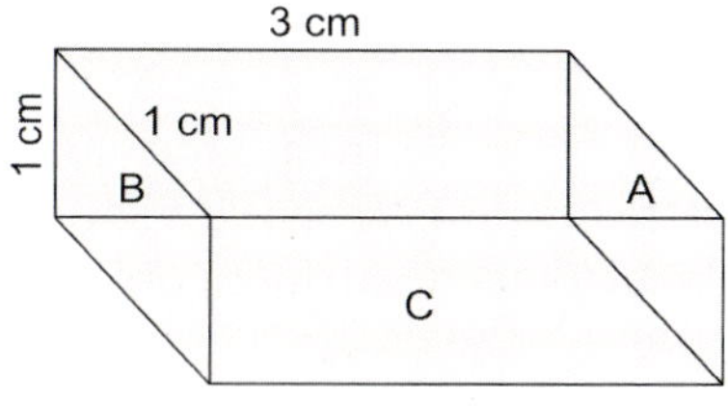

Fig. 25.2

To make the block of given size, keep 1 mm extra on all the surfaces while marking.

STEP 1

Reduce the surface A to bring the length of the block to 3.1 cm. Then level the surface A.

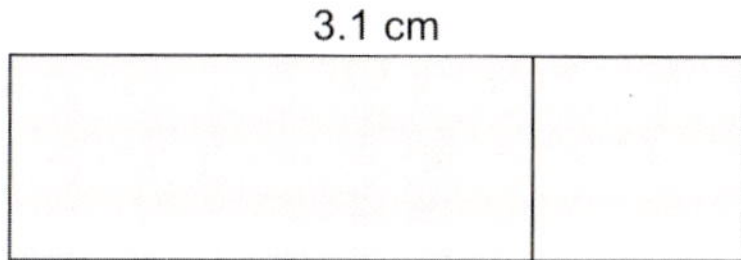

Fig. 25.3

STEP 2

- In Fig. 25.2 the block is resting on the surface C and the surface A is on your right side.
- In Fig. 25.4 and Fig. 25.5 the block is resting on the surface B, and surface C is on your right side and surface D is facing you.

On the surface A and B mark a point at a distance of 1 cm on the sides a and b of both the surfaces. Join the points (Fig. 25.4).

Reduce the surface C up to the lines marked.

Level the surface C.

A is top surface

B is bottom surface

C and D are adjacent surfaces.

To maintain the levels and smoothness, instead of reducing all 6 surfaces we are reducing only 3 surfaces A, C and D.

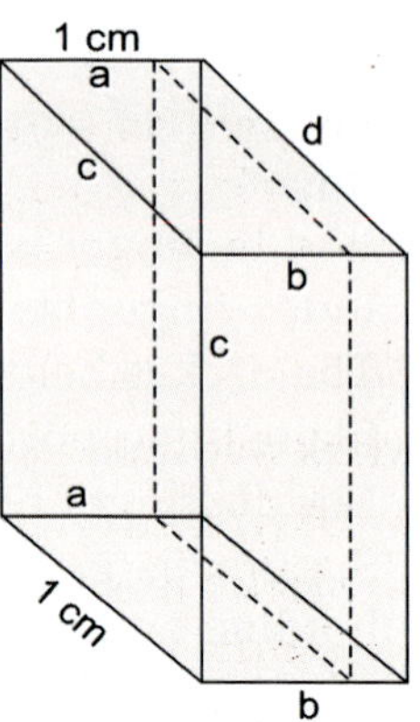

Fig. 25.4

STEP 3 (FIG. 25.5)

Mark 1 cm on the sides c and d of both the surfaces A and B.

Join all the points.

Reduce the surface D up to the lines marked.

Level the surface D.

- The given block is bigger is size.
- It has 6 surfaces.
- To make the block of required size we reduce the three surfaces A, C, D.

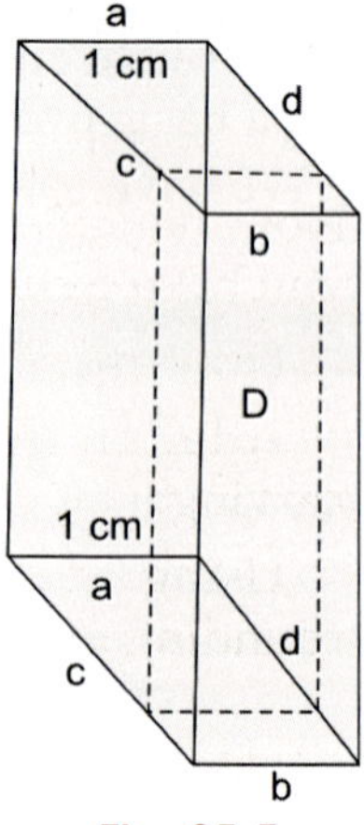

Fig. 25.5

OR

Single Step

Reduce the length of the block to 3.1 cm by reducing the surface A. Level it. Then on the surface A and B mark two points to make a square of 1 cm each side. Join all the points. Reduce two adjacent surfaces only (Fig. 25.6).

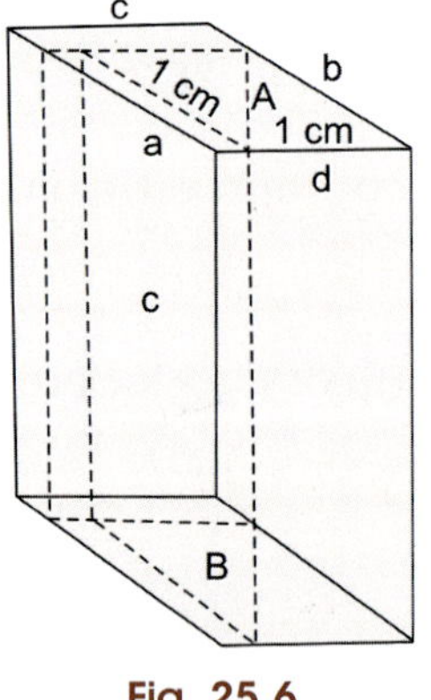

Fig. 25.6

EXERCISE–2

SINGLE DUMBBELL

To carve a sphere or a ball 1 cm in diameter centered over a cylinder (bar, rod) of length 1.5 cm or 1 cm and diameter of 8 mm (Fig. 25.7).

STEP 1

Draw two horizontal lines at a distance of 1 cm and 1.5 on all the four surfaces of the block. Each surface is divided into three parts 1 cm for sphere, 1.5 cm for the cylinder and remaining is the base.

1 cm
1.5 cm
Base

Fig. 25.7

STEP 2

Mark midline (vertical) on two opposite surfaces.

- Draw a circle with 1 cm diameter on upper part.
- Mark 4 mm on either side of the midline and draw two lines on the middle part.
- Remove the wax from the shaded portion on two opposite surfaces of the block.
- The bottom part forms the base.

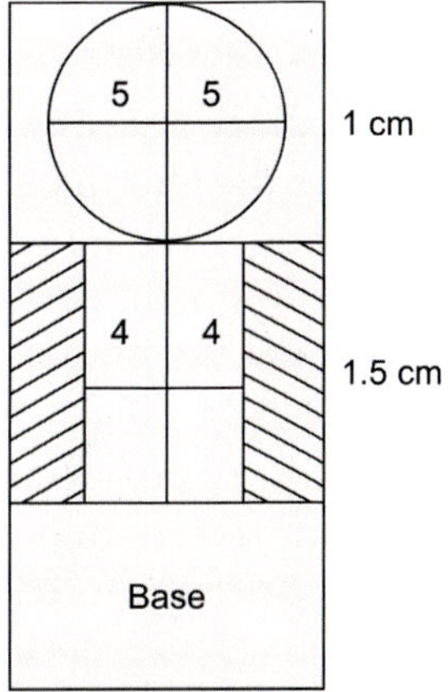

Fig. 25.8

STEP 3

Now mark the mid-line on other two opposite surfaces, i.e. the surfaces you have reduced.

Draw the circle and two vertical lines.

After all the four surfaces have been reduced you get a gross carving.

Using your judgement and while turning the block, keep on rounding off the sphere and the cylinder.

EXERCISE–3

PYRAMID

1 cm
1 cm
1 cm

Fig. 25.9

STEP 1

Divide the 3 cm block (exercise 1) into 3 parts 1 cm each by drawing two horizontal lines at a distance of 1 cm.

- Draw a mid-line on both the opposite surfaces.
- Mark equilateral triangles on the upper and lower 1 cm part of the block, on both the opposits surfaces.

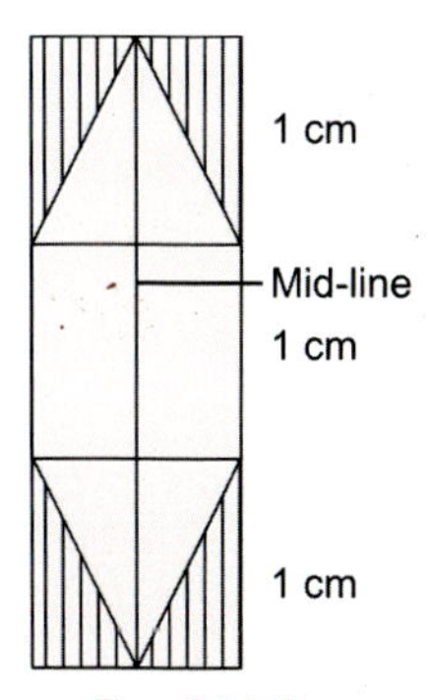

Fig. 25.10

Carve out the wax outside of the marked lines.
Repeat the same on other two opposite surfaces.

PREPARATION OF BLOCK FOR TOOTH CARVING

- Read the details of the tooth to be carved along with odontometric data and read and see the diagrams of the tooth from all five aspects.
- While carving, either keep a plaster model of the tooth to be carved or a clean extracted tooth in front of you.
- Areas in the figure where lines are drawn indicate removal of wax in that area.

TIPS FOR CARVING

1. **Maxillary anterior teeth:**
   - Let the length of the block remain as it is.
   - Reduce the four sides of the crown and root part of the block so that the top surface is a square with each side measuring 1 cm/10 mm.
   - Make the incisal ridge/cuspal ridge of maxillary anterior teeth thick and centered over the root axis.
2. **Maxillary posterior teeth:**
   - Let the length of the block remain as it is.
   - Reduce the four sides of the crown and root part of the block so that the top surface is a square with each side measuring 11 mm.
3. **Mandibular anterior teeth:**
   - Let the length of the block remain as it is.
   - Reduce the four sides of crown and root part of the block so as to get a square on the top surface with each side measuring 8 mm.
   - The incisal/cuspal ridge of mandibular anterior teeth is thin and not centered over the root axis, it is towards lingual.
4. **Mandibular posterior teeth:**
   - No reduction of the block required.

INCISORS

CLASS TRAITS

1. **Incisors have an incisal edge instead of the cusps that are found on the canines and posterior teeth.**
   - Incisal ridge is that part of the crown which makes up for the complete incisal portion.

     When the incisor is newly erupted, the incisal portion is rounded and merges with the mesial and distal incisal angles and labial and lingual surfaces. This is the incisal ridge.

     Incisal edge comes into existence only after the occlusal wear has created a flattened surface linguo-incisally, which forms an angle with the labial surface.

     Incisal edge is formed by the junction of linguo-incisal and labial surface.
2. **Mamelons are found on the newly erupted permanent incisors.**
   - Mamelons are the rounded extensions of enamel on the incisal ridge of the newly erupted incisors.
3. **Marginal ridges are located on mesial and distal borders of the lingual surface and are in vertical plane.**
4. Incisors have thin blade-like crown, La-Li dimension is less than in any other class of tooth.
5. Contact points are small and more incisally placed.

MAXILLARY CENTRAL INCISOR

PALMER NOTATION

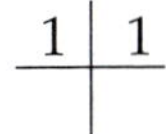

ODONTOMETRIC DATA	
Length of crown	10.5 mm
Length of root	13.0 mm
Mesiodistal width of crown	8.5 mm
Mesiodistal width of crown at cervix	7.0 mm
Labiolingual width of crown	7.0 mm
Labiolingual width at cervix	6.0 mm
Curvature of cervical line on mesial	3.5 mm
On distal	2.5 mm

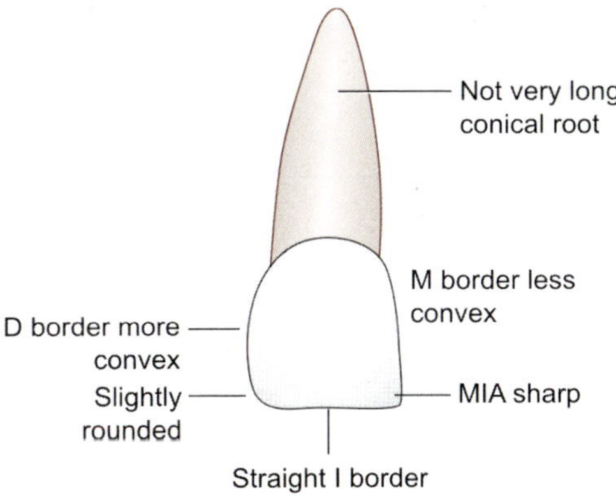

Fig. 25.11: Labial aspect

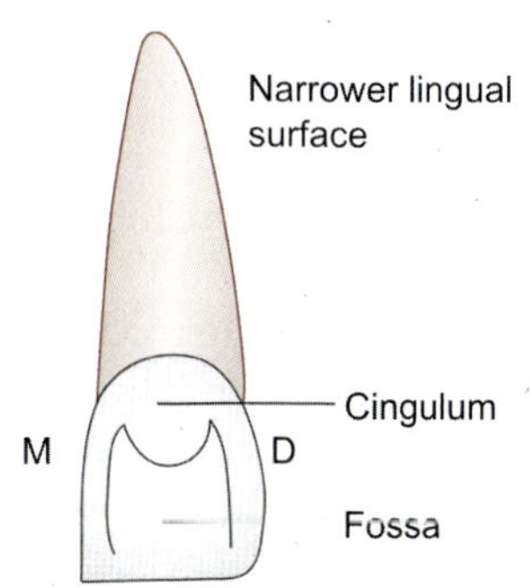

Fig. 25.12: Lingual aspect

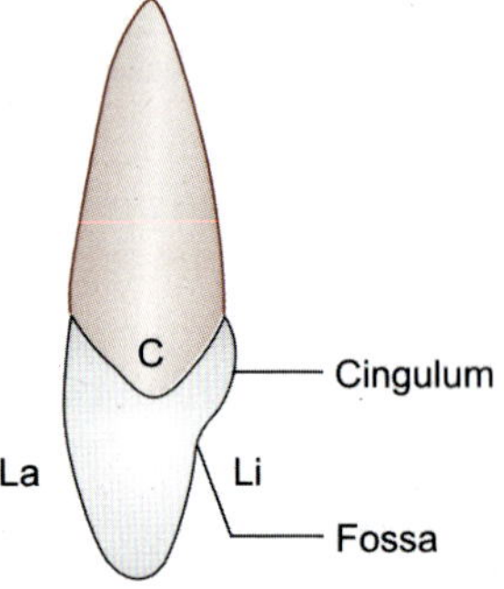

Fig. 25.13: Proximal aspect

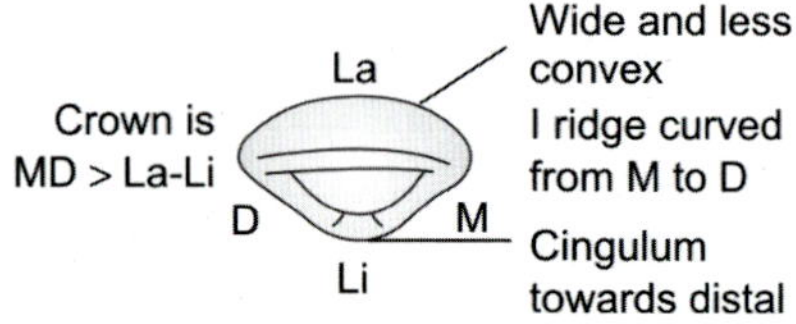

Fig. 25.14: Incisal aspect

STEPS FOR CARVING

STEP 1a

THIS PREPARATION OF THE BLOCK REMAINS SAME FOR ALL TEETH (Fig. 25.15)

For Measurements, Refer the *Chart on page 353*

- Prepare the standard size wax block for carving by making it smooth with the straight part of the blade. Rub it with a piece of gauze.
- Divide the wax block into three parts by marking two lines for crown length and root length as in the Fig. 25.15.
- Extend the two lines on all the four surfaces.
- The block is divided into 3 parts crown, root and base.
- Mark initials on all four surfaces on base part: (Fig. 25.15)

  B/L – Buccal/Labial
  Li – Lingual or P – Palatal
  M – Mesial
  D – Distal
- Draw a vertical midline on all the surfaces of the crown and root part of the block.

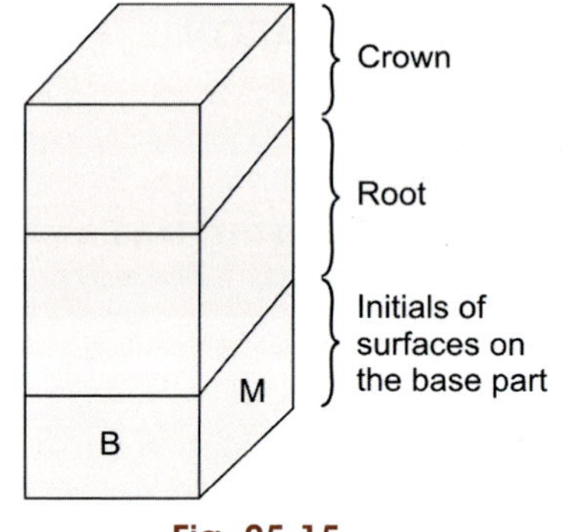

Fig. 25.15

STEP 1b

For maxillary central incisor make the block of length 24 mm, and top surface square of each side 10 mm. So that the block is centered over the base (Fig. 25.16).

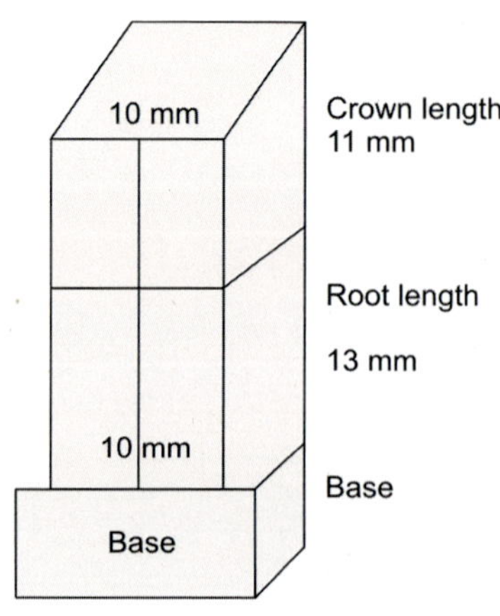

Fig. 25.16

STEP 2

Divide incisal surface (top square) into two equal halves by a single 'line 2' (midline) mesiodistally Draw two more lines on either side of the midline, line 1 and line 3 at a distance of 1 mm each from the midline to get a thick incisal ridge.

- Purpose of dividing incisal aspect into two equal parts is not to cross that line while carving the labial surface convex, because incisal ridge of the maxillary central incisor is centered over the root and it is 1.5 to 2 mm thick (Fig. 25.17).

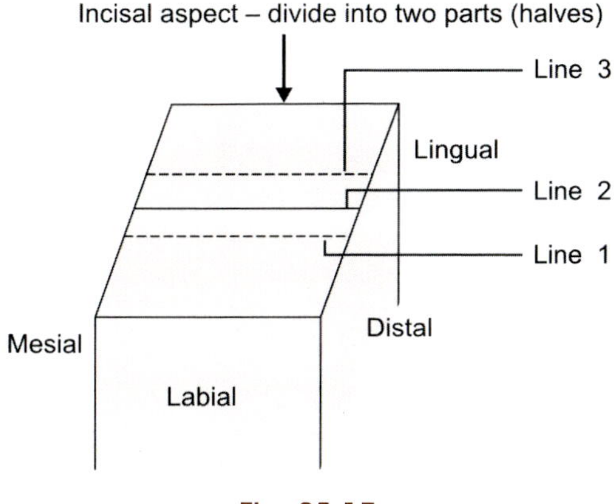

Fig. 25.17

STEP 3

THIS STEP IS COMMON TO ALL ANTERIOR TEETH

Carving of Labial Surface

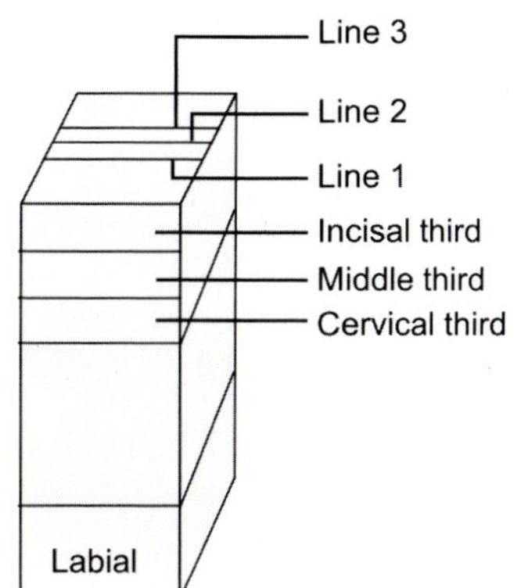

Fig. 25.18

Carve the labial surface to create convexity. Convexity is more in cervical third and tends to be less towards the incisal third.

Method

Divide the labial surface of the crown into three parts (Fig. 25.18).

1. Incisal third
2. Middle third
3. Cervical third

- Hold the carver above the cervical third and move it towards incisal ridge in upward direction and remove wax till the marked line 1 (Fig. 25.19).

Fig. 25.19

Proximal View (Fig. 25.20)

- After carving convexity in middle and incisal third **merge the incisal two-thirds with cervical third.**

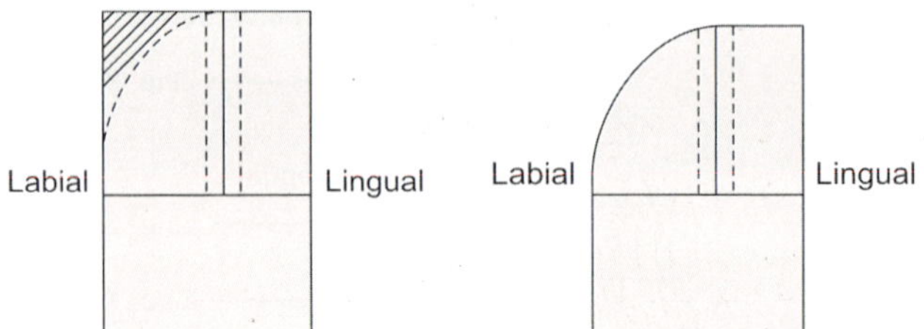

Fig. 25.20

STEP 4

THIS STEP IS COMMON TO ALL ANTERIOR TEETH

Carving of lingual surface

Method

Divide lingual surface of the crown into three parts (Fig. 25.21):

1. Incisal third
2. Middle third
3. Cervical third.

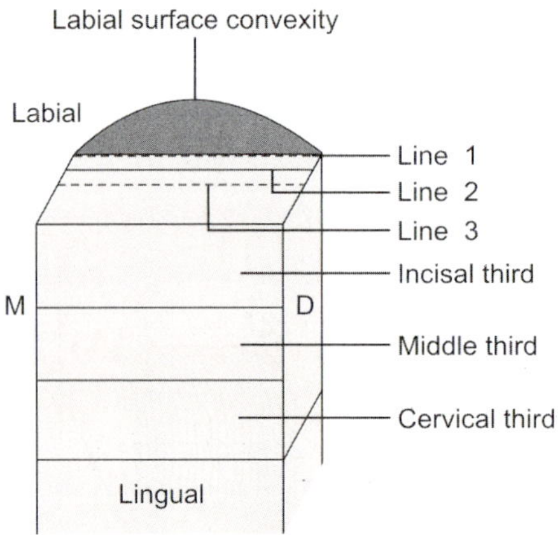

Fig. 25.21

- Hold the carver above cervical third, in the middle third and move it up and down to create concavity. Then move it in upward direction in incisal third till line 3. This will create lingual fossa (Fig. 25.22).
- Since the wax is not removed from the cervical third area it can be modified into cingulum by narrowing and rounding it.
- Remove irregularities and sharp angles from cingulum area.

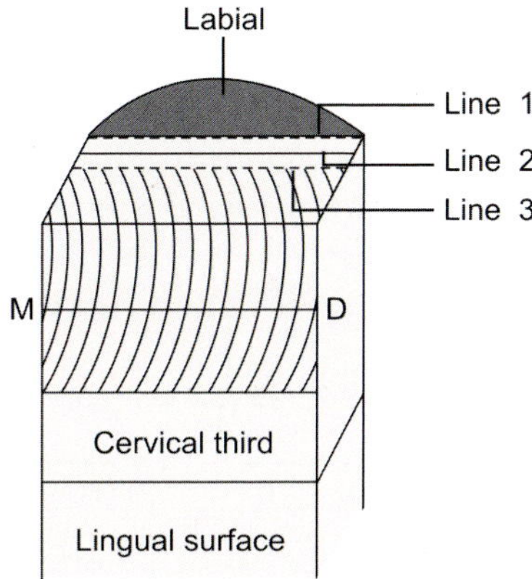

Fig. 25.22

Proximal View: (Fig. 25.23)

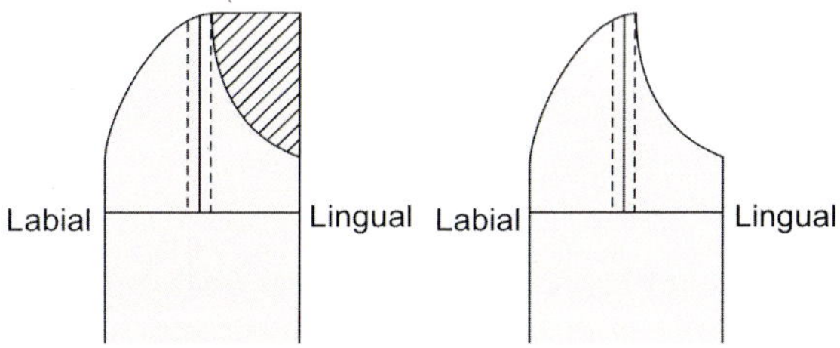

Fig. 25.23

STEP 5

THIS STEP IS COMMON TO ALL THE ANTERIOR TEETH

Giving Cervical Constriction to the Crown (Fig. 25.24)

- Give MD constriction on labial and lingual surface of the crown.
- This is done by removing wax in the cervical third of the crown on the mesial and distal surfaces as per dimensions.
- After this is done, taper the root from cervix to apex so that at cervix, crown and root are in same plane (refer Fig. 25.24).
- Make the markings on the block as shown in Fig. 25.24
- Make sure that wax is removed till the marked lines so that from cervical third of the crown to the apex of the root, the M and D surfaces are in same plane.
- This step will give constriction to the crown (from labial and lingual view) and will also show gross carving of the root.
- Since the crown and root are more narrower towards the lingual side, remove more wax on M and D surfaces towards lingual side.
- Once again mark the crown length, cervical line curvature on all four surfaces.

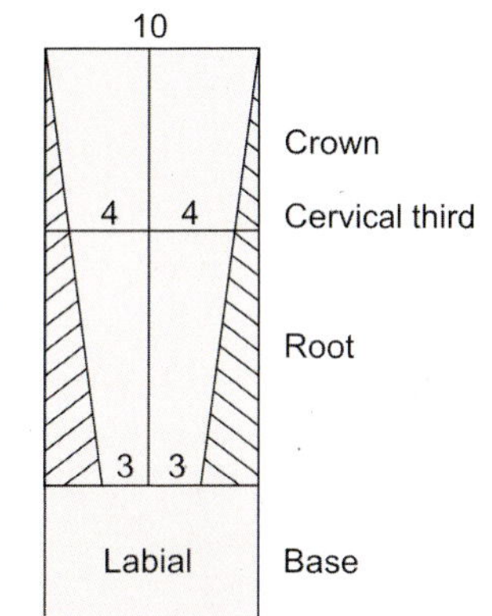

Fig. 25.24

STEP 5a

Finishing Labial Surface

- At this step complete the carving of the crown by finishing the labial surface with the M and D outlines, and the appropriate dimension of the crown at contact point and at cervix and carving the MIA and DIA.
- Make both mesial and distal angle sharp 90°. Then rub the DI with index finger to make it rounded (Fig. 25.25).

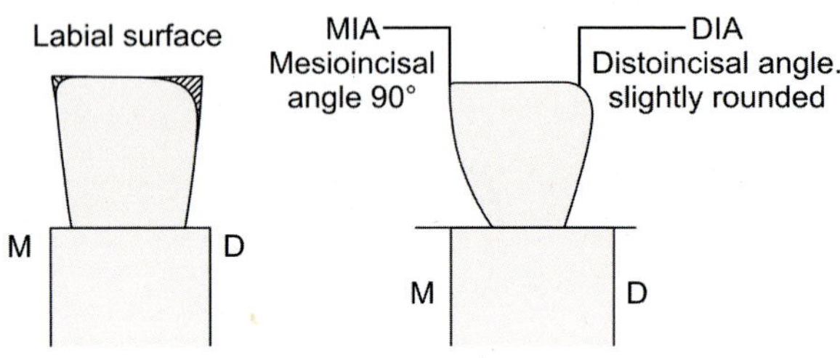

Fig. 25.25

STEP 6a

Reduction of La-Li Dimension

- Grossly the labial and lingual surfaces have been carved. Now to reduce the labiolingual dimension remove wax from base of the root upwards towards the cingulum on the lingual surface and towards the cervical third of the crown on the labial surface till the demension is 7.5 to 8 mm in the cervical third of the crown is created (Fig. 25.26).

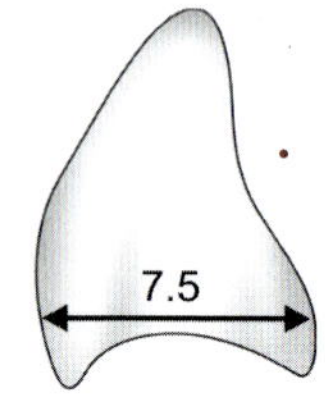

Fig. 25.26

STEP 6b

Lingual Carving of Fossa, Incisal and Marginal Ridges

- Draw the 'V' or 'W' shaped outline for fossa on the incisal two-thirds of the lingual surface by keeping 1 mm space on both sides for the M and D marginal ridges.

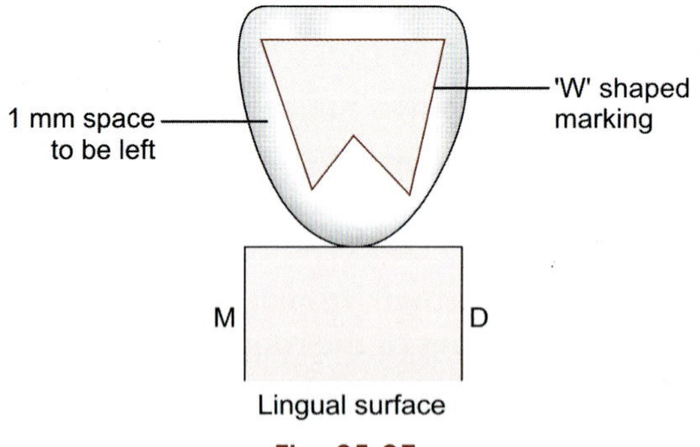

Fig. 25.27

- Remove wax within the marked 'W' shape with the carver's opposite end. (scoop)

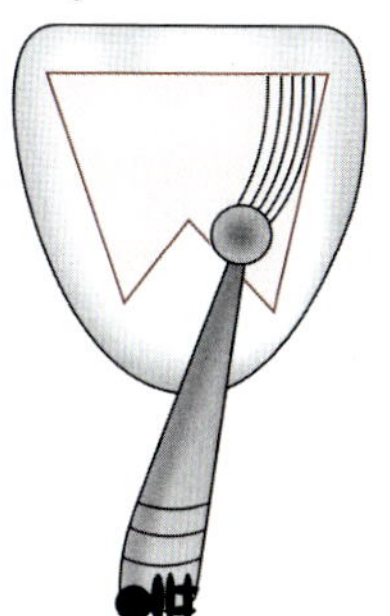

Fig. 25.28

- While making the lingual fossa deep, keep some space mesially, distally as well as incisally so as to make—mesial and distal marginal ridges and incisal ridge more prominent.

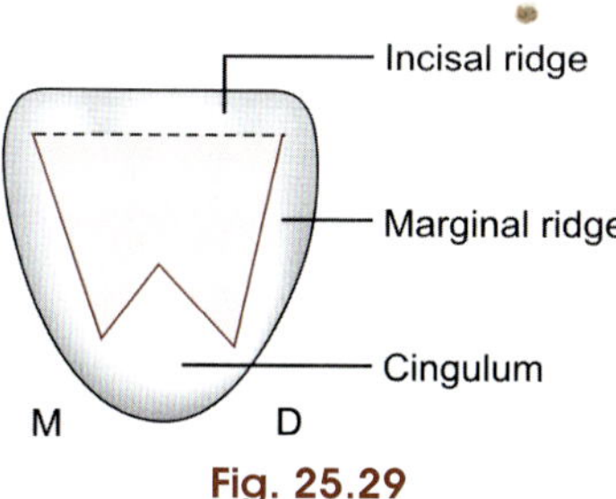

Fig. 25.29

STEP 7

THIS STEP IS COMMON TO ALL ANTERIOR TEETH

Marking of Cervical Line and Finishing

- Cervical line is more convex on mesial surface.
- By keeping morphology in mind finish the carving.
- Measure the dimensions of the finished curving.
  - Check labiolingual dimension if bulky reduce it from labial surface mainly by keeping the surface convexity proper and reduce lingual surface slightly without reducing the prominence of the cingulum.
  - Check mesiodistal width. If it is more reduce it from mesial and distal sides

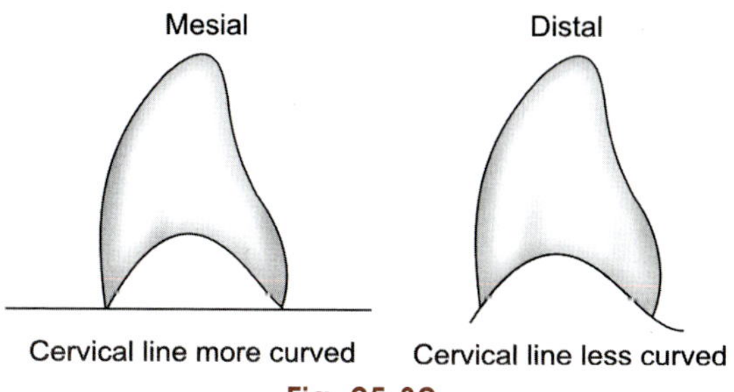

Fig. 25.30

- Finish cervical area.
- Finish lingual surface.
- Check the convexities of labial surface and cingulum from mesial, distal, incisal and labial aspect.
- Using gauze piece remove roughness on the carving.
- Polish with cotton dipped in soap water without pressure to achieve mirror like polish.

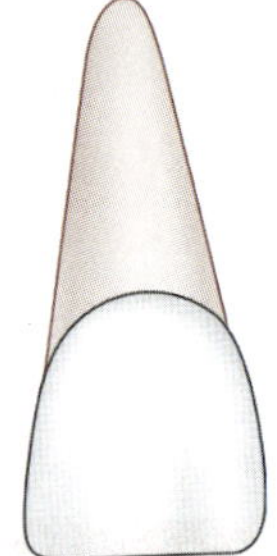

Fig. 25.31

STEP 8

Carving of Root

In step 5 the gross carving of root was done. Carve it further in proportion to the crown. So that the root is conical, gradually tapering from cervix to apex (Fig. 25.31).

While carving root or while polishing **hold the carving at the neck** (cervix) with the index finger and thumb so that it does not break.

MAXILLARY LATERAL INCISOR

PALMER NOTATION

2 | 2

ODONTOMETRIC DATA	
Length of crown	9.0 mm
Length of root	13.0 mm
Mesiodistal width of crown	6.5 mm
Mesiodistal width of crown at cervix	5.0 mm
Labiolingual width of crown	6.0 mm
Labiolingual width at cervix	5.0 mm
Curvature of cervical line on mesial	3.0 mm
On distal	2.0 mm

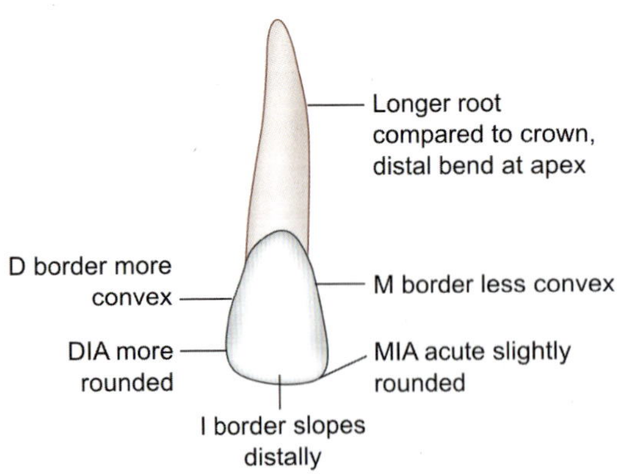

Fig. 25.32: Labial aspect

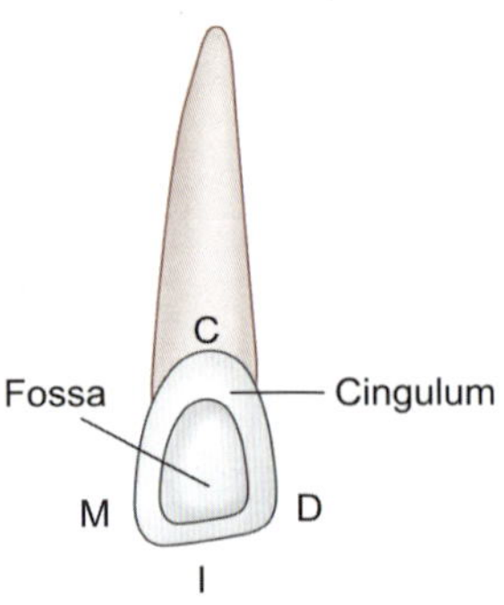

Fig. 25.33: Lingual aspect

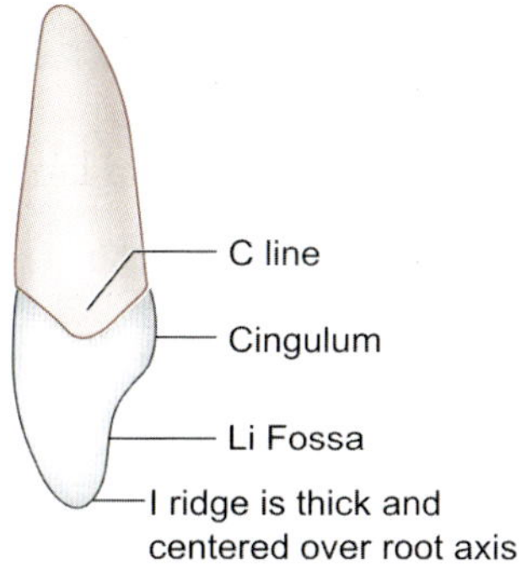

Fig. 25.34: Proximal aspect

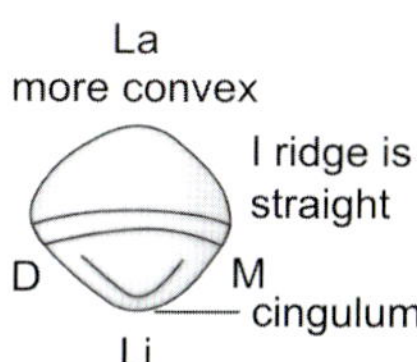

Fig. 25.35: Incisal aspect

CARVING

The method for carving maxillary lateral incisor is same as that of central incisor except for the size and few differences.

- Labial surface is more convex mesiodistally and incisogingivally than central incisor (Fig. 25.36).

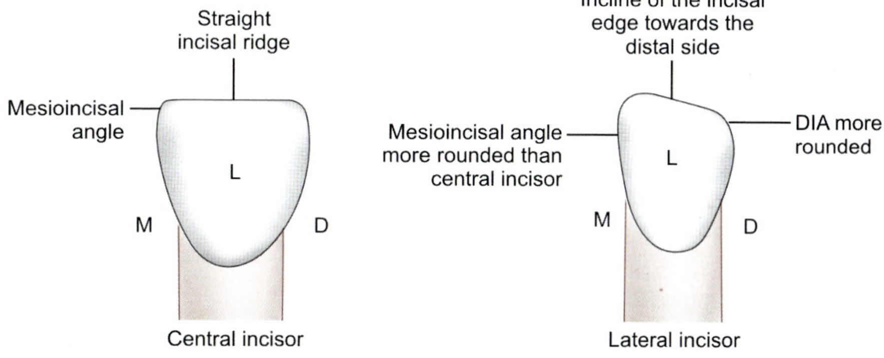

Fig. 25.36

- Mesial and distal marginal ridges and cingulum are relatively more prominent than central incisor.
- Lingual fossa is deeper and usually 'V' shaped.
- Lingual pit near the center is common finding in lateral than central incisor (Fig. 25.37).

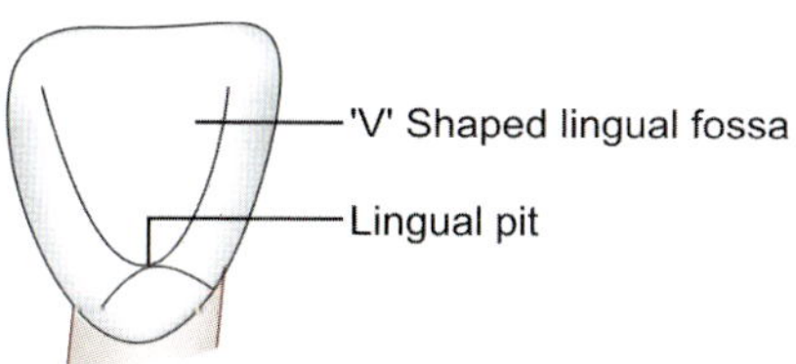

Fig. 25.37

MANDIBULAR INCISORS

MANDIBULAR CENTRAL INCISORS

Palmer Notation

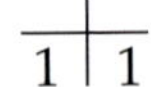

ODONTOMETRIC DATA	
Length of crown	9.0 mm
Length of root	12.5 mm
Mesiodistal width of crown	5.0 mm
Mesiodistal width of crown at cervix	3.5 mm
Labiolingual width of crown	6.0 mm
Labiolingual width at cervix	5.3 mm
Curvature of cervical line on mesial	3.0 mm
On distal	2.0 mm

MANDIBULAR LATERAL INCISORS

Palmer Notation

2 | 2

ODONTOMETRIC DATA	
Length of crown	9.5 mm
Length of root	14.0 mm
Mesiodistal width of crown	5.5 mm
Mesiodistal width of crown at cervix	4.0 mm
Labiolingual width of crown	6.5 mm
Labiolingual width at cervix	5.8 mm
Curvature of cervical line on mesial	3.0 mm
On distal	2.0 mm

MANDIBULAR CENTRAL INCISORS

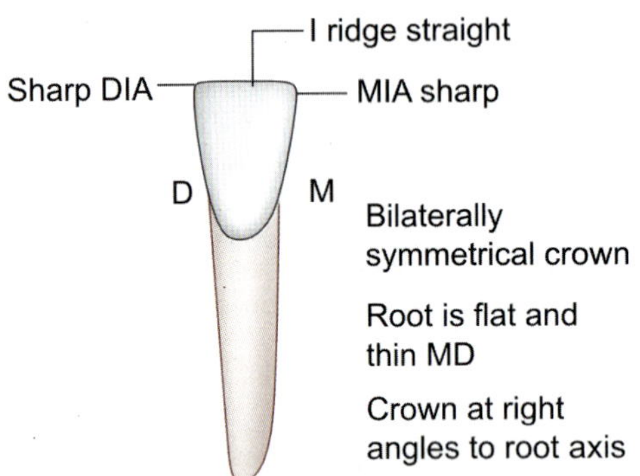

Fig. 25.38: Labial aspect

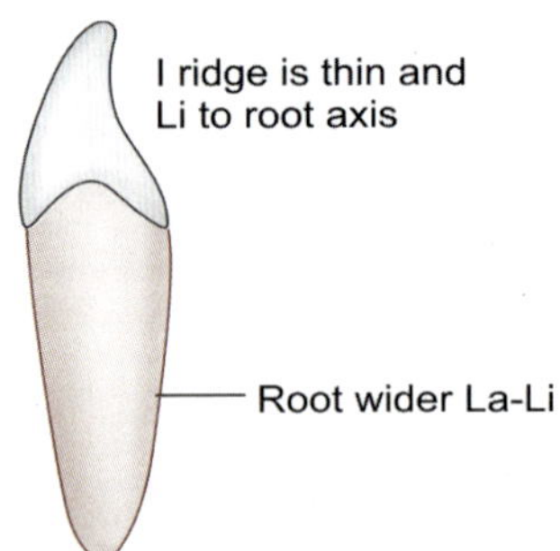

Fig. 25.40: Proximal aspect

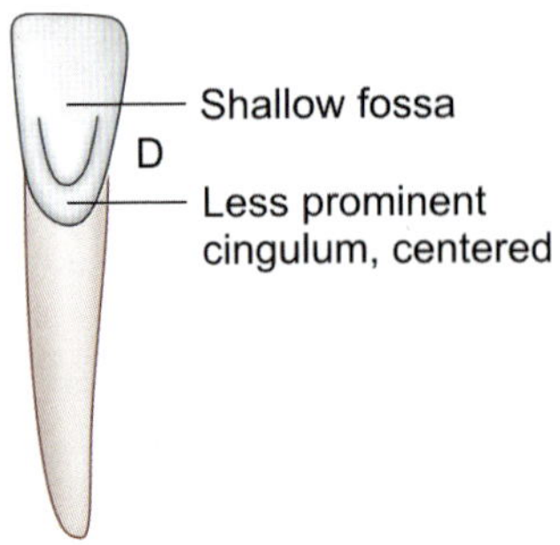

Fig. 25.39: Lingual aspect

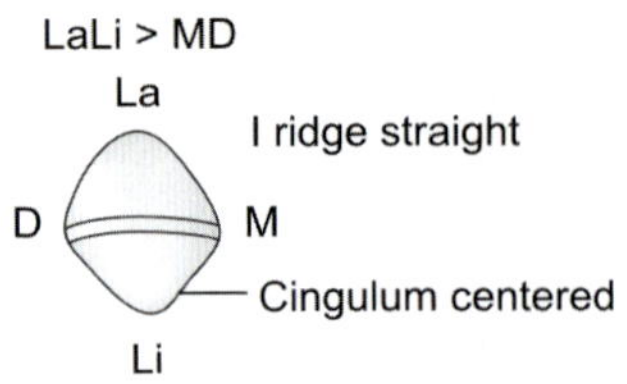

Fig. 25.41: Incisal aspect

MANDIBULAR LATERAL INCISORS

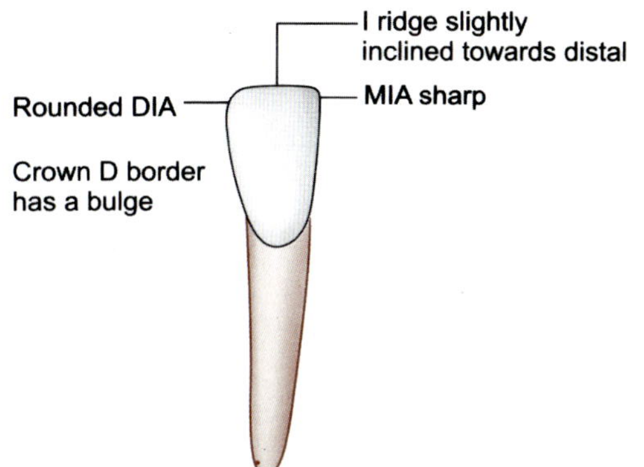

Fig. 25.42: Labial aspect

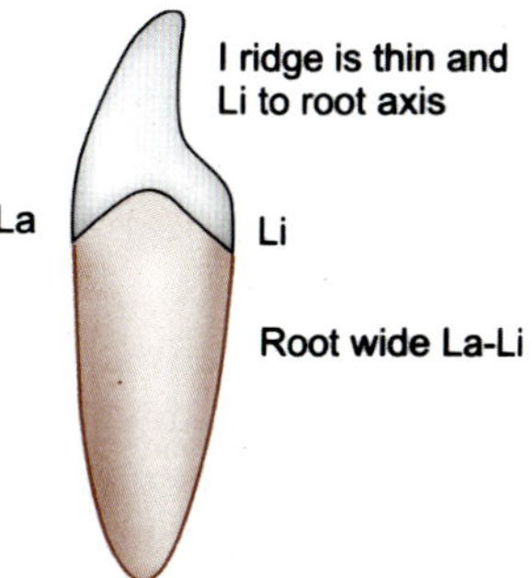

Fig. 25.44: Proximal aspect

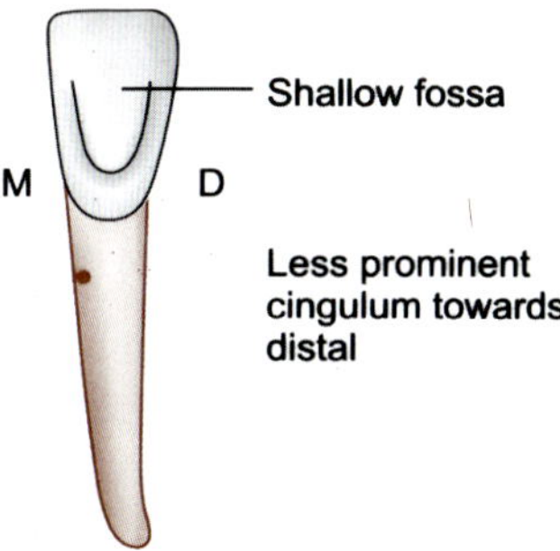

Fig. 25.43: Lingual aspect

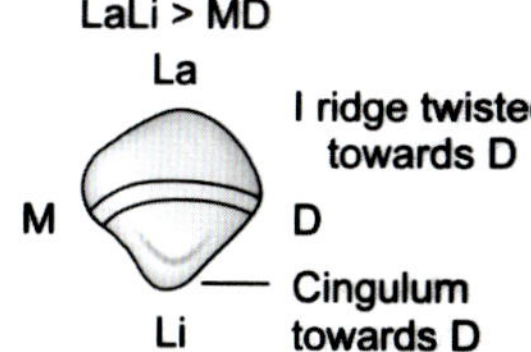

Fig. 25.45: Incisal aspect

CARVING OF MANDIBULAR INCISORS

- Method remains same as maxillary incisors except that the demensions are smaller.
- Incisal ridge (from proximal view) is little lingual to the root axis.
- Roots are flatter mesiodistally you can feel the flatness with your finger and thumb.
- From proximal view both crown and root are wider labiolingually than mesiodistally.
- In maxillary incisors we have reduced the block above the base to 10 mm square on top.
- In mandibular incisor reduce it from all four sides (after marking) so as to get the top surface as square of each side measuring 7 mm.
- Step 2 is different from that of maxillary incisor because the incisal ridge is thin, it is not centered it is slightly lingually placed.
- Since the crown and root are thin, while carving and polishing take care that the root does not break from the base.

  Hold the block (carving) at the cervix and not at the base.
- M and D root surfaces of both incisors have root depressions.

CANINES

CLASS TRAITS

- Canine has a single pointed cusp.
  Incisal ridge of canine is divided into two inclines or slopes by a cusp as opposed to a straight ridge in incisors and therefore gives crown a pentagon shape. The mesial slope is shorter than the distal slope. Canines usually do not have mamelons but have notch on either cusp slope.
- It has a single long, and strong root.
- Canine is the only anterior tooth having labial surface prominently convex in the form of vertical labial ridge.
- Canine is the longest tooth in the mouth.
- Maxillary canine has a functional lingual surface.

CARVING OF MAXILLARY CANINE

PALMER NOTATION

3 | 3

ODONTOMETRIC DATA	
Length of crown	10.0 mm
Length of root	17.0 mm
Mesiodistal width of crown	7.5 mm
Mesiodistal width of crown at cervix	5.5 mm
Labiolingual width of crown	8.0 mm
Labiolingual width at cervix	7.0 mm
Curvature of cervical line on mesial	2.5 mm
On distal	1.5 mm

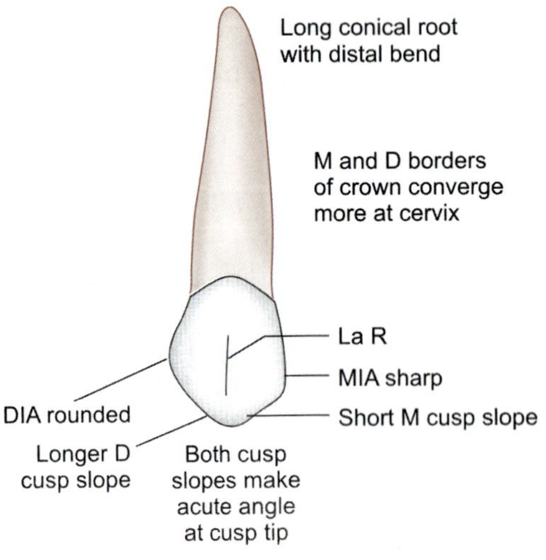

Fig. 25.46 : Labial aspect

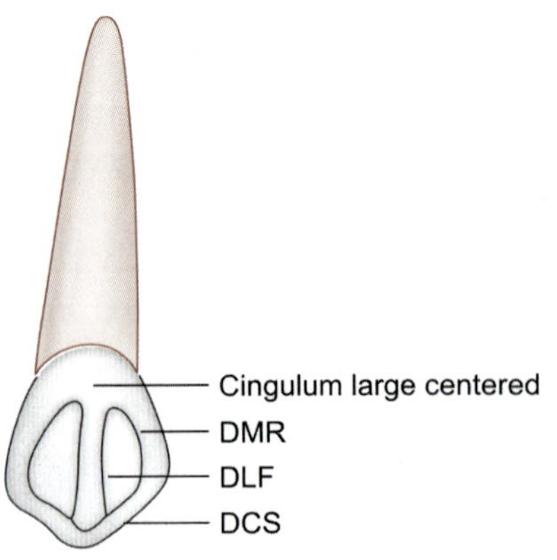

Fig. 25.47: Lingual aspect

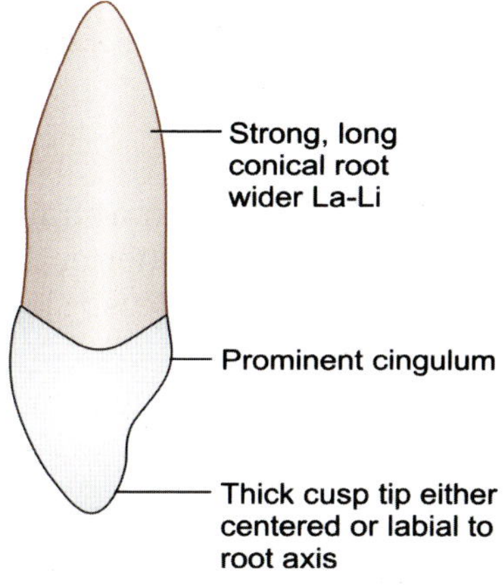

Fig. 25.48: Proximal aspect

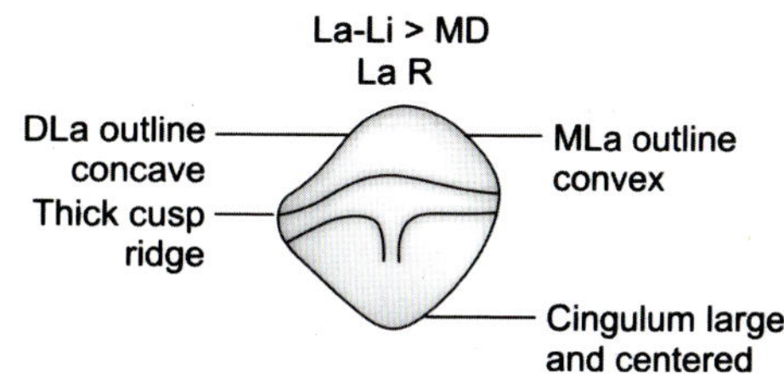

Fig. 25.49: Incisal aspect

STEPS FOR CARVING

STEP 1

THIS STEP IS COMMON TO CANINE, PREMOLAR, AND MOLAR

- Prepare the wax block and divide the wax block in three parts—crown, root, and base.
- Mark initials of each surface as labial, lingual, mesial and distal.
- Each cusp has 4 inclined planes (IP). 2 IP on B/P/la surface and 2 IP on li/occlusal surface (Fig. 1.8 page 8).
- **A cusp can be carved by making a hut-shape that is making two inclined lines meeting at a point and removing wax along the inclines.**

STEP 2 (Fig. 25.50 and 25.51)

- Divide and mark the labial surface of the crown into three parts incisal, middle, and cervical third.
- Divide and mark the incisal/top surface into two halves M and D.

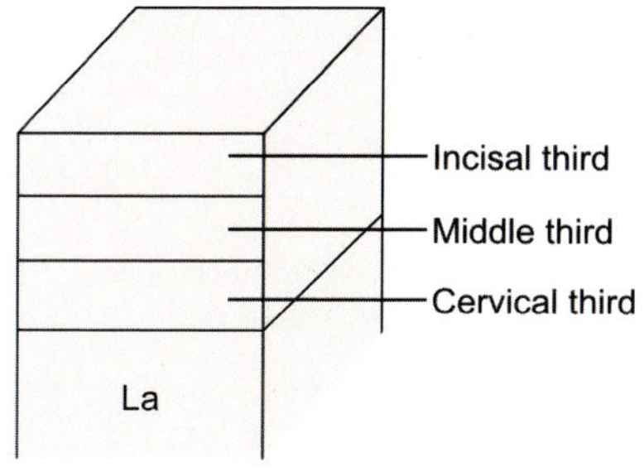

Fig. 25.50

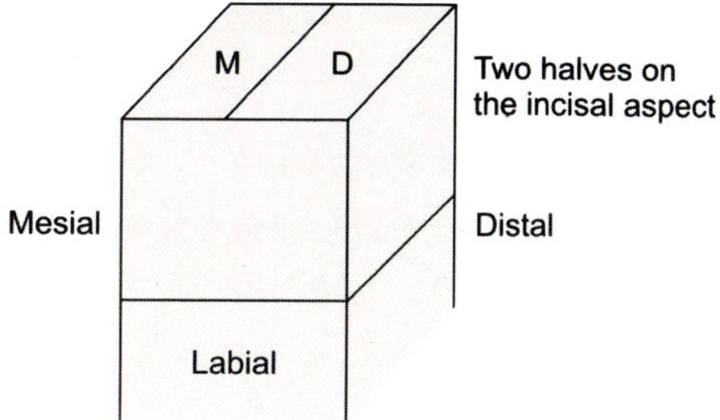

Fig. 25.51

STEP 3

Carving hut shape: (Marking two inclines for the incisal ridge) Fig. 25.52.

On the labial and lingual surface, in the incisal one-third make hut-shaped outline for carving the slopes of the cusp.

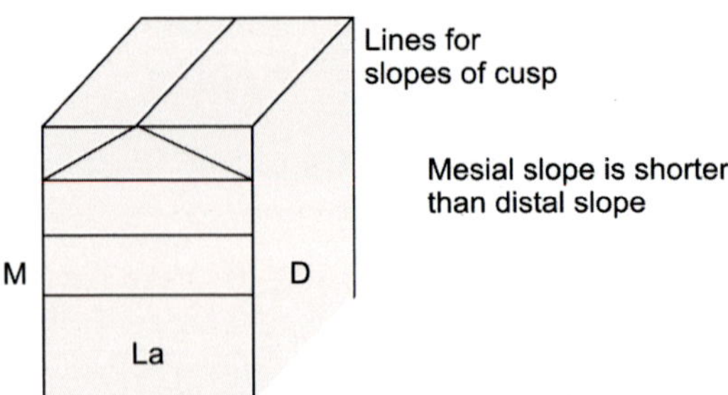

Fig. 25.52

- In maxillary canine mesial slope is shorter than distal slope. **Cusp tip is centered.**
- Remove wax along the hut-shape (Fig. 25.53 and 25.54), i.e. along the mesial and distal slopes of the hut-shape, both towards labial and lingual surfaces.

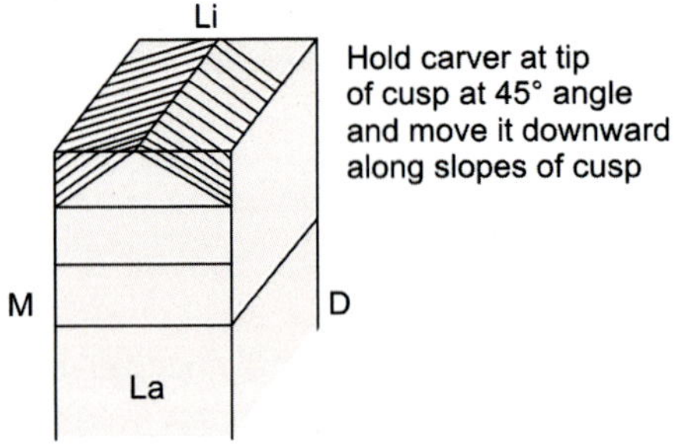

Fig. 25.53

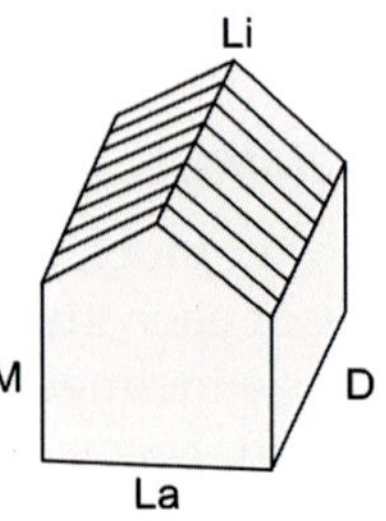

Fig. 25.54

STEP 4

Give cervical constriction to the crown on both labial and lingual surface by carving out wax from mesial and distal surfaces, **only in the cervical third** (Fig. 25.55).

- Method for giving constriction is same as Step 5 in maxillary central incisor including gross carving of root (page 363, Fig. 25.24).

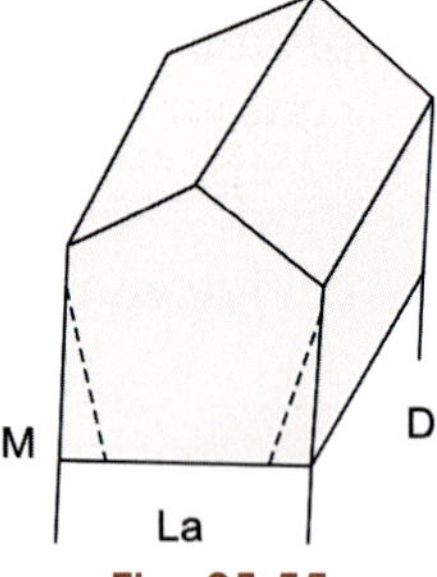

Fig. 25.55

STEP 5

Carving of Labial Surface

Make the labial surface convex so that crest of curvature on labial surface is in cervical third.

Method

1. Before making surfaces convex divide incisal surface, (top surface) into two parts labial and lingual by drawing a midline. Draw two more lines on either side of the midline as in maxillary central incisor to get thick (prominent) cusp tip and cusp ridges (Fig. 25.56).

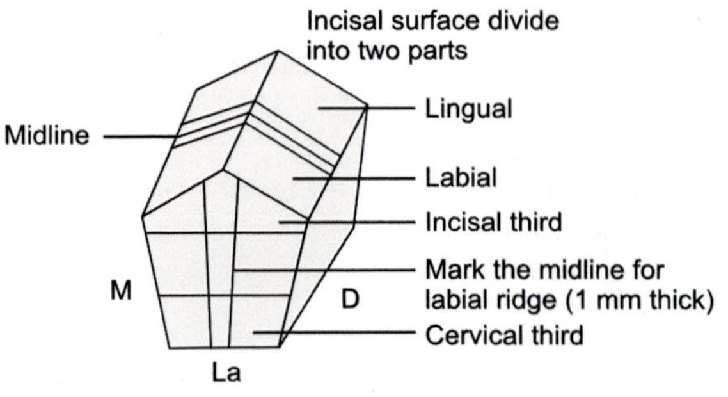

Fig. 25.56

- Purpose of making the midline is, not to cross this line while making labial surface convexity so that the incisal ridge is in the center of the crown, and it is thick when viewed from proximal aspect.

  Carving of labial surface is similar to that of central incisor except that along with making convexity in the cervical third, labial ridge and its inclined planes also need to be carved.

2. Divide the labial surface into 3 parts, incisal, middle, and cervical thirds.

   From the cusp tip to the cervical line draw a midline to carve 1 mm thick labial ridge (Fig. 25.57).

   While carving the labial surface carve only the incisal two-thirds of the labial surface of the crown on either side of the labial ridge.

   This step will give you a very prominent labial ridge and 2 inclined planes on either side of it.

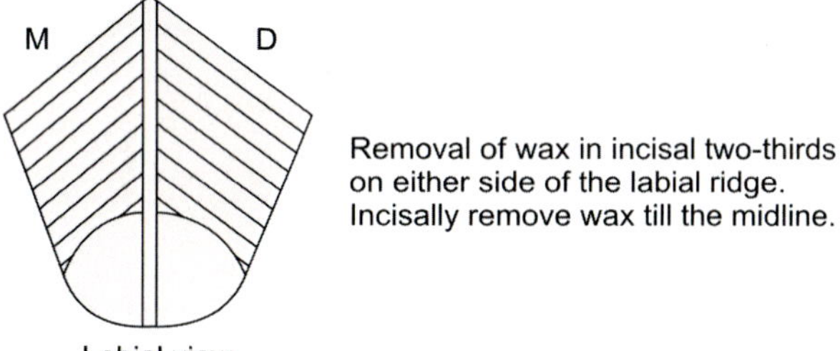

Fig. 25.57

- Merge the incisal two-thirds and the cervical third make the labial ridge less prominent in the incisal third, then merge it with cervical third.

3. When viewed from proximal, the labial ridge is less prominent in incisal third, more prominent in middle third and then merges with cervical third. You can see the height of contour in the cervical third (Fig. 25.58).

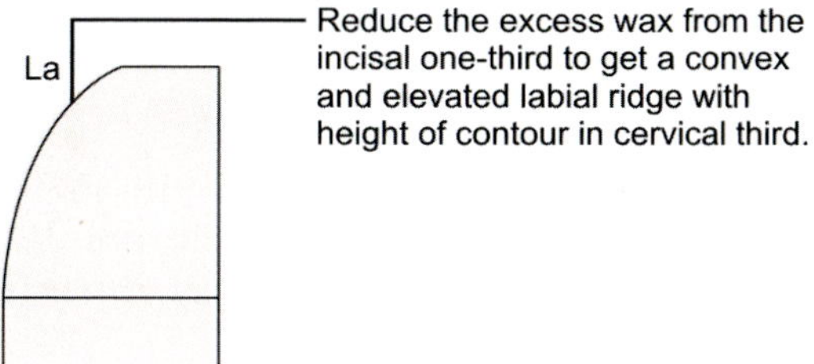

Fig. 25.58

4. Make mesioincisal sharp and distoincisal angles slightly rounded. Make the distal slope longer so that it extends to middle third of the labial surface and make distoincisal angle more rounded (Fig. 25.59).

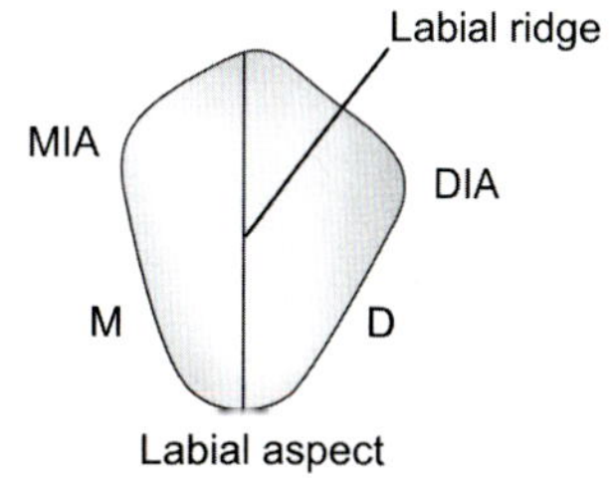

Fig. 25.59

STEP 6

Carving of Lingual Fossa

Method

1. Divide the lingual/palatal surface in three parts: (Figs 25.60A and B)
   a. Incisal third
   b. Middle third
   c. Cervical third

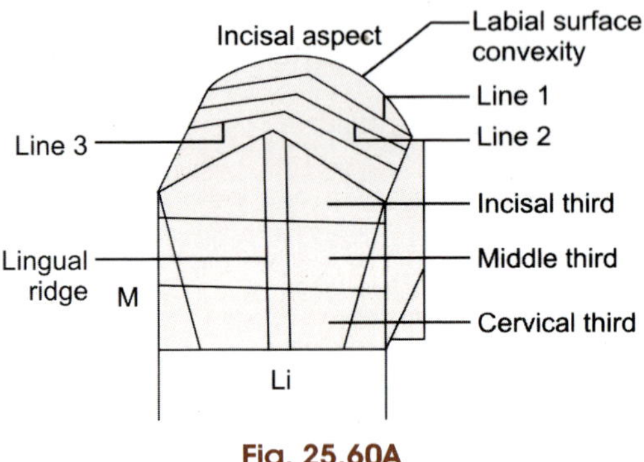

Fig. 25.60A

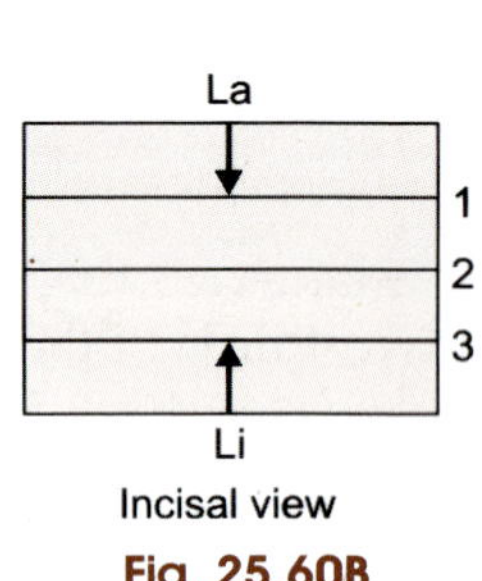

Fig. 25.60B

2. Define cervical constriction on lingual side from M and D (Fig. 25.61).

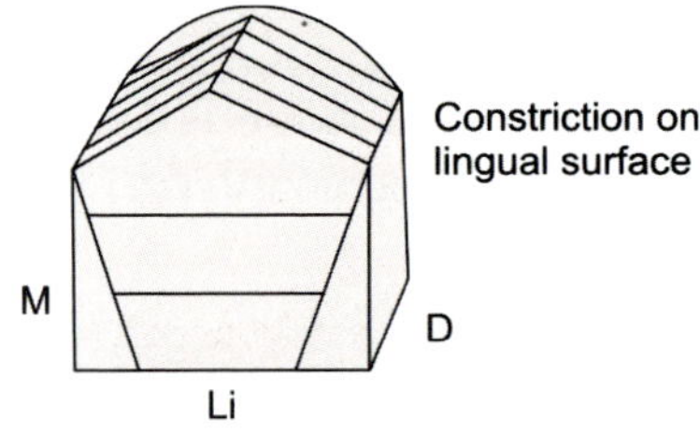

Fig. 25.61

3. After giving constrictions on lingual surface, carve out shallow concavity (as in central incisor) above the cervical line in the middle-third till the line 3 on the incisal surface (25.60B) so that when you view the crown from proximal apect, it has S-shape (Fig. 25.62).

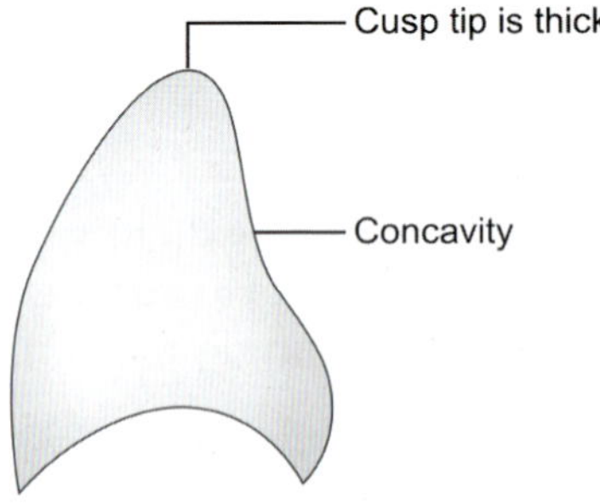

Fig. 25.62

This is gross reduction of lingual surface to make concavity.

Make this concavity in such a way that labial and lingual cusp tips and cusp ridges come closer and thickness of 1 mm is maintained (Fig. 25.60b).

At this step give roundedness to the cingulum as in maxillary central incisor.

- Before carving lingual fossae and lingual ridge further, reduce the labiolingual dimension maintaining the height of contour and proper measurements.
- Reduce the MD dimension as per the required measurement by reducing the M border of the crown by moving the carver from cervix to the sharp mesioincisal angle (MIA). Reduce the D border by moving the carver from rounded distoincisal angle (DIA) to the cervix.
- At this step carve the **root** on M and D so that at cervix both crown and root are in same plane. Gross carving of root is already done in step 4.
- Carve crown and root both more narrow towards lingual.

Carving of Lingual Fossae

- Finally, make two lingual fossae into the concavity already made in the incisal two-thirds of the lingual surface.
- Now for making the two lingual fossae, two marginal ridges and one lingual ridge (Fig. 25.63):
  - Mark one line each parallel to M and D cusp slopes at a distance of 1 mm from the cusp line.
  - Mark 1 line each parallel to M and D marginal borders at a distance of 1 mm from the borders.
  - Mark 2 parallel lines 1 mm apart from cusp tip to the cingulum as in Fig. 25.63.

Fig. 25.63

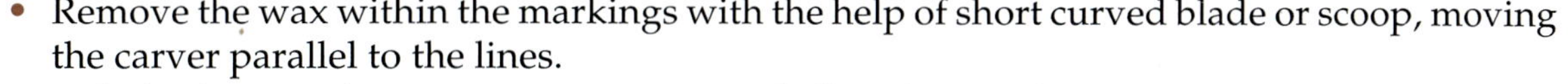

- Remove the wax within the markings with the help of short curved blade or scoop, moving the carver parallel to the lines.
- Rub the fossa with gauze piece, you get 2 shallow lingual fossae.
- Next step is rounding off the cingulum.
- Define the lingual surface. M and D marginal ridges and cusp ridges are raised and are 1 mm thick above the two lingual fossae.
- Carve the lingual ridge in such a way that when viewed proximally it is S-shaped. At cusp tip and incisal third it is raised/thick, in the middle third it is little concave and in the cervical third it merges with cingulum.

  Check the measurements.

  Carve the cervical line with the tip and short curved blade of the carver (Fig. 25.64).

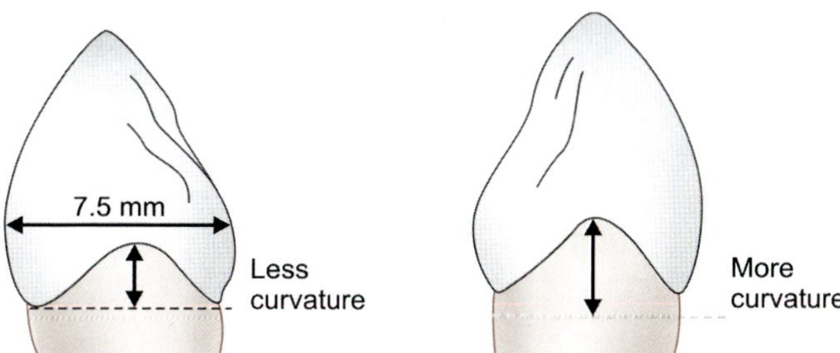

Fig. 25.64

Complete the Carving of Root

In step 4 and 6, gross carving of root is done. Shape the root further in proportion to the crown. Tapering from cervix to apex.

CARVING OF MANDIBULAR CANINE

PALMER NOTATION

$\overline{3|3}$

ODONTOMETRIC DATA	
Length of crown	11.0 mm
Length of root	16.0 mm
Mesiodistal width of crown	7.0 mm
Mesiodistal width of crown at cervix	5.5 mm
Labiolingual width of crown	7.5 mm
Labiolingual width at cervix	7.0 mm
Curvature of cervical line on mesial	2.5 mm
On distal	1.0 mm

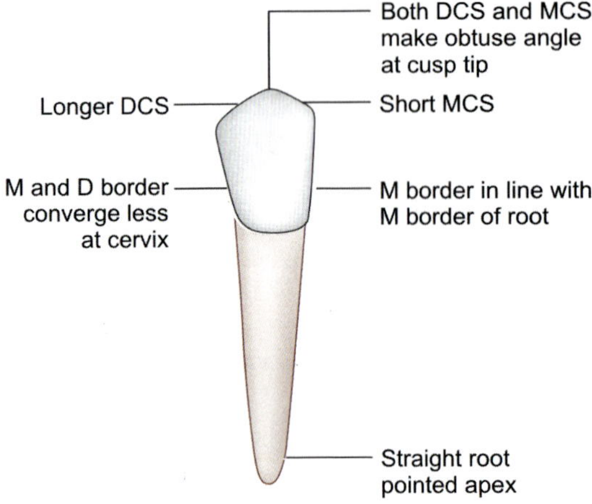

Fig. 25.65: Labial aspect

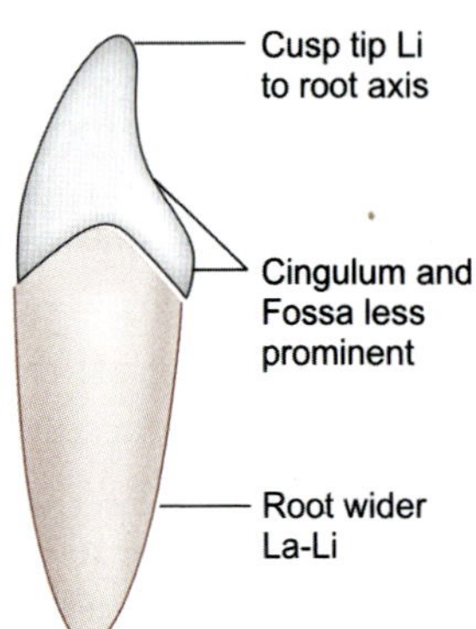

Fig. 25.67: Proximal aspect

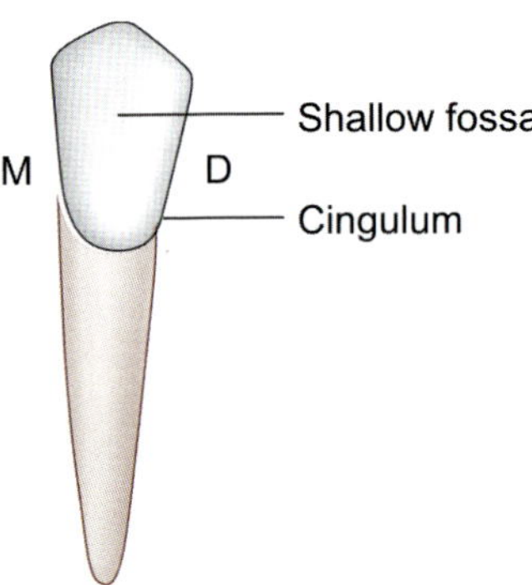

Fig. 25.66: Lingual aspect

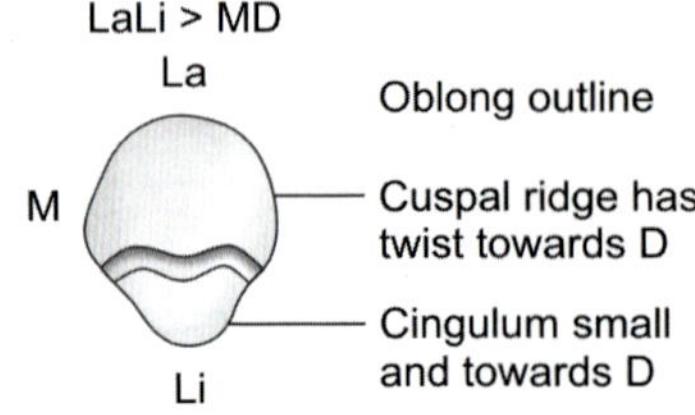

Fig. 25.68: Incisal aspect

The points to be noted during the carving of mandibular canine.

- While making hut-shape make the two slopes less inclined and make obtuse angle.
- Keep the crown length longer.
- MD width of crown is less.
- Constriction at cervix is less.

  M and D borders of the crown are more or less parallel.
- Mesial border of the crown and root are in same plane.
- Lingual ridge, lingual fossa less prominent. Cingulum less prominent and distally placed.
- Lingual inclination of the cusp ridge (as in mandibular incisors).
- Root ends in a pointed apex.

PREMOLARS

CLASS TRAITS

Premolars have a single buccal cusp.

They usually have two cusps one buccal and one lingual and are called bicuspids but the term is a misnomer because mandibular second premolars may have 3 cusps.

They may have one or two roots.

CARVING OF MAXILLARY PREMOLARS

MAXILLARY FIRST PREMOLAR

Palmer Notation

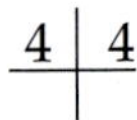
4 | 4

ODONTOMETRIC DATA	
Length of crown	8.5 mm
Length of root	14.0 mm
Mesiodistal width of crown	7.0 mm
Mesiodistal width of crown at cervix	5.0 mm
Labiolingual width of crown	9.0 mm
Labiolingual width at cervix	8.0 mm
Curvature of cervical line on mesial	1.0 mm
On distal	0.0 mm

MAXILLARY SECOND PREMOLAR

Palmer Notation

5 | 5

ODONTOMETRIC DATA	
Length of crown	8.5 mm
Length of root	14.0 mm
Mesiodistal diameter of crown	7.0 mm
Mesiodistal diameter of crown at cervix	5.0 mm
Labiolingual width of crown	9.0 mm
Labiolingual width at cervix	8.0 mm
Curvature of cervical line on mesial	1.0 mm
On distal	0.0 mm

MAXILLARY FIRST PREMOLAR

More angular crown

Buccal root

M and D borders converge more at cervix

BR prominent

Shorter DCS

Long MCS

Sharp cusp tip

Fig. 25.69: Buccal aspect

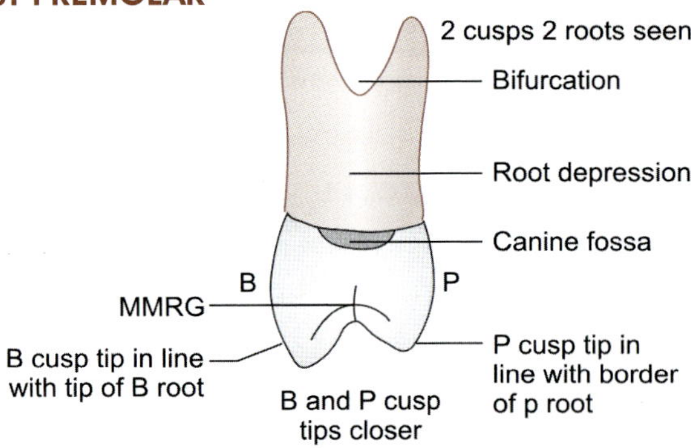

Fig. 25.71: Proximal surface

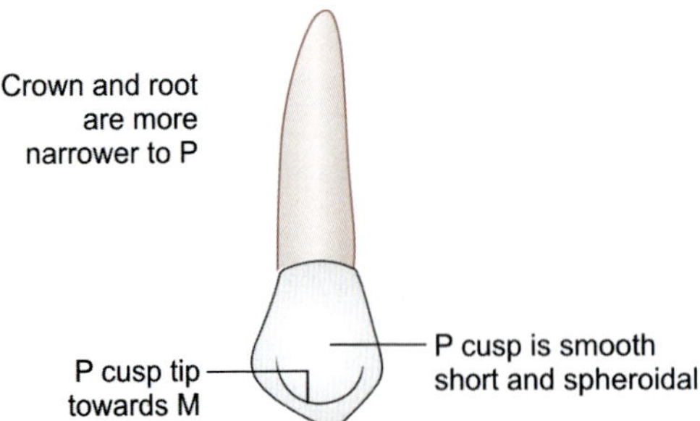

Fig. 25.70: Palatal aspect

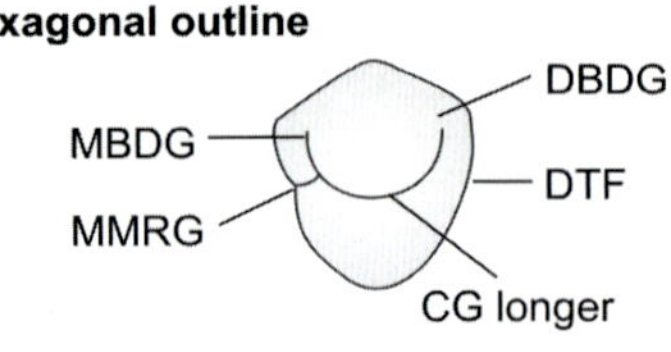

Fig. 25.72: Occlusal outline

MAXILLARY SECOND PREMOLAR

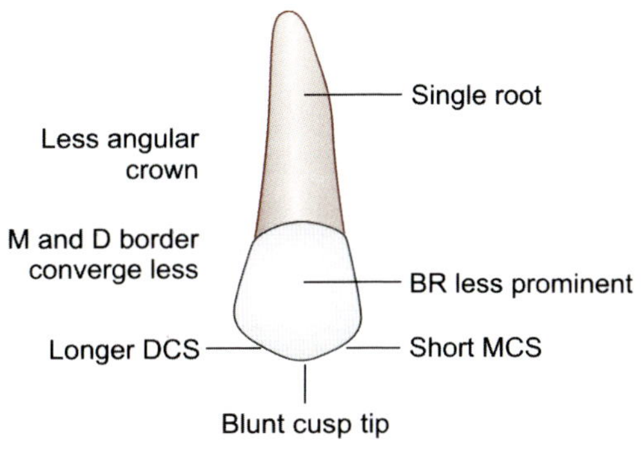

Fig. 25.73: Buccal aspect

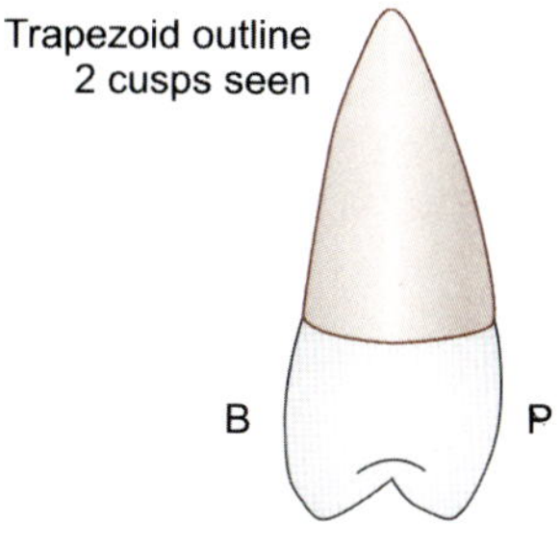

Fig. 25.75: Proximal surface

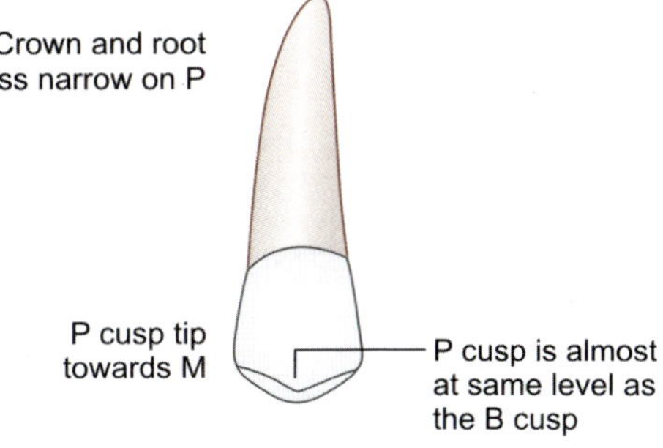

Fig. 25.74: Palatal aspect

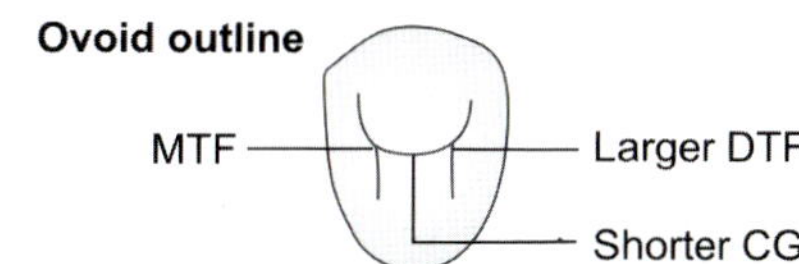

Fig. 25.76: Occlusal outline

Steps for Carving

STEP 1

Preparation of Wax Block

1. Prepare the wax block as described earlier.
2. Divide wax block in three parts.
3. Mark initials on each surface as M, D, B, and palatal (P).

STEP 2

Divide buccal surface of crown into three parts: (Fig. 25.77)

1. Occlusal third
2. Middle third
3. Cervical third

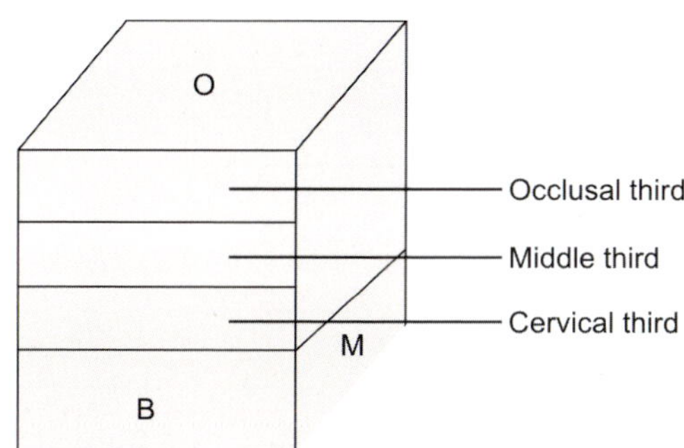

Fig. 25.77

STEP 3

Carve the occlusal surface inclined from buccal to palatal (about 1 mm) and carve it narrow from B to P also.

Proximal view: (Figs 25.78A and B)

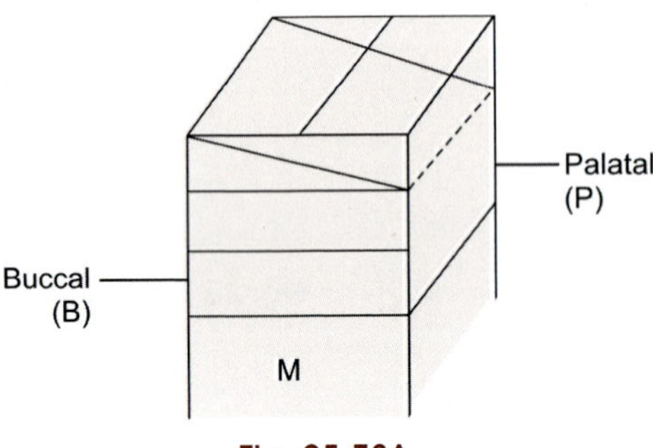

Fig. 25.78A

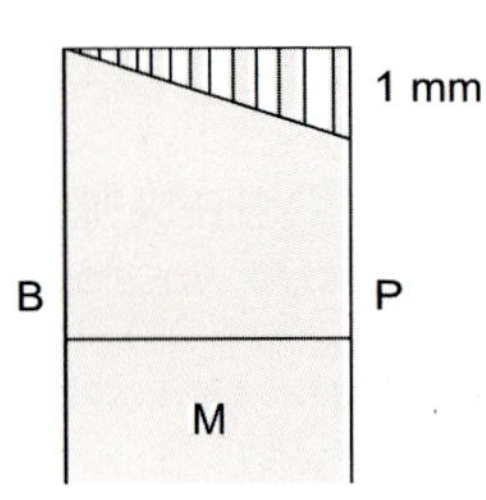

Fig. 25.78B

Occlusal View

Reduce the crown from B to P mesiodistally to narrow it towards palatal (Figs 25.79A and B).

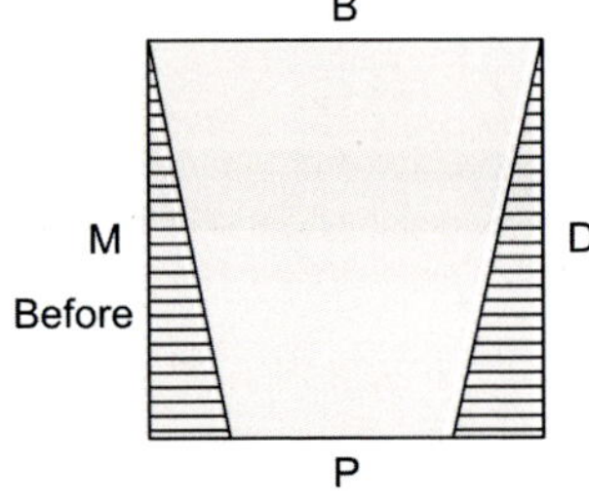

Fig. 25.79A

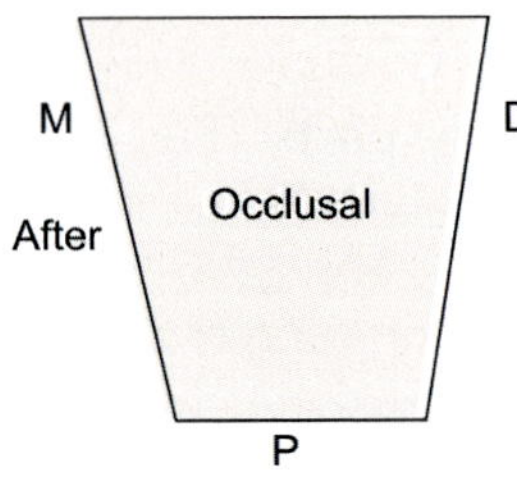

Fig. 25.79B

STEP 4

Making Inclines on Occlusal Surface

- Mark hut-shape, 2 inclines in the occlusal third of buccal surface and palatal surface (Figs 25.80A and B).

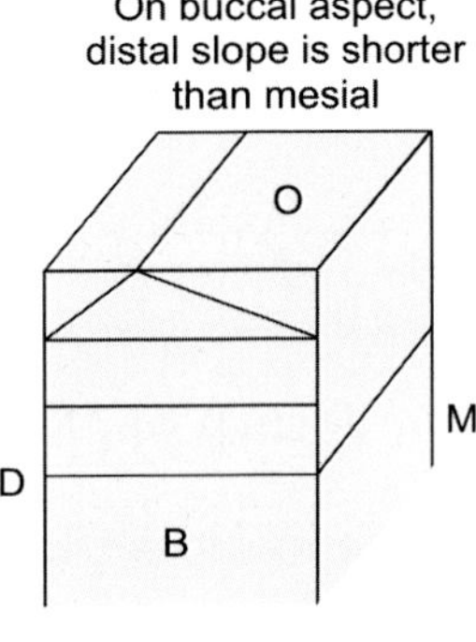

Fig. 25.80A

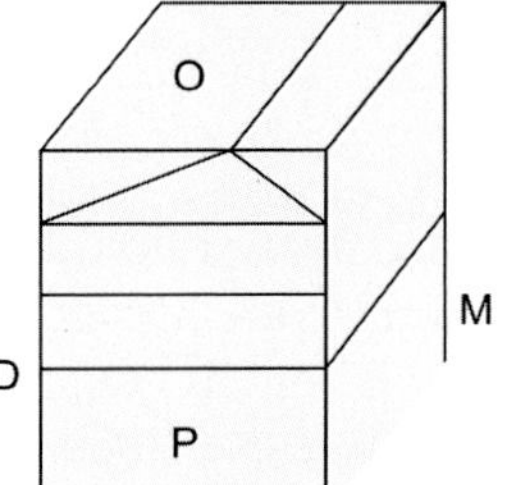

Fig. 25.80B

- On the occlusal surface, carve along the marked inclined lines from B to P. So as to get two inclined planes (Fig. 25.81).

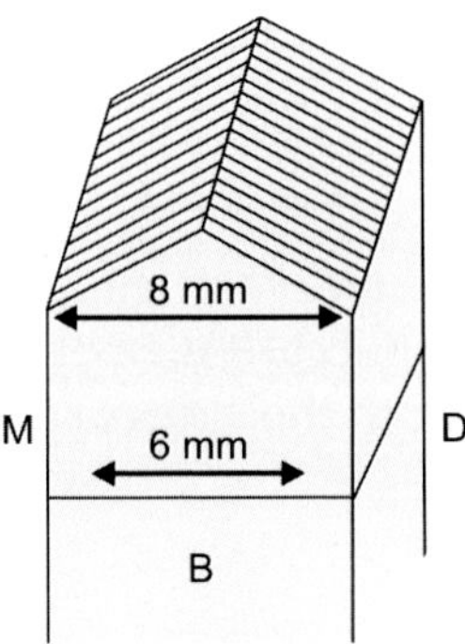

Fig. 25.81

STEP 5

Carving of Mesiodistal Constrictions

On buccal surface and palatal surface in the cervical third give constriction as in canine. So the crown is wider occlusally and narrower cervically (Fig. 25.82).

Towards palatal side give more constriction.

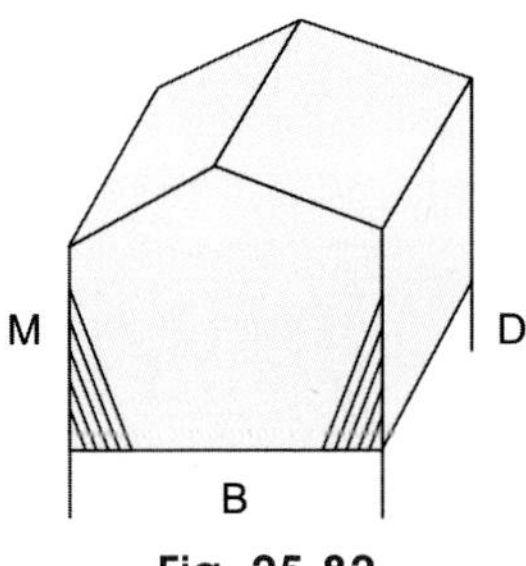

Fig. 25.82

STEP 6

Carving of Buccal and Palatal Surfaces

Method

- Before making surfaces convex divide the occlusal surface into two parts by a midline (c) and then each half into 2 parts.
- On occlusal surface draw two more lines.

Mark line 'a' 1 mm from B cusp tip and line 'b' 1 mm from P cusp tip. Remaining part between line a and b is for carving occlusal table (Fig. 25.83).

Purpose of marking these lines is to give convexities and not to cross these lines while removing the wax from buccal and palatal surfaces.

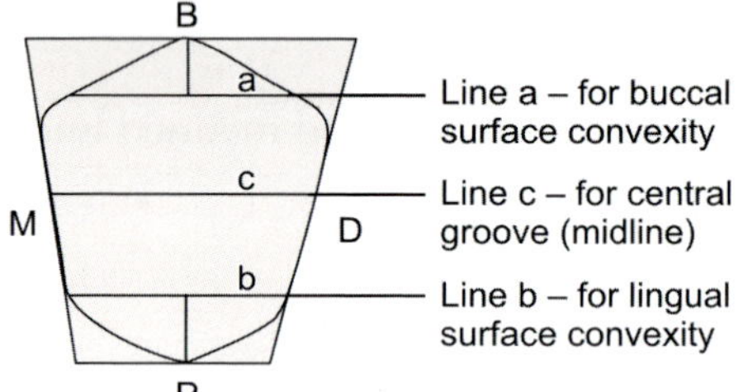

Fig. 25.83

- Carve the buccal surface as you have carved the labial surface of canine but till line **'a'** (only) on the occlusal surface for the buccal convexity. So as to give convexity on the buccal surface in cervical third. Carve on both the sides of the **buccal ridge** (Fig. 25.84).

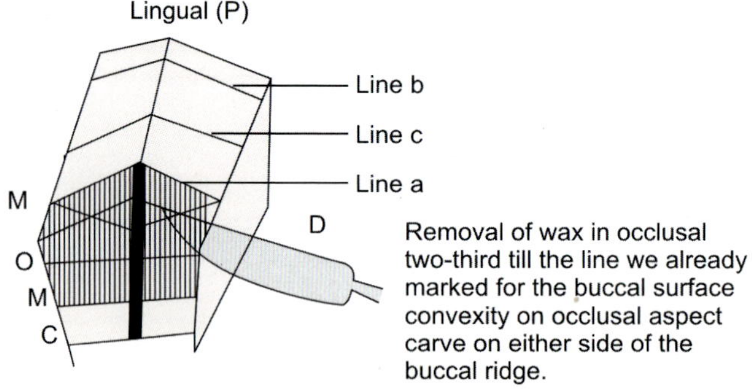

Fig. 25.84

- By using same method, remove wax from occlusal half of palatal surface till line b on occlusal surface (Fig. 25.85).

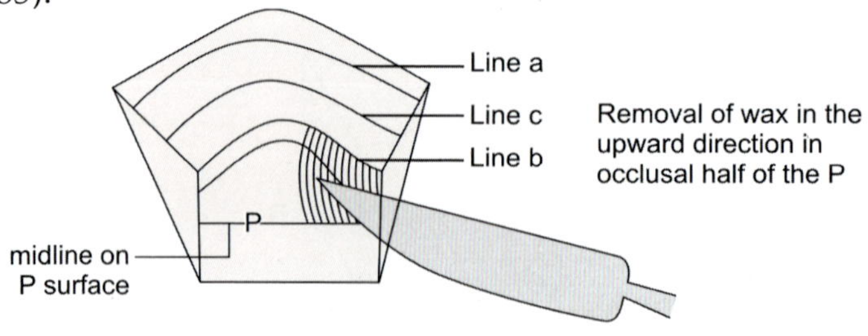

Fig. 25.85

- Since the height of contour on palatal surface is in the middle of the palatal surface, remove little wax from mid of palatal surface to the cervical line.
- Then merge occlusal and cervical half and make the palatal cusp spheroidal.

STEP 7

- Before carving of occlusal surface, check all the dimensions. (Including MD dimension at contact area, cervix, tapering of crown at cervix, and root at apex).
- Mark the cervical line and check the length of the root.
  - Carve the M and D surfaces of the root from cervix to the apex in the same plane .
  - Now rub the entire block with the gauze piece.
  - The carving will appear as in Fig. 25.86.

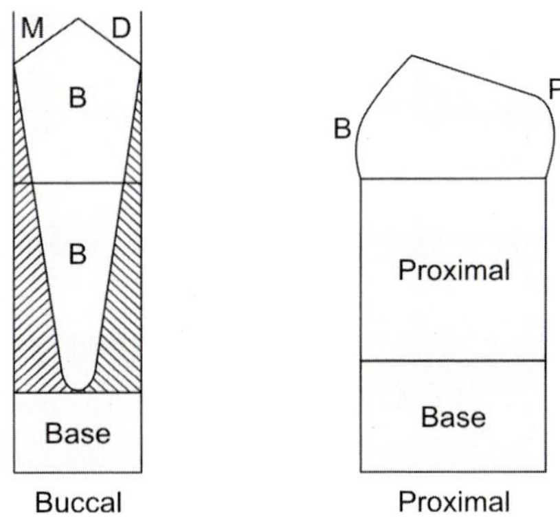

Fig. 25.86

STEP 8

Carving of Occlusal Surface

Redefine the occlusal surface, divide into two equal parts.

Before starting the inclined planes on the occlusal surface mark the outlines for triangular fossa on both mesial and distal side and the central groove (CG) dividing the buccal and palatal halves (Fig. 25.87).

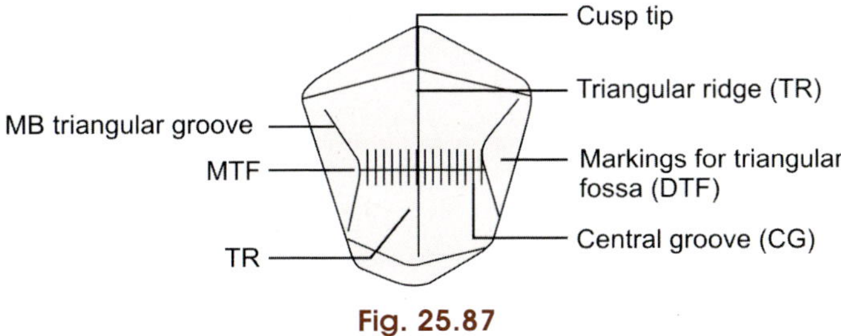

Fig. 25.87

- On either side of the central groove (CG) at shaded areas remove 1 mm wax towards groove (make a V-shaped notch).
- The inclined planes are planes that incline from cusp tip, cusp ridges, and triangular ridges to the triangular fossa marking and to the central groove marking.

- The 2 triangular ridges which form the transverse ridge also incline from cusp tip to the central groove and they are continuous (Fig. 25.88).
- As shown in Fig. 25.88 remove wax along the inclined planes.
- While carving stop at the markings so as to get prominent triangular grooves and the central groove (CG).
- In the marked triangular area remove the wax with the small part of the tip of the carver or scoop to make a triangular fossae MTF and DTF.

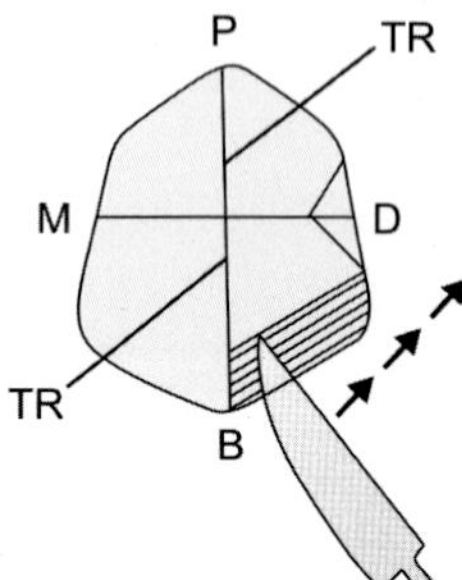

On buccal cusp take small surface area on occlusal surface and move carver from cusp tip to distal surface in downward direction.

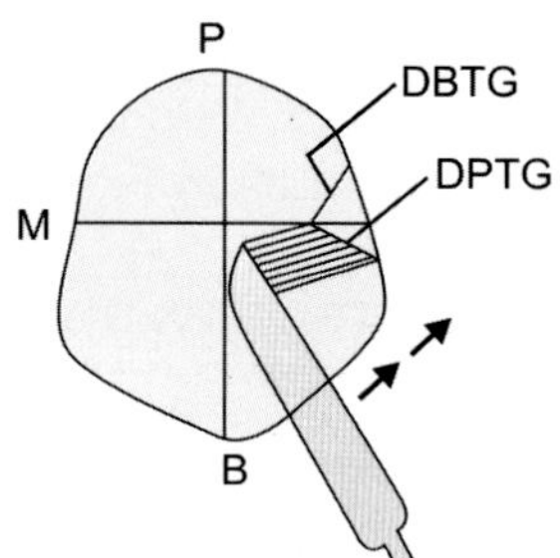

Move carver further to the central line and move in similar manner creating inclined plane and groove, i.e. distobuccal triangular groove DBTG

Fig. 25.88: Occlusal view

While carving inclined planes carve more towards the central groove so as to get prominent triangular ridges which incline towards the central groove from the cusp tips as in Fig. 25.89.

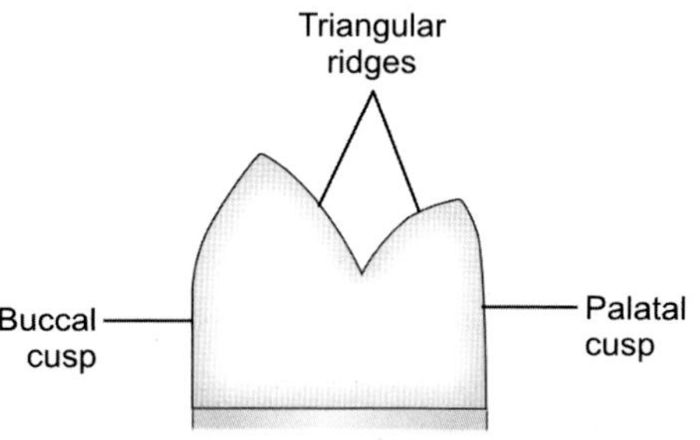

Fig. 25.89: Proximal view

Carving fine Details: (Figs 25.90 and 25.91)

1. Make triangular fossa, pits and groove pattern more defined.
2. ***Mesial marginal groove*:** It is characteristic feature in maxillary first premolar that extends from mesial pit crosses the mesial marginal ridge and reaches onto the mesial surface.

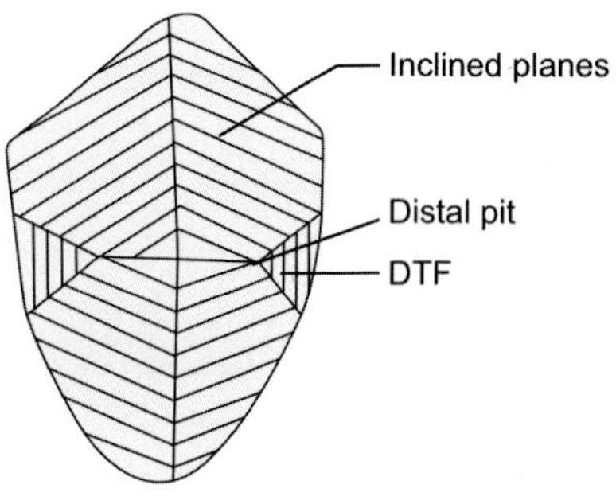

Fig. 25.90

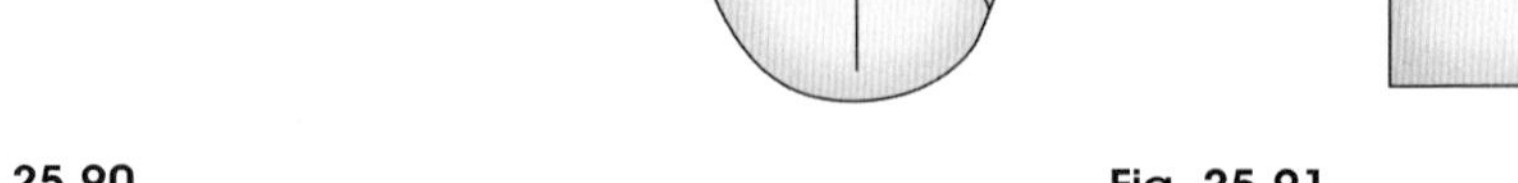

Fig. 25.91

3. Carving of **canine fossa** on the mesial surface, above the cervical line. Scoop out little wax from marked area (Fig. 25.92).

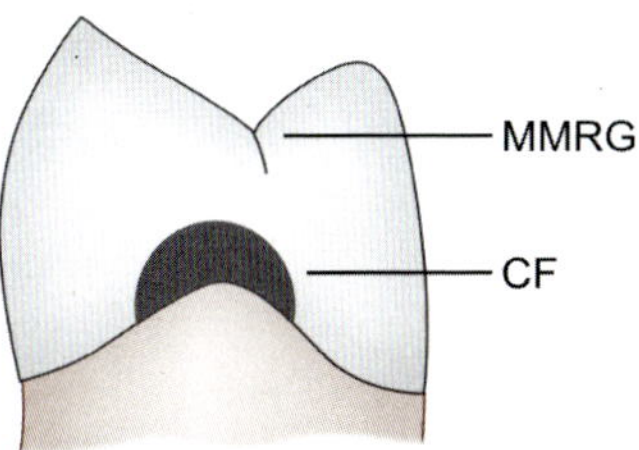

Fig. 25.92: Mesial view

CARVING OF ROOT

- In step 7 we have already done gross carving of root.
- On the proximal surface of the root mark the two curved lines from mid of the root to the apex as shown in Fig. 25.93.
- Remove wax from the shaded part on both M and D surfaces. When the carver passes through and through, clean up the empty area, smooth the margins.
- To clean up pass the rolled up corner of the gauze piece.
- Be gentle, be focused, do not break the root.

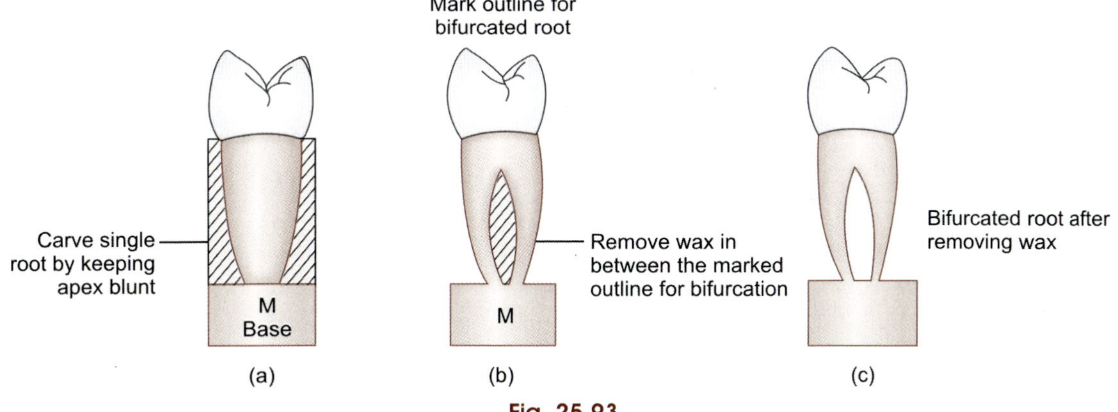

Fig. 25.93

Maxillary Second Premolar

The carving of **maxillary second premolar** is same as that of maxillary first premolar except for a few differences:

- Both the buccal and lingual cusps are at same height.
- Occlusal surface outline is ovoid.
- Buccal cusp is less sharp.
- The root is single.

CARVING OF MANDIBULAR PREMOLARS

MANDIBULAR FIRST PREMOLAR

Palmer Notation

$\overline{4 \mid 4}$

ODONTOMETRIC DATA	
Length of crown	8.5 mm
Length of root	14.0 mm
Mesiodistal width of crown	7.0 mm
Mesiodistal width of crown at cervix	5.0 mm
Labiolingual width of crown	7.5 mm
Labiolingual width at cervix	6.5 mm
Curvature of cervical line on mesial	1.0 mm
On distal	0.0 mm

MANDIBULAR SECOND PREMOLAR

Palmer Notation

$\overline{5 \mid 5}$

ODONTOMETRIC DATA	
Length of crown	8.0 mm
Length of root	14.5 mm
Mesiodistal width of crown	7.0 mm
Mesiodistal width of crown at cervix	5.0 mm
Labiolingual width of crown	8.0 mm
Labiolingual width at cervix	7.0 mm
Curvature of cervical line on mesial	1.0 mm
On distal	0.0 mm

MADIBULAR FIRST PREMOLAR

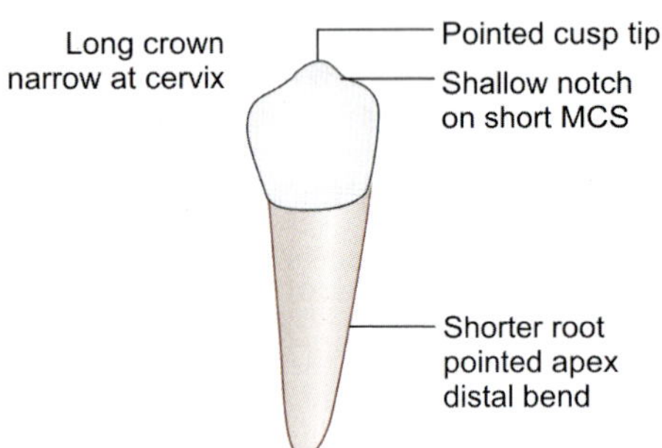

Fig. 25.94: Labial aspect

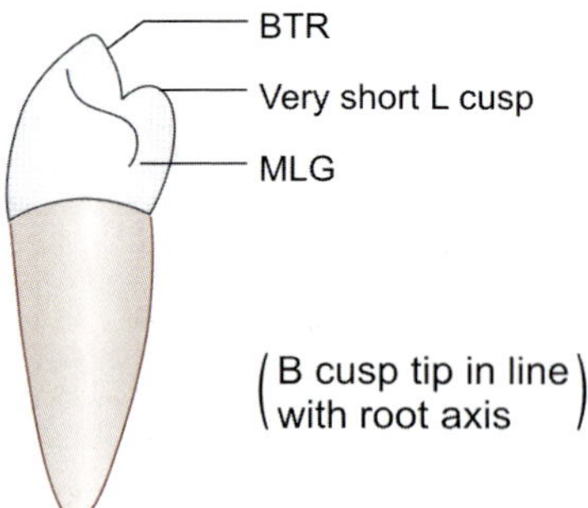

Fig. 25.96: Proximal aspect

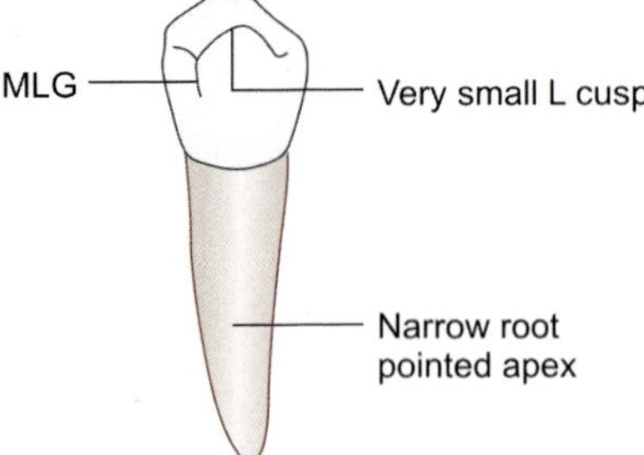

Fig. 25.95: Lingual aspect

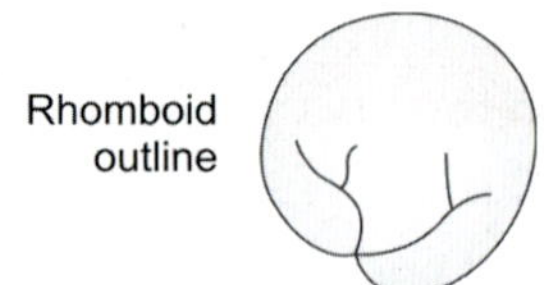

Fig. 25.97: Occlusal aspect

MANDIBULAR SECOND PREMOLAR

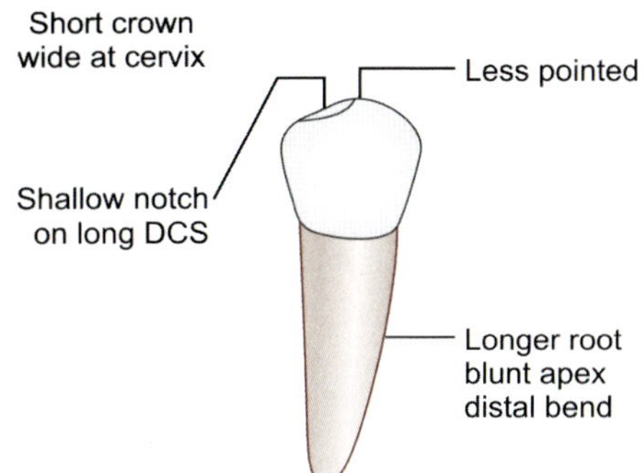

Fig. 25.98: Labial aspect

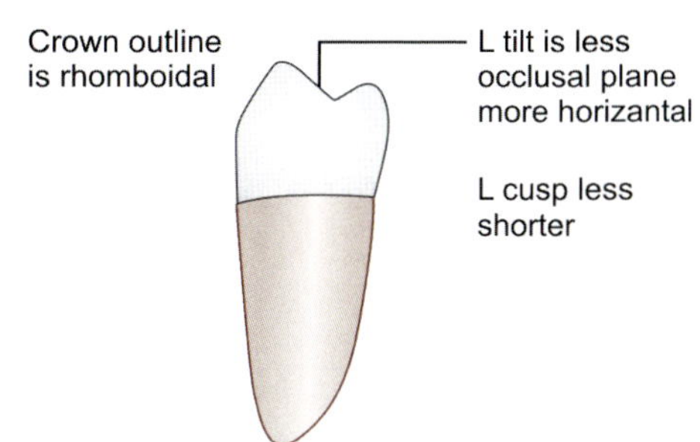

Fig. 25.100: Proximal aspect

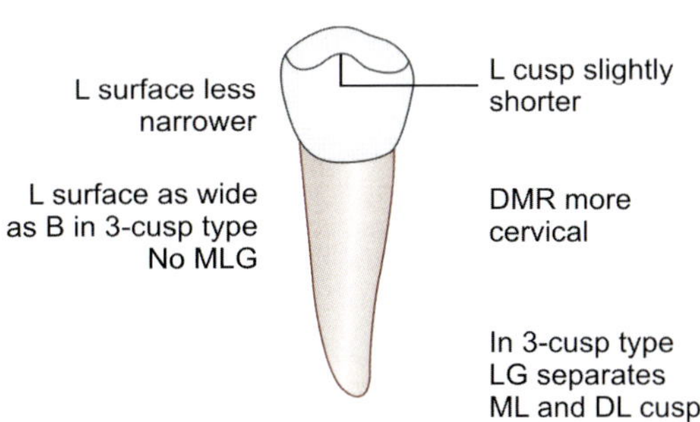

Fig. 25.99: Lingual aspect

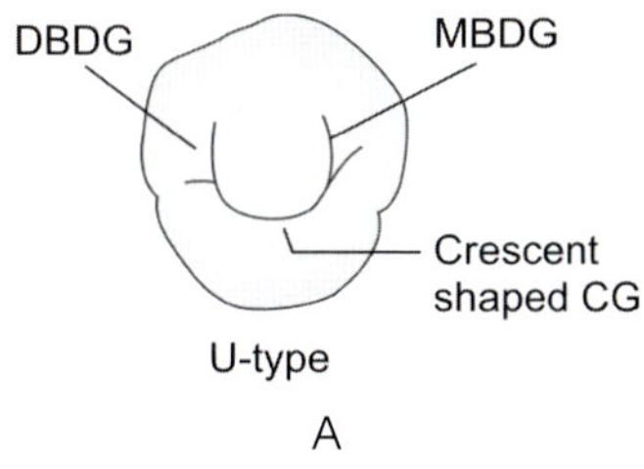

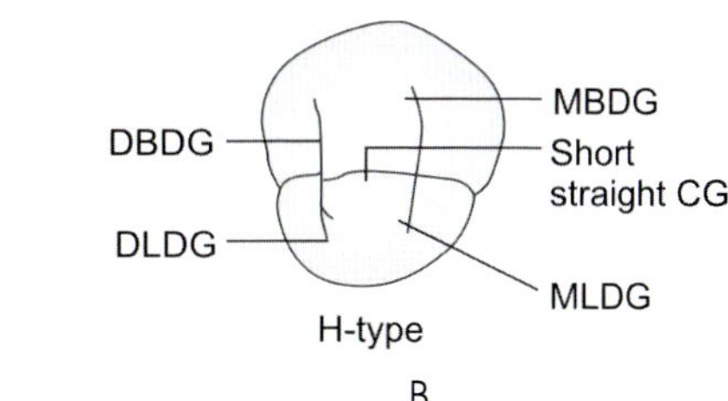

MLG = Mesiolingual groove
BTR = Buccaltriangular ridge
DBDG = Distobuccal developmental groove
MBDG = Mesiobuccal DG groove
MLDG = Mesolingual DG
MG = Mesial groove
DG = Distal groove
CP = Central pit

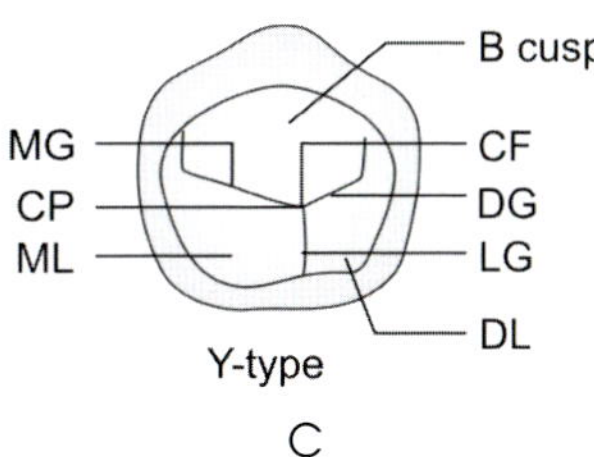

Fig. 25.101: Occlusal aspect

STEPS FOR CARVING OF MANDIBULAR FIRST PREMOLAR

STEP 1

First, carve the occlusal surface. From buccal to lingual make a slope also make the lingual side narrower (Fig. 25.102) (same as in maxillary first premolar).

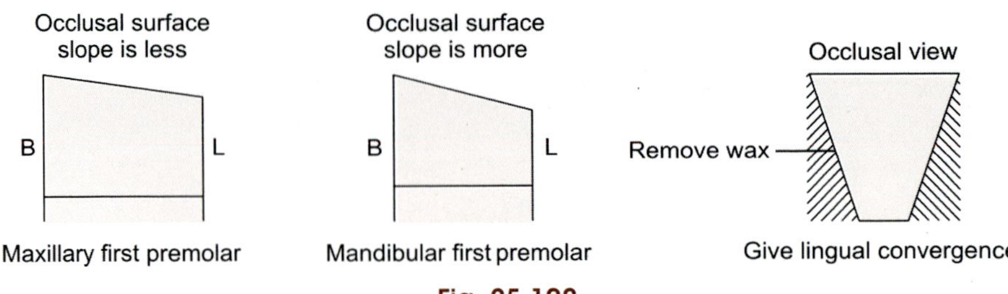

Fig. 25.102

STEP 2

Divide buccal surface into three parts (Fig. 25.103).

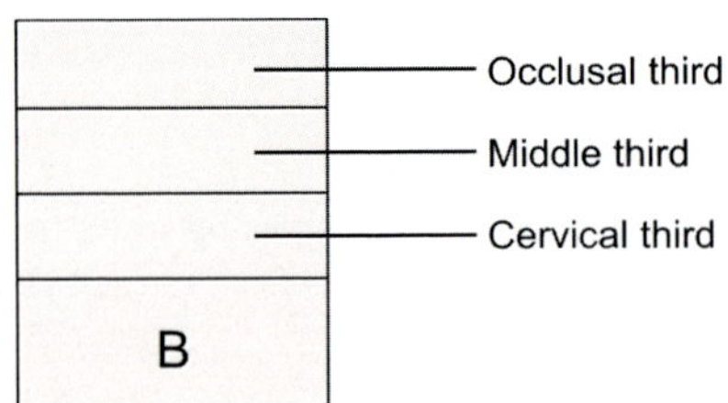

Fig. 25.103

Mark hut-shaped outline in occlusal third on buccal surface (Fig. 25.104). Carve along the hut-shape, give cervical constriction. (Steps are same as in other premolars.)

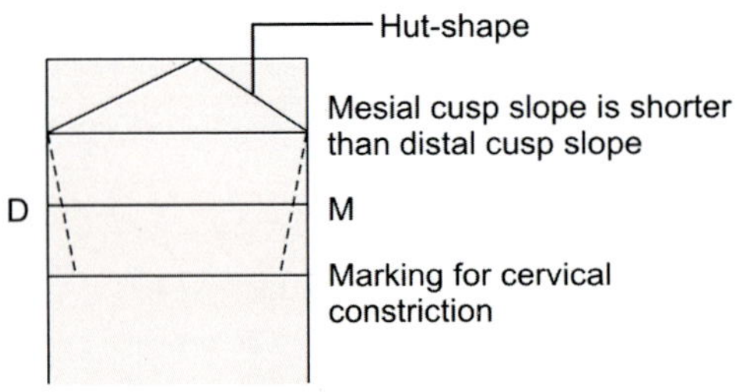

Fig. 25.104

STEP 3

For Carving Buccal Surface

- Divide the occlusal surface into 2 parts by marking a midline.
- Carve out the buccal surface in the occlusal two-thirds on either side of the buccal ridge **till you reach the midline** on the occlusal surface (Fig. 25.105). The result is, the occlusal two-thirds of the buccal surface is inclined towards lingual. You can see the buccal ridge along with both inclined planes (IP) and the buccal cusp tip, the M and D cusp slopes in the centre of occlusal surface (Figs 25.106 and 107).

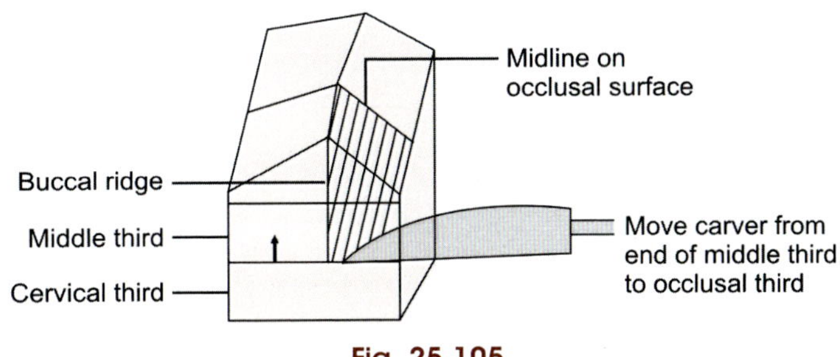

Fig. 25.105

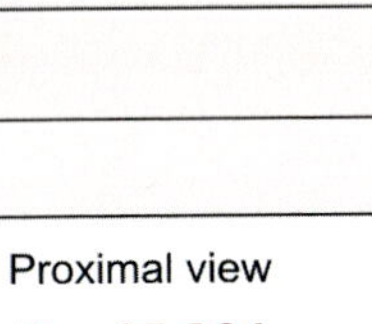

Fig. 25.106

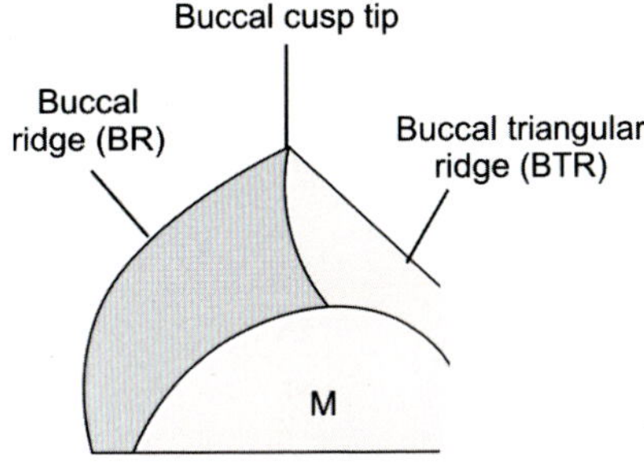

Fig. 25.107

- Define all the above features.
- Now, redefine cervical constriction on the buccal surface by reducing wax from the mesioincisal angle to the cervix and distoincisal angle (MIA and DIA) to the cervix. While giving constriction to the crown grossly carve the root, thus making it taper from cervix to apex (Fig. 25.108).

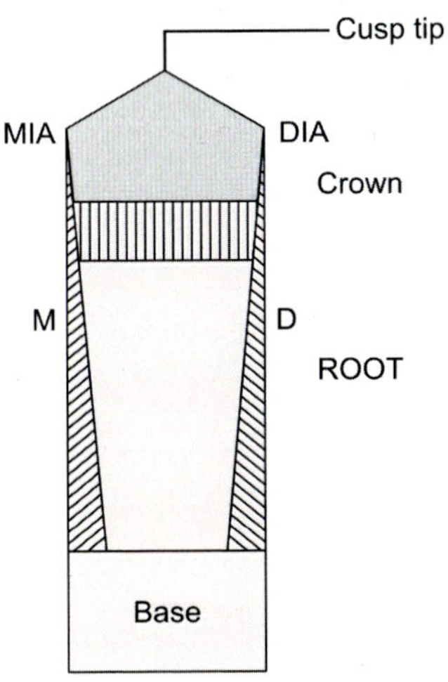

Fig. 25.108

STEP 4

Occlusal Surface

Occlusal surface has pentagon shape with mesial and distal cusp ridges, M and D borders and one narrow and rounded lingual side (Fig. 25.109).

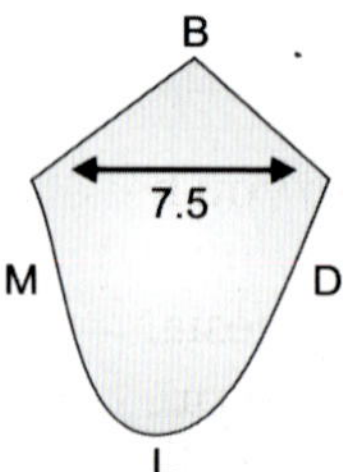

Fig. 25.109

- Now, divide the occlusal surface into 2 unequal parts the buccal two-thirds and lingual one-third and mark the triangular fossa (Fig. 25.110).

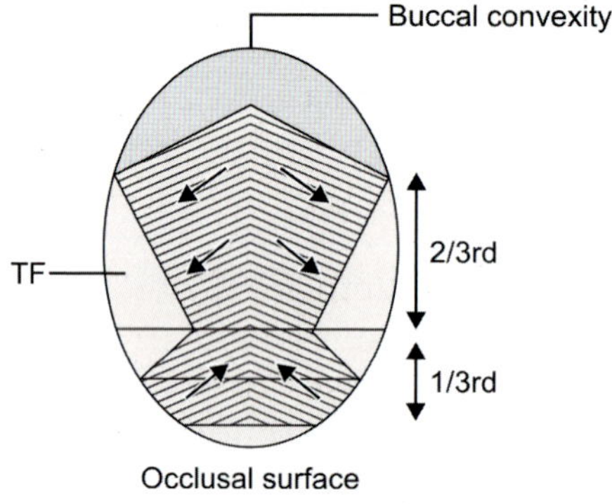

Fig. 25.110

- In the buccal two-thirds part carve two inclined planes on either side of the long prominent buccal triangular ridge (BTR) as you have carved in maxillary first premolar while doing so define the triangular fossae, marginal ridges, mesial, and distal pits.
- On the remaining one-third of the occlusal surface carve the lingual cusp tip with short and straight lingual triangular ridge and the cusp slopes and inclined planes.
- Mark the mesiolingual groove (MLG) from the mesial pit on to the lingual surface (Fig. 25.111).

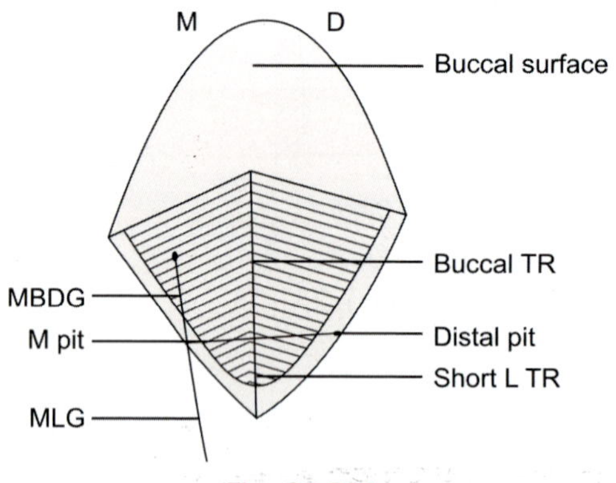

Fig. 25.111

STEP 5

Lingual Surface

- Carve the lingual surface spheroidal as you have carved for maxillary first premolar. Make the lingual cusp tip pointed.
- Define the MLG by carving both from mesial and lingual surface **towards the groove.**
- Define all the features. In mandibular first premolar the MMR is not horizontal, it is inclined and parallel to the buccal triangular ridge, therefore carve to make it inclined.
- Complete the root carving as done in other teeth.
- Carve the MMR inclined so that it is parallel to the long prominent buccal triangular ridge.
- Distal marginal ridge is horizontal and more occlusal.
- Complete the root as described before.

CARVING OF MANDIBULAR SECOND PREMOLAR

Buccal cusp of mandibular second premolar has less inclination towards lingual as compared to mandibular first premolar.

Based on groove pattern there are three types of occlusal surfaces in mandibular second premolar.

- In **3-cusp type** premolar the groove pattern is Y-shaped.
  - Occlusal outline is more or less square.
  - There is one buccal cusp which is largest. There are two lingual cusps the mesiolingual cusp is larger than distolingual cusp.

Buccal cusp highest, next high is ML and shortest is DL but difference in height is not much, ML and DL are separated by lingual groove (LG).

- In **2-cusp type** premolar the groove pattern is U and H type.
  The lingual cusp is slightly narrower and shorter than the buccal cusp.
- In **U-type groove:** The central groove forms crescent shape along with mesiobuccal developmental groove (MBDG) and distobuccal developmental groove (DBDG).
- In **H-type groove:** The central groove is short and forms H-shape along with MBDG and mesiolingual developmental groove (MLDG) and DBDG and distolingual developmental groove (DLDG).

Steps for carving Y-shaped Mandibular Second Premolar

STEP 1

Reduce the block on all sides by 2 mm.

STEP 2

Occlusal Surface

Divide the block on the occlusal surface into two equal parts (Fig. 25.112) by marking the midline.

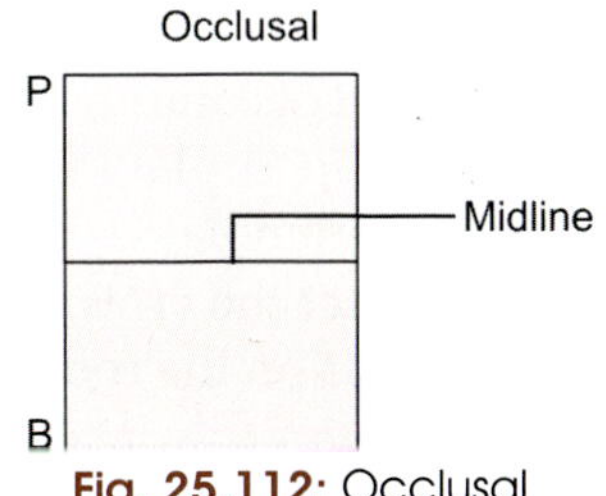

Fig. 25.112: Occlusal view

Do not narrow or slope the block from buccal to lingual.

Divide the buccal half of the occlusal surface into 2 equal parts by marking line 1 (Fig. 25.113). Mark line 2 on lingual half.

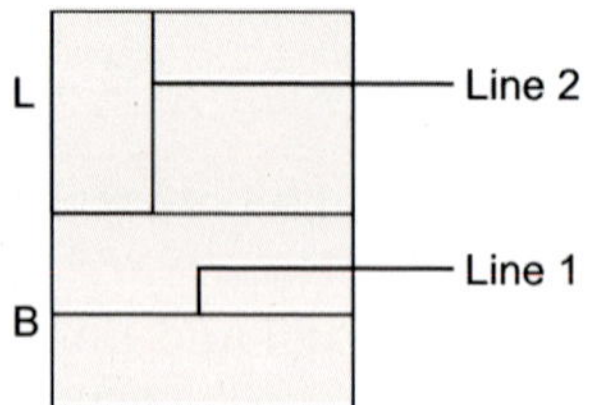

Fig. 25.113: Occlusal surface

STEP 3

Buccal Surface

Make hut-shape on the buccal surface and carve along the inclines and give height of contour by removing wax from the occlusal two-thirds of the buccal surface till the line 1. Complete the buccal surface carving along with root as done in other premolars (Fig. 25.114).

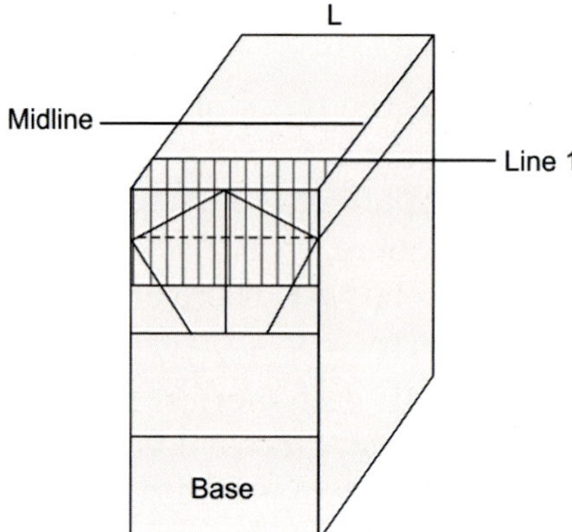

Fig. 25.114: Occlusal surface

STEP 4

Lingual Surface (Fig. 25.115)

Extend the line 2 on to the lingual surface.

Draw two huts on either side of the line. Carve along the slopes of the hut. Extend the IP on the L half of occlusal surface.

The lingual surface has 2 cusps one lingual groove, two lingual ridges, four inclined planes and height of contour in the middle of the crown, carve inclined planes and height of contour as in other premolars.

Constrict the crown in the cervical third and extend this on the root. This step is also same as other teeth.

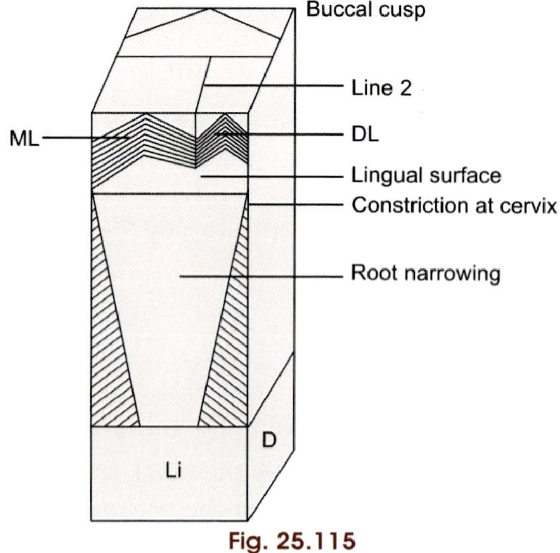

Fig. 25.115

STEP 5

Buccal Half of Occlusal Surface

Mark the triangular fossae and carve buccal cusp along with triangular-ridges and incline planes as carved in other premolars (Fig. 25.116).

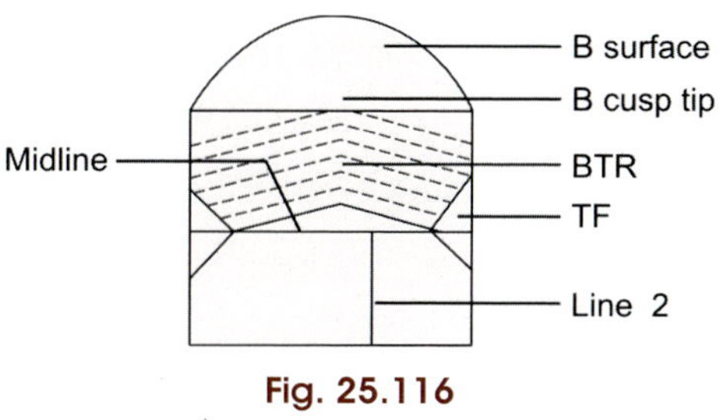

Fig. 25.116

STEP 6

Lingual Half of the Occlusal Surface (Fig. 25.117A)

Carve out the two lingual cusps along with 2 lingual triangular ridges, 4 inclined planes and lingual groove (LG) as you have carved individual cusps in other premolars.

- Define the triangular fossae, M and D pits.
- Define the midline to form 2 grooves. One longer mesial developmental groove (MG) from central pit to MTF and shorter DG from central pit to DTF.
- Redefine the LG
- The 3 grooves together form the Y-type groove pattern (Fig. 25.117A).
- U, H and Y type groove pattern (Fig. 25.117B).

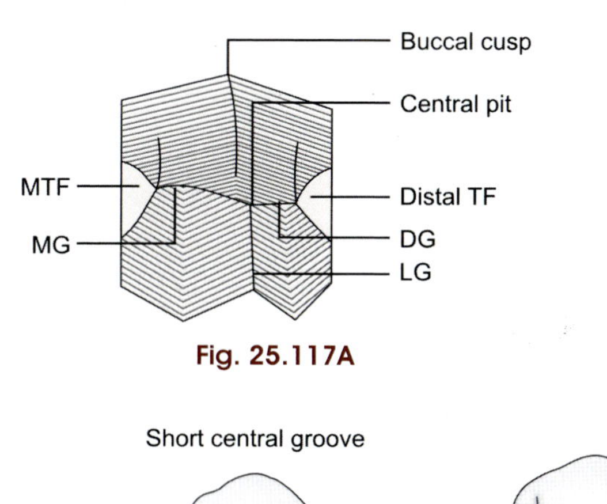

Fig. 25.117A

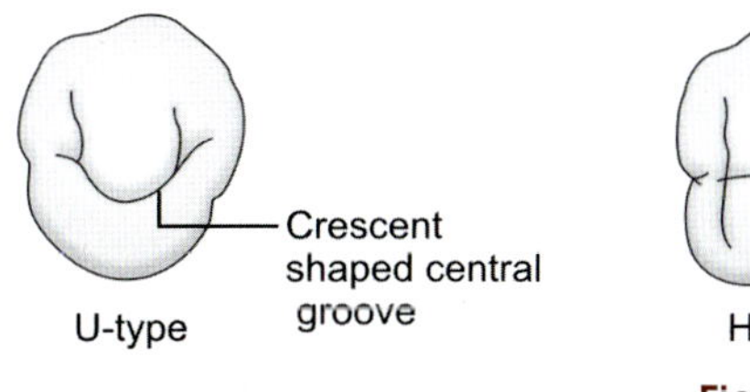

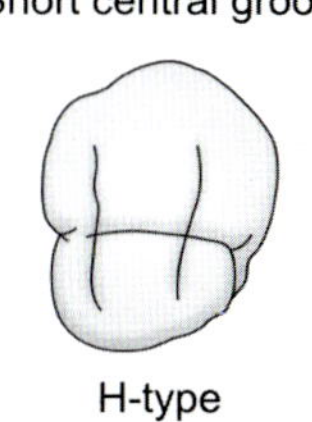

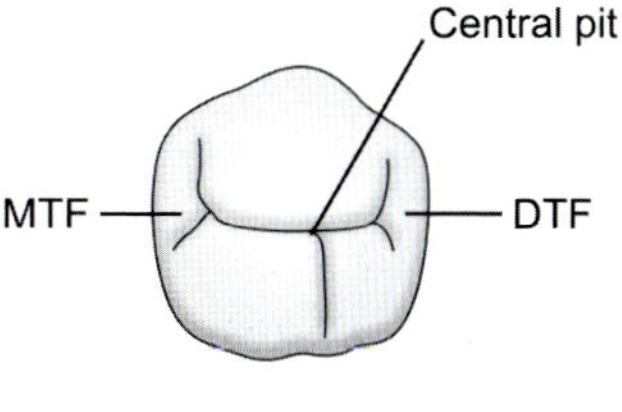

Fig. 25.117B

MOLARS

CLASS TRAITS

- Molars are largest and strongest teeth.
- They have the largest occlusal surface of all the teeth.
- They are the only teeth having two buccal cusps (more than one)
- They have three to five cusps.
- They have two to three roots.

MAXILLARY FIRST MOLAR

Palmer Notation

6 | 6

ODONTOMETRIC DATA	
Length of crown	7.5 mm
Length of root—buccal root	12.0 mm
Length of root—palatal root	13.0 mm
Mesiodistal diameter of crown	10.0 mm
Mesiodistal diameter of crown at cervix	8.0 mm
Buccopalatal diameter of crown	11.0 mm
Buccopalatal diameter at cervix	10.0 mm
Curvature of cervical line on mesial	1.0 mm
On distal	0.0 mm

MAXILLARY SECOND MOLAR

Palmer Notation

7 | 7

ODONTOMETRIC DATA	
Length of crown	7.0 mm
Length of root—buccal root	11.0 mm
Length of root—palatal root	12.0 mm
Mesiodistal diameter of crown	9.0 mm
Mesiodistal diameter of crown at cervix	7.0 mm
Bucco-palatal diameter of crown	11.0 mm
Bucco-palatal diameter at cervix	10.0 mm
Curvature of cervical line on mesial	1.0 mm
On distal	0.0 mm

MAXILLARY FIRST MOLAR

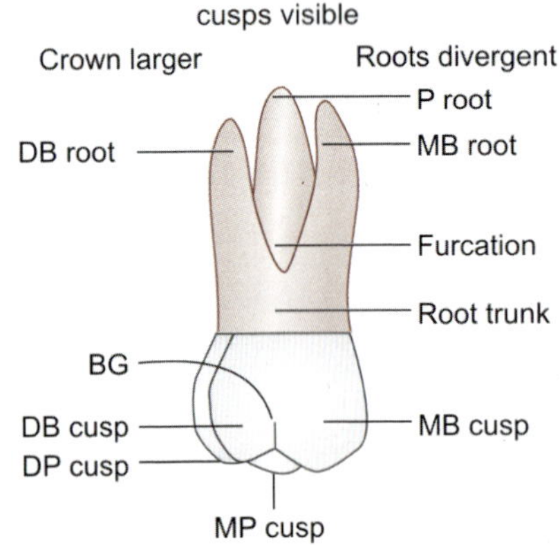

Fig. 25.118: Buccal aspect

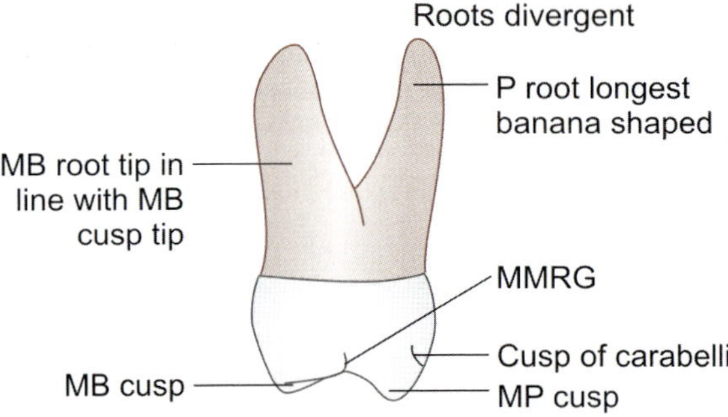

Fig. 25.120: Proximal aspect

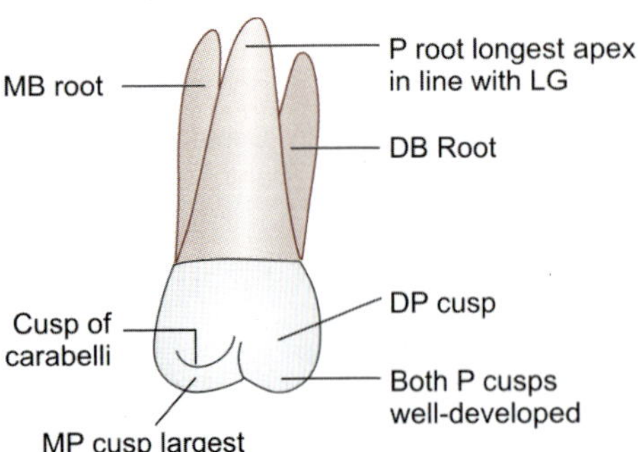

Fig. 25.119: Palatal aspect

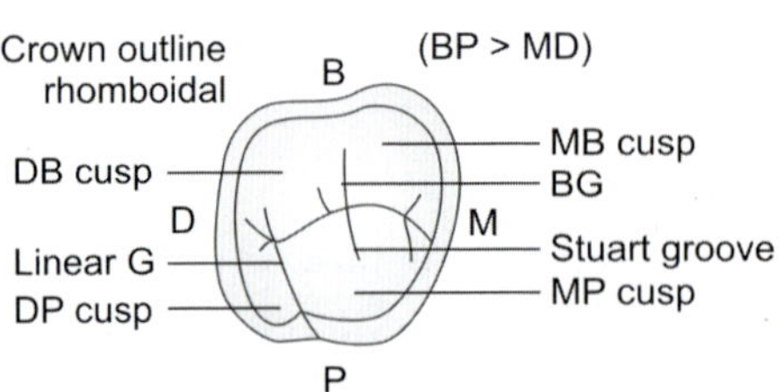

Fig. 25.121: Occlusal aspect

MAXILLARY SECOND MOLAR

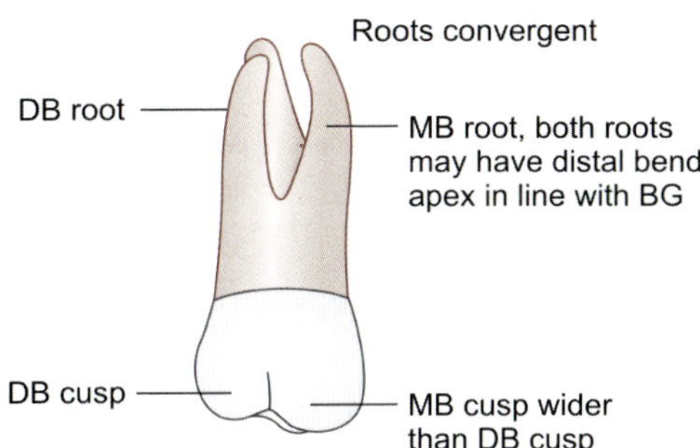

Fig. 25.122: Buccal aspect

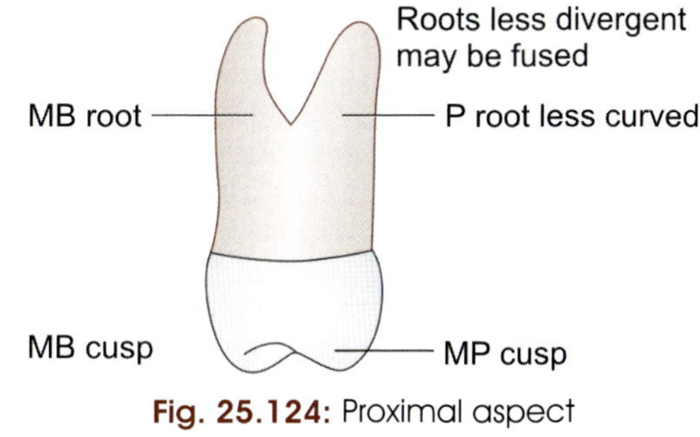

Fig. 25.124: Proximal aspect

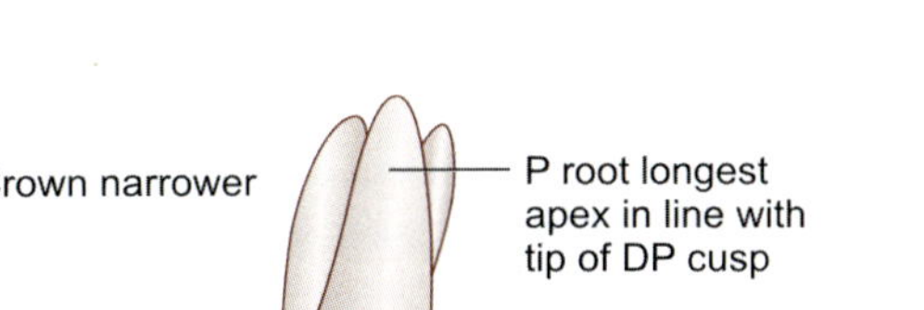

Fig. 25.123: Palatal aspect

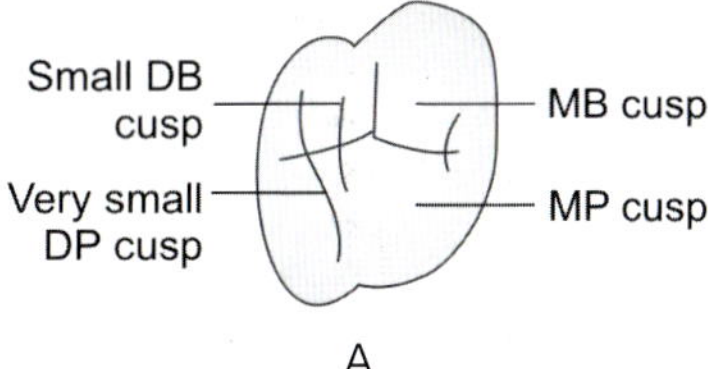

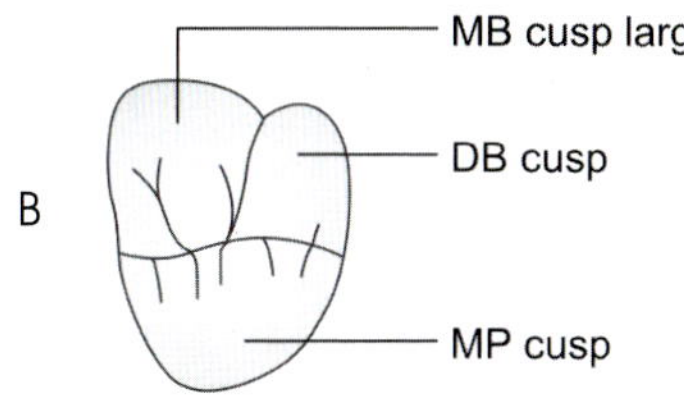

Fig. 25.125A and B: Occlusal aspect

STEPS FOR CARVING OF MAXILLARY FIRST MOLAR

STEP 1

- Do not reduce the block.
- Divide the block into crown, root, and base.
- Mark M, D, B and P on the base.
- Make sure that BP dimension is more than MD dimension (Occlusal view).
- Start with occlusal aspect.
- The occlusal outline of permanent first molar is rhomboid so make the mesiobuccal and distopalatal angles acute and distobuccal and mesiopalatal angles obtuse (Fig. 25.126).
- Divide the occlusal surface into two equal halves by a line 'C'.

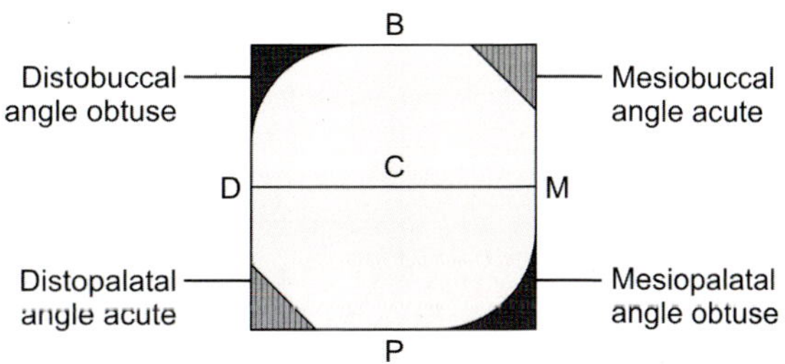

Fig. 25.126

STEP 2

- Divide buccal side of occlusal surface into 2 equal parts by a line '2' to get mesiobuccal and distobuccal parts (Fig. 25.127).
- Divide palatal side into 2 unequal parts by a line '1' to get mesiopalatal—larger and distopalatal—smaller parts (Fig. 25.127).

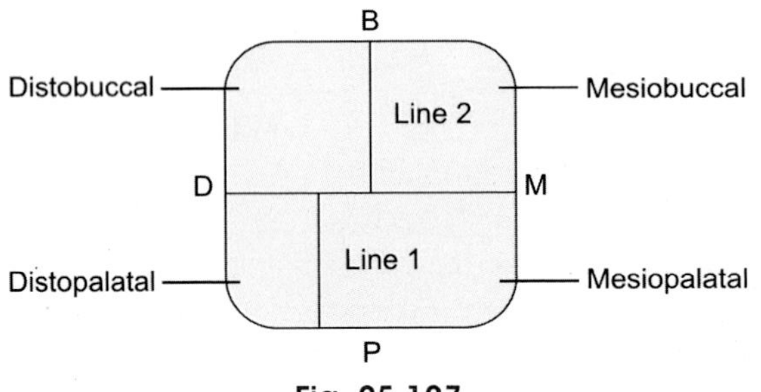

Fig. 25.127

STEP 3 AND STEP 4

STEP 3 and **STEP 4** are for gross carving of B, P, O, surfaces and giving constriction.

Divide the buccal and palatal surface of crown into three parts (Fig. 25.128):

1. Occlusal third
2. Middle third
3. Cervical third

In the cervical third give constriction, i.e. in the cervical third of M and D surfaces remove wax (towards both B and P surfaces) (Figs 25.129A and 25.129B).

(Method is same as in premolar.)

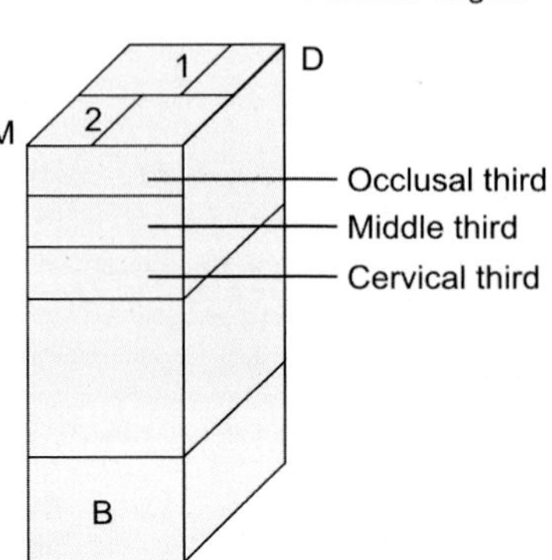

Fig. 25.128

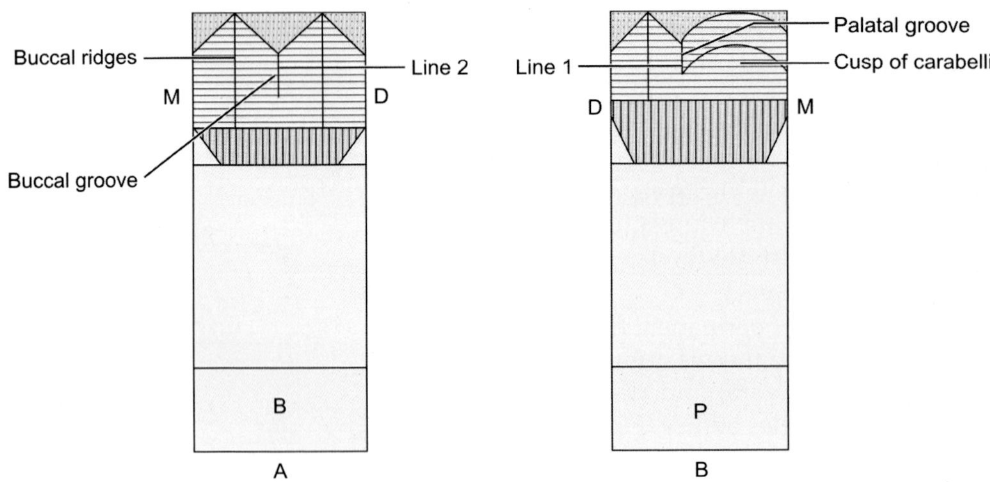

Figs 25.129A and B

STEP 4

Extend the lines 1 and 2 (which are on occlusal surface) onto the mid of palatal and buccal surfaces. Draw 2 hut shapes on either side of the extended lines on palatal and buccal surfaces.

- Remove wax along the hut shape on the occlusal surface till line 'C' (Fig. 25.127).

This gives gross carving of inclines of 2 buccal and 2 patal cusps. (Cusp inclines on occlusal as well as buccal surfaces and palatal surfaces.)

STEP 5

Buccal Surface

- On the buccal surface of the crown as in Fig. 25.129A, carve along the inclines of the two huts, only in occlusal two-thirds, (as you have carved the buccal ridge and inclines), in premolar so as to get 2 buccal ridges of 2 buccal cusps and buccal groove (BG).
- In the cervical third, remove little wax towards the cervical line and then merge the cervical third with the occlusal two-thirds so as to get the height of contour in cervical third.

STEP 6

Palatal Surface

- On the palatal surface as in Fig. 25.129B carve along the inclines of two huts in occlusal half so as to get 2 palatal ridges and the palatal groove.
- In the cervical half remove some wax towards cervical line and then merge it with occlusal half to get height of contour in the middle of the palatal surface.
  2 mm cervical to the MP cusp ridge carve a curved depression with the pointed tip of the carver to make the cusp of carabelli.

STEP 7

Occlusal Surface

- **Once again make sure that BP > MD and outline of the occlusal surface is rhomboid with MP angle and DB angle being rounded/obtuse and MB and DP angle being acute. The largest cusp is MP and smallest is DP.**
- You have already divided the occlusal surface into 4 parts. Gross carving of 4 cusps and ridges is done. Now, redefine the lines 1 and 2 as shown in Fig. 25.130. Read the labelling.
- Extend the line 2 into the MP cusp for 1 mm as line 'S'. Mark the M and D triangular pits and fossae (Figs 25.130 and 25.131).
  While carving the triangular ridge (TR) and inclined planes (IP) of each cusp move the carver from the ridge to the depression (groove), along the cusp slopes in doing so the groove and the ridge get defined (Fig. 25.131).
- First carve the DP cusp which has one straight triangular ridge (TRDP), and two inclined planes IP (Fig. 25.131). While defining the IP, define the DOG or linear groove (Fig. 25.130).
  Then carve the MB cusp which also has a straight triangular ridge TRMB with two inclines.
- Now carve the DB cusp in such a way that its triangular ridge (TRDB) runs little mesially.
- Define both triangular fossae and pits:
- We have already carved the triangular ridges of MB, DB and DP cusps, M and D triangular fossae (TF).
- MP cusp is largest. It has two triangular ridges (TR) separated by 'Stuart groove' (SG).

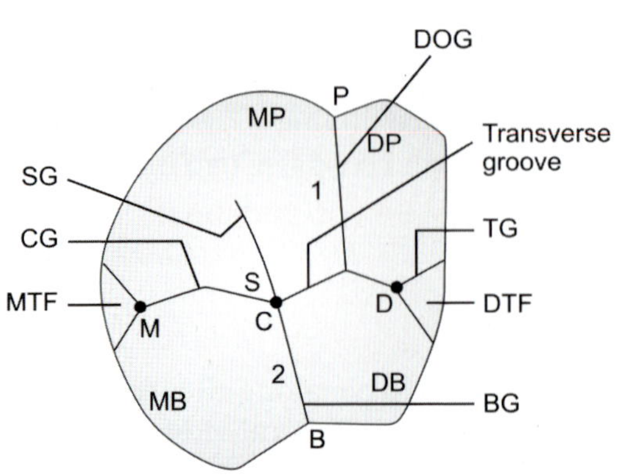

MP mesiopalatal cusp
DP distopalatal cusp
MB mesiobuccal cusp
DB distobuccal cusp

Pits:

Mesial (M), Central pits (C), distal pits (D)

Line 2 is	Buccal groove	BG
Line 5 is	Stuart groove	SG 'S'
	Central groove	CG
	Triangular grooves	TG
Line 1 is	Linear groove or DOG distal oblique groove or transverse groove	

Fossa:

Mesial and distal triangular fossae MTF, DTF

Fig. 25.130: Cusps, grooves, pits

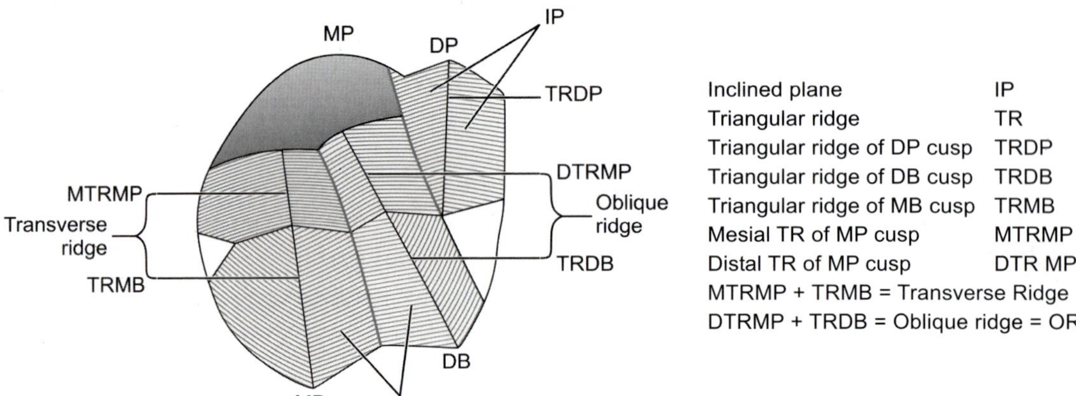

Fig. 25.131: Ridges

- The two triangular ridges are the mesial TR of MP cusp and the distal TR of the MP cusp (MTRMP and DTRMP).
- The MTRMP joins the TRMB cusp to form 'transverse ridge' and the DTRMP joins the TR of DB cusp to form the oblique ridge.

STEP 8 (Fig. 25.131)

Carve the Transverse and Oblique Ridge

- To carve the transverse ridge, extend the TR and the IP of the MB cusp into the MP cusp for about 1 mm.
- Define the Stuart groove.
- Extend the inclined planes of the DB cusp in the mesial direction into the MP cusp for about 1 mm to form the oblique ridge. While defining the IP of oblique ridge define the DOG.
- Define the OR, the Stuart groove and the distal oblique groove.
- Carve out the remaining part of the MP cusp.
- Grossly the occlusal surface is carved.
- See the Figs 25.130 and 25.131 and define the central groove, M, D and C pits, buccal and palatal groove, carve out the M and D triangular fossae keeping the M and D marginal ridges intact.

- Define the central groove by carving on both buccal and palatal side of it so that the TR and OR are inclined towards the CG.
- On the palatal surface of MP cusp, 1 mm below the MP cusp carve out a curved line to make the **cusp of carabelli (Fig. 25.129B).**

OR

Carve the oblique ridge by joining triangular ridge of DB cusp and the distal cusp ridge of MP cusp TRDB + DCRMP, as given in other texts (refer Fig. 25.132) (No Stuart groove).

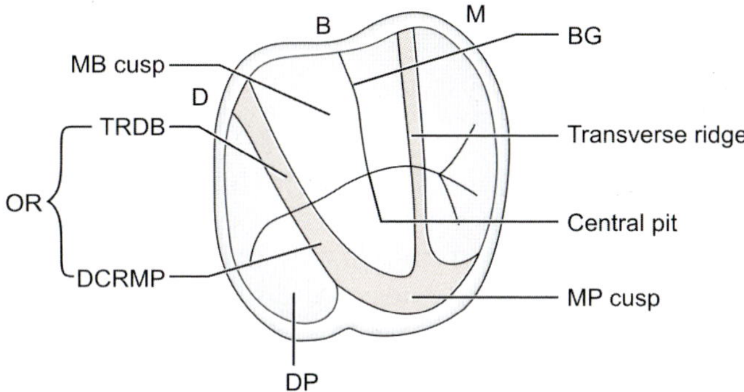

Fig. 25.132: Occlusal surface

ROOT CARVING

STEP 1

Make roughly triangular outline of root before making furcation by:

- Make the root wider mesiodistally and narrower palatally. Mark the shape of the root as follows and remove wax from shaded area.
- Mark, the outline of the buccal roots on the buccal surface (Figs 25.133A and B).
- Mark outline of palatal root on the palatal surface (Fig. 25.134).

Mark the mesial and distal root (Figs 25.135 and 2.136).

- As palatal root is flaring buccopalatal width is more.
  Remove the remaining wax other than the marked outline form of root from buccal and palatal surface. (Remove wax from shaded area.)
- By using above method we can carve the outer outline form of root.

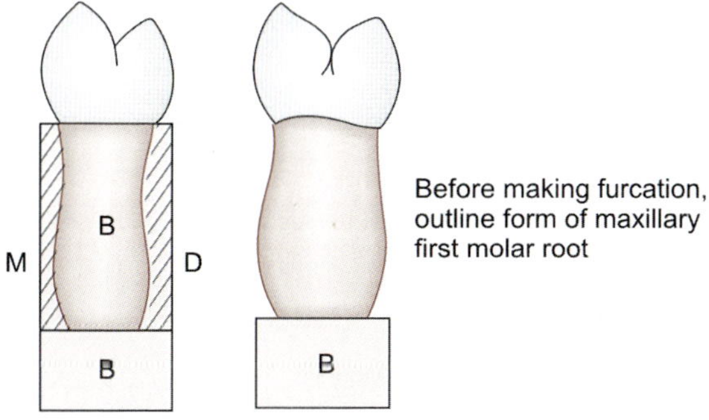

Figs 25.133A and B

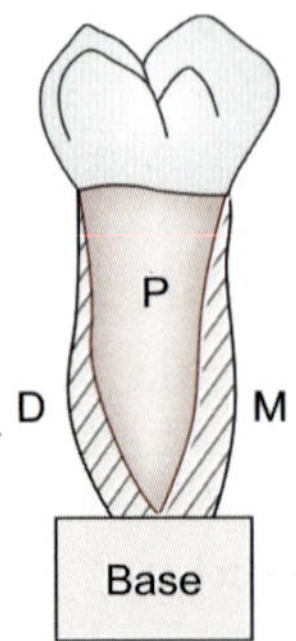

Palatal aspect
The step grossly completes the palatal root

Fig. 25.134

- After carving outer root outline on the buccal and palatal surfaces, mark outline of the individual root on the buccal, mesial and distal surface respectively. So as to carve the bifurcation on each surface (i.e. buccal, mesial and distal) (Figs 25.137– 25.139).
  Remove wax from shaded area on B, M and D surface.

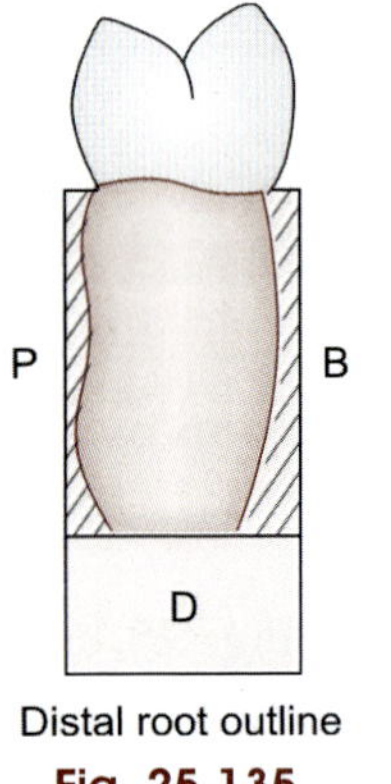

Distal root outline

Fig. 25.135

Mesial root outline

Fig. 25.136

- Continue mesial and distal bifurcation with the buccal bifurcation.
  - Remove all irregularities from carved bifurcated area.
  - Roots should be rounded and tapering towards apex.
  - Polish the roots with dry cotton first and then with cotton dipped in soap water.

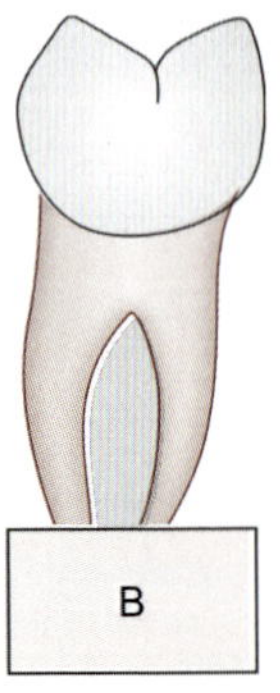

Fig. 25.137

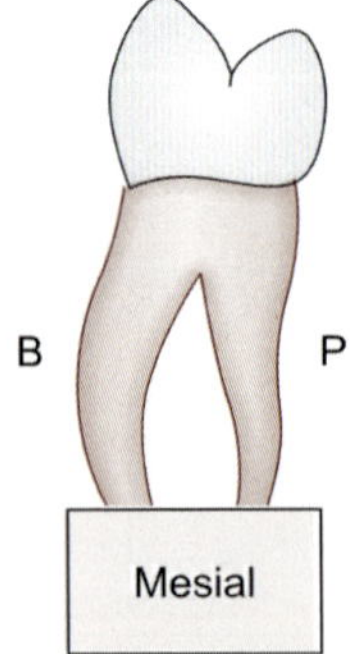

Fig. 25.138

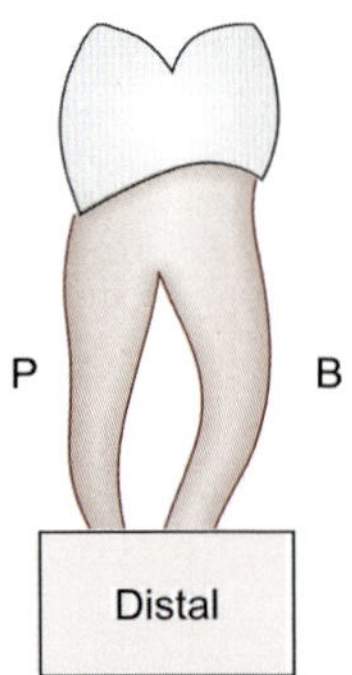

Fig. 25.139

MAXILLARY SECOND MOLAR

Maxillary second molar resembles the first molar except a few differences. Steps for carving remain same except for the occlusal surface.

Start with the occlusal surface.

Rhomboid Occlusal Surface

- BP dimension is same as that of first molar. MD dimension is 1 mm less.
- The occlusal outline is sharply rhomboid.
- MB angle is more acute. MB cusp is larger than DB cusp.
- DP angle is more acute and DP cusp is much smaller than MP cusp.
- There is no cusp of carabelli.
- Roots are not divergent.

  All steps are same as that of the first molar.

Heart-shaped Occlusal Surface

- See to it that MD dimension is less than BP dimension.
- DP cusp is absent.
- MP cusp is the largest cusp.
- MB cusp is wider and longer than DB cusp.
- To make the occlusal outline heart-shaped.
- Divide the occlusal surface into 2 equal parts.
- Divide the Buccal of occlusal into 2 unequal parts and carve the 2 buccal cusps. All the steps for carving buccal surface and occlusal part of buccal surface are same as for first M.
- MP angle make more obtuse, DB make less obtuse.
- Mark the MP cusp on the occlusal surface (Fig. 25.140).
- Remove the DP corner by rounding it off and making it the distal cusp slope of the MP cusp.
- Mark the triangular fossae. Carve the inclined planes (IP) of the MP cusp till the marked lines.
- Define the marginal ridges and the triangular fossae.

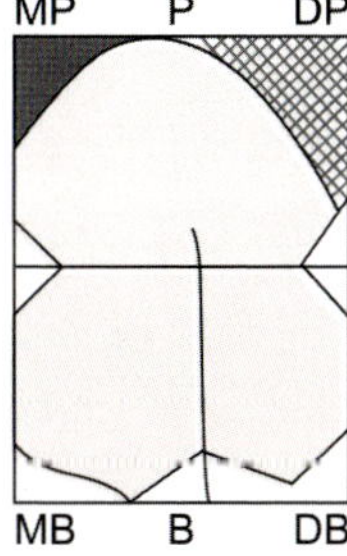

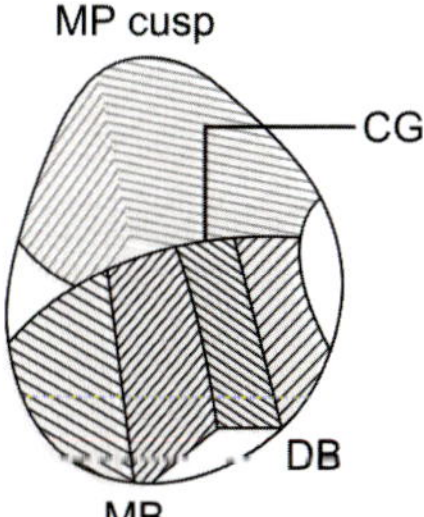

Fig. 25.140

MANDIBULAR FIRST MOLAR

Palmer Notation

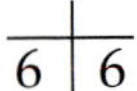

ODONTOMETRIC DATA	
Length of crown	7.5 mm
Length of root	14.0 mm
Mesiodistal diameter of crown	11.0 mm
Mesiodistal diameter of crown at cervix	9.0 mm
Buccopalatal diameter of crown	10.5 mm
Buccopalatal diameter at cervix	9.0 mm
Curvature of cervical line on mesial	1.0 mm
On distal	0.0 mm

MANDIBULAR FIRST MOLAR

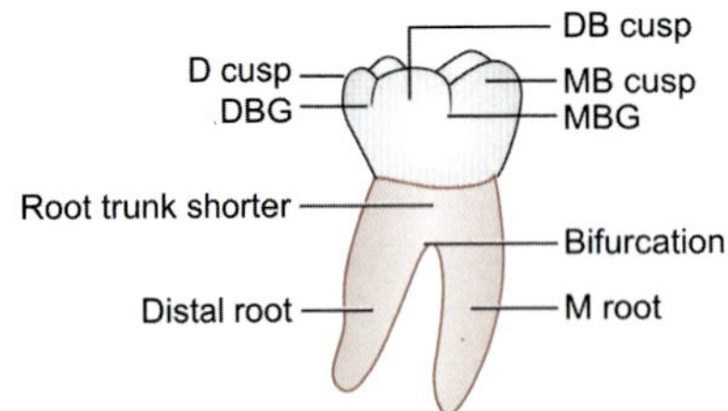

Fig. 25.141: Buccal aspect

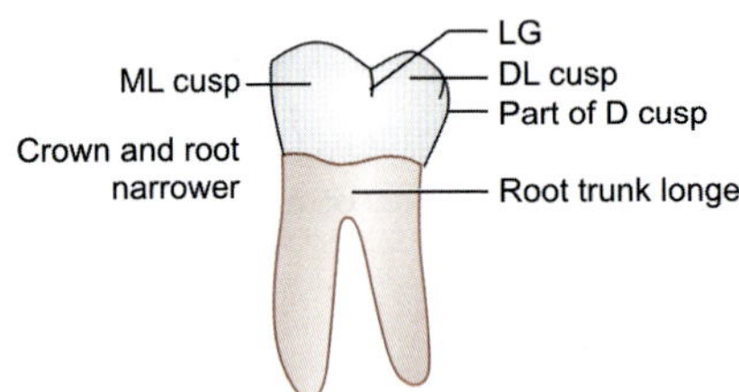

Fig. 25.142: Lingual aspect

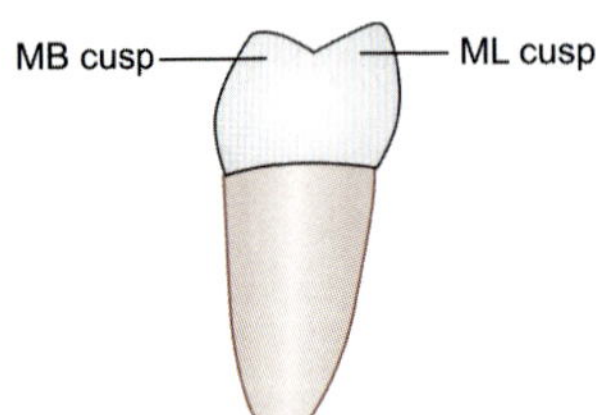

Fig. 25.143: Proximal aspect

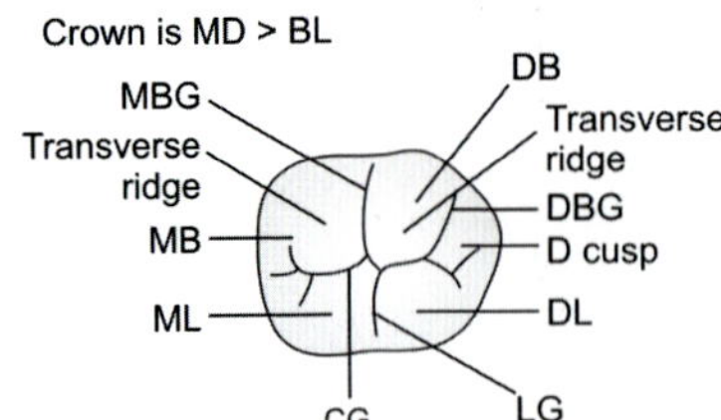

Fig. 25.144: Occlusal aspect

MANDIBULAR SECOND MOLAR

Palmer Notation

7 | 7

ODONTOMETRIC DATA	
Length of crown	7.0 mm
Length of root	13.0 mm
Mesiodistal diameter of crown	10.5 mm
Mesiodistal diameter of crown at cervix	8.0 mm
Buccopalatal diameter of crown	10.0 mm
Buccopalatal diameter at cervix	9.0 mm
Curvature of cervical line on mesial	1.0 mm
On distal	0.0 mm

MANDIBULAR SECOND MOLAR

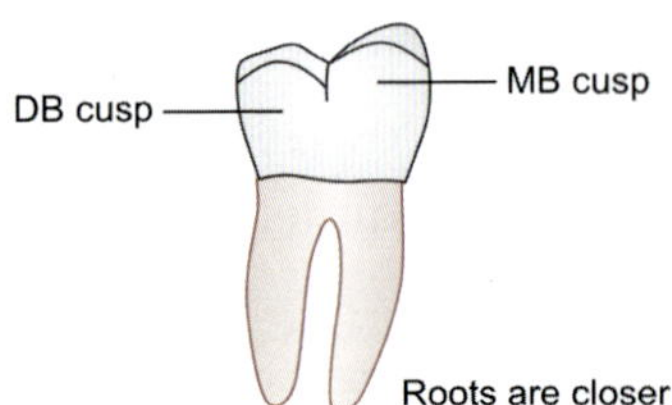

Fig. 25.145: Buccal aspect

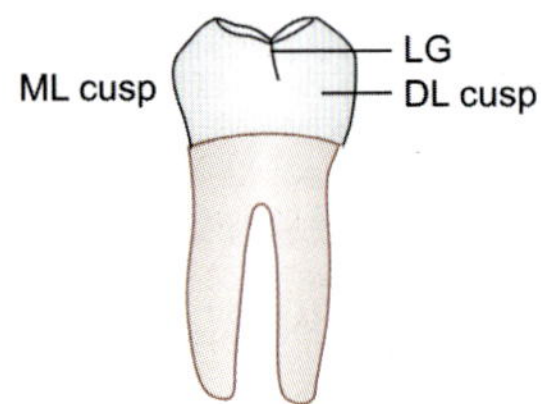

Fig. 25.146: Lingual aspect

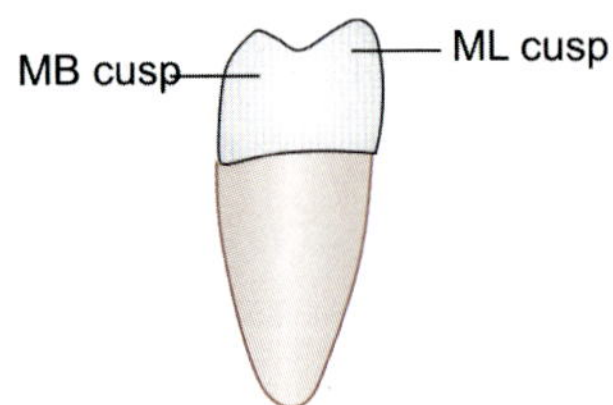

Fig. 25.147: Proximal aspect

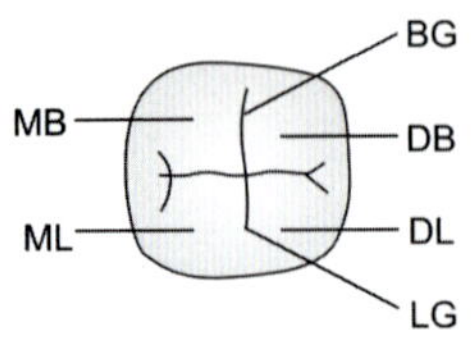

Fig. 25.148: Occlusal aspect

STEPS FOR CARVING OF MANDIBULAR FIRST MOLAR

- **For both mandibular molars make sure that MD dimension is more than BL dimension (Fig. 25.149).**
- Divide the block into crown, root and base.
  Mark the surfaces M, D, B, L on the base.

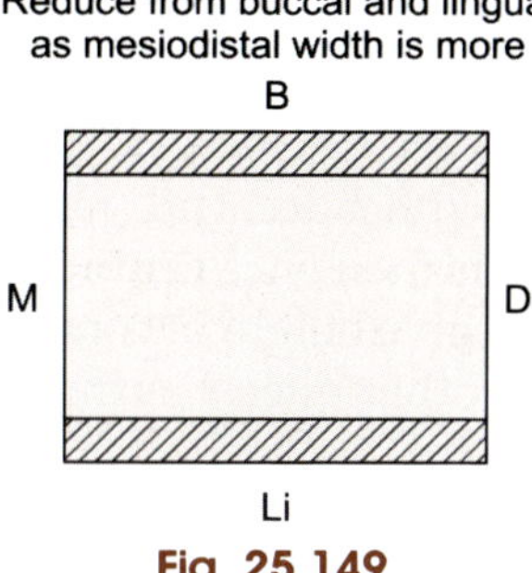

Fig. 25.149

STEP 1

Occlusal View

Occlusal aspect is pentagon in shape. From buccal aspect distal border is more rounded than mesial border, so reduce more from distal side on wax block (Fig. 25.150).

Divide occlusal surface into 5 parts: (Fig. 25.150) by line a, b, c.

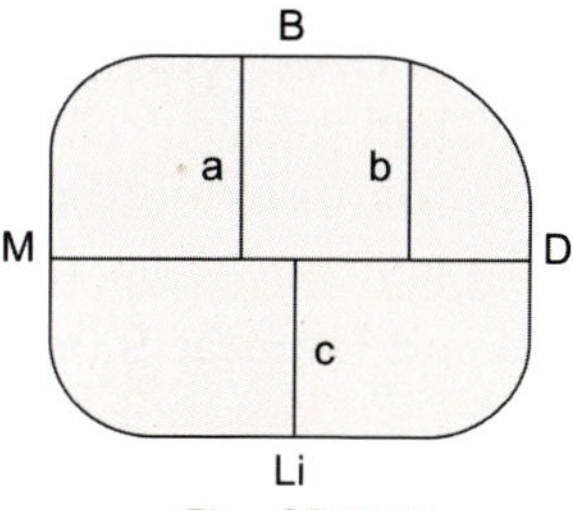

Fig. 25.150

STEP 2

Buccal Surface

- Divide the B surface of the crown in 3 parts. In the cervical third carve out some wax towards cervical line.
- Carve the occlusal two-thirds of the crown so as to give little inclination to the buccal surface towards lingual (Fig. 25.151).
- Merge the cervical third with occlusal two-thirds to give height of contour in the cervical third (Fig. 25.152).

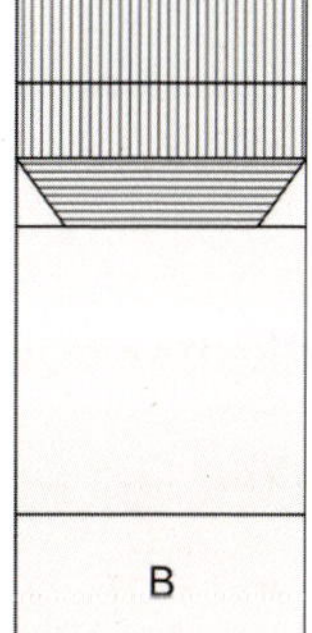

Fig. 25.151

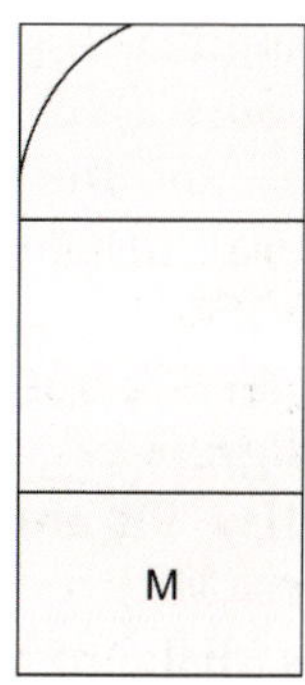

Fig. 25.152

- Give constriction in the cervical third towards both B and L. Which means remove wax from the cervical third of the M and D surfaces of the crown (Fig. 25.151).
- These two steps are same as in other teeth.

STEP 3 (Fig. 25.153)

- Extend the 2 lines a and b (Fig. 25.150) onto the buccal surface:
  - On buccal surface there are three cusps. MB, DB, D.
  - MB is widest.

    D cusp is pointed and part of it is on the distal surface.
  - Mark 3 hut shapes.

    Carve the cusps on B surface with buccal ridges and inclined planes only in occlusal two-thirds then once again merge occlusal two-thirds with cervical third to give height of contour in cervical third. (This step is same as any other buccal surface.)

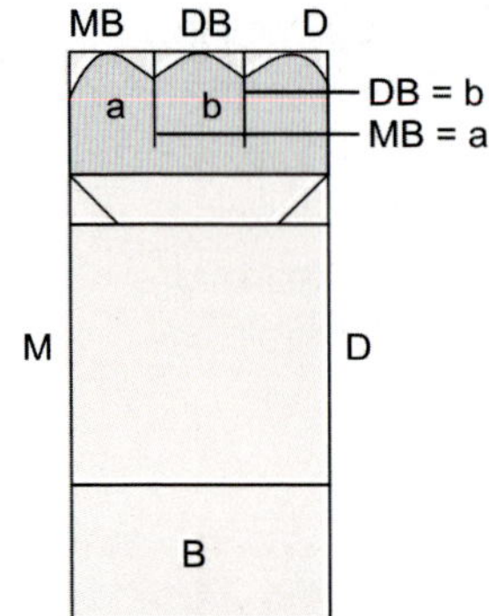

Fig. 25.153

STEP 4

Lingual Surface

- Divide the lingual surface of the crown into two parts for two lingual cusps by extending the line c drawn on occlusal surface (Fig. 25.150).
- Make 2 huts on either side of the extended line and carve two lingual cusps with their cusp tips, lingual ridges and inclined planes in the occlusal half.
- Carve out little wax in the cervical half.
- Then merge occlusal half with cervical half to give height of contour in middle of the lingual surface (Fig. 25.154).

Make the crown narrow at the cervix by removing wax on the M and D surfaces only in cervical third of the crown.

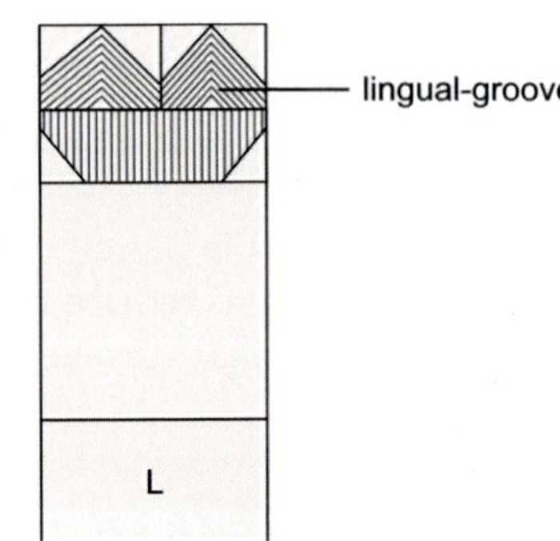

Fig. 25.154

STEP 5

Occlusal Surface: (With no Transverse Ridges)

- Because of the inclination of the buccal surface towards lingual, the midline on occlusal surface appears to be more buccally placed (Fig. 25.155).

  Mark the triangular fossa. Mesiobuccal groove MBG, distobuccal groove (DBG) and lingual groove (LG) already marked, midline is the CG.
- Carve the occlusal surface as you have carved on other molars (Fig. 25.156).

B
a
b
M
c
L
DBG
MBG
TF
LG

Fig. 25.155

- While carving the TR and IP see (Fig. 25. 157) and follow the direction of the TR so as to get zig-zag central groove.
- **Carve all the five TR and IP** inclined towards the CG define the triangular fossa TF and marginal ridges (MR).
- TRMB extends (distal to MP) linguallly.
- TRDB extends M to CP

- TRD extends M to DP
- TRML extends D to TRMB
- TRDL extends M to TRD

    TR = Triangular ridge

    MB cusp = MB

    Triangular ridge of MB cusp is TRMB

    IP = Inclined planes

    MP = Mesial pit

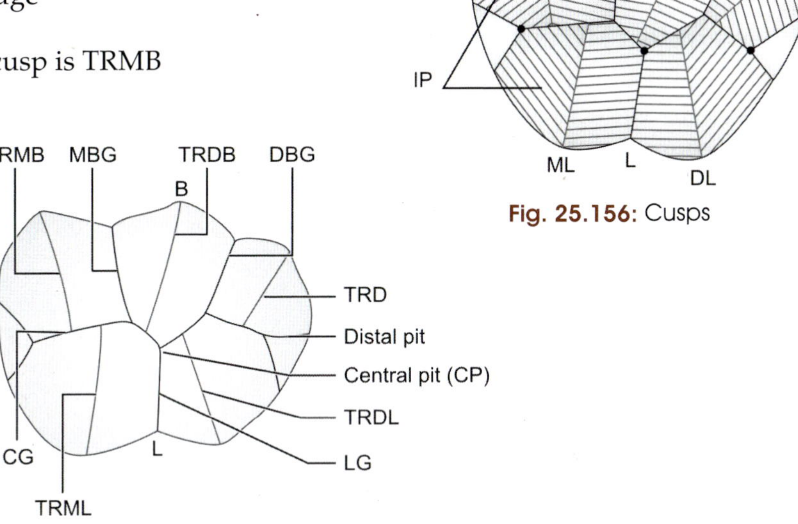

Fig. 25.156: Cusps

Fig. 25.157: Triangular ridges and Grooves

OR

Occlusal surface having two transverse ridges (Fig. 25.158).

- Mesial transverse ridge formed by joining of triangular ridge of MB cusp and triangular ridge of ML cusp. TRMB + TRML.
- Distal transverse ridge formed by joining of TRDB and TRDL cusp.

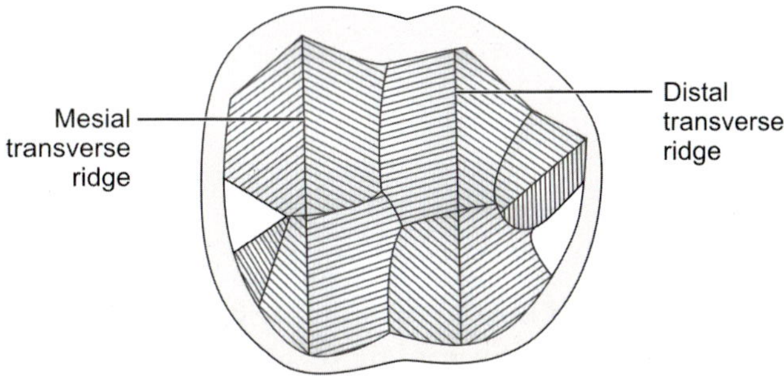

Fig. 25.158

CARVING OF ROOT

- It has a root trunk which bifurcates to form mesial and distal roots.
- Both roots are widest buccolingually.
- Two roots are usually about the same length.
- For carving root of mandibular molar use same method as given in carving of root of maxillary molar except following points:
  - For bifurcation of root, mark outline only on buccal and lingual surfaces and not on mesial and distal surface because mandibular molar has two roots.

MANDIBULAR SECOND MOLAR

Carving of mandibular second molar is very similar to carving of first molar except for a few differences.

Make sure that MD dimension is more than BL dimension.

- Divide the block into crown, root, base.
- Mark the surfaces M, D, B, L.

STEP 1

Give occlusal outline form to the wax block. Remove wax from shaded areas (Fig. 25.159).

Divide the occlusal surface into 4 parts (Fig. 25.160).

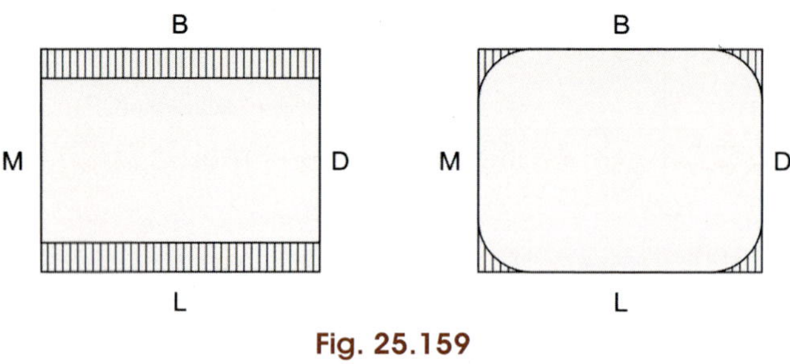

Fig. 25.159

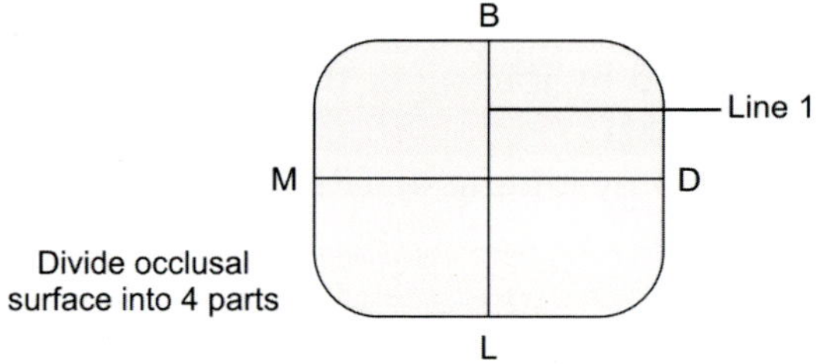

Fig. 25.160

STEP 2

Buccal Surface

- Divide the B surface of the crown into 3 parts. In the cervical third carve out some wax.
- Carve the occlusal two-thirds of the crown so as to give little inclination to the buccal surface towards lingual (Fig. 25.161).
- Merge the cervical third with occlusal two-thirds to give height of contour in the cervical third (Fig. 25.162).
- Give constriction in the cervical third towards both B and L. Which means remove wax from the cervical third of the M and D surfaces of the crown. (Same method as in other teeth.)
- Extend the line 1 in Fig. 25.160 on to the buccal surface:
  - On buccal surface there are two cusps MB and DB. MB is slightly larger than DB.
  - Mark 2 hut shapes.

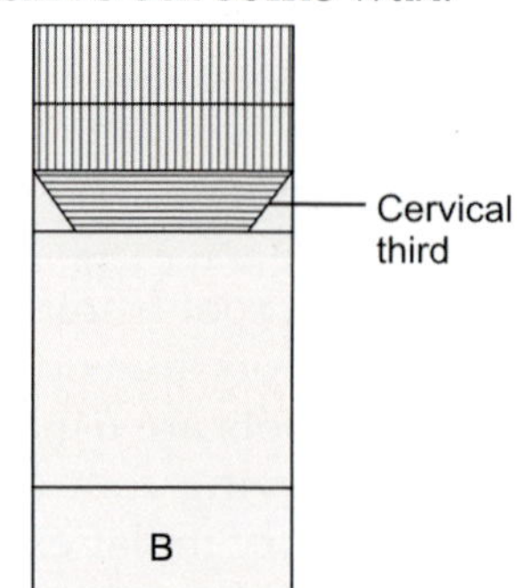

Fig. 25.161

Carve the cusps on B surface with buccal ridges and inclined planes only in occlusal two-thirds (Fig. 25.163).

Both cusps are separated by buccal groove. Cusps are not very sharp.

- Then merge the occlusal two-thirds with cervical one-third to give height of contour in cervical third on buccal surface (redefine).

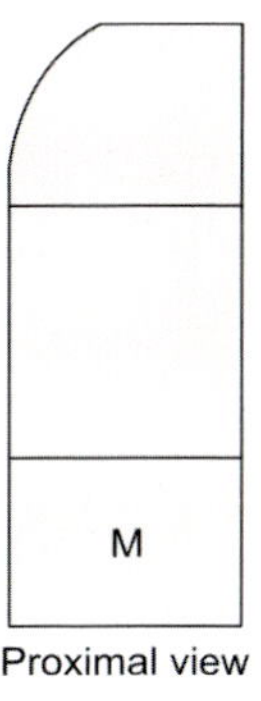

Proximal view

Fig. 25.162

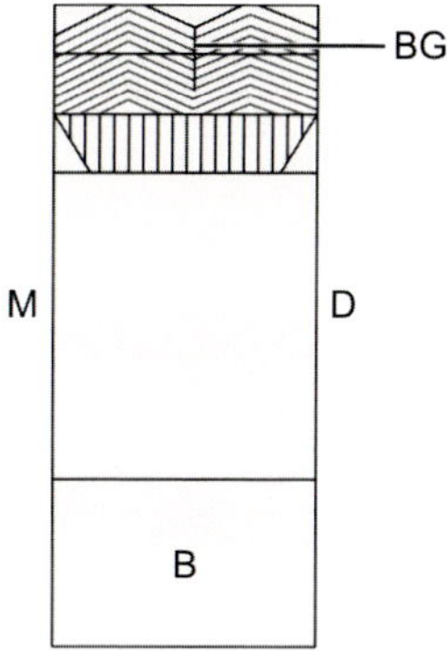

Fig. 25.163

STEP 3

Lingual Surface

- Divide the lingual surface into two parts by extending the line (1) in Fig. 25.160 on lingual surface for 1 mm.
- Carve out little wax in the cervical half.
- Make 2 huts on either side of the extended line and carve two lingual cusps with their cusp tips, lingual ridges and inclined planes in the occlusal half.
- Then merge occlusal half with cervical half to give height of contour in middle of the lingual surface (Fig. 25.164).

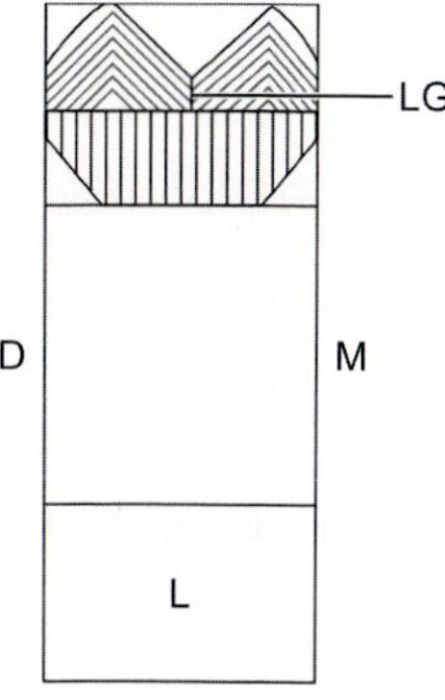

Fig. 25.164

STEP 4

Occlusal Surface

- 2 lines in cross pattern are already marked, mark the M and D triangular fossae (TF).
- Carve the occlusal surface as you have carved that of other molars (Fig. 25.165).
- Carve 4 cusps with the TR and IP. TR of MB cusp joins the TR of ML cusp to form a transverse ridge.
- TR of DB cusp joins the TR of DL cusp to form a transverse ridge.
- Define the TF, CG, BG, LG and the pits M, D and C.
- Follow the direction of the ridges and grooves (Fig. 25.165).

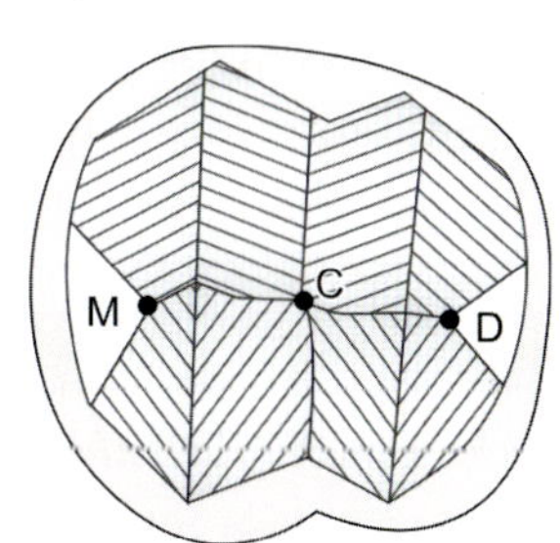

Fig. 25.165

STEP 5

Carve the root as you have carved in first molar.

The 2 roots are more or less parallel to each other.

Chapter

26

Guide for Identification of Teeth

INTRODUCTION

Identification of teeth is one of the important practical exercises in the study of 'Tooth Morphology'.

The thorough knowledge of tooth morphology can be acquired by reading about the tooth from all five aspects, by carving the tooth, by studying the plaster models, by drawing diagrams, and by collecting and studying the extracted teeth.

CLASSES OF TEETH

- In permanent dentition there are four classes of teeth incisors, canines, premolars, and molars.

Trait

A trait is a distinguishing characteristic. It helps in comparing the similarities and differences between the teeth.

- ***Set trait or dentition trait*** distinguishes the primary teeth from permanent teeth.
- ***Class trait*** distinguishes the four classes of teeth namely—incisors, canines, premolars, and molars.
- ***Arch trait*** distinguishes maxillary teeth from mandibular teeth.
- ***Type trait*** distinguishes the teeth within the same class, e.g. central incisor from lateral incisor, first premolar from second premolar.
- **Following are the guidelines to write about each permanent tooth of right side.**
- Student is expected to identify and write about the tooth as per the instructions given by the instructor.

INCISORS

MAXILLARY CENTRAL INCISOR

Identification

The given tooth is **permanent** maxillary central incisor of right side.

DECIDUOUS AND PERMANENT TEETH IN DIFFERENT NUMBERING SYSTEM						
PERMANENT TEETH	UNIVERSAL NUMBERING SYSTEM		FDI NUMBERING SYSTEM		PALMER NOTATION	
	Maxillary Teeth		Maxillary Teeth		Maxillary Teeth	
	Right side	*Left side*	*Right Quadrant 1*	*Left Quadrant 2*	*Right side*	*Left side*
	3M 2M 1M 2PM 1PM C LI CI	CI LI C 1PM 2PM 1M 2M 3M	3M 2M 1M 2PM 1PM C LI CI	CI LI C 1PM 2PM 1M 2M 3M	3M 2M 1M 2PM 1PM C LI CI	CI LI C 1PM 2PM 1M 2M 3M
	1 2 3 4 5 6 7 **8**	**9** 10 11 12 13 14 15 **16**	18 17 16 15 14 13 12 **11**	**21** 22 23 24 25 26 27 28	8 7 6 5 4 3 2 **1**	1 2 3 4 5 6 7 8
	32 31 30 29 28 27 26 25	**24** 23 22 21 20 19 18 **17**	48 47 46 45 44 43 42 **41**	**31** 32 33 34 35 36 37 38	8 7 6 5 4 3 2 **1**	1 2 3 4 5 6 7 8
	Right side	*Left side*	*Right Quadrant 4*	*Left Quadrant 3*	*Right side*	*Left side*
	Mandibular Teeth		Mandibular Teeth		Mandibular Teeth	
DECIDUOUS TEETH	UNIVERSAL NUMBERING SYSTEM		FDI NUMBERING SYSTEM		PALMER NOTATION	
	Maxillary Teeth		Maxillary Teeth		Maxillary Teeth	
	Right side	*Left side*	*Right Quadrant 5*	*Left Quadrant 6*	*Right side*	*Left side*
	2M 1M C LI CI	CI LI C 1M 2M	2M 1M C LI CI	CI LI C 1M 2M	2M 1M C LI CI	CI LI C IM 2M
	A B C D **E**	**F** G H I **J**	55 54 53 52 **51**	**61** 62 63 64 65	E D C B A	A B C D E
	T S R Q P	**O** N M L **K**	85 84 83 82 **81**	**71** 72 73 74 75	E D C B A	A B C D E
	Right side	*Left side*	*Right Quadrant 8*	*Left Quadrant 7*	*Right side*	*Left side*
	Mandibular Teeth		Mandibular Teeth		Mandibular Teeth	

Notation

Palmer notation 1|

Universal # 8

FDI 11

Set Trait or Dentition Trait

- It is a large yellowish white rectangular/square tooth.
- Cervical constriction is much less as compared to that in deciduous incisor.
- The mamelons are present on the incisal ridge of newly erupted permanent tooth.

Class Trait

1. Presence of incisal ridge.
2. Mamelons on incisal ridge in newly erupted tooth.
3. Of all the classes of teeth incisor has narraowest labio-lingual dimension.
4. Lingual surface has a lingual fossa, cingulum and marginal ridges almost parallel to the root axis.

Arch Trait

It is maxillary **central** incisor because:

1. Mesiodistal dimension is more than the labiolingual dimension. (Incisal view)
2. Incisal ridge is either centered over root axis or labially placed. (Proximal view)
3. Cingulum, lingual fossa and marginal ridges are more prominent. (Lingual view)
4. Crown is long and wide, shape is either rectangular or square. (Labial view)
5. Root is conical and not much longer than the crown.

Type Trait

The tooth is maxillary central incisor of right side because:

1. Crown is **long and wide.**
2. Incisal ridge is straight.
3. **Mesioincisal angle** is **sharp (90°)**, distoincisal angle is slightly rounded.
4. Mesial border of the crown is less convex as compared to the distal border of the crown.
5. Crown is narrower on lingual, shallow lingual fossa in incisal two-thirds of the crown.
6. Cingulum is off-centered to distal.
7. Root is conical and not much longer than the crown.

MAXILLARY LATERAL INCISOR

Identification

The given tooth is **permanent** maxillary lateral incisor of right side.

Notation

Palmer notation 2|

Universal #7

FDI 12

Set Trait or Dentition Trait

- It is a larger tooth, yellowish white in colour.
- Cervical constriction is much less as compared to deciduous teeth.
- Mamelons are present on incisal ridge of newly erupted tooth.

Class Trait

1. Presence of incisal ridge.
2. On the newly erupted incisor mamelons present.
3. Of all the classes of teeth incisors have narraowest labiolingual dimension.
4. Lingual surface has a lingual fossa, cingulum and marginal ridges are almost parallel to the root axis.

Arch Trait

1. From incisal view crown is wider **mesiodistally** than **labiolingually.**
2. From proximal aspect the incisal ridge is either labial to root axis or centered over root axis.
3. Lingual pit at the base of the fossa may be present on maxillary lateral incisor.
4. It is a more rounded tooth.
5. Root is conical, longer as compared to crown and may have a distal bend.

Type Trait

It is maxillary lateral incisor because:

1. It is short, narrower and **more rounded** tooth.
2. Incisal ridge **slopes cervically** towards distal.
3. Mesioincisal angle is rounded, **distoincisal angle** is more rounded.
4. Cingulum is centered.
   Lingual fossa is small and deep (more prominent).
5. Root is much longer as compared to the crown; it is conical and may have a distal bend.

PERMANENT MANDIBULAR CENTRAL INCISOR

Introduction

The given tooth is **permanent** mandibular central incisor of right side.

Notation

Palmer notation	1 (lower right quadrant, $\overline{1\rceil}$)
Universal	#25
FDI	41

Set Trait

- It is smaller yellowish white in color but larger as compared to deciduous tooth.
- The mamelons are present.

Class Trait

1. Presence of incisal ridge.
2. On the newly erupted incisors mamelons present.

3. Of all the classes of teeth incisors have narraowest labiolingual dimension.
4. Lingual surface has a lingual fossa, cingulum and marginal ridges almost parallel to root axis.

Arch Trait

The given tooth is a mandibular incisor because:

1. Central incisor is **much smaller** than the maxillary central incisor. It is long and narrow.
2. From proximal view **incisal ridge** is **lingual** to root axis.
3. From incisal view **labiolingual** dimension is more than mesio-distal dimension.
4. Lingual fossa, cingulum and marginal ridges are less prominent.
5. The root is flat **mesiodistally** with **mesial** and **distal** root depressions.

Type Trait

It is mandibular **central** incisor because:

1. It appears **bilaterally symmetrical** and it is a small tooth.
2. Incisal ridge is straight and at right angles to long axis of the tooth.
3. **Mesio and disto incisal angles** are sharp (90°).
4. Cingulum is centered.

MANDIBULAR LATERAL INCISOR

Identification

The given tooth is **permanent** mandibular lateral incisor of right side.

Notation

Palmer notation	2┐ (lower right quadrant)
Universal	#26
FDI	42

Set Trait

It is a permanent tooth. Deciduous teeth are much smaller and whiter in color as compared to permanent teeth.

Class Trait

1. Presence of incisal ridge.
2. On the newly erupted incisors mamelons present.
3. Of all the classes of teeth incisors have narrowest labiolingual dimension.
4. Lingual surface has a lingual fossa, cingulum and marginal ridges which are almost parallel to root axis.

Arch Trait

It is a mandibular incisor because:

1. From incisal view **labiolingual** dimension is more than **mesiodistal** dimension.
2. From proximal view, **incisal ridge** is **lingual** to root axis.
3. The root is mesiodistally flat. Root depressions are present on both mesial and distal surfaces.

Type Trait

It is mandibular lateral incisor because:

1. The crown is not symmetrical and is wider and longer than the central incisor.
2. Distal border of the crown has a **bulge.**
3. Incisal ridge is not straight, it has a **lingual twist** at distoincisal angle.
4. The cingulum is off-centered to distal.

CANINES

PERMANENT MAXILLARY CANINE

Identification

The given tooth is **permanent** maxillary canine of the right side.

Notation

Palmer notation	3⌋
Universal	#6
FDI	13

Set Trait

- It is a permanent tooth.
- It is large yellowish white tooth with a single pointed cusp.

Class Trait

It is a canine.

1. It has a **single pointed cup** with two inclines making an angle at the cusp tip instead of an incisal ridge.
2. There is **presence of a labial ridge.**
3. It has a **single, long, strong root.**
4. It has a **functional lingual surface.**

Arch Trait

1. It is a permanent maxillary canine. The inclines of the cusp make an **acute angle at the tip of the cusp.**
2. The mesial cusp slope is shorter than the distal cusp slope.
3. The crown is short, wide and **converging** at cervix (compared to mandibular canine).
4. Distoincisal angle is very much rounded. Mesioincisal angle is less rounded.
5. Mesial and distal borders of the crown converge at the cervix.
6. The **labial ridge** is more **prominent.**
7. Lingual ridge and 2 lingual fossae are prominent, cingulum is large, rounded, and centered.
8. From incisal view the distal part of the labial surface is pinched.
9. The long, stout, conical root may have a distal bend in the apical third.

There is no Type Trait

The tooth is of right side because:

1. Mesial cusp slope shorter than distal before wear.
2. **Rounded distoincisal angle** which is more cervically placed.

3. From incisal view there is **distal pinch** on the labial surface.
4. Distal bend of the root apex.

PERMANENT MANDIBULAR CANINE

Identification

The given tooth is **permanent** mandibular right canine.

Notation

Palmer notation	3⌋
Universal	#27
FDI	43

Set Trait

- It is a permanent tooth.
- It is large yellowish white tooth with a single cusp. Deciduous tooth is smaller and whiter.

Class Trait

It is a canine because:
1. It has a single cusp with two inclines instead of incisal ridge.
2. There is presence of a labial ridge.
3. It has a single, long, strong root.

Arch Trait

1. It is a permanent mandibular canine.
2. It is **long, narrow,** single cusped tooth.
3. The shorter mesial cusp slope and longer distal cusp slope meet at an **obtuse angle** at the **tip of the cusp.**
4. Mesial and distal outlines (border) of the crown **converge less** at the cervix.
5. Cingulum is off centered to distal.
6. Root is flat **mesiodistally,** wider labio-lingually and ends in a pointed apex.
7. The **labial ridge,** the **lingual ridge** and **fossa** are less prominent.

There is no type trait. The tooth is of right side because:
1. Mesial cusp slope shorter than distal cusp slope.
2. Cingulum is off-centered to distal.
3. **Mesiol border** of the crown is in line with the **mesial border** of the root.

PREMOLARS

MAXILLARY FIRST PREMOLAR

Identification

The given tooth is a maxillary first premolar of the right side.

Notation

Palmer notation $\underline{4|}$

Universal #5

FDI 14

Set Trait

Premolars have no set traits as there are no premolars in deciduous dentition.

Class Trait

- They are called bicuspid, when one buccal and one lingual cusp present. Second premolar may have 3 cusps.
- Premolars have a **single buccal cusp.**
- They may have of **one or two roots.**

Arch Trait

1. Occlusal outline of maxillary premolars is hexagonal or oval, that of mandibular premolars is square or rounded.
2. Maxillary premolars are wider buccopalatally compared to mesiodistal dimension.
3. From proximal view the maxillary premolars do not have a lingual tilt whereas mandibular premolars have a lingual tilt.
4. From proximal view the outline of maxillary premolar is trapezoidal whereas outline of mandibular premolar is rhomboidal.

Type Trait

1. **Mesial slope of the buccal cusp is longer than the distal cusp slope.** (Right from left) in first premolar. Cusp tip pointed. Angular outlines
2. From proximal view, **lingual cusp** is about 1 mm shorter than the **buccal cusp** in first premolar.
3. On the **mesial surface** of the crown of maxillary first premolar there is presence of mesial concavity **(canine fossa)** which is **continuous with the concavity on root.**
4. There is presence of **mesial marginal groove crossing** the mesial marginal ridge from the occlusal to the mesial surface. This MMRG is not present on second premolar (right from left).
5. Occlusal surface **sharply hexagonal** in shape in maxillary first premolar, in second premolar it is oval in shape.
6. In maxillary first premolar more often there are **two roots, one buccal** and **one lingual.** Maxillary second Premolar has single root.

MAXILLARY SECOND PREMOLAR

Identification

The given tooth is maxillary second premolar of the right side.

Notation

Palmer notation $\underline{5|}$

Universal #4

FDI 15

Set Trait

Premolars have no set traits as these are no premolar in deciduous dentition.

Class Trait

- They are called bicuspid, when one buccal and one lingual cusp present. Second premolar may have 3 cusps.
- Premolars have single buccal cusp.
- There is presence of one or two roots.

Arch Trait

1. Occlusal outline of maxillary premolars in hexagonal or oval, that of mandibular premolars is square or round.
2. Maxillary premolars are wider buccolingually compared to mesiodistal dimension and mandibular premolars are almost equal buccolingually and mesiodistally.
3. From proximal view maxillary premolars do not have a lingual tilt, while mandibular premolars have a lingual tilt.
4. From proximal view the outline of maxillary premolars is trapezoidal whereas outline of mandibular premolar is rhomboidal.

Type Trait

1. Less angular outlines. Crown is shorter compared to that of 1st premolar.
2. **Mesial cusp slope** of buccal cusp is shorter than the **distal cusp slope.**
3. From proximal view **both buccal** and **lingual cusps** are almost at same level.
4. There is no **mesial marginal groove,** no **canine fossa** on the mesial surface of the crown.
5. **Tip of the lingual cusp** is towards **mesial (right from lift).**
6. Mesial marginal ridge is more occlusal compared to distal marginal ridge (R from L).
7. **Occlusal surface** has **oval outline.**
8. In maxillary second premolar there is **single root.**

MANDIBULAR FIRST PREMOLAR

Identification

The given tooth is mandibular first premolar of the right side.

Notation

Palmer notation	4┐
Universal	#28
FDI	44

Set Trait

Premolars have no set traits as there are no premolars in deciduous dentition.

Class Trait

- They are called bicuspid, when one buccal and one lingual cusp present. Second premolar may have 3 cusps.
- Premolars have single buccal cusp.
- They may have one or two roots.

Arch Trait

- Occlusal outline of mandibular premolars is more or less square or rounded and that of maxillary premolars is hexagonal or oval.
- From proximal view mandibular premolars have a lingual tilt, the maxillary premolars do not have a lingual tilt.
- From proximal view the outline of mandibular premolar is rhomboidal whereas in maxillary premolars, it is trapezoidal.

Type Trait

- In mandibular **first** premolar the **buccal cusp tip** is more pointed and the **lingual cusp** is very small and non-functional.

  In mandibular **second premolar** the **buccal cusp tip** is **less pointed** and the lingual cusp is not very small and it is **functional.**
- There is presence of **mesiolingual groove** in the **first** premolar, separating the mesial-marginal ridge from the mesial cusp slope of the lingual cusp.
- From proximal view the buccal cusp tip is in line with the root axis.
- The occlusal surface of the first premolar is diamond shaped and that of second premolar, 2 cusp type is more or less rounded and 3 cusp type is more or less square.

RIGHT FROM LEFT

- The presence of mesiolingual groove on lingual surface.
- The mesial-marginal ridge not straight but inclined lingually and parallel to buccal triangular ridge.

MANDIBULAR SECOND PREMOLAR

Identification

The given tooth is mandibular second premolar of the right side.

Notation

Palmer notation	5┘
Universal	#29
FDI	45

Set Trait

Premolars have no set traits as there are no premolars in deciduous dentition.

Class Trait

- They are called bicuspid, when one buccal and one lingual cusp present. Second premolar may have 3 cusps.

- Premolars have single buccal cusp.
- There is presence of one or two roots.

Arch Trait

1. Occlusal outline of mandibular premolars is square or round. Maxillary premolars is hexagonal or oval.
2. Mandibular premolars are almost equal mesiodistally and buccolingually (MD and BL) whereas maxillary premolars are wider buccolingually compared to mesiodistal dimension.
3. From proximal view mandibular premolars have a lingual tilt, the maxillary premolars do not have a lingual tilt.
4. From proximal view the outline of mandibular premolar is rhomboidal while that are maxillary premolars is trapezoidal.

Type Trait

Y-type groove pattern

- There are 3 cusps, one buccal cusp and 2 lingual cusps. Mesiolingual cusp is larger than distolingual cusp (right from left).
- A lingual groove separates the two lingual cusps.
- The long mesial groove, the short distal groove, and the lingual groove together form a Y-shaped groove pattern.
- The occlusal outline is square-shaped.
- The mesial marginal ridge (MMR) is more occlusal compared to distal marginal ridge (right from left).

H-type groove pattern

- There are two cusps, one buccal and one lingual. Lingual cusp is not as short as that of first premolar.
- The straight short central groove along with mesiobuccal, mesiolingual, distobuccal, and distolingual developmental grooves form H-shaped groove pattern.
- Lingual tilt of the crown is less as compared to that of first premolar.
- MMR is more occlusally placed compared to DMR.

U-type groove pattern

- There are two cusps, one buccal and one lingual. Lingual cusp is not as short as that of first premolar.
- The occlusal outline is more or less rounded.
- The crescent shaped central groove along with mesiobuccal developmental groove and distobuccal developmental groove form a U-shaped groove pattern.
- Lingual tilt of the crown is less as compared to that of first premolar.
- Mesial marginal ridge is more occlusally placed than the distal marginal ridge (right and left).
- Lingual cusp tip may be towards mesial or may be just opposite to the buccal cusp tip.

GROOVES ON PREMOLARS

- Mesial marginal ridge groove (MMRG) is present on the **mesial surface of maxillary** first premolar (both from mesial and occlusal view).

- Mesiolingual groove (MLG) is present on the lingual surface of mandibular first premolar.
- Lingual groove (LG) present between ML and DL cusps of mandibular second premolar Y-type.

MOLARS

MAXILLARY FIRST MOLAR

Identification

The given tooth is **permanent** maxillary first molar of the right side.

Notation

Palmer notation	6┘
Universal	#3
FDI	16

Set Trait

Permanent first molars are larger than and similar to deciduous second molars.

- Primary first molars are smaller than the primary second molars.
- Primary maxillary and mandibular second molars are similar to permanent maxillary and mandibular first molars and also smaller than the permanent first molars, which erupt distal to the primary second molars.

Class Trait

1. They are the only teeth having at least two **buccal cusps.**
2. Molars are largest and strongest teeth.
3. They have largest of all the occlusal surfaces.
4. They are multicusp teeth with 3–5 cusps.
5. They have 2–3 large roots.

Arch Trait

1. Maxillary molars are narrower mesiodistally and wider buccolingually whereas mandibular molars are wider mesiodistally and narrower buccolingually.
2. **Occlusally,** shape of the crown is **rhomboidal** in maxillary molars. In mandibular molars it is rectangular or hexagonal.
3. There is presence of **oblique ridge** on the occlusal surface of maxillary molars.
4. In **maxillary molars 3 roots** are present; in **mandibular molars** 2 roots are present.
5. In maxillary molars, the lingual cusps are unequal, whereas in mandibular molars, the lingual cusps are more or less equal in size.
   Lingual cusps are longer than buccal cusps in mandibular molars.
6. Maxillary molars do not have lingual tilt.

Type Trait

- The **cusp of carabelli** is present on palatal surface of mesio palatal cusp of first molar.
- In first molar the **distopalatal cusp** is well developed whereas in second molar, distopalatal cusp is very small or absent.

- In first molar, the mesiobuccal and distobuccal cusps are more or less of same size. In second molar the distobuccal cusp is much smaller than the mesiobuccal cusp.
- The roots are **more divergent** in first molar.

RIGHT FROM LEFT SIDE

- The distopalatal cusp is smallest cusp.
- Cusp of carabelli present on palatal surface of mesiopalatal cusp of first molar.
- Mesial marginal ridge is more occlusally placed compared to distal marginal ridge.

MAXILLARY SECOND MOLAR

Identification

The given tooth is permanent maxillary second molar of the right side.

Notation

Palmer notation	7⏌
Universal	#2
FDI	17

Set Trait

- Primary first molars are smaller than the primary second molars whereas permanent first molars are larger than permanent second molar.
- Primary maxillary and mandibular second molars are similar to permanent maxillary and mandibular first molars and also smaller than the permanent first molars which erupt distal to the primary second molars.

Class Trait

1. They are the only teeth having at **least two buccal cusps.**
2. Molars are **largest** and **strongest teeth.**
3. They have **largest** of all **occlusal surfaces.**
4. They are multicusp teeth with **3–5 cusps.**
5. They have **2–3 large roots.**

Arch Trait

1. Maxillary molars are **narrower mesiodistally** and wider buccolingually whereas mandibular molars are wider mesiodistally and narrower buccolingually.
2. **Occlusally,** shape of the crown is **rhomboidal** in maxillary molars. In mandibular molars it is rectangular or hexagonal.
3. There is **presence of oblique** ridge on the occlusal surface of maxillary molars.
4. In maxillary molars **3 roots** are present; in mandibular molars 2 roots are present.
5. In maxillary molar, **the lingual cusps** are unequal, whereas in mandibular molars the lingual cusps are more or less equal in size.
6. Lingual cusps are longer than buccal cusps in mandibular molars.
7. Mandibular molars have a lingual tilt (Proximal view).

Type Trait

As compared to first molar

- From occlusal view the shape of the crown is more twisted (accentuated rhomboid shape) in second molars or may have heart-shape.
- The mesiobuccal cusp is wider than the distobuccal cusp.
- The **distopalatal cusp** is very small in rhomboid shape and absent in heart-shaped second molar mesiopalatal cusp is longer and larger.
- The crown is narrow on the palatal side.
- The roots are less spread and within the confines of the crown.
- Oblique ridge is less prominent.

In rhomboid shape, to distinguish right from left:

- **Mesiobuccal cusp** is wider than the distobuccal cusp.
- Distopalatal cusp is very small.
- Mesial marginal ridge is more occlusal.

In heart-shape to distinguish right from left:

- MB cusp is wider than DB cusp.
- Mesiopalatal cusp is more towards mesial due to absence of distal cusp.
- MMR is more occlusal as compared to DMR.
- DMR is longer than MMR.

MANDIBULAR FIRST MOLAR

Identification

The given tooth is permanent mandibular first molar of the right side.

Notation

Palmer notation	6┐
Universal	#30
FDI	46

Set Trait

- Primary first molars are smaller than the primary second molars whereas permanent first molars are larger than permanent second molar.
- Primary maxillary and mandibular second molars are similar to permanent maxillary and mandibular first molars and also smaller than the permanent first molars, which erupt distal to the primary second molars.

Class Trait

1. They are the only teeth having at least two buccal cusps.
2. Molars are largest and strongest teeth.
3. They have largest of all occlusal surfaces.
4. They are multicusp teeth with 3–5 cusps.
5. They have 2–3 large roots.

Arch Trait

1. Mandibular molars are **wider mesiodistally** and narrower buccolingually. Maxillary molars are narrower mesiodistally and wider buccolingually.
2. **Occlusally,** shape of the crown in mandibualr molars is **rectangular** or **hexagonal.** It is rhomboidal in maxillary molars.
3. In mandibular molars the **oblique ridge** is absent. There is presence of oblique ridge on the occlusal surface of maxillary molars;
4. In mandibular molars **2 roots** are present. In maxillary molars 3 roots are present.
5. In mandibular molars, the **lingual cusps** are more or less equal in size. In maxillary molars, the lingual cusps are unequal.

   Lingual cusps are longer than buccal cusps in mandibular molars.
6. From proximal view, the **mandibular molars** have a lingual tilt.

Type Trait

- Mandibular **first molars** have 5 cusps. 3 buccal cusps and 2 lingual cusps. Second molars have 4 cusps, 2 buccal and 2 lingual cusps.
- First molars have zig-zag groove pattern. Second molars have cross shaped groove pattern.
- First molars are larger than the second molars.
- The 2 roots of first molars are widely separated and curve distally whereas the roots of second molars are closer and parallel.

RIGHT FROM LEFT SIDE

- The distal cusp on the buccal surface is the smallest.
- The mesial marginal ridge is more occlusal as compared to distal marginal ridge.

MANDIBULAR SECOND MOLAR

Identification

The given tooth is permanent mandibular second molar of the right side.

Notation

Palmer notation	7┐ (lower right quadrant)
Universal	#31
FDI	47

Set Trait

- Primary first molars are smaller than the primary second molars whereas permanent first molar is larger than the permanent second molar.
- Primary maxillary and mandibular second molars are similar to permanent maxillary and mandibular first molars and also smaller than the permanent first molars.

Class Trait

1. They are the only teeth having at least two buccal cusps.
2. Molars are largest and strongest teeth.

3. They have largest of all occlusal surfaces.
4. They are multicusp teeth with 3–5 cusps.
5. They have 2–3 large roots.

Arch Trait

1. Mandibular molars are wider mesiodistally and narrower buccolingually. Maxillary molars are narrower mesiodistally and wider buccolingually.
2. Occlusally shape of the crown in mandibualr molars is rectangular or hexagonal. It is rhomboidal in maxillary molars.
3. There is no oblique ridge on mandibular molars. There is presence of oblique ridge on the occlusal surface of maxillary molars.
4. In mandibular molars 2 roots are present. In maxillary molars 3 roots are present.
5. In mandibular molars the lingual cusps are more or less equal in size. In maxillary molar, the lingual cusps are unequal.
6. Lingual cusps are longer than buccal cusps in mandibular molars.
7. From proximal view the crown has a lingual tilt.

Type Trait

Compared to first molar

- The cervical ridge on the mesiobuccal cusp is more prominent (occlusal view).
- The second molar is smaller in size.
- It has 4 cusps and cross-shaped groove pattern, 4 cusps are more nearly equal.
- The roots are closer and parallel.
- The roots are less wide buccolingually.

Right from Left Side

- Prominent cervical ridge on the buccal aspect of mesiobuccal cusp.
- Mesial marginal ridge more occlusal as compared to distal marginal ridge, which has a V-shape notch and it is often crossed by mesial marginal groove.
- Crown tapers from mesial to distal (occusal aspect).
- Crown is shorter from mesial to distal (buccal aspect).

Chapter

27

Age Determination of Dental Casts

CHRONOLOGY OF THE HUMAN PRIMARY DENTITION					
Tooth	*Hard tissue formation begins*	*Amount of enamel formed at birth*	*Enamel completed*	*Eruption*	*Root completed*
		Maxillary			
Central incisor	4 mos. *in utero*	Five sixths	1½ mos.	7 ½ mos.	1½ years
Lateral incisor	4 ½ mos. *in utero*	Two-thirds	2½ mos.	9 mos.	2 years
Cuspid	5 mos. *in utero*	One-third	9 mos.	18 mos.	3¼ years
First molar	5 mos. *in utero*	Cusps united	6 mos.	14 mos.	2½ years
Second molar	6 mos. *in utero*	Cusp tips still isolated	11 mos.	24 mos.	3 years
		Mandibular			
Central incisor	4 ½ mos. *in utero*	Three-fifths	2½ mos.	6 mos.	1½ years
Lateral incisor	4 ½ mos. *in utero*	Three-fifths	3 mos.	7 mos.	1½ years
Cuspid	5 mos. *in utero*	One-third	9 mos.	16 mos.	3¼ years
First molar	5 mos. *in utero*	Cusps united	5½ mos.	12 mos.	2¼ years
Second molar	6 mos. *in utero*	Cusp tips still isolated	10 mos.	20 mos.	3 years

CHRONOLOGY OF THE HUMAN PERMANENT DENTITION					
Tooth	*Hard tissue formation begins at or after birth*	*Amount of enamel formed at birth*	*Enamel completed*	*Eruption*	*Root completed*
		Maxillary			
Central incisor	3–4 mos. —"—	....	4–5 years	7 – 8 years	10 years
Lateral incisor	10–12 mos.	....	4–5 years	8 – 9 years	11 years
Cuspid	4–5 mos.	....	6–7 years	11–12 years	13–15 years
First bicuspid	1½–1¾ years	....	5–6 years	10–11 years	12–13 years
Second bicuspid	2–2¼ years	....	6–7 years	10–12 years	12–14 years
First molar	At birth	Sometimes a trace	2½–3 years	6–7 years	9–10 years
Second molar	2½–3 years	....	7–8 years	12–13 years	14–16 years

(Contd.)

CHRONOLOGY OF THE HUMAN PERMANENT DENTITION (*Contd.*)					
Tooth	*Hard tissue formation begins at or after birth*	*Amount of enamel formed at birth*	*Enamel completed*	*Eruption*	*Root completed*
		Mandibular			
Central incisor	3–4 mos.	....	4–5 years	6–7 years	9 years
Lateral incisor	3–4 mos.	....	4–5 years	7–8 years	10 years
Cuspid	4–5 mos.	....	6–7 years	9–10 years	12–14 years
First bicuspid	1¾–2 years	....	5–6 years	10–12 years	12–13 years
Second bicuspid	2¼–2½ years	....	6–7 years	11–12 years	13–14 years
First molar	At birth	Sometimes a trace	2½–3 years	6–7 years	9–10 years
Second molar	2½–3 years	....	7–8 years	11–13 years	14–15 years

SEQUENCE OF ERUPTION OF TEETH IN DECIDUOUS DENTITION			
Maxillary teeth	*Age of eruption in months*	*Mandibular teeth*	*Age of eruption in month*
Central incisor	7	Central incisor	6
Lateral incisor	9	Lateral incisor	7
First molar	14	First molar	12
Canine	18	Canine	16
Second molar	24	Second molar	20

SEQUENCE OF ERUPTION OF TEETH IN PERMANENT DENTITION			
Maxillary teeth	*Age of eruption in years*	*Mandibular teeth*	*Age of eruption in years*
First molar	6–7	First molar	6–7
Central incisor	7–8	Central incisor	6–7
Lateral incisor	8–9	Lateral incisor	7–8
First premolar	10–11	Canine	9–10
Canine	11–12	First premolar	10–12
Second premolar	10–12	Second premolar	11–12
Second molar	12–13	Second molar	11–13
Third molar	17–21	Third molar	17–21

CAST IDENTIFICATION AND AGE DETERMINATION

- Cast identification and age determination is an important practical exercise in dental Anatomy. It further helps to learn and revise the classes of teeth and different traits of teeth.
- Before attempting this exercise, the student is expected to read and learn the tooth anatomy from all aspects and numbering system and also learn the age and sequence of eruption of teeth.
- The age of the cast should be assessed on the basis of **eruption status** of deciduous and permanent dentition.

- The identification of teeth on the cast becomes easy after learning tooth morphology and carving of teeth.
- The following points/features need to be analysed for assessment of probable age of the **Normal dentition cast.**
  1. **Arch:** Maxillary or mandibular cast.
  2. **Dentition:** Deciduous, mixed or permanent.
  3. **Position of teeth.**
  4. **Last erupted** tooth in the dentition.

1. Arch Identification

For identification of arch, refer the Figs 27.1–27.3.

- To view the cast hold it as shown in Fig. 27.1.
- Maxillary cast has rugae on palate. Mandibular cast has tongue space.
- To identify the cast, to identify the side, to name the teeth, hold the maxillary cast with pointed narrow anterior surface away from you and the flat, wide posterior surface towards you.

  Hold the mandibular cast with narrow, pointed anterior surface towards you and flat, wide, posterior surface away from you.
- By viewing the cast as in Figs 27.1–27.3, it becomes easy to write the correct side (right or left) of the tooth and write the correct tooth number.

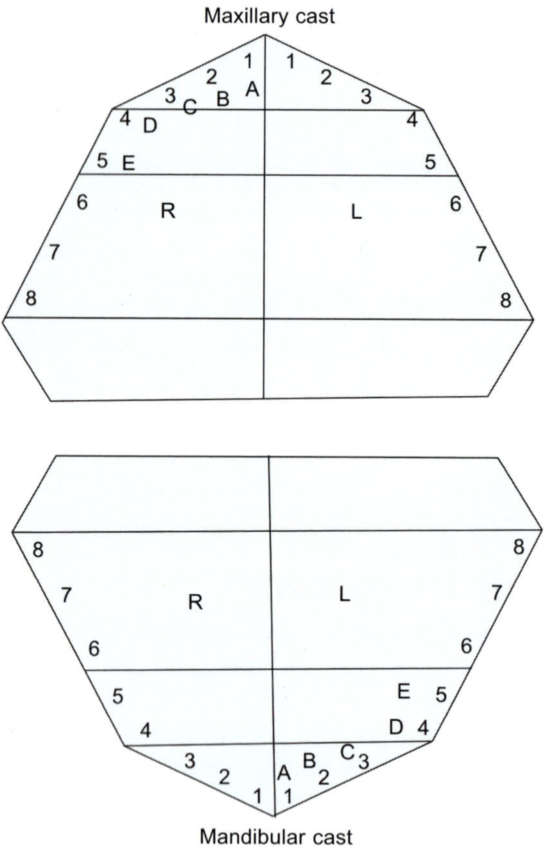

Fig. 27.1

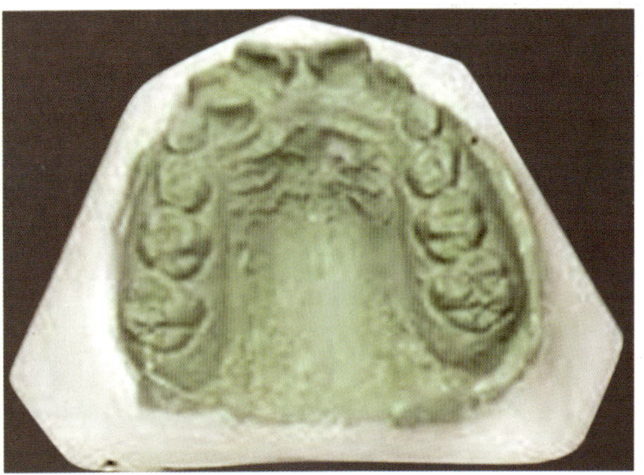
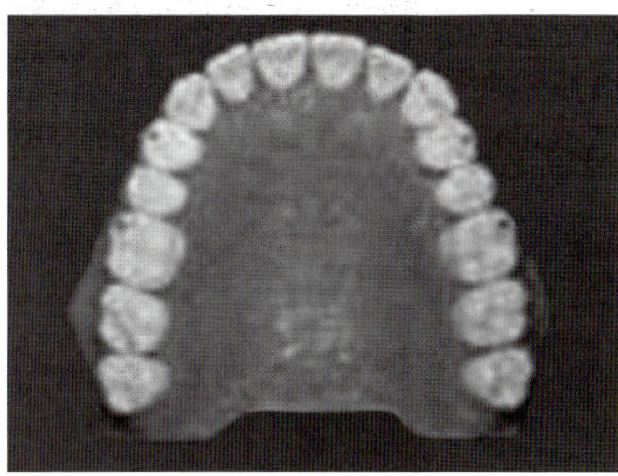

Maxillary cast

Fig. 27.2

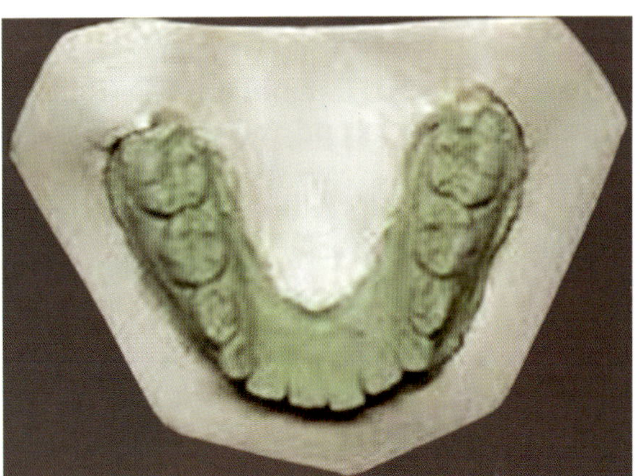
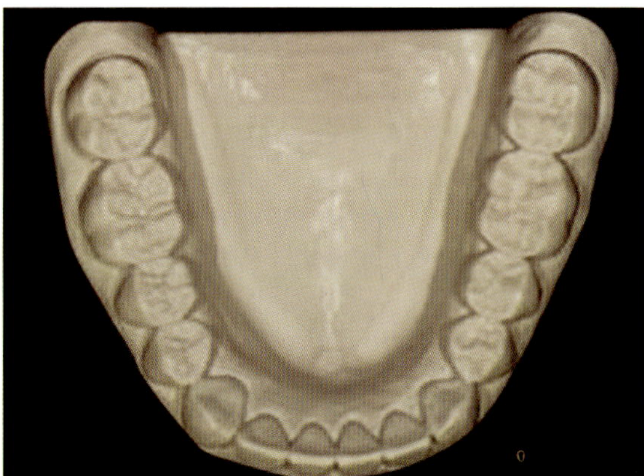

Mandibular cast

Fig. 27.3

2. Dentition (Figs 27.4ñ27.6)

- ***Deciduous cast*** is smaller in size with smaller teeth.
  - In each quadrant of the **normal deciduous dentition cast** 5 or less than 5 teeth are present.
  - The teeth present are incisors canine and molars.
- ***Mixed and permanent dentition cast:***
  - If more than 5 teeth are present in each quadrant of a **normal dentition cast** then it is either mixed dentition cast or permanent dentition cast.

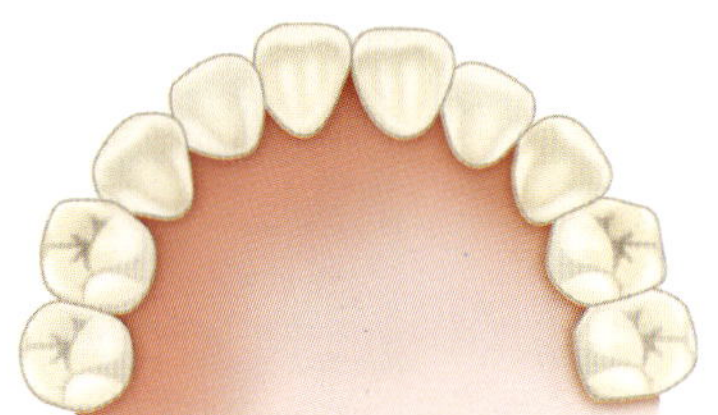
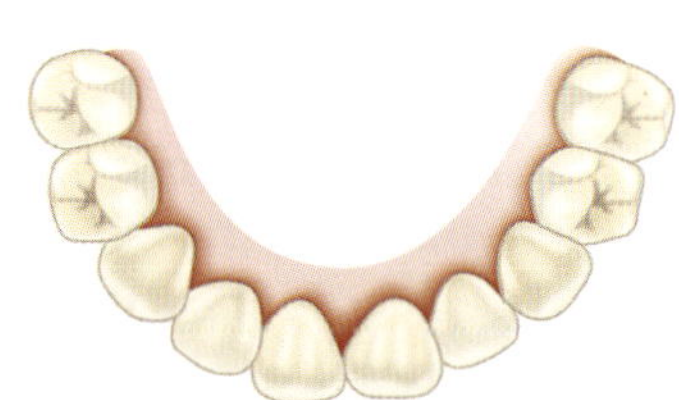

Fig. 27.4: Deciduous dentition

3. Position of Teeth (Figs 27.1 and 27.6)

The followig explanation is given to understand the position, name and number of teeth in a **Normal Dentition Cast**

- **From the midline:**
  - The first and second teeth would be central and lateral incisors.

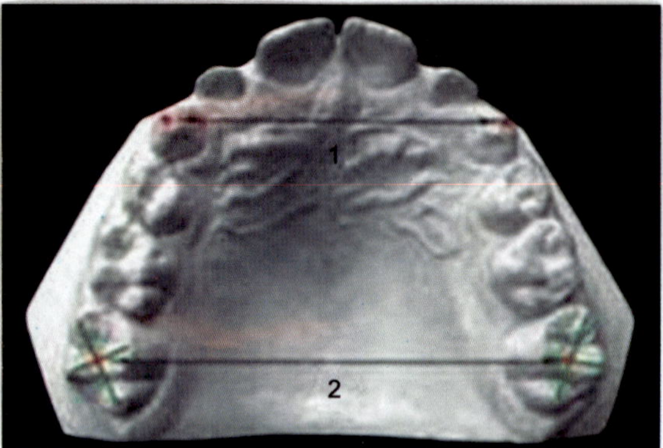

Fig. 27.5: Mixed dentition

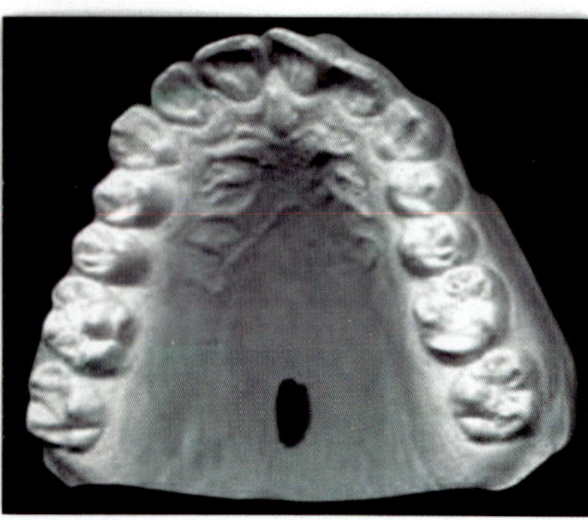

Fig. 27.6: Permanent dentition

- The third tooth would be canine.
- The Fourth tooth could be either deciduous first molar D or first premolar.
- The Fifth tooth could be either deciduous second molar E or second premolar.
- **The sixth tooth in a normal dentition would be permanent first molar.**
- The seventh and eight teeth in a normal dentition would be second and third permanent molars.

- **Deciduous incisors and permanent incisors in the first and second positions can be identified on the basis of size and presence of mamelons** (Fig. 27.7).
  - Deciduous incisors are smaller in size as compared to permanent incisors.
  - Deciduous incisors are short and wider as compared to permanent incisors which are longer and narrower.
  - The newly erupted permanent incisors would have mamelons on their incisal ridges whereas the incisal ridges of deciduous incisors could be attrited.

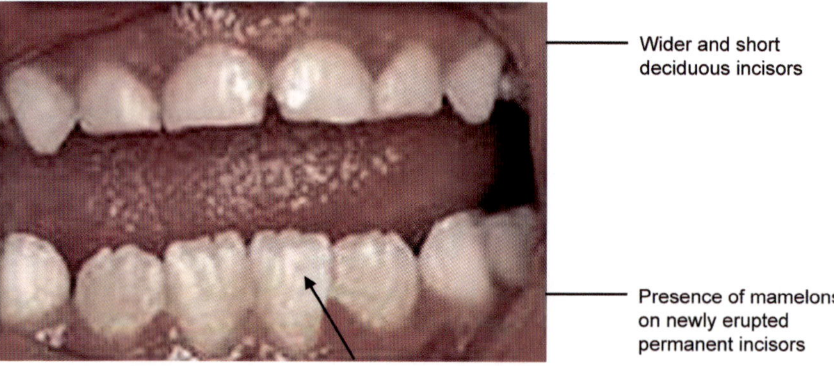

Fig. 27.7

- **Deciduous and permanent canines in the third position can be identified on the basis of their size and sharpness of their cusp tip.**
  - The **deciduous canine** is smaller and narrower as compared to permanent canine.
  - The newly erupted permanent canine would have a sharp-pointed cusp tip as compared to the attrited cusp tip of deciduous canine.

- Usually, permanent mandibular canine would erupt before the eruption of mandibular first and second premolars (9–10 years).
- Usually, permanent maxillary canine would erupt after the eruption of maxillary first and second premolars (11–12 years).

- **Deciduous molars and premolars in fourth and fifth position could be identified on the basis of the width, buccal aspect and occlusal outline of the crown** (Fig. 27.8).
  - To distinguish deciduous first molar D from the first premolar in the fourth position following points may be noted;

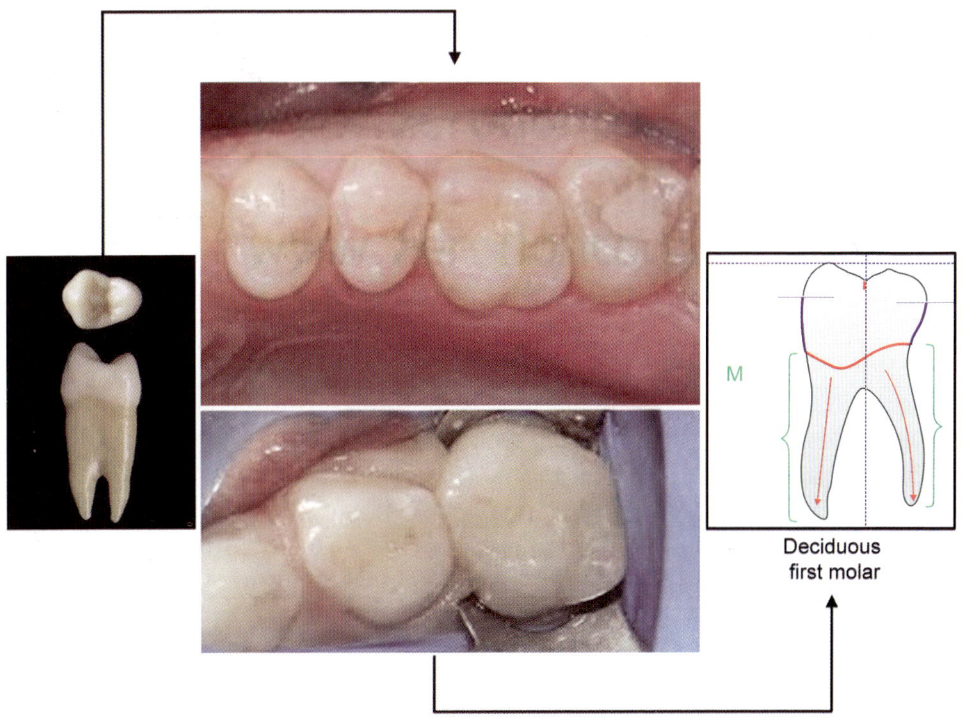

Fig. 27.8

- **Deciduous maxillary first molar** when viewed from **buccal aspect:**
  - Would have a crown wider MD than cervicoincisally,
  - Would have not so sharp two cusps MB cusp being longer than DB cusp.
  - Cervical line would be more curved towards mesial **whereas occlusal aspect** would show rectangular outline, MB corner shows a bulge.
- **Maxillary first premolar** when viewed from **buccal aspect:**
  - Would have a crown longer cervicoincisally than MD.
  - Would have a single pointed cusp.
  - Cervical line would be uniformaly curved **whereas occlusal aspect** would show **hexagonal** outline.

- **Deciduous mandibular first** molar when viewed from **buccal aspect:**
  - Would have a crown wider MD than cervicoincisally.
  - Would have two cusps MB > DB.
  - Cervical line would be more curved towards mesial **whereas occlusal aspect** would show a rhomboidal otline.
- **Mandibular first premolar** when viewed from **buccal aspect:**
  - Would have a longer crown.
  - Would have a single, long, pointed cusp.
  - Cervical line would be uniformly curved **whereas occlusal aspect** would show **diamond-shaped outline** and a **very small lingual cusp.**
- **To distinguish deciduous second molar E from the second premolar in the fifth position** is not at all difficult because the deciduous second molar (E) does not resemble a premolar at all. It resembles the **first permanent molar** in the sixth position.
  - It is larger than the tooth in the **fourth position.**
  - It is smaller and similar to the **tooth in sixth position.**
- ***In normal dentition in the sixth position it is always permanent first molar:***
  - which is similar in morphology to the deciduous second molar E in fifth position and larger than E.
  - and in the seventh position it is always the permanent second molar.

4. The Last Erupted Tooth

- *Following points would help to identify the last erupted tooth.*
  - It is the tooth which has not reached its occlusal or functional position.
  - If the last erupted tooth is anterior tooth it may be lingually placed (Fig. 27.10).
  - If it is a posterior tooth, only cusp tip may be seen.
  - Sometimes the last erupted tooth may be associated with deciduous tooth which has not yet exfoliated and is overretained then it needs to be mentioned.

Following points would help the student to present the write-up for age determination of the cast.

1. Identify the arch and dentition.
2. Write the teeth present, in palmer notation.

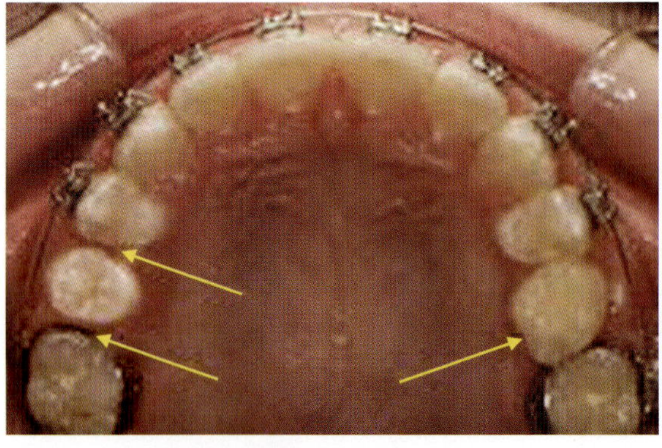

Fig. 27.9

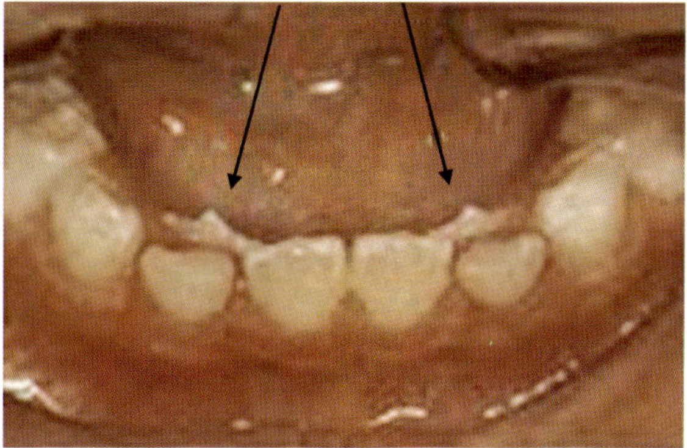

Fig. 27.10

3. If the tooth is erupting write it in palmer notation with (↑) up arrow.
4. If permanent tooth is erupting and deciduous tooth is overretained write both in palmer notation. $\overset{3}{\underline{C|}}$
5. If the tooth is missing write it as—in palmer notation.
6. If there is any discrepancy in eruption on both sides, of the arch, e.g. Fig. 27.9. $5\,\underline{4|4}\,E$. Age of the cast will be 10–12 years.
7. Write the specifications (over retained, rotated, erupting) in palmer notation as well as in sentence form.
8. Write age of the cast giving reason also.
9. Write other specifications in a sentence form.

For example,

CAST 1: *(Fig. 27.11)*

- The given cast is maxillary cast showing mixed dentition.

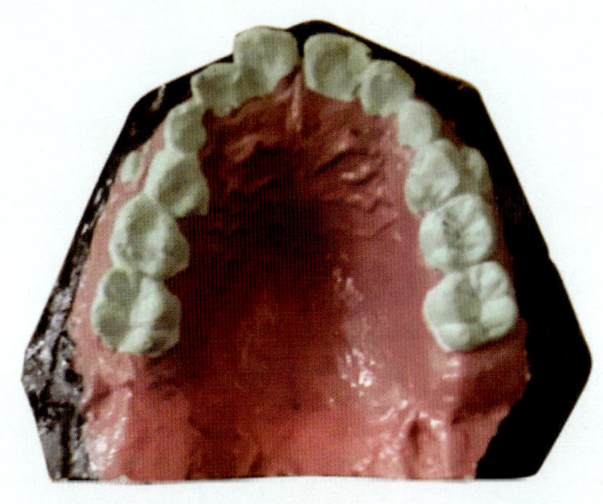

Fig. 27.11

- Teeth present are:

Palmer Notation

4	4
6 E D C 2 1	1 2 C D E 6

FDI Notation

		14				
16	55	54	53	12	11	R
21	22	63	64	65	26	L
		24				

- Permanent teeth right and left first molars central and lateral incisors have erupted.
- Deciduous first molars have not exfoliated and first premolar is erupting buccally.
- The approximate age of eruption of maxillary first premolar is 10–11 years.
- Since the first premolars are the last erupting teeth the approximate age of the cast is 10–11 years.

CAST 2 *(Fig. 27.12)*

- The given cast is maxillary cast with mixed dentition.
- Teeth present are:

Palmer Notation

↑ 5 3	
7 6 E 4 C 2 1	1 2 3 4 5 6 7

FDI Notation

		↑		15		13	
17	16	55	14	53	12	11	R
21	22	23	24	25	26	27	L

- On the left side, permanent first molar, central and lateral incisor, canine first and second premolars and second molar have erupted.
- On right side, permanent first molar, central and lateral incisor first premolar have erupted. Deciduous canine is over retained due to which permanent canine is erupting palatally. Deciduous second molar is over retained due to which second premolar is erupting buccally.
- The approximate erutpion age of maxillary canine and second premolar is 10–12 years and second molar is 12–13 years.
- Permanent canine second premolar and second molar on right side are erupting teeth. Therefore, age of the cast is 11–13 years.

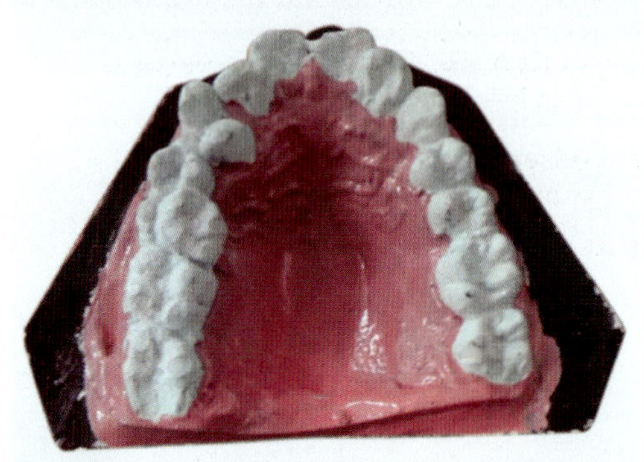

Fig. 27.12

Bibliography

1. Avery JK, Chigo Jr DJ. Essentials of oral histology and embryology: a clinical approach, ed. 3, Canada, Mosby Elsevier, 2006.
2. Bath-Balogh M, Fehrenbach MJ. Dental embryology, histology and anatomy, ed. 2, St. Louis Missouri, Saunders, 2006.
3. Berkovitz BKB, Holland GR. Moxhan BJ. Oral anatomy, histology and embryology, ed. 3, Mosby Elsevier, 2009.
4. Fuller JL, Denehy GE, Schulein TM. Concise dental anatomy and morphology, ed. 4, 2001, Michigan, University of lowa Publications Dept.
5. Kumar GS. Orban's histology and embryology, ed. 4, 2015, India, Elsevier.
6. Nanci A. Ten Cate's oral histology, development, structure and function, ed. 7, St. Louis Missouri, Mosby Elsevier, 2008.
7. Nelson SJ, Ash Jr M. Wheeler's dental anatomy, physiology, and occlusion, ed. 9, St. Louis Missouri, Saunders, 2010.
8. Scheid RC, Weiss G. Woelfels Dental Anatomy, ed. 9, Wolters Kluwer, 2016.

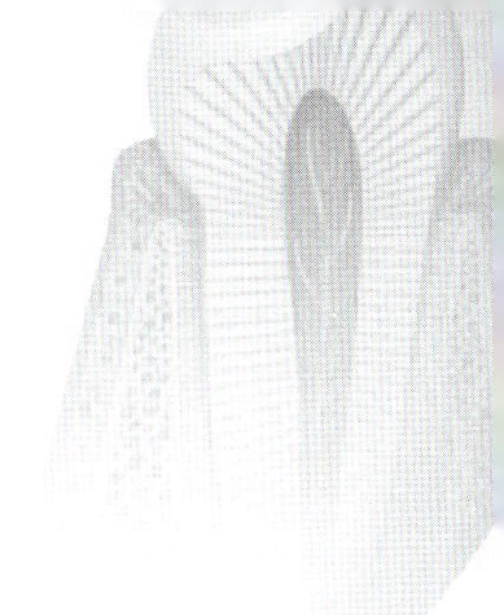

Index

Reader’s Notes

Reader's Notes